the other children

Under the editorship of Wayne H. Holtzman

the other children
an introduction to exceptionality

John B. Mordock

Astor Home for Children

Harper & Row, Publishers

New York, Evanston, San Francisco, London

Sponsoring Editor: George A. Middendorf
Project Editor: Cynthia Hausdorff
Designer: Frances Torbert Tilley
Production Supervisor: Bernice Krawczyk

THE OTHER CHILDREN: AN INTRODUCTION TO EXCEPTIONALITY

Library of Congress Cataloging in Publication Data
Mordock, John B   1938-
    The other children: an introduction to exceptionality.

    Bibliography: p.
    1. Communicative disorders in children.   2. Excep-
tional children.   I. Title.
RJ496.S7M66   618.9'28'55   74-18400
ISBN 0-06-044611-0

To the daughters in my life—
the Daughters of Charity
and my own two daughters,
Kalay and Kaylin.

Contents

Preface

Unlike edited texts where an authority in each area of exceptionality contributes a chapter, this book was written by a practicing school psychologist originally trained as an experimental child psychologist. The school psychologist is perhaps the only professional whose occupation brings him into contact with all types of atypical development. Consequently, although he can never hope to be an expert in any one area, his practical experience with many types of exceptionality enables him to see beyond their differences and notice their similarities. He is usually the first to offer help to the child and his family and is experienced in helping teachers come to grips with the exceptional child in the classroom. Hopefully, this experience equips him to write a text that will stimulate a student's curiosity in a manner similar to the way in which his interest was stimulated by the exceptional child.

The orientation of the book is an interdisciplinary one. Although the school psychologist may initiate child study in the school, his work is only the first step in a child's treatment. He is usually the family's advocate, helping them to seek help for their child; other professionals then contribute to the helping process. Because of this multidisciplinary emphasis, the student from each profession will find references to articles published in journals representing his field.

No effort is made to catalog all the different types of exceptionality. Some are treated in depth; others are merely mentioned. The reason for such coverage is simple: exposing the reader to the complexities of one type of atypical development may stimulate his curiosity more than superficial coverage of a variety of types. If this book is the only book on exceptionality that a student ever reads, it will have failed in its purpose.

The author is aware that many instructors will require students to supplement this text by writing a term paper in an area of exceptionality that is of interest to them. Many students do not know how to begin such a task and fail to realize that reviews of the literature should attempt to integrate disparate findings. The manner in which Down's syndrome and phenylketonuria are covered in Chapter 3 or stuttering in Chapter 5 can serve as models to follow when writing about other types of exceptionality. This text also makes reference to a large number of articles that can serve as departure points for students from almost any discipline. The glossary includes not only terms used in this book but also those that the student might encounter in his supplementary readings.

The author would like to thank the individuals who assisted in the preparation of the manuscript: Wayne Holtzman and George Middendorf for their support and encouragement; Cynthia Hausdorff for her able assistance in clarifying points and editing this author's specific spelling and writing disabilities; Frank Dwyer and Jim Torpy, special educators at the Astor Home for Children, for their critical reading of several chapters; Bernice Hutchison for her helpful suggestions from the layman's viewpoint; Erna Wilcox for typing the first draft of the manuscript; and Rosali Zimmerman, the Astor Home's librarian, for her assistance in obtaining reference materials. The author would also like to thank his wife, Judie, and oldest daughter, Kalay, for their patience and understanding when he had less time to be a husband and father. Special thanks go to the Daughters of Charity and to the other child care and teaching staff at the Astor Home. Because of their untiring energies on behalf of children, the author was able to find the time for this scholarly pursuit.

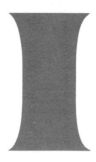

Hide them
or help them?

A variety of agencies are needed to help the exceptional child and his family, and these agencies should cooperate with one another to provide continuity of care. As we will see, most communities lack such continuity.

There are often gaps among existing agencies. For example, there may be an agency that looks after the child when he is at one age-stage, but none to help him or his family when he reaches another. A retarded child may become eligible for vocational training when he reaches 16, but until then must remain in a regular school program that does not include prevocational training.

At other times agencies operate in ignorance of each other. For example, a family in an urban renewal project may refuse to meet with relocation staff but meets regularly with the staff of a child guidance clinic, and neither agency may be aware of the efforts of the other.

Friction between agencies and among staff within agencies sometimes prevents adequate delivery of comprehensive services.

Chapter 1 describes the services that exist in most communities as well as those that might exist in the future. How soon the future will become the present depends largely upon eliminating the resistance to change that exists in many communities. Hopefully, communities that overcome this resistance will show others the way.

Each service expected a troubled child to adapt to the service's requirements. There was little provision to adapt the service to the child's needs.

—Barbara Blum

1
Multidisciplinary relationships

Mrs. Jones reports that William misbehaves on the playground, throws food in the cafeteria, fights and interrupts in class. Academic problems do not seem to be responsible for this behavior. On a behavior rating scale Mrs. Jones indicates that William is disrespectful and defiant, causes classroom disturbances, and frequently blames others for his behavior.

Mrs. Smith has been contacted by Susan's mother. The mother reports that Susan has been threatening to run away or kill herself and has been demanding a great deal of attention. Mrs. Smith suggests Susan meet with the school psychologist.

Miss Ames reports that Bob makes continual errors orienting his papers and workbooks, usually placing them upside down, that he assembles puzzles rotated 45 degrees, and that he works from the bottom of the paper upward.

Miss Green reports that Mary is simply not making any progress. She is totally withdrawn in class and never does the work assigned. She frequently complains of stomach aches and is absent from school a great deal.

Each brief statement above was made by a teacher when she referred a child for psychoeducational evaluation. Most school systems employ the services of a school psychologist, remedial reading teacher, and speech therapist. In addition to these professionals, school systems sometimes employ social workers, crisis teachers, and learning disabilities specialists. When a teacher experiences difficulty with a child, she can ask any one or all of these specialists to evaluate the child or to help her to pinpoint reasons for the child's difficulties. Sometimes the difficulty lies within the child, sometimes it is the result of conditions within the classroom, or sometimes the child brings into the classroom difficulties that originate in the home.

The most appropriate way to obtain information about a child is to refer him to a child study team rather than to one professional. A teacher may refer a child for a speech evaluation, hoping speech therapy will correct his poor speech patterns, when the child's real problem lies elsewhere. If the various professionals in the school work in isolation, then the child may be given speech therapy when speech is only a part of his problem. When the child is referred to a child study team, each professional can listen to the teacher's report on the child and then decide the role his discipline will play in the child's evaluation.

Throughout this book we will be engaged in child study. We will examine what each discipline has to say about children who have difficulty in school or within their community, and we will learn about programs designed to help these children. Several of the chapters will begin by describing a child as he presents himself to his teacher, the person who is often the first to verbalize that some of the child's behavior is not like that of other children or that usual behavior patterns are displayed in exaggerated form. We will then provide the reader with more information about the child, much in the manner as is done by the various professionals who make up a child study team. In other chapters we will first give the reader some background information and then present a case. Just as the classroom teacher needs to reexamine her impressions about a child after he has been evaluated by others, so will the reader need to review the cases presented in order to identify aspects of the child's behavior that become understandable in the light of the information gathered. In order to prepare the reader for the chapters that follow and to acquaint him with the manner in which child study proceeds, the case of Andrew will serve to launch us into the child study process.

ANDREW: AN EIGHT-YEAR-OLD NONREADER

Andrew was not learning to read. He was now in the latter half of his fourth year in school, and was essentially a nonreader. In the fall of the year Andrew had been referred for remedial reading. At that time the reading teacher's evaluation revealed that Andrew could name only nine letters of the alphabet in both lower and upper case. He could give the sounds of only eight consonants when in the initial position and none when in the end position. He could recognize only 55 percent of the words on a preprimer list and was untestable on the Gilmore Oral Reading Inventory. Following this evaluation, Andrew was given daily half-hour remedial reading sessions with the reading teacher.

After seven months of remedial work, Andrew was reevaluated. At this time he recognized all but three letters in upper case and five in lower case. He could give both the initial and ending sounds of all 18 consonants and could recognize 90 percent of the words on a preprimer list and 55 percent on a primer list. He also achieved a grade level of

1.5 on word attack skills on the Gilmore Oral Reading test, but could not comprehend material read to him at that level. Andrew's progress was attributed more to his daily half-hour sessions with the reading teacher than to his classroom instruction, since in the classroom setting he was extremely hyperactive and inattentive.

Both teachers felt that Andrew should be evaluated by other members of the child study team and the findings discussed at a formal conference, for such a conference might reveal additional factors and result in a different approach toward Andrew's instruction. Although he had made initial progress in remedial reading, he seemed to have reached a plateau. Each team member met with the two teachers and was acquainted with Andrew and his progress in their remedial program.

Andrew's evaluation by team members

The psychologist administered an individual intelligence test, the Wechsler Intelligence Scale for Children (WISC), the Bender Visual-Motor Gestalt Test (Koppitz, 1964), and the Goodenough-Draw-a-Man Test (Goodenough, 1926; Harris, 1963).

Andrew's total IQ score (full scale IQ) of 91 placed him on the low end of the average range (90–110). His verbal IQ, a summation of five subtests of verbal skill and reasoning, placed him in the borderline retarded range (70–80). On the basis of his verbal IQ alone he would qualify for placement in a class for the educable retarded (50–75). However, his performance IQ of 110 (summation of five or six subtests which measure reasoning with pictorial, figural, and manipulative material) approached the high average range (110–120).

On the Bender, where Andrew was asked to copy nine figural designs, he achieved a score equivalent to a 5-year-old. His drawing of a human figure on the Goodenough test was poorly proportioned and revealed spatial disorientation. Although the test protocol revealed signs of emotional difficulties, the psychologist considered the emotional problems to be Andrew's reaction to rather than the cause of his learning difficulties.

The remedial reading teacher administered the Illinois Test of Psycholinguistic Abilities (ITPA), a test of channels of communication, levels of organization of material received, and psycholinguistic process. Andrew's test profile revealed deficiencies in the processing of auditory stimuli.

The social worker visited Andrew's home and talked with his parents. Her report suggested that emotional factors were not the primary reason for Andrew's difficulties.

The staff conference

The work of the child study team was coordinated by the school system's director of special education. His role was to focus the investigation

Figure 1.1 *Andrew's profile. (As designed and utilized by the Instructional Resources and Assistance Center of the Ulster County Board of Cooperative Educational Services for the schools of Ulster County.)*

STUDENT'S NAME Andrew **SCHOOL** Sunset Ridge **AGE** 7-4 **GRADE** 2 **DATE** 4/21/72

Diagnosis (specific)	Recommendations (general)	Procedures and materials (specific)
Classroom Teacher		
Pleased by individual attention. Does not attend to directions.	Needs individual attention.	Must receive individual help no matter what program used.
Good coordination. Often answers verbal questions with wrong answers. Speech impairment (rambles on). Language deprivation.	Needs opportunities to express himself verbally.	
Likes to grow things (science).	Needs involvement in projects.	
Brings home library books, often too difficult.		Inform librarian about helping with selection of books.
Does not retain information. Does not know spelling or number patterns. Grossly below grade level in all areas. Capable of recognizing whole words.		Tutor to work on math. See teacher for math needs.
Nutrition below par. Hygiene problems.	Balanced lunch. Hygiene information.	No one made a commitment to follow through on this.
Remedial Reading		
Displaying interest in learning. Will come to reading on his own. Motivated—wants to learn. Reversals—*d, b, p, q.* Can write letters. Knows sounds and shapes but cannot name letters. Uses phonic attack as opposed to whole word. Two years behind grade level.	Needs one-to-one instruction. Should be given small bits of information. Should overlearn. Do not bombard with materials. Use multisensory approach	Working with Barnell-Loft? Programmed reader like Sullivan. Work with manipulative materials, e.g., sand. Kinesthetic approach. Taste and touch experiences. Concrete experiences: picture and actual representation, e.g. "Here is a dog" (real) and child expresses this in words. Put into writing and then expand. Oral language approach. In-depth medical. Visual acuity and hearing check-up.

Figure 1.1 (*Continued*)

Diagnosis (specific)	Recommendations (general)	Procedures and materials (specific)
Psychological Dec. 1971—WISC: 76 verbal, 110 performance. Bender and figure drawing: immaturity, more than a motor problem, speech defect.		Instead of marking papers with number wrong (−5), write how many correct (+5).
Makes errors in subtraction. Makes systematic errors in 2-column math examples.	Do not mix addition and subtraction problems on same page. Have volunteer aide make up sheets with one type of problem.	Get aide to provide basic materials.
Rigid-inhibited learning style.		
Primary deficit is in processing of auditory information; strengths in recognizing visual patterns, noting details, eye-hand coordination, concepts.	For further recommendations see full report submitted earlier.	Explore possibility of a split program, e.g., modified Joplin plan—(half day in 2nd grade section, half day in 3rd grade section) or similar approach.
Home Unaffected, cooperative, closely knit family. Marital and child-parent relationships seem good. Parents have limited education and income. Mother (now convalescing from meningitis) works. Children attended by neighbor. Little time to give children individual attention although need for it is recognized. Father strong masculine figure. Gas company service man. Hobby, stockcar racing, provides family recreation. Both parents have farm background. Gardening encouraged. Siblings: William, 12, learning problems, hyperactivity, improving; John, 11, quiet studious; Keith, 6, learning problems; Michael, infant.	Simplification of school environment needed for child from very unsophisticated background.	Inform parents of basis for Andrew's difficulties. Recommend medical evaluation (as above). Impress upon father that Andrew's interest in cars is desire to identify with him. Encourage father to take Andrew with him to races.

of the team members, to facilitate communication among them, and to prepare a profile on the referred child which included the highlights of each team member's contribution at the conference. The summary of Andrew's conference appears in Figure 1.1. In addition, the psychologist who had special training in learning disabilities prepared a comprehensive report following the conference which gave specific teaching suggestions.

In Andrew's case the key team members were the classroom teacher and remedial reading specialist. The social worker helped rule out family difficulties as the chief cause of Andrew's problems, and the psychologist's finding of a 34-point difference between verbal and performance IQ supported the impression of the two teachers that Andrew had an unusual language handicap. The finding that Andrew could not easily process auditory stimuli, particularly those that are rapidly processed by other children, explained why it took him so long to learn relatively easy material. For some reason, his brain was unable to retain and integrate verbally presented material, particularly symbolic material. Chapter 8 will include a discussion of children with problems similar to Andrew's.

CHILD STUDY IN THE SCHOOL

Thorough child study may involve considerably more specialists than were involved in Andrew's case. There are essentially twelve areas of assessment in a thorough child study. These areas are presented in Table 1.1.

Social and developmental assessment (Table 1.2) may reveal family difficulties, either past or present, traumatic events, or parental pathology that frequently cause developmental difficulties in children. The case history may also reveal factors which may have produced brain injury or cerebral dysfunction.

Table 1.3 summarizes historical-etiologic clues frequently responsible for brain injury (see Chapter 3), and Table 1.4 summarizes behavioral

Table 1.1 AREAS OF ASSESSMENT

1. Educational assessment	8. Auditory processing and language assessment
2. Social development assessment	
3. Case history	9. Dominance and left-right orientation assessment
4. General physical examination	
5. General psychological assessment	10. Gross and fine motor assessment
6. Emotional and behavioral assessment	11. Ophthalmologic-optometric assessment
7. Visual-perceptive and visual-motor assessment	12. Neurological examination

Table 1.2 SOCIAL DEVELOPMENT ASSESSMENT (BY SOCIAL
WORKER, PSYCHIATRIST, PSYCHOLOGIST)

1. History from parents	4. Behavior rating scales
2. School reports	5. Sociometric measures
3. Vineland Scale of Social Maturity	6. Self-concept measures

clues which are often signs of minimal cerebral dysfunction (see Chapter 8). The general physical examination can also reveal signs of cerebral dysfunction. Table 1.5 presents the clues which can be picked up by the pediatrician or family physician.

Gross disorders from brain dysfunction are usually detected prior to school entrance. Disorders such as cerebral palsy, severe mental retardation, aphasia, and childhood psychosis fall into this category (see Part II). However, many developmental disorders go unnoticed until the child reaches school. The teacher's observations of the child's classroom productions may lead her to suspect that the child is not adequately equipped for a conventional learning experience.

Members of the child study team

The psychologist In many schools the first person to receive a teacher's request for assistance is the school psychologist. Although the training and certification requirements of psychologists vary from state to state, most psychologists trained to function in school settings hold a master's degree. Their academic training includes courses in child development, learning theory, psychopathology, tests and measurement, educational foundations, group and individual counseling, and research design. A

Table 1.3 CEREBRAL DYSFUNCTION: HISTORICAL-ETIOLOGIC CLUES

Pregnancy	Duration, spotting, false labor, drugs, infections, skin eruptions, exposure to childhood diseases, weight gain, toxemic symptoms, intrauterine activity, premature rupture of membranes
Labor	Duration and severity
Delivery	Birth presentation, instruments used, anesthesia
Perinatal	Birthweight (especially in relation to duration of pregnancy), resuscitative efforts, excessive moulding or other evidence of trauma, abnormal concentrations of biochemicals in the urine, infections, maternal and infant weight loss, birthmarks
Infancy	Meningitis, high fever (especially with convulsions), skin eruptions, hallucinations, developmental regression following illness, head trauma, dehydration, head size
Childhood	Rare; causes are obvious
Family history	Parental age, obstetrical history, blood types, skin lesions or other stigmata, familial dyslexia, "late bloomers" or problems similar to those of patient

Table 1.4 **MINIMAL CEREBRAL DYSFUNCTION: HISTORICAL-BEHAVIORAL CLUES**

Pregnancy	Abnormal intrauterine activity
Newborn nursery	Poor temperature regulation, inadequate sucking efforts, jittery activity, excessive somnolence, respiratory irregularity, poor coloring
First year	Alteration of sleeping patterns, colicky symptoms, "too good," excessive mucus, early hand dominance, hypo- or hypermuscle tone, excessive startle, delayed motor and verbal development, absent creeping phase, delayed fontanelle closure, delayed teething, minor squints, febrile convulsions
First year preschool	Overactivity, extreme temper tantrums, gratification immediacy, minor speech problems, excessive drooling, hearing inattention, toeing in, toe walking, seizures, paradoxical drug responses
Kindergarten	Short attention span, "fidgety," poor impulse control, distractibility, "immaturity," dominance ambivalence, low frustration threshold, poor coloring, poor body concepts, "can't tie shoes"
First–second grade	Poor penmanship, letters and words backwards, dyslexia, poor athletic ability, can't finish assignments
Secondary reactive patterns	Aggressivity, withdrawal, poor peer relationships, nighttime bedwetting, school phobias, negativisms

knowledge of research design equips the psychologist to make an important contribution to the child study team, since he is usually the only individual with such training employed within the school. This skill is an essential part of the evaluation of any program offered to a child for it enables the team to determine whether changes in children are the result of their efforts or dependent upon factors not related to the program.

Some states require a doctoral degree (Ph.D.) for certification as a school psychologist, while others require 60 graduate hours. Graduate training includes a full-time internship experience which varies in length from three to six months (Cardon & French, 1968–1969). The doctorate usually includes a full year's internship in both clinic and

Table 1.5 **CEREBRAL DYSFUNCTION: CLUES ON GENERAL PHYSICAL EXAMINATION**

Congenital stigmata	Pigmentations or depigmentations, vascular lesions (especially in scalp) high palate, abnormal width between two paired organs, abnormal skin folds, palm creases, abnormal surface markings of skin, deflection of one or more fingers, abnormal ear placement, midline defects
Head	Circumference compared to standards for age, shape, facial asymmetry, orbital elevation
Eyes	Squint, reduced or dim vision, abnormal eye position, developmental lesions, retinal spots or pigmentations, retinal inflammations
Body	Limb or nail asymmetry, range of motion of ankles

school settings. Ideally, the training of the school psychologist should include supervised experience in a variety of educational settings, such as Head Start, day treatment and child study centers, special class settings, therapeutic schools, resource rooms, open and traditional classrooms, and in a variety of community agencies, such as family counseling centers or child guidance clinics.

The psychologist frequently acts as an advocate for each child referred to him and coordinates the activities of those providing the child with special services.

The teacher asks the psychologist to evaluate the child and suggest a manner in which she might approach him in class. Typically, she is asked to fill out a referral form in which she states the reasons for referral as well as her own view of the child. This form serves several purposes. It alerts the psychologist to the type of problem, forces the teacher to think about the child before referral, and serves as a base for comparison should the child be referred again when he is older. Figure 1.2 presents a typical referral form. Examples of reasons for referral were given at the start of this chapter.

The psychologist usually observes the child in class and sees him individually. At this stage he may give the child some brief screening instruments, such as the Wide Range Achievement Test, which is a brief test measuring word recognition and pronunciation, spelling and arithmetic, a brief IQ measure, and drawings. He will also examine the child's classroom work. His evaluation then proceeds according to his tentative conclusions about the child's difficulties. If he believes they stem primarily from factors existing within the classroom, he will attempt to help the teacher manage the child according to his findings. If he suspects the child is not equipped for learning at a normal rate, either because of emotional factors, mental retardation, a specific learning disability, or a visual or hearing deficiency, he would evaluate the child further (see Tables 1.6 and 1.7) or refer him to the proper specialist.

Whatever form his evaluation takes, the psychologist usually schedules a parent conference to assess their view of the child and to disseminate his findings in a manner he hopes will ensure their cooperation in endeavors to assist the child.

In almost all instances the parents have the right to determine the welfare of their child. They can reject any special services the school may offer and in many states can refuse to give permission to have their child evaluated. Frequently, parents who give the school permission to evaluate their child do not follow through when further evaluations are requested. Some do not cooperate because the evaluation represents a threat to their self-image, especially if it involves a trip to a child guidance or mental health center; others do not follow through because of disinterest in the child. Sometimes parents neglect to take their child for relatively unthreatening evaluations, such as ophthalmologic or

Figure 1.2 *Psychoeducational referral form.*

PSYCHOEDUCATIONAL REFERRAL FORM

Child's Name: _____ Teacher: _____

Age: _____ Grade: _____

Have parents been informed: _____ Priority: Urgent _____

No hurry _____

1. What are the main behaviors which lead to referral? _____

   _____

2. What do you think the reasons are for these behaviors? _____

   _____

3. What role do you feel the child's parents play in these behaviors? To what

   degree are they aware of his behavior? _____

   _____

   _____

4. What procedures have you employed in an attempt to handle or ameliorate

   these behaviors? _____

   _____

5. What is this child's social standing among peers and how does he currently

   relate to them? _____

6. List the positive behaviors this youngster performs in class as well as those
   things he enjoys doing or has interest in.

   1. _____

   2. _____

   3. _____

Comments:

Table 1.6 GENERAL PSYCHOLOGICAL EVALUATION (BY THE SCHOOL OR CLINICAL PSYCHOLOGIST)

1. Psychometric testing: IQ, achievement, learning profile
   Cattell Infant Intelligence Scale
   Stanford-Binet Intelligence Scale (2½–adult)
   Wechsler Preschool-Primary Scale of Intelligence (4–6)
     or Wechsler Intelligence Scale for Children (5–16)
   Gray-Votaw-Rogers oral reading paragraphs
   Wide-Range Achievement Test (5–adult)
2. Projective testing: emotional makeup, conceptual reasoning
   Thematic Apperception Test
   Sentence completion tests
   Rorschach ink-blot test
   Goodenough Draw-a-Man Test

speech and hearing examinations. The psychologist hopes to avoid such occurrences and tries to set resistive parents at ease.

The psychologist sees the parents also to assess family factors. To obtain relevant material he may take a detailed case history or request that a social worker do so, if one is employed to perform this function.

Figure 1.3 presents a continuous behavioral record employed by one psychologist in order to highlight the essential characteristics of each child he studies.

The social worker The social worker helps the school staff to appreciate the family's influence on the child's attitudes. It is often difficult to determine whether a child's learning difficulties are the result of emotional problems (Chapter 7) or emotional reactions to failure. In some cases, a child has both a learning disability and an unhappy home life. Some children who are preoccupied with problems at home do poorly in school, although others do surprisingly well. Frequently, a child doing poorly with one teacher does well when transferred to another, even though "home problems" have remained the same (see Chapter 12). Teachers are usually aware that a child's family life can have a negative influence on learning. Nevertheless, they are not always aware of the exact manner in which this influence takes place.

Table 1.7 VISUAL-PERCEPTIVE AND VISUAL-MOTOR EVALUATION (BY THE PSYCHOLOGIST, OCCUPATIONAL THERAPIST, OR PHYSICAL THERAPIST)

1. Goodenough Draw-a-Man Test, House-Tree-Person Technique (4–adult)
2. Bender-Gestalt Test (5–adult)
3. Beery-Buktencia Developmental Test of Visual-Motor Integration (2–15)
4. Frostig Developmental Test of Visual Perception (3–8)
5. Benton Visual Memory for Designs (8–adult)
6. Graham-Kendell Memory for Designs (8–adult)

Figure 1.3 *Continuous behavioral record.*

CONTINUOUS BEHAVIORAL RECORD

NAME _____ SEX _____ DATE _____

ADDRESS _____ SCHOOL _____

GRADE _____ TEACHER _____ BIRTHDATE _____

PLACE _____ AGE: YRS. _____ MOS. _____

REASON FOR REFERRAL _____
_____

FAMILY: PARENTS(S) _____ OCCUPATION _____

NO. OF CHILDREN _____ POSITION THIS CHILD _____

DIFFICULTIES IN HOME _____

PARENT CONFERENCES _____
_____

SCHOOL ATTENDANCE: HEALTH:

    Regular _____   Hearing: Normal _____ Other _____

    Irregular _____   Vision: Normal _____ Wears glasses _____ Other _____

    Truant _____   Pertinent medical history _____

EDUCATIONAL DEVELOPMENT: Earliest grade in school _____ Grades retained _____

Reason: _____

Indicate child's involvement with specific departments by placing check mark if child has

been referred to or is being worked with. Speech and hearing: _____ Guidance _____

Reading: _____ LDC _____ Other (specify) _____

SCHOOL ABILITY (indicate by grade): Reading _____ Writing: creative _____ cursive _____

Arithmetic: concepts _____ problem solving _____ Spelling _____ Social Studies _____

Science _____ Music _____ Art: creative _____ drawing _____ Conversation _____

Following directions _____ Attention span _____

SPECIAL HABITS: Nail biting _____ Thumb sucking _____ Tics _____ Hair pulling _____

Teeth grinding _____ Restless _____ Other _____

WORK HABITS: Attitude toward work and/or school _____

SOCIALIZATION:
1. Independent activities and assignments: completes on own _____ with prodding _____

   does not complete _____

2. Group and classroom activities: initiates activities _____ contributes ideas when

   asked _____ follows others _____ can't work with others _____

3. Prefers to work and/or play: alone _____ with one another _____ in a small group _____

   in large group _____ with younger children _____ with older children _____ children of

   same age _____ remain on sidelines _____

4. Play: intelligent and self-motivated _____ vigorous _____ imitative _____ aimless _____

   lethargic _____ other (specify) _____

DIFFICULTIES IN SPECIFIC SKILLS: (check)

1. Visual: confusion or reversal of letters _____ confusion of words _____ choppy eye

   movements in reading _____ poor eye focus in close work _____ in distant work _____

   other (specify) _____

2. Auditory: confusion of sounds _____ difficulty in understanding conversation _____

   difficulty in expressing ideas ___ unable to produce rhythmic taps or simple melody ___

   difficulty in memory _____ other (specify) _____

3. Vocabulary: limited _____ misuse of words _____ adequate _____ above average _____

   speech difficulty _____ other (specify) _____

4. Motor skills: difficulty in fine coordination _____ in gross coordination _____

PREVIOUS TEST DATA (name and date):

The social worker's responsibility is to help elucidate the particulars in each child's problem. Such information can help the teacher to maximize her influence rather than to give up because of the seemingly hopeless family situation.

Permanent certification as a school social worker requires 60 hours of graduate study in the field of social work. Academic preparation includes courses in individual and family assessment, family counseling, group work, community organization, and social work administration. The social worker usually makes home visits and serves as a liaison with other community agencies involved with a particular child.

The special teacher The reading teacher's evaluation is usually confined to a thorough assessment of basic reading skills and is, therefore, considered an educational evaluation. Figure 1.4 presents a typical check list employed by a remedial reading teacher to summarize the skills of a particular child.

The speech teacher evaluates the child's articulation patterns, language development, voice inflections, and language usage (see Chapter 5). Since speech defects are often the result of faulty hearing, the speech teacher is usually trained to evaluate hearing efficiency as well. In some settings the differences between the reading and speech teacher dissolve and each functions as a language therapist. Table 1.8 presents the evaluation procedures of the language therapist concerned with assessing the channels of communication open to a child.

Other specialists In Andrew's case an educator, reading teacher, social worker, and psychologist were the primary participants in child study. It was recommended that Andrew receive a thorough speech and hearing

Table 1.8 AUDITORY PROCESSING AND LANGUAGE ASSESSMENT (BY THE AUDIOLOGIST, LANGUAGE THERAPIST, OR PSYCHOLOGIST)

1. Peripheral hearing competence
   Audiogram

2. Central auditory processing
   Speech discrimination testing (e.g., Wepman Auditory Discrimination Test)
   Auditory figure-ground discrimination
   Auditory sequencing, perceptual and motor
   Auditory memory (e.g., Wepman Auditory Memory-Span Test)
   Sound localization

3. Central language formulation
   Illinois Test of Psycholinguistic Abilities (3–9)
   Slingerland Screening tests (6–10)

4. Motor speech patterns
   Clinical examination
   Templin-Darley Screening and Diagnostic Tests of Articulation

Table 1.9 GROSS AND FINE MOTOR AND PERCEPTUAL-MOTOR
ASSESSMENT (BY THE PHYSICAL THERAPIST,
OCCUPATIONAL THERAPIST, PSYCHOLOGIST,
PHYSICAL EDUCATOR, OR NEUROLOGIST)

1. Clinical examination
2. Quantitative testing
    Purdue Perceptual Motor Survey (Kephart) (5–12)
    Oseretsky Motor Ability Scale (Scott revision) (5–adult)
    Devereux Test of Extremity Coordination
    Halstead neuropsychological test battery (Reitan modification) (5–adult)

evaluation at the clinic associated with the local hospital, so the team was extended to include professionals from outside the school. In other instances the team might include the school physician, the guidance counselor, the school nurse, or the school's physical educator. Often the physical educator is asked to assess the child's gross and fine motor coordination when he is trained in this area or when physical or occupational therapists are not available.

Table 1.9 presents some of the methods used to evaluate motor functioning. The Halstead battery requires special training to administer and interpret and its use is confined to those psychologists specializing in neuropsychological assessment. The clinical examination typically performed by the neurologist includes an assessment of motor reflexes and coordination, as well as assessment of cerebral dominance or left-right orientation (Table 1.10).

A child is often referred for a visual examination (Table 1.11) or an emotional and behavioral assessment (Table 1.12). Frequently, the latter assessment is required in order for the child to be placed in a class for the emotionally disturbed.

The pediatric neurologist Children with a profile of strengths and weaknesses similar to Andrew's are often referred for a neurological evaluation. The pediatric neurologist, a medical doctor trained in neurological disorders of childhood, administers a series of tasks to elicit

Table 1.10 CEREBRAL DOMINANCE AND LEFT-RIGHT ORIENTATION
(BY THE PSYCHOLOGIST, NEUROLOGIST, PHYSICAL
THERAPIST, OR OCCUPATIONAL THERAPIST)

1. Clinical examination
2. Quantitative testing
    Harris Tests of Lateral Dominance
    Halstead neuropsychological test battery (Reitan modification)
    Wechsler Intelligence Scale for Children (maze test)
    Roadmap test
    A-B-C Vision Test for Ocular Dominance

Figure 1.4 *Reading teacher's check list. (Courtesy of B. Moran.)*

INDIVIDUAL READING SKILLS CHECK LIST

Mark (+) for strengths and (−) for weaknesses. Marking begins first year of school.

NAME: _____

Birthdate _____ Year _____ Age _____

LEVELS

	1	2	3	4	5	6
Visual strength						
Auditory strength						
Receptive ability						
Expressive ability						
Gross motor skills						
1. Fine motor skill						
2. Directionality						

WORD ATTACK SKILLS

LEVELS

	1	2	3	4	5	6
3. Sight vocabulary development						
4. Alphabet recognition						
a. upper						
b. lower						
5. Alphabet writing						
a. upper						
b. lower						
6. Character writing (i.t.a.)						
7. Symbol-sound association application						
a. initial consonants						
b. final consonants						
c. initial blends						

LEVELS

	1	2	3	4	5	6
d. final blends						
e. initial consonant digraphs						
f. final consonant digraphs						
g. short vowels						
h. long vowels						
i. final *e*						
j. vowels— *l* and *r*						
k. vowel digraphs						
l. vowel diphthongs						
8. Blending—*a–l*						
9. Use of context						
10. Structural analysis						
11. Syllabication skills						

LANGUAGE DEVELOPMENT	1	2	3	4	5	6
1. Follow simple directions						
2. Follow compound directions						

COMPREHENSION SKILLS	1	2	3	4	5	6
3. Follow complex directions						
4. Communication ability						
a. conversation						
b. gestures						
5. Interpretative—Reading						
a. basal readers						
b. basal reader work books						
c. content areas						
1) main idea						
2) specific facts						
3) sequence of ideas						
4) cause-effect relationships						
5) critical analysis						

Table 1.11 CHILD STUDY OPHTHALMOLOGIC-OPTOMETRIC EVALU-
ATION (BY THE OPHTHALMOLOGIST, OPTOMETRIST)

1. Retinal examination
2. Visual acuity, fields, refractive error
3. Convergence ability, retinal congruence, depth perception
4. Ocular dominance
      A-B-C Vision Test
      Keystone visual tests

sensory and reflex reactions and then observes for abnormalities in response. He also asks the child to perform a series of voluntary perceptual-motor acts and judges the quality of performance displayed. Table 1.13 lists the major areas of evaluation. The neurologist may also ask for ancillary examinations, such as an electroencephalogram (EEG) or skull X-rays, as well as the results of ophthalmologic and audiometric testing. The child's responses are then subjectively compared to what the neurologist knows about both normal and atypical development (Touwen & Prechtl, 1970).

The team in Andrew's school had worked closely with a neurologist for several years and knew how to make the best use of his time. They suspected that he would find no gross neurological abnormality and would probably concur with their opinion and make a diagnosis of language deficiency caused by a disorder of the central nervous system. Because the neurologist usually was unable to translate his diagnosis into an educational prescription, the team limited their use of the neurologist to those cases where they suspected the presence of seizures, where medication might be useful, or where repeated testing revealed loss of function. The team's findings, however, were always shared with the family's physician who might choose to refer the child to another medical specialist (see Chapter 5). The majority of team members felt the diag-

Table 1.12 EMOTIONAL AND BEHAVIORAL ASSESSMENT (BY THE
PSYCHIATRIST, PSYCHOLOGIST)

1. Play evaluation
2. Formal psychiatric interview and evaluation
3. Informal projective tests
      Three wishes
      Earliest memory
      Meanest person in the world
      What animal would you like to be?
      Draw-a-car
4. Behavior rating scales
5. Formal projective testing
6. Personality inventories

Table 1.13 NEUROLOGICAL EXAMINATION

1. Formal neurological examination: includes cranial nerves, deep and superficial reflexes, muscles strength, primary modalities of sensation
2. Fine motor coordination
3. Gross motor coordination
4. Motor praxis (extremities, speech, eye movements)
5. Visual, tactile, auditory recognition of objects
6. Visual-perceptual, visual-motor abilities
7. Cerebral dominance, body image, left-right orientation
8. Temporal sequencing, rhythm
9. Involuntary movements, motor overflow
10. Language structure and formation
11. Mental status examination
12. Behavioral attributes, interaction with parents, examiner, environment

nosis of brain dysfunction since birth (chronic brain syndrome) to be of limited usefulness educationally since the effects of the disorder were often revealed in academic performance and in behavior rather than in formal neurological assessment (Tucker, 1970).

Sometimes the neurologist can help to localize the area of a brain deficiency. His results can help explain a particular cognitive disorder isolated by psychological testing. For example, parietal lobe damage frequently results in an inability at spatial construction. A child's very poor handwriting may be due to parietal lobe dysfunction but also may be due to lack of practice. Should the neurologist find other signs of parietal lobe disorder, then there is greater certainty that the poor writing is the result of brain dysfunction. Both the child, his parents, and his teachers would be told that his poor writing is not "his fault" and to ease up on pressures for neat writing. Frequently, the neurologist's diagnosis of minimal cerebral dysfunction (see Chapter 8) is nothing more than a summary statement resulting from examination of the reports of other team members. Table 1.14 presents the contribution of each area of assessment.

The nonprofessional Although we have placed our discussion of the role of the nonprofessional following our discussion of the role of professional, this order by no means implies that the nonprofessional is of lesser importance. To the contrary, the teacher aide, the community volunteer, and the college or high school volunteer may be the most critical members of a child study team, since it is they who help carry out the recommendations of the team. Teenagers who tutor younger children, college students who counsel adolescents or preadolescents, high school students who "rap" with junior high students about drugs, dating, and other teenage problems, parents who tutor other parents'

Table 1.14 MINIMAL CEREBRAL DYSFUNCTION: SYNTHESIS OF AREAS OF ASSESSMENT

1. Etiologic history—50 percent false negatives
2. Behavioral history—important and often neglected
3. Physical examination—helpful if positive
4. Formal neurological examination—not often helpful
5. Supplementary neurological examination—20–30 percent false negative
6. EEG—abnormal in 50–60 percent; 15–20 percent false positives
7. Skull X-rays—5–10 percent yield
8. Audiologic testing—30–40 percent yield
9. Ophthalmologic consultation—small yield
10. Psychological (psychometric and projective) evaluation—the most revealing
11. Diagnostic trial of drugs, e.g., amphetamines, anticonvulsants
    (barbiturates vs. hydantoins)—limited usefulness

Adapted from S. H. Tucker. The difficulties of making an early diagnosis in children with minimal cerebral dysfunction. Paper presented at the annual conference of the American Physical Therapy Association, Washington, D.C., July 1970.

children in return for tutoring of their own, and aides who tutor or form relationships with withdrawn or deprived children are all delivering a service that the busy professional has little time to give.

Sometimes the nonprofessional is better than the professional at delivering some of the services the professional has always regarded as within his domain. The tutor often reaches the hard-to-reach child better than does the teacher, and the college student often makes a better counselor of the teenager than does the guidance counselor. There is no academic credit given for training in life; if there were, many of the "untrained" would be perhaps better trained than the professional. The ex-addict, for example, gets no credit for his life experiences, but works well in drug abuse treatment centers or in school counseling programs.

Roles other than child study   Because this book focuses on exceptional children, it may appear as if the psychologist, social worker, or psychiatrist's roles are confined to the assessment of individual children. Although beyond the scope of this book to describe the various activities in which these professionals engage, it would be remiss to leave the impression that the psychologist only tests, the psychiatrist only interviews, and the social worker only takes case histories.

In the school both the psychologist and the social worker frequently develop inservice training programs for teachers, help teachers to develop more effective classroom management procedures, and clarify the relation between family style and learning style. They also consult with school administrators about school policy, help select teachers, hold jam sessions with students, train student monitors, run parent guidance groups, or provide individual and group counseling to children. In many instances, these two professionals serve to ease tensions which arise in the school and in this way prevent problems from developing.

Outside the school psychologists and psychiatrists in clinics consult with other community agencies such as urban renewal, daycare centers, family court, or neighborhood youth centers. Those employed in hospitals or residential centers do intensive child study. They also do psychotherapy, consult with child care and educational staff, and perform research and program evaluation. Research, as we will see throughout this book, is necessary in order to learn more about exceptional children. Unfortunately, what is learned through research is not always put into practice.

The tools of evaluation

The psychiatrist and social worker employ no real tools when they evaluate a child. By real tools we mean standardized tests or mechanical devices for measurement or examination. The social worker interviews the family and asks a series of questions which elicit information about family background and the current family situation. Some ask families to fill out a questionnaire before they are seen and use the answers as a place to begin further inquiry. The psychiatrist interviews the child, usually in a playroom, but does so in a very unstructured manner. He observes how the child responds to his presence and the manner in which he uses the toys in the room. It is his training and clinical experience with many children that enable him to make a judgment about the kind and degree of emotional immaturity present in the child. For example, if the child immediately goes to the dolls, takes off their clothes, and makes them kiss, this behavior would suggest sexual preoccupation and anxiety about sexuality.

The pediatric neurologist takes a developmental history (see Chapter 2) and performs a neurological evaluation, testing reflex and voluntary movements. His tools are only a reflex hammer, tape measure, ophthalmoscope, applicator sticks, coins, pellets, match sticks, a visual target, bell, pencil and paper, a chair, and a table. His knowledge of abnormal development is what enables him to make a valid assessment.

The reading teacher employs standardized tests. These tests consist of graded reading passages, graded word lists, and standard questions to determine if a child performs as well as most children his age. A third grade child who makes more errors in reading a passage than the average third grader cannot read at his grade level. Sometimes a child can read a passage without error but comprehends less material than other children his same age. In this fashion the reading teacher learns a child's vocabulary, reading, and comprehension levels and the types of errors made in reading.

The psychologist, particularly those interested in intellectual and language development, utilizes standardized tests to assess a child. It is not within the scope of this chapter to discuss psychometric theory or test development. The reader is referred to any of the introductory texts on psychological testing (Anastasi, 1968; Cronbach, 1970; Freeman, 1962). Some brief comments are in order, however, to familiarize the reader with tests mentioned in the following chapters.

Intelligence tests The most widely used individual tests of intelligence are the Stanford-Binet Intelligence Scale and the Wechsler Intelligence Scale for Children (WISC). The Binet is an age-scale test and the WISC a point-scale test.

The Binet employs verbal, pictorial, and manipulative material at younger age levels and primarily verbal material at older levels. The test gives a mental age equivalent which is converted into an IQ score. The child is given problems which are grouped by age levels. A problem passed by approximately 70 percent of 6-year olds and 90 percent of 7-year olds is considered a problem for the 6-year level. There are usually six problems at each age level, each worth two months credit. The child is given problems until he can pass all six at one age level (basal age) and then testing proceeds until all six items are failed at another age level (ceiling). For example, if a child passes all items at the 6-year level, passes four at the 7-year level, two at the 8-year level, two at the 9-year level and none at the 10-year level, his mental age is 7 years, 4 months. If his chronological age is 6 years, 3 months, his IQ is determined by the formula $IQ = MA/CA \times 100$. The type of items the child fails and passes provides some clues about his strengths and weaknesses. For example, a child who can define abstract words well beyond his chronological age level, but cannot unscramble sentences, may have difficulty in sequencing of ideas but not in abstraction or comprehension. Of course, such analysis is limited because of the limited number of items of a particular type.

The WISC was developed somewhat differently. There are six subtests which purport to measure verbal intelligence, or reasoning with words, and six which measure performance intelligence, or reasoning with manipulative and pictorial material. Each subtest is composed of a number of items. The number the child gets correct is scored and compared with scores received by children of various ages. For example, there are 20 questions in the information subtest; 7-year olds pass 8 items, while 12-year olds pass 16. The subtests of the WISC and what each purports to measure are listed in Table 1.15. Because six tests are considered verbal and six performance, a child obtains three IQ scores: verbal IQ, performance IQ, and full scale IQ (a kind of average of the two).

Psychologists sometimes prefer the WISC to the Binet because they feel it allows for a better assessment of strengths and weaknesses. (Chapter 10 presents an analysis of a gifted child's WISC subtest scores.) The WISC is also preferred because it gives both a verbal and performance

IQ score, while the Binet is more heavily weighted with verbal items. Psychologists particularly interested in verbal functioning sometimes use the Binet and later administer a performance test if they suspect that the Binet has unduly penalized the child.

Factor analytic techniques (intercorrelation studies) have indicated that verbal and performance subtests can measure a similar trait. For example, a child may do poorly on both the similarities and block design subtests of the WISC because he lacks abstract thinking skill. He may, however, do poorly on similarities because he relates words on the basis of physical similarities (low order of abstraction) but do well on block design because he has good analyzing and synthesizing ability, another aspect of block design performance. For this reason, only a trained examiner should administer and interpret intelligence test results.

Particular problems in using intelligence tests with certain types of exceptionality will be discussed in the chapters to follow. In general, intelligence tests were developed by ascertaining how a typical population at each age level performed on test items. Using such tests with certain types of exceptionality may not be justified. If the test is modified in some fashion (obviously a timed motor test would be invalid on a poorly coordinated child with motor tremors), then research is necessary to demonstrate that scores obtained can still be compared with the original norms.

Personality tests Psychologists, particularly those employed in clinics, sometimes use projective tests of personality. The Rorschach ink-blot and the Thematic Apperception Test (TAT) are the two most popular.

The Rorschach consists of ten cards containing ink blots. The cards are shown to the child one at a time in a prescribed order and the child states what they look like to him. Different children "see" different things and their responses are evaluated in a number of ways. The assumption is made that the predominating aspects of personality are projected onto the ambiguous blots when the child is encouraged to associate to them freely. The Rorschach responses of a severely disturbed boy are presented in Chapter 4. In this boy's case it is relatively easy to see that he is disturbed, since he perceives hostile and frightening images in areas of the blot where others typically do not see such images. In other cases the responses are not as bizarre and only a trained examiner can interpret them. Although various quantitative methods have been applied to score Rorschach responses (e.g., area of blot, number of responses, form level), its clinical use primarily involves qualitative analysis and, therefore, is subject to the examiner's theoretical and personal bias. Consequently, some psychologists consider descriptions of personality that are based on Rorschach responses to be of questionable validity.

In the Thematic Apperception Test the child is shown a standard series of pictures and asked to make up a story about each one. The

Table 1.15 PRESCRIPTIVE-TEACHING GUIDE BASED ON PERFORMANCE
(See key at bottom of page for interpretation of codes in parentheses.)

Information	Comprehension	Arithmetic	Similarities	Vocabulary	Digit span
Memory	Concepts	Concentration Visualization	Concepts	Memory Visualization	Attention Concentration
Details (Ed.) (A)	Common sense Social awareness (A)	(Ed.) (A)	Perception Verbalization Part-to-whole (A)	Experience and exposure (A)	Anxiety (A)
Associative techniques Multisensory approach	Exposure and experience Gestalt development through part-to-whole	Kinesthetic-associative Concrete experiences Auditory attention and visualization	Language development Gestalt development through part-to-whole Visualization training	Language development Associative techniques Visual memory	Auditory training Patterns and part-to-whole Visualization techniques

(Ed.) Influenced by education, (A) Auditory-vocal, (V) Visual, (VM) Visual-motor.
From N. Banas & I. H. Wills. The vulnerable child and prescriptive teaching. *Academic Therapy,*
1969, 4, p. 217.

assumption underlying this test is that the meaning obtained from, or injected into a picture, reveals feelings, attitudes, and motives. For example, a child in residential treatment told the following two stories about a picture of a boy sitting by a violin. The interval between the two stories was two years.

He's making up that he wants to hit someone in the head with the violin. (Q. What does he do?) He runs away. (Q. Where does he go?) He goes to his grandmother's house. (Q. Why?) He didn't like the school, they treat him bad. (Q. What happens?) He dies. (Q. How?) In an accident. (Q. How?) Run over. (6/11/70)

A boy staring at a violin he got for his birthday. He knows he can't play it. He just stares and stares at it. (Q. What happens?) He learns how to play it. (Q. How?) Teacher teaches him. (6/20/72)

In the first story we get a picture of a boy who is angry at adults and who would like to strike out at them in anger but can only run away and

ON THE WECHSLER INTELLIGENCE SCALE FOR CHILDREN

Picture completion	Picture arrangement	Block design	Object assembly	Coding	Mazes
Perception	Concepts	Perception	Concepts Perception	Visual-motor coordination Perception	Perception Visual-motor coordination
Noting details (Ed.) (V)	Part-to-whole Planning Attention to details (V) (VM)	Part-to-whole Analyze and synthesize (V) (VM)	Gestalt (V) (VM)	Anxiety Memory (V) (VM)	Anxiety Planning (V) (VM) (A)
Education and exposure Manipulation Meaningful context	Experience and exposure Manipulation Sequential awareness	Part-to-whole development Working to a model (key) Organization: puzzles, other	Patterns and part-to-whole Gestalt visualization Visualization of minimal clues	Eye-hand training Visual-memory and perception Directionality	Eye-hand training Visualization of the gestalt Organization and planning

get protection from a benevolent figure. For even this assertive act, he anticipates severe punishment.

The second story gives quite a different picture. The boy still lacks assertion but feels less aggressive and perhaps more positive toward adults. He might, however, feel somewhat resigned to his passive situation and angry that he needs adults to help him. To clarify the situation, more stories would need to be analyzed and information from other sources added.

Psychologists use TAT stories not only to get a picture of personality, but also to measure means-ends thinking, a prerequisite for reading comprehension and for fulfilling many of the demands made upon the child in class.

Criticisms of the TAT are basically the same as those directed at the Rorschach. Very few psychologists, however, employ any one test in isolation. Typically, they pool all available data before formulating a decision about the nature of a child's problems.

Other projective tests used are the Children's Apperception Test (pic-

tures of animals performing human behaviors, used with young children),
the Symonds Picture-Story Test (pictures of adolescents engaged in various activities, used with older children), and the Michigan Picture Stories
(pictures of children involved in school activities).

Some psychologists use personality inventories to learn about a child,
but their use is relatively infrequent. An inventory is a printed form
composed of various statements about children. The child is asked to
indicate whether the statement applies to him. The inventory is then
scored and compared to normative data.

The Illinois Test of Psycholinguistic Abilities (ITPA)   Speech and reading
specialists, as well as psychologists, use the ITPA to evaluate a child's
psycholinguistic development. Psycholinguistic abilities consist of language or communication skills. These include all the ways in which
children gain information from others and the environment, organize
and manipulate information and concepts mentally, and communicate
information and ideas to others. The rationale and structure of the ITPA
is based on a functional framework proposed by Osgood (1957). According to Osgood, the basic processes of communication can be incorporated
into two levels of language organization, three processes of communication, and two channels of communication.

The first level of language organization is the *representational level*.
At this level mediation takes place between a stimulus and a response;
stimuli take on meaning for the child and he can think about them in
their absence. At the *automatic level,* behavior is less voluntary but
highly organized and integrated. Habits are formed from repetitive exposure to similar situations so that responses are automatic (for example,
using correct grammatical forms or repeating poems from memory).

Three processes of communication are utilized in the ITPA. The first
is *reception,* which involves recognizing, understanding, or memorizing
what is seen or heard. The second process is *association,* which involves
an organizing process in which abstract, conceptual understanding, and
symbolic manipulation take place. The associational process exists at
both the representational and automatic levels of organization, although
at the automatic level association consists only of an unconscious conditioned stimulus-response link. The third process is *expression,* which involves the communication of ideas or information through words or
gestures.

Two channels or routes of flow of communication are utilized by the
ITPA. Channels of communication refer to the sense modalities through
which stimuli are received and the modes of expression of the resulting
response. Theoretically, many channels exist. Helen Keller used tactile-
motor and tactile-verbal channels of communication. It would be possible
to construct a gustatory-motor subtest in which the subject had to discriminate between salty, bitter, sour, and sweet tastes and then push the

Table 1.16   THE ILLINOIS TEST OF PSYCHOLINGUISTIC ABILITIES

Level	Subtests	Tasks involved
Representational	Auditory reception	Answer Yes or No to questions such as "Do airplanes fly?"
	Visual reception	Observe a pictured item and then find the same item on another page after stimulus is covered
	Auditory association	Finish an incomplete analogy, such as "A daddy is big; a baby is _____."
	Visual association	Select one of four peripheral pictures most closely associated with a central picture, such as a central picture of a pillow and a peripheral picture of a bed
	Verbal expression	Talk about objects presented
	Manual expression	Demonstrate use of pictured object, such as a hammer
Automatic	Grammatic closure	Complete incomplete statement guided by pictures that represent content of verbal expression, such as "Here is a bed. Here are two _____."
	Visual closure	Find hidden pictures, such as "See these dogs? Put your finger on one. Show me another."
	Auditory sequential memory	Repeat increasingly longer sequences of numbers.
	Visual sequential memory	Observe a sequence of ordered chips and replicate the order from memory
Supplementary	Auditory closure	Supply missing parts of incomplete words
	Sound blending	Pronounce whole word or nonsense word after being given successive sounds or syllables, such as "d . . . og. What word is that?

appropriate button to indicate his decision. The ITPA utilizes only the *auditory-vocal* and *visual-motor* channels of communication simply because they are the crucial ones for learning and communication.

No attempt is made to separate the receptive, associative and expressive processes at the automatic level. The four subtests at this level are essentially "whole level" tests. However, the ITPA is founded on the supposition that the three processes can be separated and individually assessed at the representational level. For example, suppose a child is unable to answer questions about a story that has just been read to him. There is no way of knowing whether he just didn't understand the story (receptive process) or was unable to express his ideas (expressive process). The ITPA is structured so that it can pinpoint whether a child's problems are receptive, associative, expressive, or any combination of the three.

Just as specific deficits in processes of communication can be singled out by the ITPA, so can deficits in either the auditory-vocal or visual-motor channels of communication. Perhaps a child cannot assimilate

Figure 1.5 *Andrew's ITPA profile.* (Illinois Test of Psycholinguistic Abilities, *Revised Edition Record Form, Profile of Abilities.* Urbana: University of Illinois Press. Reproduced by permission.)

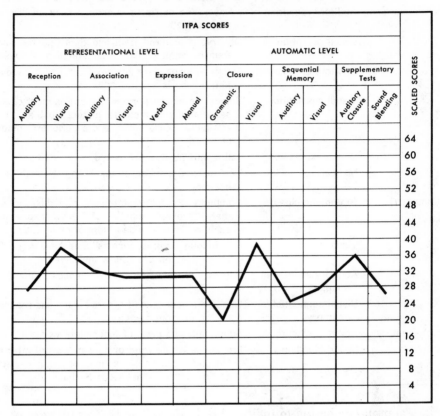

information presented verbally. In this case, he has an auditory-vocal channel disability. He might also have trouble expressing his thoughts verbally, but this need not be the case.

Similarly, it is possible to distinguish discrepancies in performance between the representational and automatic levels of organization. A child might be very proficient in automatic tasks such as rote memorization of a series of digits or visual symbols, but be seriously deficient in tasks requiring abstract conceptual understanding.

Analyzing the child's subtest scores by utilizing the concepts of processes, channels, and levels, it is possible to evolve a picture of the child's psycholinguistic functioning and then to prescribe appropriate remediation.

The model for the ITPA provides a total of ten separate subtests, six at the representational level and four at the automatic level. There are also two supplementary tests measuring auditory closure and sound blending. At the representational level the subtests are auditory and visual

Table 1.17 OPTIMAL ASSESSMENT—TEAM APPROACH*

Aspect	Time (Min.)	Cost
1. Case history and physical examination	45	$30.00
2. Neurological examination	45	30.00
3. EEG	90	35.00
4. Psychological testing	120	50.00
5. Audiogram and language evaluation	60	25.00
6. Visual- and perceptual-motor examination	45	20.00
7. Motor assessment	45	20.00
8. Ophthalmologic examination	30	25.00
9. Social development assessment	45	20.00
10. Psychiatric assessment	60	30.00
11. Educational assessment	30	15.00
	10 hrs. +	$300.00 +

* This does not include team conference, preparation of reports, parental counseling, follow-through with school.

Adapted from S. H. Tucker. The difficulties of making an early diagnosis in children with minimal cerebral dysfunction. Paper presented at the annual conference of the American Physical Therapy Association, Washington, D.C., July 1970.

reception, auditory and visual association, and verbal and manual expression. At the automatic level the subtests are grammatic closure, visual closure, auditory sequential memory, and visual sequential memory. Remember that tests on the automatic level are whole level subtests, that is, there is no attempt to distinguish between reception, association, and expression at the automatic level of organization. (The subtests are described in Table 1.16.)

The ITPA was administered to Andrew, whose case was presented earlier. Let us examine how it contributed to understanding his problem. Figure 1.5 gives Andrew's profile. Andrew's chronological age was 8 years, five months. The subtest scaled score at his chronological age level is 36. As can be seen, Andrew scored below age level on all but two subtests. His greatest deficiencies were on auditory memory (a scaled score of 25 corresponds to a language age of 4 years, 2 months), grammatic closure (22 = 5 years, 0 months), and sound blending (27 = 5 years, 0 months). These scores along with other information supported the impression that an auditory language disorder prevented Andrew from learning efficiently. The ITPA is discussed more fully in Bateman (1968) and Parakevopoulas and Kirk (1969). Remediation based on ITPA scores is presented in Kirk and Kirk (1971). One major drawback of the ITPA is that it lends itself to "cookbook" approaches to remediation. As we will learn in Chapter 8, children with specific deficits do not necessarily respond to remediation programs designed to circumvent these deficits, that is, a visual approach for a child with an auditory deficit.

Table 1.18 DIFFICULTIES IN EARLY DIAGNOSIS OF CHILDHOOD
DISORDERS

1. Insufficient abnormality for recognition
2. Failure of parent, teacher, or physician to recognize abnormality
3. Lack of referral facility
4. Cost of assessment prohibitive to parents
5. Failure of assessment team to distinguish disorder from normal developmental
   variability
   a. Range of normal variability
   b. Incomplete expression of developmental potential in early years
   c. Difficulty in obtaining valid exam; child not cooperative
   d. Lack of appropriate normative standards for early ages
   e. Failure of standards to discriminate well in early ages
6. Failure of team to translate diagnosis into a meaningful educational or remedial
   prescription

Speech and hearing evaluation Speech and hearing specialists use an
audiometer to measure hearing. This instrument produces a variety of
controlled tones that vary in pitch and loudness. The simplest procedure
is one where the child raises his finger when he hears sounds in earphones. The Snellen chart is used to test visual acuity and the perimeter
to measure field of vision. More will be said about audiometry and visual
testing in Chapter 5.

Reasons for the limited use of thorough child study

Although child study can include assessment in all areas, usually such
assessment is employed only when a neurological disorder is suspected.
The cost of a thorough child study runs in excess of $300 (see Table
1.17). In addition, it is often difficult to determine the exact nature of
a child's difficulty if he lives in an impoverished or chaotic environment.
The differentiation of minimal cerebral dysfunction from emotional
difficulties is difficult, particularly when there is family strife. Table 1.18
summarizes the major difficulties in early diagnosis of childhood disorders.

MULTIDISCIPLINARY TEAMS IN OTHER SETTINGS

While psychiatrists are rarely consulted in public school settings, they
usually are the chief figures in teams in child guidance clinics, psychiatric
hospitals, and institutions for the retarded. These centers are partially
supported by funds from state departments of mental hygiene who usually stipulate that psychiatrists be in charge of such agencies and that
they assume chief responsibility for a patient's welfare. As a consequence,

they usually lead team meetings and oversee the treatment of all cases. In most agencies operated by psychiatrists, the overriding philosophy of treatment derives from an illness model of dysfunction; the child is "sick" and needs medical treatment. The relative emphasis on illness varies from institution to institution depending upon the background of the physician in charge.

When psychiatrists function in institutions operated by physicians without training in psychiatry, they usually find themselves allied with their nonmedical colleagues. As we will see in Chapter 6, psychiatrists employed in general hospitals or even in children's hospitals often find that their medical colleagues in pediatrics or general medicine ignore the child's emotional needs and concentrate only on his physical needs. In such settings the psychiatrist looks for support from psychologists and social workers, professionals who have traditionally emphasized social and environmental factors as causes of emotional distress.

Regardless of who directs agencies for exceptional children, professionals from a variety of disciplines are represented on their staff. We will now examine some of these agencies and the underlying philosophies that guide their functioning.

The mental health concept

Institutions for the retarded Individuals with unusual behavior, behavior which cannot be tolerated by the community at large, have traditionally been removed from the community and placed in institutions designed to provide for their care. Retarded children were and still are enrolled in large state run institutions where they are isolated from society. While this situation is changing, with more retarded being cared for within their community, parents of the more profoundly retarded are still encouraged to institutionalize their children. Most institutions for the retarded are filled beyond capacity and have long waiting lists. The profoundly retarded are characterized by gross retardation, minimal capacity for functioning, and inability to profit from training in self-help. Consequently they need complete care and supervision. The IQ ranges from 0–20. These children remain at home until such time as an institution has an opening.

There are approximately 200,000 residents of more than 150 state institutions for the mentally retarded, and thousands more are on the waiting lists to be admitted. A 1968 survey of 44 states revealed that the total number awaiting admission was 27,048. Fifteen states indicated 500 or more applicants awaiting admission, 13 reported having a list of between 100 and 500 individuals, and only 7 states reported having no waiting list (Pinder, 1969).

Although institutions for the retarded are called training schools or state schools, they often function more like hospitals than like schools.

Physicians, rather than educators, usually direct these "schools," as well as the different units within the institution. While this situation is rapidly changing, the change has been brought about as much by the disinterest of physicians in working in such settings as it has by a genuine belief that other professionals may be better trained to operate these centers.

The early institutions for the retarded, although directed by physicians, were perhaps more like the model institutions of today. Their designers did not intend to isolate individuals from others; they hoped that their programs would enable retarded children to return to society better equipped to function in a normal manner. To understand why present-day institutions vary from state to state requires that we present a brief history of institutional practices.

The original founders of institutions for the retarded envisioned a "cure" for mental retardation. They believed that educative, moral, and medical measures would improve intelligence; the exercise of mental functions would facilitate their functioning. As late as 1877 Seguin, a pioneer in the field of institutional care of the retarded, noted that educating the brain results in noticeable enlargement of the cranium (Kanner, 1964).

When children did not make the anticipated gains after years in residence, the original notion of curability was rejected. Amelioration, rather than normalcy, became the new goal; the retarded would be trained to develop good study and work habits as well as self-respect. Each new institution started with a small number of pupils who were the center of zealous efforts to improve their functioning. It did not take long, however, for admissions to multiply. It also became clear that a considerable portion of the retarded showed no prospects of return to the community. Thus, the institution lost its initial unitary character. Different types of services were needed, and the retarded were assigned to different sections of the institution based on the severity of their disorder.

At the same time the public, as well as some professionals, began to emphasize more concern for the needs of society than for the needs of the retarded. Because of their peculiarities, society began to regard the retarded as potentially dangerous. They were viewed as a menace to civilization, incorrigible at home, burdens to schools, sexually promiscuous, breeders of defective offspring, and spreaders of poverty, degeneracy, crime, and disease (Davis & Ecob, 1959; Wallin, 1955). People demanded the segregation of all mental defectives so that society could be purified by building a solid wall around its contaminators. The movement began in about 1900 and by 1910 it had become as unanimous an opinion as had been ever held about the retarded (Kuhlmann, 1940).

Institutions, begun in the mid-nineteenth century to benefit the mentally retarded, fifty years later became places to isolate what were considered the undesirable elements of society. The physicians who were the heads of these institutions found themselves isolated from the medical world outside the institution. Mental deficiency was not a subject of medical research nor was it even mentioned in medical circles.

Two events brought about the dawn of a new era. First, in 1934 Fölling discovered that one form of retardation was the result of a metabolic disturbance and might be reversible by means of dietary regulation (see Chapter 3). This discovery made the subject of mental deficiency respectable as a field of research for the medical and biological professions. Second, the mental hygiene movement, led by Clifford Beers in 1909, resulted in the establishment in 1922 of child guidance clinics. Although help for retarded children was given only token attention in these early clinics, they helped pave the way for a more positive approach toward all children who showed difficulties in adjustment.

In spite of these changes in attitude, actual changes in practice were slow in coming. When cure for retardation was dismissed as impossible and custodial care became the rule rather than the exception, well-trained professionals could see no challenge to working with the retarded and sought employment elsewhere. The treatment team was actually a misnomer. Staff from the various disciplines would meet to discuss a child's reaction to his placement, his current ward behavior, or his transfer to another ward, but rarely was it envisioned that he would leave the institution. When the concept of treatment returned to habilitation, the physical therapist, occupational therapist, and vocational rehabilitation counselor were added to the team.

In spite of attractive financial offers, well-trained professionals still avoid employment in the field of retardation. Without skilled professionals to foster change and to deliver services, institutions will continue to offer limited assistance to retarded children and their families.

For example, in spite of the current push to keep retarded children in their community, many states have no written criteria on which to base the admission of children into their institutions. Most admit children on the basis of chronological order by earliest date of application. In 1968 only nine states had written criteria for placing applicants on a waiting list in order of relative need and presenting problems. These states were Delaware, Florida, Georgia, New Mexico, Pennsylvania, Washington, Wisconsin, Wyoming, and Utah (Pinder, 1969). Texas has developed computer-assisted management of their waiting list (Levy & Pinder, 1971). Their system is worth describing in some detail.

All applications for state school admission in Texas are screened to determine legal eligibility and evaluated for assurance that all community placement opportunities have been explored and exhausted. If state school placement is considered necessary, a standard data collection form is compiled which consists of the following descriptor variables: sex, date of birth, adaptive behavior level, IQ, self-help skills, toilet training, ambulation, speech, impairment of special senses, psychiatric impairments, presence of physical handicaps, and presence of health problems. Each item is coded to yield discrete response categories which can be processed by computer. In addition to the applicant profile, an index of urgency is established for each applicant. This index is based upon the various indicators of placement urgency which appear in Table 1.19.

Once the children are admitted, they are assigned to living units which are relatively homogeneous with respect to the twelve descriptor variables. There are approximately 250 living units within the Texas state school. An applicant needing immediate placement, according to the index of emergency, is assigned to the first unit that has a vacancy congruent with his profile. He is later transferred to a second congruent unit nearer his home if the first assignment was at a distant institution.

Parents of profoundly retarded children in rural communities are less fortunate than those in more populated areas. Because of the lack of community facilities, many vacancies in institutions are filled by children who would not be institutionalized if they lived in urban areas. This phenomenon is a nationwide trend. Talkington (1970) found a general trend toward the admission of increasingly lower ability levels in more urban institutions, whereas rural institutions still admitted children with relatively high ability levels but who needed special education or vocational training not available in their community. Obviously, the recent trend toward the development of community resources for mildly and moderately retarded has not yet extended into many rural communities.

The recommendations of the President's Panel on Mental Retardation (1962) called for extension of institutional boundaries into the community. Texas responded to this challenge and developed the Outreach Team (Talkington, 1971). The Outreach Team is a group of institutionally based staff who travel throughout the state not only to evaluate children and counsel parents, but also to facilitate the development of community facilities for the retarded. One service is to help develop trainable level classes for those retarded who are on the institution's waiting list.

Those states that have developed better community based facilities to help the retarded child and his family are not necessarily those states that are the most forward looking in other areas. Often they are those that lacked institutional facilities to begin with and could, therefore, devise a plan whereby smaller residential units could be spread throughout the state and retarded children kept closer to home (for example, Maryland and Nebraska). States with a considerable investment in large institutions find it difficult to abandon these facilities in favor of newly constructed smaller units (New York and Pennsylvania). Later in this

Table 1.19 INDEX OF URGENCY

I. Urgent ratings

Medical

1. Specialized medical and nursing procedures required which are unavailable.
2. Uncontrolled convulsive seizures.
3. Tube feeding required.
4. Rapidly expanding hydrocephalus.
5. Open spina bifida.
6. Non-ambulatory and weighs over 35 pounds.
7. Other—specify.

Family

1. Complete inability of parents or guardian to function in parental roles.
2. Applicant completely dependent with no known relative or substitute persons or agencies to provide necessary care and supervision.
3. Overt signs of family disintegration with the applicant's presence in the home severely threatening the destruction of marital and family relationships.
4. Applicant is severely neglected, rejected or abused by the family or persons caring for him.
5. Other—specify.

Community

1. Aggressive and violent behavior placing self and/or others in imminent danger.
2. Extremely destructive, deviant, antisocial behavior, intense social maladjustment necessitating institutional care and supervision.
3. Grossly unacceptable sexual behavior.
4. Other—specify.

II. Moderate ratings

Medical

1. Specialized medical care and supervision required but minimum services available.
2. Other—specify.

Family

1. Parents or guardian minimally able to function in parental roles and temporarily able to assume responsibility but in need of relief.
2. Applicant's presence in the home is disrupting family relationships, causing marital disharmony or problems in sibling relationships.
3. Neglect and rejection of applicant by parents and family.
4. Parents under emotional and/or physical strain due to applicant's presence in the home.
5. Other—specify.

Community

1. Pattern of occasional extreme aggressive and destructive behavior toward self and/or others.
2. Other—specify.

III. Minimal ratings

Medical

1. No significant medical problems.

Family

1. Applicant's presence in home creating no significant problems.

Community

1. Applicant has made a borderline adjustment in family and community.

Explanation: The Index of Urgency consists of a three-digit code in which the first digit indicates the number of situation categories (Medical, Family, and Community) contributing toward an Urgent rating; the second digit indicates the number of situations contributing toward a Moderate rating; and the third digit indicates the number of situations contributing toward a Minimal rating. As an illustration, an Index of 210 would represent at least one Urgent indicator in any two situation categories, at least one Moderate indicator in any one category, and no Minimal indicators.

From J. Levy & S. Pinder. Computer-assisted management of state school waiting lists and admission procedures. *Mental Retardation*, 1971, **9**, p. 31.

chapter we will discuss more ideal arrangements for servicing retarded children.

Inpatient psychiatric facilities   The birth and growth of psychiatry in America coincided with the birth and growth of hospitals designed to care for the insane. With the exception of Benjamin Rush (1745–1790), the father of American psychiatry, the early American psychiatrists were all directors of mental hospitals. Following the lead of Phillippe Pinel (1745–1826) in France and of William Tulce (1732–1826) in England, early nineteenth-century psychiatry rejected the system of restraint treatment and adopted a more humanitarian treatment of the mentally ill. During the nineteenth century the term *madhouse* was replaced by *asylum* in recognition of a new therapeutic attitude toward the insane. Prior to this period the mentally deranged were viewed as evil, guilty, and worthy of punishment. They were often mechanically restrained because of fears of their demonic powers or their aggression toward others. When they were unchained, many were found to be reasonable and tractable, and many were able to leave the asylum for community living.

Unfortunately, the emancipation of patients was short-lived. With the rise in population and the accumulation of chronic cases in the asylums, moral treatment, the treatment which stressed compassionate understanding in peaceful and relaxing surroundings, vanished, except in some expensive private hospitals. Mechanical restraint reappeared, now under psychiatric supervision. To the general population, the word asylum became as frightening as the word madhouse had been before it. Dorothea Dix's (1802–1887) tireless crusade to get the insane out of prisons, dungeons, and cellars and into a humane and promising environment ultimately led only to their being set apart from the rest of society in institutions that had lost their ability to achieve their stated purpose.

As patients in mental hospitals increased, particularly patients from foreign countries speaking a foreign tongue, the problems outgrew the capacity of hospital psychiatry. The moral therapist disappeared and the watchful, custodial psychiatrist took his place. Psychiatric thinking had swung from a social stress theory of mental illness to one stressing an organic causation and a pessimistic prognosis for cure.

A better outlook reappeared when emphasis switched from organic to dynamic psychiatry. Both Adolph Myer (1866–1950) and Sigmund Freud (1856–1939), with their studies of the life histories of patients and their emphasis that a patient's experiences, feelings, and thoughts are essentially similar to those of all human beings, kindled a renewed interest in treatment of the mentally ill. The concept that other people are involved in both the origin and healing of mental illness became an accepted belief. This knowledge was soon applied to major social problems and the field of social psychiatry emerged. As a result, there developed an interest in the human personality as it develops in social settings.

After Myer and Freud's influence, hospital psychiatry changed very little between 1900 and 1960. Understaffed and poorly funded, hospitals tried to offer treatment to those who might profit from it and served as detention centers for the remainder. When psychopharmacological methods were introduced in the late 1950s, many more patients were able to leave the hospital. Nevertheless, the organization at the hospital remained more or less the same during this period and the mode of treatment still stressed need for change within the patient rather than within his community. When a patient did recover in the hospital, he was usually returned to the community without adequate community support. As a consequence the readmission rate was high. Let us examine the roles of the various professionals during this era.

Roles of professionals in psychiatric hospitals Because of the early relationship between the hospital and the church, hospitals were and still are organized after a model that communicates downward. Psychiatric hospitals follow the model of the general hospital. Treatment decisions are made by the psychiatrist-physician and care is provided through the nurse who supervises the hospital attendant or nurse's aide.

A clear caste system exists within the hospital. Unless he leaves the hospital for further schooling, the attendant cannot become a nurse nor the nurse a physician. Consequently, employees cannot move upward within the system. Readers interested in sociological studies of the psychiatric hospital are referred to Caudill (1958), Goffman (1961), and Stanton and Schwartz (1954).

During the era when psychotherapy was viewed as the main treatment, it made little difference whether such a caste system existed or not. The nurse's or attendant's role was simply to provide routine care between the patient's visits to his psychiatrist. The psychiatrist encouraged the patient to explore his past in an effort to reveal the roots of his disturbing behavior. Because there were never enough psychiatrists to provide every patient with psychotherapy, some decision had to be made about whom to concentrate efforts upon. In general, psychiatrists recognized that certain patients responded more favorably to insight oriented psychotherapy. If these individuals could be identified upon admission, then much valuable time could be saved which might otherwise be wasted. This need for differential diagnosis resulted in the addition of the psychologist to the hospital staff.

Since 1905 psychologists have been concerned with intelligence testing. The psychologist could evaluate each patient intellectually and pass this information on to the psychiatrist. Once the psychologist gained experience with mental patients, he discovered that different patterns of answers appeared in the test results of patients with differing symptomatology. Such discoveries led to the development of tests specifically designed to reveal these patterns. These tests to measure personality have been called projective tests. More recently, self-inventories also have been developed to assess a patient's image of himself.

As psychiatry became more aware of a family's influence upon a patient, they desired more information about family background and current family conditions. For this reason they acquired the services of social workers whose experiences in family and community organization they considered an asset. The social worker was required to take a detailed case history and to keep the family abreast of the psychiatrist's treatment activities. When the family visited the patient, the social worker talked with them and helped clarify their feelings. It soon became clear that many families needed extensive guidance and counseling. Because the social worker was not trained in psychopathology, much of his learning was provided through supervisory sessions with the psychiatrist. In order to meet the needs of institutions, schools of social work revamped their training to include courses in psychiatric case work, individual psychotherapy, and psychoanalytic theory.

Although psychiatry's leaders once worked in state-run institutions, very few highly qualified professionals now choose to work in state hospitals. A large proportion of psychiatrists employed in such settings are foreign-trained physicians who receive the majority of their psychiatric training within the state hospital system. Many, called resident psychiatrists, are not licensed to practice medicine in the state in which they reside and live on hospital grounds, isolated both physically and culturally from the community at large.

Although salaries for doctoral-level psychologists are often high in state hospitals, relatively few seek such employment. Well-trained social workers, nurses, and other professionals also avoid employment in state hospitals. As inpatient units become associated with community mental health centers, to be discussed later, this staffing pattern should change. As a consequence, better or differently trained professionals will work with inpatient populations.

When psychiatry became interested in children, many children who in the past would have been placed in institutions for the retarded were instead placed in psychiatric institutions.

The pattern established in adult psychiatric hospitals was followed in those established for children. The physician-psychiatrist utilized the testing skills of the psychologist and the interview skills of the social worker to assist him in formulating a treatment plan. To this team was added the educator who taught the institutionalized child, the recreation worker who provided care after school hours, and the child care worker or attendant who looked after the child's basic needs. Each person's role was considered clear, as were the lines of authority. As psychotropic drugs were introduced into treatment programs, it became the nurse's role to administer the drugs and to keep progress charts.

Every state has a state-funded psychiatric hospital, but not all have separate facilities for children and many place adolescents in adult sections of the hospital. Florida, for example, opened its first children's psychiatric hospital in 1969.

A new concept of residential service   Both a 6000-bed institution, such as Willowbrook State School in Staten Island, New York, and a small group home or halfway house are considered residential services. The first, however, is more likely to be labeled an institution. Most citizens would define an institution on the basis of features that emphasize isolation from the community at large. Wolfensberger (1971) feels that a more useful definition is one based on the deindividualization that pervades most institutional communities. Most of the features associated with institutions are corollaries of deindividualization rather than of separation from the "outside," and he lists four such features.

1. *A community where all members are subjected to a program designed to handle the behavior of its worst members.* Because a few residents are destructive or aggressive, all residents are subjected to an environment necessary to handle these few.
2. *Congregation of individuals into residential groups larger than those found in the community.*
3. *Reduced autonomy and increased regimentation of residents,* including mass movement and mass action.
4. *Continuous residence on one continuous campus.* Most of us sleep, study, work, and play in different settings and interact with different people in each setting. In most residential facilities interacting repeatedly with the same group of individuals reduces opportunities for individualization.

He states (1971, p. 15):

Thus, when I distinguish between institutions and other group residences . . . the term institution refers to a deindividualizing residence in which . . . persons are congregated in numbers distinctly larger than might be found in a large family; in which they are highly regimented; in which the physical or social environment aims at a low common denominator; and in which all or most of the transactions of daily life are carried out under one roof, on one campus, or in a largely segregated fashion.

Wolfensberger (1969, 1971) predicts that the concept of the institution will be replaced by a broader concept of residential service. The concept of care, as in the phrase "institutional care," will acquire new meaning. If the concept of care survives at all, it will apply only to those services which specialize in the maintenance of life of the most severely handicapped or the infirm aged. The widely prevalent institutional practices, historically derived from perceptions of the atypical as sick or dangerous, will be replaced by practices which emphasize the developmental capacity of all children. The widely used concept of "treatment" of institutional residents will be subsumed under a broader concept of "management," a concept that will refer to a wide range of actions and practices.

Newly established centers will be small, specialized, dispersed, and integrated into the community at large. By small, Wolfensberger means residences for 6 to 20 persons. Specialization means the identification of a single, overriding function associated with a residence. For the mentally retarded, optimal specialization will probably result in the creation of 10 to 12 types of facilities. These are summarized in Table 1.20. Units of types 3, 4, and 8 will be the most common. More detailed descriptions of these service types are described in Menolascino, Clark, and Wolfensberger (1968, 1970).

Services now provided by institutions will be provided by other agencies within the child's community. Community recreational facilities will be shared by the exceptional and normal. Shopping will be in ordinary community stores rather than in institutional canteens.

The return to small, dispersed, community residences will be accompanied by an increase in the use of live-in house parents, whose role will differ considerably from that of the institutional attendant who returns to his own residence each evening. The use of community-integrated residences will result in an increase in short-term residential placements and a decrease in long-term placements. There will be more overnight and extended home visits by both short- and long-term residents.

A number of other trends will result in a reduced incidence of children

Table 1.20 TYPES OF SPECIALIZED RESIDENTIAL SERVICES OF THE FUTURE

Type	Primary function	Ages served	Maximum number of persons per residential		Profession in charge
			Residence	Complex	
1	Maintenance of life	All	12	24	Medicine
2	Infant nursery	0–5	7	14	Pediatric nursing
3	Child development	3–12	8	16	Child development
4	Prevocational education	10–16	8	16	Special education
5	Behavior shaping	All	8	24	Psychology
6	Structured correctional training	15 +	8	16	Correction
7	Habilitation training	16–25	8	12	Rehabilitation
8	Sheltered living	16 +	8	20	Social work or rehabilitation
9	Minimal supervision	18 +	6	20	Social work or rehabilitation
10	Crisis assistance	All	8	12	Social work or rehabilitation
11	Five-day per week residential school*	6–15	10	40	Special education
12	Combination of Types 3, 4, and 11*	3–16	10	40	Special education

* For rural areas only.

From W. Wolfensberger. Twenty predictions about the future of residential services in mental retardation. *Mental Retardation*, 1969, **7**, p. 52.

needing institutionalization, such as preventive advancements in medicine, improvement of health services and the quality of life of disadvantaged, high-risk mothers, increased use of contraception by high-risk mothers, and legalization of abortion in high-risk pregnancies. Extension of early childhood education to those children exposed to adverse environmental influences, as well as increased adoptive and foster home placement of atyptical children when the public comes to accept deviancy among its members, should also reduce the need for institutionalization (Wolfensberger, 1969).

Gaps in existing institutions Although several states have made plans toward actualizing the predictions made by Wolfensberger, others are a long way from even considering such plans. Many states, although considerably ahead of others, still lack even institutional placements for particular types of children.

Rose, a girl of 12, had been institutionalized in a children's treatment center at age 10. After two years in the center, she had made considerable progress but still needed a sheltered environment. Her mother was on welfare and could not afford the cost of private institutionalization. The New York Bureau of Child Welfare was willing to pay the cost of further treatment, provided the setting was approved by their agency. The following telephone referrals were made, but no center would accept her application.

1. A private residential school—it was not certified by the Bureau of Child Welfare.
2. A home-school for girls on Long Island—the school program started at seventh grade.
3. Letchworth Village and Wassaic State School, two state-operated facilities for the retarded—her IQ was too high; they took none higher than 70–75.
4. The joint planning board for Jewish institutions—Rose did not fit into any of their institutions.
5. The state childrens' hospitals—they would take only psychotic children.
6. A private day school—it was open only five days a week, ten months a year.
7. Normal child care institutions—they felt she was too disturbed.

Because Rose was minimally brain-damaged but not retarded or psychotic, her functioning was too good for enrollment in state institutions. Because her reading and academic abilities were deficient and she had a history of behavioral disturbance, she was too impaired for institutions for dependent and neglected children. She was too old for the special classes in her local school district and, even if she hadn't been overage, she could not live with her severely depressed mother who could not care for her. An out-of-state placement in a private residential facility with a prevocational training program was also attempted, but they too rejected her.

A fortunate turn of events resulted in Rose's placement in a foster home and a Catholic school that had funds available for tutoring. She did well for a year and was then transferred to a public school that had developed a resource room for children and youths with learning disabilities.

Other children like Rose are not so fortunate. Foster homes for pre-teen and teenage youngsters are difficult to find and are not always successful. Many are placed in group homes, but even if adjustment there is adequate, the communities in which the homes are located often lack an educational program adequate to meet the children's needs. In Rose's case, all the high-powered experts failed to appreciate the strengths in this girl and the positive effect that the foster parent and school would have upon her future development.

Outpatient psychiatric services Child psychiatry developed from the common interests and ideas of different groups. Clinical psychology as the specific study of the individual was initiated by Lightner Witmer in his psychoeducational clinic opened in 1896 at the University of Pennsylvania. In this era university scholars became interested in school systems as a result of John Dewey's emphasis on education as the fundamental method of social progress. Nevertheless, the field of education at this time was not concerned with the training of exceptional children (Witmer, 1915). Witmer, influenced by the work of the pioneers in mental retardation, made an effort to introduce scientific principles into common school practice, not only for exceptional children, but for all children. He felt that the study and training of the exceptional child "constituted the most favorable point of approach for a psychology applied to educational practice" (Witmer, 1915, p. 537).

Witmer was an academician and scientist interested in practical problems. His clinic, and those that immediately followed, were closely involved with the public schools. Clinic staff provided training to teachers through the use of demonstration classes in addition to consultation. Teachers trained in these demonstration classes were placed in schools as "visiting teachers" to serve as examples to others. In short, Witmer's clinic was an integrated school and clinic effort. By 1914 there were more than 100 such clinics functioning in the United States, mostly directed by psychologists (Mora, 1954).

Unfortunately, most of Witmer's work was forgotten and clinics, under the influence of psychiatry, became less interested in the child in his environment and more interested in direct efforts to modify the child through individual psychotherapy. This movement grew out of increasing awareness that psychopathology had its origins in childhood. As a result, hospitals established both inpatient and outpatient services for children. St. Elizabeth's Hospital in Washington, D.C., Iowa Psychopathic Hospital, Philadelphia General Hospital, and Boston Psychopathic Hospital were the first well-known mental hospitals to work with children. Other hospitals followed suit, and communities without hospitals set up outpatient services for children either separately or as part of services to adults.

In 1926 the National Committee for Mental Hygiene opened a special office to coordinate the work done in different clinics, to make them more efficient, and to help communities to establish new clinics. Gradually, clinics established through the efforts of this committee outnumbered those run by university programs, and the medical approach to treatment eventually dominated the child guidance movement. Child guidance centers became isolated from other community agencies, even from the schools with which the original clinics were intertwined. The result was that clinics had almost no meaningful contact with the teachers and principals of the children they were asked to treat.

The contemporary child guidance clinic offers individual, group, and family therapy, either on a short- or long-term basis, and has little investment in working closely with community agencies or schools. Only a small proportion of clinic time is spent in community education (Witmer's original intent) and virtually no time is spent in attempting to influence local and state government to improve the social conditions which cause or exacerbate mental health problems (Levine & Levine, 1970). This isolation is not so critical in treatment of the middle-class patient whose problems are usually single-faceted. Treatment of the lower-class patient, however, requires close cooperation with other agencies. The patient's father may need job training and his family may need better housing, public health services, or legal advice. The outpatient clinic was not set up with the disadvantaged patient in mind.

In 1969 there were approximately 2,000 outpatient clinics in the United States (National Center for Health Statistics, 1971). In 1969, 819,000 patients terminated their treatment in these outpatient services. In contrast, there were 313,000 terminations in 1960. The number of cases under care is close to twice that amount since many cases are carried longer than one year. Children under 18 comprise 34 percent of the total case load of these clinics.

Each year about 700,000 children under 18 years of age receive some service in a psychiatric facility in the United States (National Institute of Mental Health, 1971). Of those seen in outpatient clinics, only one in three receive more than a diagnosis. In addition, clinics tend to be in suburban and urban areas. Of the 2,000 clinics open in 1965, only 234 of those located in rural areas served children. A total of 25,000 children were served in these rural clinics in 1965, only 8 percent of all children under clinic care in the United States. Also, only slightly more than half of the rural clinics were open full time and only 60 percent had the full orthopsychiatric team of psychiatrist, psychologist, and social worker.

Although psychiatric clinics had been concentrated in urban areas for a number of years, their services were not always available to the poor who lacked both the awareness of such services and the funds to travel to them. Also, psychotherapy by itself had little affect on solving their multifaceted difficulties. Traditional insight-oriented therapeutic techniques were of limited use for patients not used to introspection and self-examination. Out of work, chronically depressed, and angry, the poor saw no purpose in talking about their problems.

Of the 15 million youngsters in the United States who are reared in poverty, one in three are considered to have serious emotional problems that need attention. More than 500,000 youngsters are brought before the courts each year for antisocial acts. Many are from disadvantaged communities. Consequently, estimates are that only 5 percent of the children in the United States who need psychiatric help are getting it, and of those treated, less than one-half receive the kind of help that is needed (National Institute of Mental Health, 1968).

These figures indicate that the Community Mental Health Centers Act of 1963 was a timely one. Because of this act, which provides federal support for the construction and staffing of community mental health centers, comprehensive centers are being made available throughout the country. Federal assistance for construction and staffing of these centers requires the overall center program to include five essential elements of care: outpatient service, inpatient service, partial hospitalization, emergency service, and education and consultation service. The centers serve their community in cooperation with other community agencies and groups. Their education and consultation service can strengthen the mental health of children through work with schools, well baby clinics, and other agencies which serve the young (*American Journal of Psychiatry*, 1972).

At the time of the act it was projected that 2,000 such centers would be established by 1980, one for every 200,000 people. Federal cutbacks during the late 1960s and early 1970s, however, brought a halt to their growth. In 1971 there were approximately 290 such centers (National Coalition for Mental Health Manpower, 1971). At that time, therefore, the majority of psychiatric outpatient clinics still operated independently from other agencies.

Even if mental health services are greatly expanded, it is doubtful if they will meet the needs of all disability groups. For example, mental health workers have been relatively uninterested in the mentally retarded and have, therefore, limited their services to these patients primarily to diagnosis (Burton, 1971).

With the current emphasis on community mental health, some clinics are slowly getting more involved with other community agencies. They are doing so, however, as if such an approach was a contemporary one (Mora, 1972). Few professionals are aware that we are returning to a model of clinical services that was practiced between 1896 and the mid-

1920s. Let us hope that professionals will acquaint themselves with the struggles of these early clinics, since there is a well-known maxim that those who forget the past are doomed to repeat it (Levine & Levine, 1970).

Roles of professionals in mental health clinics Because of their ability to gather background material, social workers eventually became responsible for maintaining case records and for the management of clinic operations. As they gained skill in administration, many became the administrators of child guidance clinics, while the psychiatrist remained the medical director. In essence, the social worker carried out the wishes of the medical director who had final say in most matters. The psychologist continued in his role as tester and was eventually allowed to do psychotherapy under psychiatric supervision, as was the social worker.

In many mental health clinics the roles of each profession have become less distinct. Each engages in individual, group, and family psychotherapy. Each does intake interviews and consults with other agencies. Nevertheless, a distinction still remains. Because maladjusted children are considered ill, the physician-psychiatrist is still considered necessary for their treatment. Because the physician is scarce, he demands a high salary, a salary nearly twice as high as the psychologist or social worker. Consequently, the caste system remains in most mental health facilities.

The disordered behavior concept

Social work agencies Many social workers never joined forces with the psychiatrist but continued to operate their own agencies funded either by state departments of social welfare or the local community chest. Child welfare agencies, such as child care institutions for dependent and neglected children, foster homes, and family counseling services are examples. Social workers consider many families to be disorganized and their children to be disturbed in response to this chaos. Since illness is not an essential component of the disturbance, the social worker is considered competent to provide assistance to such families. In 1970 almost three million children were receiving social services from public welfare and voluntary child welfare agencies operated by social workers (U.S. Department of Health, Education, and Welfare, 1972). Although child welfare agencies employ psychologists and psychiatrists, the social worker has ultimate responsibility and guides the direction the agency will take in the future.

Psychologists: a profession without a home The psychologists, so prominent in the early child guidance movement, now direct no community agency of their own. If they lead team meetings in psychiatric or social work agencies, it is through the grace of the other professional. The medical lobby keeps them from setting up their own community agencies, since, by definition, illness is the province of the medical practitioner and paramedical staff are allowed to practice only under medical supervision. State departments of mental health will not provide them with funds because they do not have a license to practice medicine, and departments of social welfare stipulate that agencies receiving welfare funds be directed by social workers. Many universities have reestablished child study and psychological service centers, but no agency operated solely by psychologists has yet to be supported by community, county, or state funds. Psychologists can become administrators of such centers, but a psychiatrist must be a member of their staff and is usually listed as the clinical director.

In 1970 the California School of Professional Psychology was established as the first educational institution operated by psychologists to train individuals to provide psychological services at various levels of proficiency. The school confers A.A., B.A., M.A., and Ph.D. degrees. The New York Society of Clinical Psychologists has established a center approved by the State Education Department to provide psychological assistance to needy persons. Psychological services are now reimbursable under many insurance policies, and in New York State psychologists can engage in private practice without having to be associated with a psychiatrist, a situation that exists in many states. Nevertheless, these agencies can receive no state funds without a psychiatrist on their staff.

When psychological science began to demonstrate that many forms of maladjustment were due to faulty development, inadequate learning, or restrictive environments rather than to disease, society allowed psychologists to apply their methods to ameliorate maladjustment independently of other professions. However, this independence is currently restricted to operating in the private rather than in the public sector.

This brief background of interdisciplinary relationships perhaps makes psychiatrists look like the "bad guys" and psychologists the "good guys," particularly when mental health concepts have swung to a model more in keeping with the views of early psychologists. Actually, forces operating on both groups in the early 1900s set the stage for the power struggles that followed and neither is free from blame.

The early clinics that operated out of university psychology departments never had the strong backing of the psychology departments themselves or of the universities that sponsored them. Many psychologists, bent on gaining acceptance for psychology as a science, felt that the profession should concentrate on research into basic fundamental human processes rather than prematurely applying untested assumptions. In addition, the university itself was not considered an institution where treatment should take place, and university leaders stressed that practical matters should be left to other community agencies. Consequently, the staff of these early university clinics found themselves lacking the emotional and financial support necessary to continue their type of service.

Psychiatrists, too, were engaged in a struggle with their colleagues in other branches of medicine. To convince the medical profession that psychiatry was indeed a medical science and not a mixture of folklore, religion, mysticism, and philosophy, psychiatrists had to fight for acceptance of the idea that "crazy" people were actually ill. Once this idea was accepted, it followed that only physicians were qualified to lend assistance or to treat individuals so afflicted.

Freud had always maintained that, although he himself was a physician, his method of treatment could be applied by nonphysicians. Consequently, psychologists turned their research efforts toward scrutinizing various aspects of psychoanalytic theory while they taught the theory to their students. Without a working knowledge of psychoanalytic theory, the psychologist would have been ill-prepared to work in those psychiatric institutions that needed his testing and research skill. Witmer and his orientation toward the community rather than the individual was to be forgotten for over fifty years.

WHAT ALL COMMUNITIES SHOULD HAVE

Andrew, a youngster with rather severe learning disabilities, needed certain facilities to help him learn efficiently. These facilities are included among those identified in Figure 1.6. Andrew needed extensive remedial reading, placement in a resource room, and perhaps even special class placement within the public school setting. Because Andrew's family was relatively stable, the school staff could support them throughout

Figure 1.6 *Facilities needed to service children and families.*

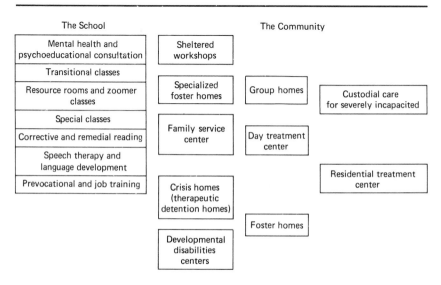

Andrew's remediation. Had there been severe family conflicts, the school would have referred the family to the child guidance center within the family service center.

Andrew would eventually need a work-study program. Continual academic failure, for that's what it is to any youngster aware that he's behind and in a special program, only reinforces feelings of inadequacy. Such feelings precipitate depression, and depression, usually too heavy a burden to bear in full force, results in behavior designed to dull its affect, behavior such as an attack on others or a search for an exhilarating experience. Placement in an appropriate educational program can sometimes prevent such an occurrence. Let us examine each of the services listed in Figure 1.6.

Services within the school

Mental health and educational consultation have already been mentioned in reference to child study teams and will be discussed in greater detail in Chapter 12. Perhaps one psychologist and one social worker for 3000 children would be a realistic figure. Less than that leaves little time for adequate consultation. Consultation is of less value when it exists in the absence of alternatives to regular class instruction with a single teacher. To service exceptional children adequately within the public school a variety of special programs are necessary. Perhaps the first is the transitional class.

The transitional class

Dear Parent:

As you know, we have been concerned about your child's readiness in kindergarten. It is our feeling that he will be unable to succeed in our regular first grade. Therefore, we are placing him in our pre-first grade so that he will be given an extra year to mature and prepare himself for our regular first grade program.

The curriculum offered in our pre-first grade will, by its very nature, be different from both the kindergarten program and that offered in our regular first grade. Hopefully, we will meet the students at their level and guide them through a program that will encompass both kindergarten and early first grade work with much emphasis on the development of visual, perceptual, and listening skills.

Unless unusual circumstances arise, your child will be placed in a regular first grade the following year.

Respectfully,

John J. Johnson

John J. Johnson
Elementary Principal

The transitional class was designed for the immature child who after a year in kindergarten is not considered ready for placement in the first grade but who is not retarded, emotionally disturbed, or educationally handicapped (Oberlin, 1965). Table 1.21 gives the attempts of one group of kindergarten teachers to delimit the characteristics of children who should be placed in such a class. Perhaps 15 to 20 percent of the children entering kindergarten are unable to obtain the full benefits of the instructional program. The transitional class was designed to assist that portion considered developmentally immature. A number of immature children are those who are slow to develop in early childhood and were either premature or of low birth weight. To differentiate such children from those with mild mental retardation or learning disorders is not always easy, and many are inappropriately placed.

Initially, educators assumed that concentrated instruction would enable a child to "catch up" within one year so that he would be ready for the second grade at the same time as his first grade classmates. In practice, this rarely happened. As stated in the principal's letter, most children go to the first grade after a year in the transitional class and, therefore, remain a year behind their equal-age classmates.

For children who are developmentally immature, it might be more beneficial to delay their school entrance than to place them in the transitional class. The transitional class is actually a repetition of kindergarten. To justify its effectiveness, three groups of developmentally immature children would have to be compared: those who delay their school entrance one year, those who repeat kindergarten, and those who are assigned to a transitional class, or, as some schools call it, "junior first grade."

Some educators hope that identification of immature children could take place prior to kindergarten, that more individualized instruction at that time would enable the child to catch up. But, developmental immaturity may not be made up in one year. If a child's developmental time clock runs more slowly than other children, then environmental changes . will probably have no appreciable affect. Perhaps the need for differentiation of instruction might be necessary throughout a child's entire school career rather than for one or two years. This need is suggested by research that demonstrates no significant differences between immature kindergarten children placed in a special program and those placed in a regular kindergarten (Spollen & Ballif, 1971). Both groups were still inferior to developmentally normal children at the end of the kindergarten year.

Perhaps individualization of instruction for kindergarten children has not been sufficiently different in scope or intensity from the regular kindergarten curriculum. Perhaps more specific short- and long-range objectives for each unit of instruction and more careful use of instructional materials may result in more positive results in future investiga-

Table 1.21 CRITERIA FOR ADMISSION TO THE PRE-FIRST GRADE

The slow child	The immature child

1. Poor self-concept
    Fearful of changes in routine
    Fearful of new situations
    Cries or sulks when defeated or opposed
    Poor social adjustment
    Cannot judge when to talk or when to stop talking
	Not as frequently (though does occur)
	Has stronger emotional stability

2. Poor perceptual skills
    Visual—difficulty seeing likenesses and differences in pictures and matching letters, words
    Auditory—difficulty hearing rhymes and words that have the same beginning sounds
	Poor skills, but more apt to be due to lack of experience than to intellectual inefficiency

3. Marked space-form deficiency Visual-motor tests suggest immaturity markedly below age level	Better understands relationships of up and down, top and bottom, little and big

4. Disorganized
    Difficulty finding the main idea in situations
    Difficulty giving reasons for opinions or acts
	More capable of structuring his work (even though he cannot carry a very heavy load)
	Understands classifications of words that represent people, places, or things

5. Lacks communication skills
    Small vocabulary
    Difficulty retelling a story or telling a story of his own
	Has better vocabulary
	Can express main idea of story better
	Can remember important details
	Can give reasons for his opinions

6. Speech problems (poor auditory perception or physical impediment)	May also have speech deficiency, but not as frequently (may be extended "baby talk" or lack of careful listening)

7. Less endowed physically
    Poor sensory-motor skills
    Lack of dexterity in running, skipping, jumping, balancing, bouncing ball
    Poor control of smaller muscles—writing, cutting
    Hyperactive—cannot stay still, has need of much physical activity
	Poor coordination usually due to lack of physical growth rather than slow motor response
	Gross coordination better than fine
	Lack endurance

8. Poor work habits
    Easily distracted
    Short attention span
    Unable to follow directions
    Needs concrete examples
    Needs to be taught "how"
    Cannot work independently
	Better motivated and more alert
	Better able to keep sequence of directions
	Short attention span, but more capable of developing longer continuity
	More apt to recognize abstract terms
	Wants to know "why" and to discover things for himself
	Cannot work independently, but need for adult not so great

9. May be chronologically old for grade	May have fall birthdays

Courtesy of the Red Hook School System, Red Hook, New York.

tions. Chapter 9 presents a discussion of programs designed to offset the poor school readiness of economically disadvantaged children, many of whom are considered "immature."

Should immature children need special instruction throughout their education, they might best be taught in a resource room rather than being grouped together in a self-contained class.

Resource room Resource rooms are specially equipped rooms staffed by a coordinating teacher well trained in instructing children with learning problems, perhaps a second teacher, and some teacher aides (Dunn, 1968). Small group and individual instruction are the featured services. The child's strengths and weaknesses are evaluated through child study. He is then assigned to the resource room for a particular period or periods during the day. If the child needs assistance for more than half of the day, then he is assigned to a special class rather than to a resource room. Several resource rooms are described by Gardner (1971), Reger and Koppmann (1971), and Valett (1970).

Evidence is beginning to accumulate which suggests that the resource room can be a viable approach to educating the exceptional child (Bruininks, Rynders, & Gross, 1974; Walker, 1974). Philosophically speaking, any method that keeps the child in the mainstream of education without substantial loss in self-esteem is preferable to isolation in special classes, because that isolation appears to have a crippling effect on self-esteem (Dunn, 1968). Research is needed to substantiate the superiority of the resource room approach over other approaches. More than likely, a significant number of children will continue to need special class placement and many of the children now floundering academically, being retained, or being socially promoted will make up the bulk of those profiting from a resource room experience. Many retarded children as well as those with severe learning and emotional disorders will continue to need a full day of special programming. Follow-up studies, to be reviewed in Chapter 8, indicate that many neurologically impaired children, limited cognitively, fail to acquire age-appropriate social behaviors. It is naive to assume that retarded teenagers, many of whom will never read beyond the fourth grade level, will be accepted by normal adolescents.

The zoomer class Originally designed as a "catch-up" class for children returning to public school from a special residential program (Project Re-Ed, see Chapter 12), the zoomer class may have implications which go beyond this restricted use. This class was billed as a high status, high expectation class where four high-status public school children were placed with four re-ed students. The class met for three months of teacher-student planned educational activities. At the end of this period, the re-ed children displayed 1½ months of academic gain per month of zoomer class instruction, while the public school children gained 2⅔ months for each month in class (Weinstein, 1971). While the zoomer class concept would probably be of little help in the education of children with marked deficiencies, it could have a significant impact on children or adolescents with underachievement due to poor self-esteem.

Special classes   School systems are not immune to trends originating in other quarters. Perhaps we should not expect them to be so, although we would hope the "enlightened" were more far seeing. Schools, however, have followed, if not actively participated in, the trend to isolate those who do not fit into programs for normal children. To "fit in" means capable of being taught by conventional methods, that is, by group instruction in classes numbering from 20 to 30. The first children isolated were the blind, the deaf, and retarded children with IQs below 50. These children were usually excluded from public schools altogether and whatever education they received was acquired within special institutions designed for their care.

While the moderately retarded are allowed to attend public schools, they are often educated apart from others. Sometimes this education takes place in classrooms within the regular school, but often it takes place in separate buildings set aside for exceptional children. To qualify for these classes, the child must give evidence of only moderate retardation. This means that, while he may have poor social awareness, he must have fair motor development, be able to communicate, be expected to function at the fourth grade level by his late teens, and have an IQ between 50–75. Those at the upper end of this IQ range may achieve at the sixth grade level, but need considerable help in secondary school.

More recently, special classes have been established for the emotionally disturbed and minimally brain-injured child (a child with a potentially average IQ but with perceptual or conceptual disorders that impair learning). Because of the proliferation of special classes for various disabilities, it has been laughingly said that soon the special class will be the one that contains normal children.

Past and present efforts to classify and segregate children   In the early part of the nineteenth century, society began to show increasing concern with its obligation to the blind, deaf, and moderately retarded child. Public school teachers lacked the training to provide for these children, so special schools were established to educate them. In 1829 the Massachusetts School for the Blind was incorporated, and in 1832 the New York Institute for the Education of the Blind was opened in New York City. Children were sent to these schools from various parts of the state. By 1862 there were 19 state schools for the blind in the United States, but some blind were housed with the deaf. Every territory that became a state through 1920 had established some type of residential facility for some group of exceptional children prior to or shortly after statehood.

As the population increased and more people congregated in urban areas, schools could be set up to serve the local community. These schools could, therefore, operate on a day rather than residential basis.

Concepts of classification of handicapping conditions were introduced between 1920 and 1930. Binet's classification of the retarded on the basis of scores on his test led to the development of the concept of individual differences. Residential schools began grouping children on the basis of intelligence test scores after Goddard introduced Binet's test to the United States in 1914. Professionals began to realize that certain retarded children could be taught academic skills. These youngsters, children with IQs between 50 and 75, were labeled "educable." A second group, those with IQs below 50, could probably never learn to read and write, but could be taught rudimentary social skills. These were labeled "trainable."

Teachers trained in the residential schools were asked to teach similar classes in public school settings or in settings funded by local communities. These teachers also were asked to train other teachers, and a number of teacher training institutions began to offer courses in the education of the exceptional child. Berry, in 1914, set up the first teacher training program at the Lapeer State Home and Training School in Michigan. This was a summer training program for the teachers at this residential school for educable and trainable retardates. Shortly thereafter the first college program was established at what now is Eastern Michigan University at Ypsilanti (Cruickshank, 1967). This program provided special training in the instruction of the deaf, hard-of-hearing, blind, retarded, and those with special health problems.

Teachers with special training were shared by small school districts who didn't have enough students to start a class of their own. Very few school districts had enough deaf or blind children to have special classes for each of these groups. Consequently, day schools were set up and funded by the joint efforts of several school districts.

Other children, besides those with obvious handicaps, also did not seem to profit from regular class placement. They were either disruptive and aggressive or extremely withdrawn and apathetic. These children were considered to be socially or emotionally maladjusted. Consequently, special classes for such youngsters were set up in many school districts. Because of the prevailing notion that maladjusted children were "sick," evaluation by a psychiatrist was frequently a requirement for placement.

It is estimated that the number of children enrolled in special programs for the emotionally disturbed is now about 100,000, in addition to the more than 65,000 children under the age of 18 who are enrolled in public and private residential schools (Schultz, Hirshoren, Manton, & Henderson, 1971).

In the early 1960s, based largely on the work of Cruickshank with brain-injured children, educators began to realize that many children with emotional disorders are not socially maladjusted because of chaotic family conditions or "mental illness," but are reacting to subtle neurological dysfunctions that affect their ability to learn. Cruickshank and his colleagues (Cruickshank, Bentzen, Ratzeburg, & Tannhauser, 1961) emphasized that children with minimal brain damage require specialized educational procedures in order to overcome attentional and perceptual deficits accompanying their disorder (see Chapter 8).

Because these children were classified as neurologically impaired, evaluation by a neurologist became a requirement for placement. Enter the era of the educator's reliance upon the physician to make what is essentially an educational decision. As will be pointed out in Chapter 8, current research has established that neurologically impaired children do not differ substantially from those with emotional disturbances. Many times there are no positive signs of neurological impairment. Nevertheless, on the basis of symptomatology, a symptomatology varying little from that displayed by children from chaotic families, neurologists classify the child as minimally brain-impaired. Frequently, the decision of whether a child should be placed in a class for the emotionally disturbed or for the brain impaired depends on whether the neurologist or psychiatrist is more available or on which class the parent will accept. Hopefully, educators will discover for themselves what type of child responds favorably to what type of educational program. Placement in special classes will be made, therefore, on the basis of educational diagnosis rather than on physical, neurological, or psychiatric nosology, nosologies which have little bearing on responsiveness to educational practices.

An approach that may be a viable alternative to grouping children according to their disability has been described by Hewett (1970). Hewett helped develop a generalist strategy for special education based on his concepts of the hierarchy of educational tasks (1964) and the engineered classroom (1968). Children are grouped regardless of disability according to their educational attainment. Thus, blind or partially seeing, deaf, and retarded or disturbed children can be in the same class if all are functioning academically at the same level. The first level of class is the most basic. Placed here are children lacking attention and concentration abilities. Instruction is on an individual basis, with concentrated effort on increasing attention and concentration. Tangible reinforcers may be employed to shape and maintain desired behavior. From this highly structured classroom, the child moves to the second level where group instruction is employed on a limited basis and the number of children in the class is increased. Instruction at the third level includes approximately the same degree of group instruction as found in the regular classroom but with fewer children in the class. As the child masters the educational tasks at each level, he is moved to the next. This is a developmental strategy for educating children and each child proceeds through each level at his own pace and according to his own educational growth. Unlike the typical special class, a child can be moved from one level to the next whenever he is ready rather than at the end of each academic year or semester.

Pressure to integrate Recently the Pennsylvania Association for Retarded Children, a parent organization, brought suit in a federal district court on behalf of the right of every retarded child to a free public school education regardless of IQ classification. Victory would mean that a retarded child could no longer be excluded from the public school system because he is unable to meet his state's requirements that he have a minimum IQ of 25, a mental age of five, or whatever.

In Dutchess County, New York, the Association for Children with Learning Disabilities brought pressure on the local Board of Cooperative Educational Services to cease grouping learning disabled children in classes in a centrally located building and instead to establish resource rooms in each local school from which the children were referred. In 1972 in Dutchess County 369 children with learning difficulties due to emotional or neurological problems were grouped in two buildings especially set aside to educate them. Approximately 708 children were in some sort of special class in the county. The approximate cost of educating each learning disabled child was $2950 in 1971–1972 and anywhere from $1400 to $2250 for educating the educable retarded. Parents in various parts of the country are beginning to question the legality of exclusion from regular classes (Ross, DeYoung, & Cohen, 1971). Mac-Millan (1973) attempts to identify the issues and trends that have contributed to the current concerns in special education.

Corrective and remedial reading In nearly all first grade classes, there are children who are not equipped to begin reading. Yet begin they do, and many fall quickly behind their equal-age peers. As discussed in Chapter 9, many economically disadvantaged children learn at slower rates than their advanced peers. Similarly, the immature, the hyperactive, or the disturbed child may learn at a slower rate. At each grade level these children are considerably behind their faster-learning peers and are required to learn material without having mastered the prerequisites. But they stumble along, knowing some consonant sounds and not others, knowing words by sight but unable to analyze them phonetically, reading through use of contextual clues or educated guesses based on the accompanying pictorial material. Reading becomes a chore, a labor without love; various ways are found to avoid the embarrassment of reading aloud poorly, ways which annoy others or the teacher. By fourth grade they cannot "get by" through the use of these strategies. Because they are not allowed to learn at their own pace, they never acquire a sound foundation of basic reading skills.

Most schools employ specially trained teachers to help each poorly reading child learn material missed at earlier levels. Such reading instruction is referred to as *corrective*, after Betts (1954), who used the term to categorize reading problems of children whose mental age is less than their reading age, who show no significant indication of an inability to profit from visual or visual-auditory learning techniques, who have no severe disturbances in memory functioning, and whose reading and spelling is less developed than oral language.

Many corrective reading cases could be prevented if children could learn to read at their own rate. Others might be avoided if children were tutored as soon as they experience difficulty. Perhaps a reading teacher's time would be better spent if she consulted with teachers about corrective cases, so that individualized instruction could take place within the classroom. She could then supervise a tutoring program which would supplement classroom instruction.

Remedial reading is instruction provided to children who have shown inability to learn from traditional visual or visual-auditory learning techniques. They do poorly on associative learning tasks, have poor memory for visual or auditory materials, and are often considered neurologically abnormal in spite of adequate functioning in nonreading tasks. These children are discussed in Chapter 8. Some reading teachers are especially trained to teach such children to read and either tutor them individually or supervise their tutoring. Being tutored by other students can often result in more academic gain than small group instruction by a teacher in a resource room (Jenkins, Mayhall, Peschka, & Jenkins, 1974).

Speech therapy and language development Any child who speaks so that he distracts attention from what he is trying to say to how he is saying it, assuming age is considered, has defective speech. Approximately 5 percent of school-age children have such speech. In order to help these children, speech therapy should be available within the public school setting.

Group and individual counseling Many children experience difficulty relating appropriately to peers and adults. This inability usually results from family factors, some of which are discussed in Chapter 7. While a child guidance center is better equipped to provide counseling services, many parents are reluctant to take their child to such centers or to embark on a course of treatment for themselves. The child, therefore, remains untouched unless the school can offer him help. Often children, particularly at the secondary level, need advice on matters they feel they cannot ask their parents or teachers about. Time-limited counseling, either for children, teachers, or parents, on either a group or individual basis, should be offered at both the primary and secondary levels. In Chapter 12, psychotherapy is discussed in more detail.

Prevocational and job training The majority of our public schools consider their role simply as providing academic training. Although shop, art, and home economics are offered in the junior and senior high school, these courses could hardly be conceived of as prevocational or vocational training.

School systems usually have a trade or technical school for those who perform poorly in the academic curriculum. Many children, frustrated with school and lacking good work habits, do no better in technical schools. They quickly realize that society considers technical or trade school graduates as second-class citizens. If prevocational and vocational training were a part of the regular curriculum and all students were required to take basic courses in prevocational areas, then perhaps choices of vocation would be based on the student's rather than someone else's interest. The introduction of such a program might improve our philosophy of work and thereby help diminish behavior problems which result from low self-esteem.

Cooperation with other agencies   Regardless of how many changes are made in educational programs, it is doubtful if schools can habilitate a child alone. Kotting and Brozovich's (1969) follow-up study of emotionally disturbed children who were enrolled in special classes demonstrated that family stability is related to the child's later adjustment. They suggest that increasing efforts should be devoted toward improving the home environment of children placed in special programs. Hopefully, schools will work more closely with other community agencies when they develop future programs. Some of these agencies will now be described.

Services outside the school

In many communities a number of social service, health, and mental health agencies exist to provide a variety of services to community residents. Stable, well-organized families are crucial for the normal development of the child. The secure family provides the warmth and acceptance needed for optimal growth. Various community supports are needed, however, to enable many family members to cope effectively with our complex society.

All families face the stress produced by an automated, depersonalized society. About one-fifth of the nation's families move each year. Such movement adds to existing strains through the loss of support from friends and the extended family. About one-fourth of all families live on incomes of less than $5000 per year. Isolation, mobility, and economic problems, along with other factors, have placed considerable strain on families. Thirteen percent of our children are now reared in one-parent families and because of earlier divorces a large number are raised with stepparents (Joint Commission on Mental Health of Children, 1969). The problems of minority group children warrant immediate attention. Poverty and prejudice combine to hinder development.

The specialized services present in some communities can be of aid to many families. The Joint Commission on Mental Health of Children reports (1969, p. 23), however, that

these services have become so overly specialized, frequently so expensive, so poorly coordinated, and so centered on individuals rather than on families, that very few parents have the resources needed to mobilize these services for the well being of each family member or for the family as a unit. There are enormous gaps, especially in day care, relevant education, and physical and mental health facilities.

Our discussion of facilities will be confined to those needed to service the exceptional child (see Figure 1.6). Keep in mind that many children come from families whose other members need support and that agencies for children need to coordinate their activities with those of other agencies which might be of service to families.

The family service center   The family service center is the agency to which a family first turns for assistance regardless of the problem. If the problem revolves primarily around the child, then child guidance experts within the center handle the problem. If later it develops that the actual problem is the mother's alcoholism which results in the child's neglect, then those experts trained in alcoholism take part in the case. If the parents already realize that they need marital counseling, then this help is provided. Each family contacts the center, is seen by a central intake team, and is referred to the appropriate staff for assistance.

In practice, no such center actually exists. The closest approximation to such a model is the multiservice center. Approximately 200 such centers now exist throughout the country, and within them families can obtain at a single physical location a variety of services. Even though these centers have not achieved an optimal level of comprehensiveness, they are a step in the right direction (Schulberg, 1972).

The family service center would differ from the community mental health center in several ways. First, families and family members would not be considered "patients," since they would consult the center for many reasons such as family planning, child rearing advice, marital counseling, financial or legal counseling, relocation because of urban renewal projects, or welfare assistance. They could request homemaker services, after-hours emergency children's services, day care, or emergency loans. Consequently, the stigma of being "mental" or "psycho" would be avoided by those seeking help for disturbed family members.

Second, the center would be operated as a social service agency rather than as a hospital. Mental health centers are costly to operate since they assume highly trained medical and paramedical personnel are needed to service "ill" people. The salary of one beginning psychiatrist is usually three times that of a beginning social worker and five or six times that of the family service aide, a community college graduate with an associate of arts degree. Many people who need help in managing their lives are not sick. To imply that they are is a costly assumption!

Therapeutic detention homes   The staff of the family service center may decide that temporary removal of one or several family members is essential for the eventual well-being of the particular member or of the family itself. Should a parent become severely ill or temporarily disturbed, the children may be better off if they leave the home temporarily. Runaway adolescents often need a place to "cool off" before returning home. The detention home serves as a neutral place where teenager and parent can be guided by a neutral party. The home may also "come to the family" by sending staff to assist in the home while a parent is away.

Occasionally, families do not survive a crisis. Children are deserted by one or both parents and remaining family members are left unable to provide for their basic needs. When this occurs, the detention home refers the children to a staff trained in foster home services and the children are placed under foster care. When such services exist many children can avoid institutionalization (Burt & Balyeat, 1974).

Group homes   Approximately 63,000 children in the United States live in children's institutions for the dependent and neglected (U.S. Department of Health, Education, and Welfare, 1972). Another 27,000 live in state mental hospitals (Rosen, Kramer, Redick, & Willner, 1971) and 14,000 in residential treatment centers (National Institute of Mental Health, 1971). Large institutions are no place to grow up. Rapid staff turnover prevents the development of intimate relationships between children and adults, relationships needed to foster normal growth and identification with adult standards. If current trends continue, one out of every nine children will appear before a juvenile court before age 18 (National Institute of Mental Health, 1968). Many of these youngsters were reared in large, impersonal child care institutions after being abandoned or neglected by their parents.

An alternative to institutional care for disturbed as well as retarded children is small group care where from six to eight children live in homes interspersed throughout the community. Children attend regular school and socialize with community families. They differ from large families in that the children are not all related and their live-in house parents are not their own parents. While turnover of house parents is quite high, attachment to other adult figures in the community may help offset these separations. In addition, the child can visit his natural parent or parents more often because of his proximity to them. If the salaries and working conditions of house parents improve, the turnover may decrease.

Group homes with therapeutic supports are an alternative to the psychiatric hospital. Many institutions operate what are called "halfway homes." These homes are halfway points back into the community for those who have been institutionalized. One large private institution has established the College House. This group home is designed to provide semisheltered living for seriously disturbed youth who have the potential to attend college on either a full- or part-time basis. Staff are trained to cope with disturbed youth and supportive psychotherapy is provided by professionals.

The importance of having group homes cannot be overestimated. The number of children and adolescents admitted to and resident in mental hospitals and other psychiatric facilities is on the increase in spite of increased outpatient services. Since 1950 the number of boys in the population has doubled, while their number in mental institutions has quadrupled (National Institute of Mental Health, 1968). Many children are placed in hospitals because no other resources are available. The development of group homes would help decrease both the number of hospital admissions and the length of stay. Nevertheless, in 1970 there were only 3500 children in group homes in the United States operated by public welfare agencies in contrast to the 104,000 living in some type of institution. The latter figure does not include those in correctional facilities for delinquents.

Foster homes The rapid migration to cities of rural families unprepared for urban life often results in a breakdown of family life. Because these new city dwellers are largely minority group members, a large proportion of the children needing foster home placement are children from these minority groups—children for whom foster and adoptive family resources are least available because of the lesser affluence of these groups. Of the 243,000 children in foster family homes in 1970, only a small proportion were blacks, Mexicans, or Puerto Ricans.

Before children are placed in a foster home, many have already experienced neglect and abuse. Consequently, they are suspicious and distrustful of adults. These attitudes make it difficult for foster parents to provide consistent care. As we will see in Chapter 9, children are often placed in a succession of foster homes, each as unsuccessful as the first.

Children who are placed away from home, regardless of the quality of life they experience there, go through successive stages of protest, despair, and detachment. If the placement is unsuccessful, the child becomes detached, hard-to-reach, and emotionally blunted.

Unsuccessful placements are not simply the result of the child's prior experiences. Motives of foster parents are varied. Some desire to extend to other children the satisfactory experience of mothering that they gave their own children. Others want a foster child to get another chance to succeed as a mother, to gain pleasure from a child to make up for the displeasure experienced with their own, but without the risks of bearing another. They can return the foster child if their needs are not met! Still others want a child as a companion to their own child or as a means to make extra money.

Many children need only temporary foster care until the crisis which brought about the breakdown of their family is over. Others can never return home and need care only until placed for adoption. A large and increasing number, because of their age, behavior, intellectual status, or family status, face long-term temporary care. This group includes those whose families will not permit foster placement and prefer their child to remain in a child care institution or group home. Only in cases of extreme neglect can the court recommend foster home placement against parental wishes, and in these cases placements can be unsuccessful because natural parents often interfere with the placement (Goldstein, Freud, & Solnit, 1973).

Other children facing long-term temporary care include those who could have returned home if appropriate services had been available to their family and children who might have been placed for adoption but became too old or emotionally unstable. Too often staff shortages, staff turnover, and other administrative difficulties, such as failure to examine agency practices, have hindered a child's chances for family life (Garett, 1966; Goldstein et al., 1973).

The child's natural parents usually have strong feelings about placement. Often they feel relieved and at the same time ashamed, hurt, angry, and empty. Guilt often is unbearable. Mothers whose children are placed because of neglect feel empty and numb, as if everything was beyond their control. They would now have to prove themselves all over again (Jenkins, 1967). Others feel isolated, lonely, and inadequate, expecting punishment for having allowed placement away from home. Some express the fear that when their children are grown they will return to destroy them in retaliation for this wrong (Mandelbaum, 1962).

A successful foster home service should take all these factors into consideration when planning a program. The majority of communities do not have an adequate foster home service and make only sparing use of interdisciplinary collaboration in selection and training of foster home parents and in providing back-up support once placement is made. When a foster home program is well run even retarded children can be successfully placed (De Vizia, 1974).

Day treatment Day treatment is intended primarily for children who are too disturbed to profit from special classes operated by the public schools, but whose behavior is not so disruptive of the family's life that they cannot be cared for at home. Each child's day is programmed both educationally and therapeutically, but each returns home at night. Family counseling and guidance is offered at the day treatment center and is sometimes made a prerequisite for a child's admission. Centers vary as to their orientation, some placing great emphasis on enhancing the skills of the child so as to make him more able to cope with his family, while others stress intensive family counseling and individual psychotherapy. Ideally, the day treatment center should have a limited number of beds for emergency placements. Sometimes, a family cannot handle their child on weekends or during times of crisis. Having limited residential facilities allows the same agency to continue servicing a family until such time as the child can return home. Continuity of care is essential for successful treatment.

Most day treatment centers are interdisciplinary in approach and employ child study practices identical to those described earlier. More recently, considerable overlap between the professions has occurred in some settings. Child care staff frequently serve as co-therapists in family therapy sessions or see children in individual play therapy. Psychologists and child care workers accompany the social worker into the home to help the family manage their child more successfully. Staff morale is usually higher in such settings than in those where strict lines are drawn between professional roles and where subprofessionals are left with routine tasks.

The child in day treatment usually returns to the public school or to special classes, and the family continues to receive help from the family service center staff. Sometimes conditions worsen and residential treatment is indicated. Nevertheless, most children in residential treatment come from communities that lack day treatment facilities. Where such facilities do exist, fewer referrals are made to residential centers. One study suggests that with some children day treatment is as effective as residential (Goldfarb, Goldfarb, & Pollack, 1966). In 1965, 120 day treatment centers in the United States serviced children under 17; however, only 72 of these serviced children under 12 (Rosen et al., 1971). More are expected to develop, however, because of the funds available through the Community Mental Health Centers Act.

Residential treatment centers A residential treatment center is a live-in service where children are given a planned program of milieu therapy and other therapy modalities (see Chapter 12). The center differs from the state hospital primarily in size of staff and in philosophy. The setting is open, meaning that children are free to move around the grounds and are not "locked in" at night. This means that the children have to be capable of understanding rules of group living and the dangers of running in the street or roaming off into the woods. Seriously disturbed children, such as the autistic or severely psychotic described in Chapter 4, are usually treated in state hospitals where there is more confinement to living quarters and less danger of self-injury.

So-called borderline children, those who distort reality only under certain conditions, make up the largest portion of children treated in residential centers. Although these children frequently lose control of their emotions and attack others or run out into the street oblivious to danger, most of the time they participate in treatment programs without causing undue alarm.

Individual child study is the main feature of residential treatment. The staff plan activities for groups of youngsters, but each child's needs are considered in group planning. The better residential centers are sub-divided into living groups of about ten children each. Some have cottages for groups of about twenty youngsters, but even these are usually divided into wings for five to ten children.

Most children referred to these centers have experienced difficulty in making and maintaining friendships with peers and adults. By living in small units, they are not overwhelmed by large numbers of different chil-dren. In due time they develop a feeling of group unity and identity, and each group member eventually seeks a closer relationship with one or two of the ten children with whom he lives. In the small living unit children cannot avoid relating at some level to one another. In the large state hospital children can get "lost in the crowd" or can remain in a state of withdrawal for long periods. In the living unit of the residential center they have to participate in activities and do their chores. Rarely can they avoid involvement in the arguments and fights of others and are almost forced to learn new styles of coping. Staff are reluctant to use high dosages of sedative medication, because they are oriented toward encour-aging the children to assume responsibility for themselves and to learn to control their own behavior. In understaffed hospitals, where larger groups of children cannot be well supervised, medication and isolation from others are methods used to control the children. Even in well-staffed children's hospitals, the prevalent medical orientation conveys to the children an image of themselves as "mental" or "sick," that is, not capable of self-control. The atmosphere in the residential center conveys a much different message, both to staff and children alike.

In 1968 there were 269 residential centers in the United States, servicing approximately 14,000 children (National Institute of Mental Health, 1971). It is unlikely that there will be a rapid growth of such centers because of the recent emphasis on developing services which will keep children in their own community. Many residential centers are now developing day treatment programs and are attempting to admit children from particular geographical areas so as to better serve the family as well as the child.

The development disabilities center Child development centers, at-tached to children's hospitals or mental health centers, were originally set up to provide training and education for preschool children suffering from developmental disorders. Physical therapy services were available for the cerebral palsied (Chapter 2) and physically handicapped. The severely retarded preschooler also received training in these centers by attending a day school attached to the center. Pediatric neurologists or pediatricians were usually in charge of the centers but other professions were represented. When the children reached school age, they were referred to agencies which handled older children.

With the passage of the Mental Retardation Facilities Act of 1963, funds were made available to develop more of these centers and to expand the services of existing ones. Special classes were set up for the trainable retarded and the cerebral palsied, and, in some cases, the language or visually impaired. Diagnostic services were available and families were charged fees based on their ability to pay. In 1970 the Developmental Disabilities Services and Facilities Construction Act expanded and extended the services provided by the earlier act. The federal government shared in the cost of improving a state's services, with urban and rural poverty area projects receiving the most federal support.

In essence, the Developmental Disabilities Act made the earlier child development center a comprehensive agency. Diagnosis, evaluation, treatment, personal care, day care, domiciliary care, special living arrangements, training, education, sheltered employment, recreation, counseling of individuals and families, protective and other social services, information and referral services, follow-up services, and transportation were all included. A developmental disability is a disability attributable to mental retardation, cerebral palsy, or other neurological handicapping condition that originated before the individual reached 18 years of age and which is expected to continue indefinitely. Consequently, the child development center was submerged within a more comprehensive center, perhaps more appropriately named the development disabilities center.

These centers also are eligible for funds available through the Handicapped Children's Early Education Assistance Act. This act makes funds available for the establishment of model preschool programs for handicapped children. In addition, the development disabilities center will undoubtedly work more closely with public schools as a result of the Children with Specific Learning Disabilities Act of 1969 which provides funds to state education departments to establish learning disabilities child service demonstration programs. The act stipulates that these centers can be administered by a local school or community agency in a cooperative effort with the state education agency. Ideally, like the community mental health center, the development disabilities center in each community would be tied in with the family service center.

Sheltered employment Within the network of human service agencies in a community, there should be a sheltered workshop. A sheltered workshop is a setting where retarded, cerebral palsied, or disturbed adolescents and young adults who cannot function in our competitive job market can earn some money and perform a needed service. These workshops, under federal support, usually do subcontract work for other businesses. Sign painting, package assembly, furniture repair, and collation of printed material are examples of the work performed. Workers receive hourly pay for these services, and as a consequence they gain the pleasure of taking home a paycheck. As a result of the Developmental Disabilities Act more sheltered workshops will be established.

CONCLUDING REMARKS

We have discussed both what exists and what should exist if exceptional children are to be helped to develop to their fullest potential. Currently, most agencies operate independently, sometimes coordinating their services around the needs of clients, other times operating in ignorance of one another. Perhaps the community of the future will have multipurpose family service centers where families in crisis, regardless of the reason, can be helped to resolve their difficulties. Perhaps churches, schools, health clinics, welfare agencies, and legal organizations will coordinate their services under one roof, with a series of satellite centers established to reach rural areas.

If we continue to define the exceptional as sick, however, we will be doing them a great disservice. Such a conception not only increases the cost of services, but also produces caste systems within agencies and implies "treatment" instead of "management." In the early 1970s community colleges initiated programs to train community service assistants and mental health technologists (Atty, 1972). Although the "professional establishment" has not readily accepted the graduates of these programs (Maloney, 1972), the die has been cast. Without these individuals, whose training costs considerably less than that of the physician, the psychologist, and the social worker, the needs of the exceptional child and his family will never be met. Hopefully, the resistance to change which exists in most agencies can be overcome, enabling this new group of professionals to take their place alongside other members of multidisciplinary teams.

References

American Journal of Psychiatry. Special section, community mental health centers: Emerging patterns. *American Journal of Psychiatry,* 1972, **129,** 173–210.
Anastasi, A. *Psychological testing.* (3rd ed.) New York: Macmillan, 1968.
Atty, L. M. A new technician in the mental health field. *Perspectives in Psychiatric Care,* 1972, **10,** 12–18.
Bateman, B. D. *Interpretation of the 1961 Illinois Test of Psycholinguistic Abilities.* Seattle: Special Child Publications, 1968.
Betts, E. A. *Foundations of reading instruction.* New York: American Book, 1954.
Bruininks, R. H., Rynders, J. E., & Gross, J. C. Social acceptance of mildly retarded pupils in resource rooms and regular classes. *American Journal of Mental Deficiency,* 1974, **78,** 377–383.

Burt, M. R., & Balyeat, R. A new system for improving the care of neglected and abused children. *Child Welfare*, 1974, **53**, 167–179.

Burton, T. A. Mental health clinic services to the retarded. *Mental Retardation*, 1971, **9**, (5) 38–40.

Cardon, B. W., & French, J. L. Organization and content of graduate programs in school psychology. *Journal of School Psychology*, 1968–1969, **7**, 28–35.

Caudill, W. *The psychiatric hospital as a small society.* Cambridge, Mass.: Harvard University Press, 1958.

Cronbach, L. J. *Essentials of psychological testing.* (3rd ed.) New York: Harper & Row, 1970.

Cruickshank, W. M. The development of education for exceptional children. In W. M. Cruickshank & G. O. Johnson (Eds.), *Education of exceptional children.* Englewood Cliffs, N.J.: Prentice-Hall, 1967.

Cruickshank, W. M., Bentzen, F. A., Ratzeburg, R. H., & Tannhauser, M. T. *A teaching method for brain-injured and hyperactive children.* Syracuse, N.Y.: Syracuse University Press, 1961.

Davis, S. P., & Ecob, K. Q. *The mentally retarded in society.* New York: Columbia University Press, 1959.

De Vizia, J. Success in a foster home program for mentally retarded children. *Child Welfare*, 1974, **53**, 120–125.

Dunn, L. M. Special education for the mildly retarded—Is much of it justifiable? *Exceptional Children*, 1968, **35**, 5–22.

Freeman, F. S. *Theory and practice of psychological testing.* (3rd ed.) New York: Holt, Rinehart & Winston, 1962.

Gardner, S. O. The birth and infancy of the resource center at Hauula. *Exceptional Children*, 1971, **38**, 53–58.

Garett, B. L. Meeting the crisis in foster family care. *Children*, 1966, **13**, 2–8.

Goffman, E. *Asylums.* Garden City, N.Y.: Doubleday, 1961.

Goldfarb, W., Goldfarb, N., & Pollack, R. C. Treatment of childhood schizophrenia: a three year comparison of day and residential treatment of schizophrenic children. *Archives of General Psychiatry*, 1966, **14**, 119–128.

Goldstein, J., Freud, A., & Solnit, A. J. *Beyond the best interests of the child.* New York: Free Press, 1973.

Goodenough, E. L. *The measurement of intelligence by drawings.* New York: Harcourt Brace Jovanovich, 1926.

Harris, D. B. *Children's drawings as measures of intellectual maturity.* New York: Harcourt Brace Jovanovich, 1963.

Hewett, F. M. A hierarchy of educational tasks for children with learning disorders. *Exceptional Children*, 1964, **31**, 207–214.

Hewett, F. M. *The emotionally disturbed child in the classroom.* Boston: Allyn & Bacon, 1968.

Hewett, F. M. The learning center: the children and instructional strategies. Paper presented at the annual international convention of the Council for Exceptional Children, Chicago, April 1970.

Jenkins, J. R., Mayhall, W. F., Peschka, C. M., & Jenkins, L. M. Comparing small group and tutorial instruction in resource rooms. *Exceptional Children*, 1974, **40**, 245–250.

Jenkins, S. Filial deprivation in parents of children in foster care. *Children*, 1967, **14**, 8–12.

Joint Commission on Mental Health of Children, Inc. *Digest of crisis in child mental health: challenge for the 1970's.* Washington, D.C.: Joint Commission on Mental Health of Children, Inc., 1969.

Kanner, L. *A history of the care and study of the mentally retarded.* Springfield, Ill.: C. C Thomas, 1964.

Kirk, S. A., & Kirk, W. D. *Psycholinguistic learning disabilities: diagnosis and remediation.* Urbana: University of Illinois Press, 1971.

Koppitz, E. M. *The Bender-Gestalt Test for young children.* New York: Grune & Stratton, 1964.

Kotting, C., & Brozovich, R. A descriptive follow-up study of a public school program for the emotionally disturbed. (Final Report, Project No. 8-5068, U.S. Department of Health, Education, and Welfare) Unpublished manuscript, U.S. Office of Education, Bureau of Research, Washington, D.C., 1969.

Kuhlmann, F. One hundred years of special care and training. *American Journal of Mental Deficiency,* 1940, **45,** 8–24.

Levine, M., & Levine, A. *A social history of the helping services.* New York: Appleton, 1970.

Levy, J., & Pinder, S. Computer assisted management of state school waiting lists and admission procedures. *Mental Retardation,* 1971, **9,** (5) 30–34.

MacMillan, D. L. Issues and trends in special education. *Mental Retardation,* 1973, **11,** (2) 3–8.

Maloney, E. M. How to play the territorial game. *Perspectives in Psychiatric Care,* 1972, **10,** 31–33.

Mandelbaum, A. Parent-child separation: its significance to parents. *Social Work,* 1962, **7,** 26–24.

Meloy, J. The motives and conflicts in foster parenthood. *Children,* 1962, **9,** 222–226.

Menolascino, F., Clark, R. I., & Wolfensberger, W. (Eds.) *The initiation and development of a comprehensive, county-wide system of services for the mentally retarded of Douglas County.* Vol. 1. (2nd ed.) Omaha, Neb.: Greater Omaha Association for Retarded Children, 1968.

Menolascino, F., Clark, R. I., & Wolfensberger, W. (Eds.) *The initiation and development of a comprehensive, county-wide system of services for the mentally retarded of Douglas County.* Vol. 2. (2nd ed.) Omaha, Neb.: Greater Omaha Association for Retarded Children, 1970.

Mora, G. Child psychiatry in the United States: Its development and present status. *Acta Paedopsychiatrica,* 1954, **21,** 18–26.

Mora, G. The relevance of history for the community mental health approach to children. *American Journal of Psychiatry,* 1972, **129,** 408–414.

National Center for Health Statistics. *Health resource statistics.* (U.S. Department of Health, Education, and Welfare. Publication No. (HSM) 72-1509) Rockville, Md.: National Center for Health Statistics, 1972.

National Coalition for Mental Health Manpower. *Mental health manpower for the seventies: a national concern.* Washington, D.C.: Coalition for Mental Health Manpower, 1971.

National Institute of Mental Health. *Mental health services for children.* (Public Health Service Publication No. 1844) Washington, D.C.: U.S. Government Printing Office, 1968.

National Institute of Mental Health. *Residential treatment centers for emotionally disturbed children, 1969–1970.* (U.S. Department of Health, Education, and Welfare Publication No. (HSM) 72–9022) Rockville, Md.: National Institute of Mental Health, 1971.

Oberlin, D. S. The case for the transitional first grade. *Psychology in the Schools,* 1965, **2,** 129–133.

Osgood, C. E. *Contemporary approaches to cognition.* Cambridge, Mass.: Harvard University Press, 1957.

Parakevopoulas, J. N., & Kirk, S. A. *The development and psychometric characteristics of the Revised Illinois Test of Psycholinguistic Abilities.* Urbana: University of Illinois Press, 1969.

Pinder, S. Criteria for priority admission to state residential facilities for the mentally retarded. *Mental Retardation,* 1969, **7,** (5) 17–21.

President's Panel on Mental Retardation. *A proposed program for national action to combat mental retardation.* Washington, D.C.: U.S. Government Printing Office, 1962.

Reger, R., & Koppmann, M. The child oriented resource room program. *Exceptional Children,* 1971, **37,** 460–462.

Rosen, B. M., Kramer, M., Redick, R. W., & Willner, S. G. *Utilization of psychiatric facilities by children: current status trends, implications.* (Public Health Service Publication No. 1868) Washington, D.C.: National Institute of Mental Health, 1971.

Ross, S. L., DeYoung, H. G., & Cohen, J. S. Confrontation: special education and the law. *Exceptional Children,* 1971, **38,** 5–12.

Schulberg, H. C. Challenge of human service programs for psychologists. *American Psychologist,* 1972, **27,** 566–573.

Schultz, E. W., Hirshoren, A., Manton, A. B., & Henderson, R. A. Special education for the emotionally disturbed. *Exceptional Children,* 1971, **28,** 313–319.

Spollen, J. C., & Ballif, B. L. Effectiveness of individualized instruction for kindergarten children with developmental lag. *Exceptional Children,* 1971, **38,** 205–209.

Stanton, A. H., & Schwartz, M. S. *The mental hospital.* New York: Basic Books, 1954.

Talkington, L. W. *Admission trends in rural states: an unfulfilled prediction.* (Mental Retardation Research Series No. 11) Austin, Tex.: Austin State School, 1970.

Talkington, L. W. Outreach: delivery of services to rural communities. *Mental Retardation,* 1971, **9,** (5) 27–29.

Touwen, B. C. L., & Prechtl, H. F. R. *The neurological examination of the child with minor nervous system dysfunction.* (Clinics in Developmental Medicine No. 38) London: Spastics International Medical Publications, Heinemann, 1970.

Tucker, S. H. The difficulties of making an early diagnosis in children with minimal cerebral dysfunction. Paper presented at the annual conference of the American Physical Therapy Association, Washington, D.C., July 1970.

U.S. Department of Health, Education, and Welfare. *Children served by public welfare agencies and voluntary child welfare agencies and institutions. March, 1970.* (U.S. Department of Health, Education, and Welfare Publication No. (SRS) 72–03258) Rockville, Md.: National Center for Social Statistics, 1972.

Valett, R. E. The learning resource center for exceptional children. *Exceptional Children,* 1970, **36,** 527–530.

Walker, V. S. The efficacy of the resource room for educating retarded children. *Exceptional Children,* 1974, **40,** 288–289.

Wallin, J. E. W. *Education of mentally handicapped children.* New York: Harper & Row, 1955.

Weinstein, L. The zoomer class: initial results. *Exceptional Children,* 1971, **38,** 58–65.

Witmer, L. The exceptional child: at home and in school. In *University lectures delivered by members of the faculty in the Free Public Lecture Course, 1913–1914.* Philadelphia: University of Pennsylvania Press, 1915.

Wolfensberger, W. Twenty predictions about the future of residential services in mental retardation. *Mental Retardation,* 1969, **7,** (6) 51–54.

Wolfensberger, W. Will there always be an institution? I: the impact of epidemiological trends. *Mental Retardation,* 1971, **9,** (5) 14–20.

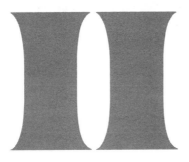

Identifiable
incapacitating
disorders

In this part we will discuss children whose development is usually so atypical that they are raised apart from society. Either brain tissue damage or structural malformation of the brain is generally responsible for the atypical development. While we will concentrate on highlighting the behaviors which set these children apart from others, keep in mind that there is more to the exceptional child than his deficits. Even the severely disabled child is more child than disability. In most cases development is arrested, so that he thinks and acts like children younger than he. What seems bizarre in his behavior might not appear so if he were younger. Hand regard, for example, is perfectly normal in the infant, but looks bizarre when displayed by the 5-year old. Similarly, low frustration tolerance, rapid mood swings, and demanding behavior are normal in the preschool child and are therefore tolerated by loving parents. However, these same behaviors in the 7-year old are not likely to be tolerated.

The fact that children are disabled does not mean that they can't be helped to function more effectively. If special assistance is provided to these children, many of whom will remain "children" throughout their development, they can lead more productive lives than has been characteristic in the past.

A civilization is judged by the way it treats its weakest members. Let us be certain that our civilization earns high marks at the bar of history.

—Pearl Buck

2
Brain damage

In this and the following chapter we will discuss children whose brain structures do not function normally because of brain tissue damage or improper interuterine development of brain structure. This chapter will present children whose dysfunctions are attributed to actual brain tissue damage. Before proceeding to this topic, however, a brief overview of the central nervous system (CNS) will be presented.

THE BRAIN AND BEHAVIOR

For over a century scientists have been performing investigations into the structure and function of various parts of the brain. Much of their research has been directed toward answering the question "What parts of the brain are responsible for controlling the various behaviors displayed by man?" In other words, are various human behaviors controlled by discrete areas of the brain?

The first successful studies of brain function were carried out in the late 1800s by a Russian anatomist, Betz, and by two German physiologists, Fritsch and Hitzig. Betz demonstrated that motor behaviors were controlled by what he called the giant pyramidal cells that were located just prior to the center of the brain. Fritsch and Hitzig showed that stimulation of localized areas of the cerebral cortex led to involuntary contractions of particular muscles on the opposite side of the body. Since that time, experiments have demonstrated that stimulation of particular areas of the brain lead to particular movements, and stimulation of other areas lead to visual, auditory, or tactile sensations. These findings clearly established that different areas of the brain are associated with different mental functions.

Clinical observation of patients with localized brain lesions also revealed the heterogeneity of different parts of the brain. In 1861 Paul Broca identified an area in the frontal lobe of the left hemisphere as an area responsible for speech. This area has become known as *Broca's area.* About ten years later Carl Wernicke discovered that destruction of the cortex of the left temporal lobe below Broca's area (area 44 in Figure 2.1) resulted in inability to understand spoken language. This area has come to be called *Wernicke's center* (areas 41 and 42 in Figure 2.1). Since then, considerable research has been designed to map areas of the brain responsible for different functions.

The observations of Broca and Wernicke convinced neurologists that study of the effects of circumscribed brain lesions would reveal the location of other, more complex mental processes. Studies were made of the disturbance in mental activity that accompanied particular local brain lesions. Lesions in the occipital regions of the brain caused disturbances in the perception of visually presented objects (optic agnosia), those in the parietal region caused a loss in the ability to construct an objective action (apraxia). Soon disorders of arithmetic (acalculia), of writing (agraphia), of reading (alexia), of musical ability (amusia), and of constructive activity (constructive apraxia) were associated with lesions in narrowly localized areas of the brain. Some of the areas associated with language appear in Figure 2.1.

This research clearly established that lesions in different areas of the brain result in different symptoms. These early efforts to map the areas of the brain were based upon the notion that isolated faculties could be localized in well-defined areas of the brain. The map given in Figure 2.1 implies that the functions listed are subserved only by the particular areas of the brain indicated, and that each specified area is the cortical center for each function. This view implies that destruction of a specified area in the brain will lead to a loss in the specific function controlled by this center. Such specificity, however, does not exist. Numerous observations of patients with gunshot wounds or tumors have revealed that disturbance of a particular complex function does not arise as a result of a narrowly circumscribed lesion in one part of the brain, but can occur as a result of lesions in many different areas. Disorders of writing, for example, can result from lesions in the temporal, postcentral, premotor, and occipitoparietal regions of the brain. Consequently, attempts to relate the complex act of writing to one localized area, such as Exner's writing center (areas 17 and 18, Figure 2.1), would be fruitless (Luria, 1966). Similarly, patients with brain lesions in many different parts of the brain have difficulty in sound recognition. The same statement can be made about arithmetical operations, reading, and other behaviors.

Furthermore, a lesion in a narrowly circumscribed area of the brain almost never leads to the loss of any single isolated mental function, but rather to a disturbance of a group of mental and behavioral processes, forming a symptom-complex, or syndrome. For example, a lesion of the

Figure 2.1 *Brain areas and language functions. (From A. Agranowitz.* Aphasia handbook, *1964. Courtesy of Charles C Thomas, Publisher, Springfield, Ill.)*

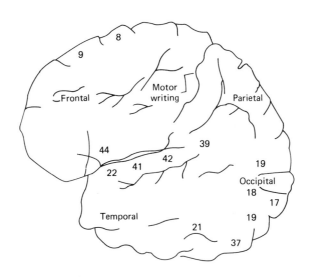

Area	Function	Language defects caused by destructive lesions
41 and 42 (Wernicke's center)	Recognition of spoken language	Auditory verbal agnosia
21 and 22	Recall and interpretation of spoken language	
44 (Broca's area)	Memory of motor patterns of speech	Motor aphasia (speech)
37	Recall of names and words; language formulation	Anomia Amnesic aphasia
39 (angular gyrus)	Symbols for reading, writing, and arithmetic (letters and numbers)	Alexia Agraphia (spelling) Acalculia
8 and 9 (Exner's writing center)	Knowledge of how to make movements of hand and fingers	Agraphia (motor)
17 and 18	Visual perception and recognition	Visual-verbal agnosia without agraphia*

* This is caused by subcortical lesion between 17 and 39.

external portions of the left temporal region of the cortex causes a disturbance of speech that is accompanied by an inability to analyze speech sounds, faulty repetition and memorizing of words, gross defects of writing, and impaired cognitive functioning, but the lesion leaves intact orientation in space, discrimination of direction, and written arithmetical operations (Luria, 1966).

Also disputing the notion of specified areas for highly specified functions was the finding that patients who have lost particular functions as a result of brain lesions frequently regain these functions. Since neurons in the cerebral cortex are incapable of regeneration, other areas of the brain must come to subserve these functions. Further work demonstrated that elementary sensory and motor functions (sight, hearing, touch) cannot be restored after destruction of particular zones in the cortex, but that complex behaviors are sometimes capable of full restoration (Lashley, 1960). This restoration, however, does not take place by a simple transfer of control to another part of the brain; rather it is the result of a functional reorganization. In general, a lesion in the occipital region of the brain impairs analysis and synthesis of visual symbols (areas 17 and 18, Figure 2.1). After a time, reading comes to be carried out through tactile and motor tracing of letters and through sounding words out. In other words, acoustical-motor skill substitutes for visual skill. All this evidence suggests that the brain is not a conglomeration of individual organs, each the center for a certain isolated mental or behavioral function, but is a network of interrelated systems that work together to produce a behavioral act. The brain thus consists of dynamic structures or "constellations" of neurons that work together to produce different functions so that the brain as a whole carries out complex behaviors.

The brain is now considered a highly complex, differentiated structure in which highly specialized areas work in harmony with areas subserving more general functions. Among the specialized areas there are centers that subserve various analyzers: visual, located in the occipital; auditory, in the temporal; cutaneous, in the postcentral; motor, in the central and premotor regions (motor writing area, Figure 2.1). These centers, however, do not function in isolation from other parts of the brain, as was originally proposed, but work interdependently with them. Furthermore, zones that subserve specific functions account for only half the surface of the human cortex. The nonspecific zones, which are poorly developed in other animals, are considered responsible for complex forms of integrative activity that require constant interaction between analyzers located in different zones of the brain. Lesions in these areas lead to disturbances in functions that require the combined participation of various cortical regions.

In the early 1950s research focused not only on the structure and function of specific divisions of the brain but also on the function of a nonspecific system of the brain, a system that plays a role in maintenance and regulation of bodily states and in the reception of signals that provide feedback about an organism's activity. Magoun (1958) and his colleagues studied the role of the system now called the *reticular activating system* (RAS). This system is involved in maintaining states of alertness and in selecting and filtering information emanating from the environment. For example, one experiment demonstrated that when a mouse crosses the path of a hungry cat, the cat's brain no longer responds to other stimuli in the environment. In this experiment it was first established that the cat's brain was registering a sound signal, as measured by EEG tracings of electrical activity in the area of the cerebral cortex that receives auditory stimuli. Then, in the presence of the sound, a mouse was seen by the cat. EEG tracings revealed that the auditory signal was no longer received by the cortex. Evidently the sound signal never reached the hearing center of the brain; since the auditory signal was of no importance to the cat, the visual signal of the mouse was given preeminence. The reticular system is considered responsible for this decision making about what stimuli are important at what time.

Although it is beyond the scope of this chapter to discuss the various nonspecific systems and their interdependent relationships with each other and with the specific systems, the preceding review should serve to emphasize that higher psychological functions are *"complex functional systems, based on the combined working of individual and sometimes far remote parts of the brain, each of which performs its own specific role and makes its own specific contribution to the integrated functional system"* (Luria, 1966, p. 38).

We can see, then, why any lesion that destroys the central portions of a particular analyzer does not cause just the loss of that single function, but results in a disturbance of a whole complex of behavioral processes that depend upon the integrity of the particular analyzer. Consequently, a *primary* disturbance of certain forms of analyzers and synthesizers (vision in lesions of the occipital, auditory in lesions of the temporal, etc.) leads to *secondary* consequences by disturbing the normal working of all functional systems linked to this analyzer. Disturbances differ in character and assume different forms depending upon which link is affected. Nevertheless, every local lesion of the cerebral cortex has a far more extensive secondary effect than may be originally realized. The primary defect arising in any local lesion does not disturb all functional systems equally; it affects only those systems that include the damaged link in their composition. Behavioral processes not including the link remain unaffected (Luria, 1966).

For example, a lesion of the cortical segments responsible for analyzing sound does not affect the ability to copy or to write highly automatized words, words that have been converted into kinetic skill. It does affect writing words from dictation. Similarly, a lesion in the audio-speech area makes impossible the clear identification of phonemes from the flow of sounds. Being unable to distinguish between closely similar phonemes or pick out individual phonemes from a stream of consonants results in gross mistakes in writing. Luria (1966) describes the manner in which focal lesions in different areas of the brain can all produce writing difficulties. Careful study of the types of errors can sometimes demonstrate the nature of the underlying defect.

Brain damage in children

We have been discussing the brain from a static viewpoint. Disturbances of individual functions in early stages of mental development will have quite different consequences than disturbances in later stages. Brain damage early in a child's life can prevent the acquisition of skills necessary for adequate functioning. We know that the formation of complex types of behavioral activity is dependent upon a well-developed system of simpler, concrete forms of mental activity (Piaget, 1953). Voluntary attention, logical thinking, and memory are all derived from more elementary forms of mental activity and will not attain perfect development if the elementary forms have not developed adequately (hierarchical concept of development). For example, disturbances in auditory perception may cause only minor problems when they occur in an adult, but may make it impossible for the child to acquire perfect speech and, therefore, to have adequate writing and expressive skills. In some instances, however, damage occurring in infancy results in less severe consequences than the same damage occurring in the adult. The conclusion from these facts is that *a lesion of the same area of the brain at different stages of development may lead to completely different consequences* (Luria, 1966). This topic will be discussed again at different points in the text.

Diffuse brain damage Up to this point we have been discussing damage that occurs to particular areas of the brain. Although tumors, structural abnormalities, or ruptured blood vessels can produce circumscribed brain lesions, most brain damage is diffuse rather than specific. The effects of diffuse damage can be demonstrated by partially filling a balloon with water and striking it sharply on one side. We can clearly see that the water is forced to the other side of the balloon. The harder the balloon is hit, the greater the force of water against the other side and the wider its dispersion. Although clean lesions can be made in animals through operative techniques, damage to humans usually occurs in the manner demonstrated with the balloon. Blows to the head can cause damage throughout the brain. Anoxia, high fevers, or shock also can cause diffuse damage. In general, children with diffuse damage show a wide variety of functional disorders, with many having conceptual and intellectual deficiencies. Lashley's (1929) work has demonstrated that loss of function may be more dependent on the amount of damage than on the exact location.

. This chapter focuses on children whose tissue damage is confined largely to one area of the brain. In the next chapter we will discuss children in whom either diffuse brain damage, damage to "critical" areas, or abnormal brain development results in pronounced perceptual, conceptual, and intellectual deficiency.

Causes of brain damage Brain tissue damage can be the result of factors operating before (prenatal), during (perinatal), or after (postnatal) birth. Genetic or inherited conditions can result in structural malformation of the brain. Metabolic disturbances in the mother and Rh incompatibility can cause cerebral tissue damage *in utero*. Most cerebral tissue damage occurring at birth results from asphyxia incurred from placental abnormalities, pathological labor, pulmonary diseases, or cardiac arrest. Childhood diseases such as meningitis, encephalitis, and influenza, and high fevers in typhoid, diphtheria, and pertussis (an acute infectious disease often called whooping cough) can result in brain tissue damage, as can head injuries from accidents, poisoning and toxic conditions (lead, carbon monoxide), or strangulation (McDonald & Chance, 1964). The most common postnatal cause is inflamation of brain tissue (encephalitis) due to viral infections or other disease (Blake & Wright, 1963).

Considering what has been said about the brain, we will now examine brain damage that results in loss of specific functions (localizable) but which, of course, will produce general, or nonfocal, alterations in behavior. Two conditions will be presented: cerebral palsy, a condition resulting in motor abnormalities, and aphasia, a condition resulting in a failure to acquire or comprehend language.

Cerebral palsy

The term cerebral palsy is used to categorize children who display motor abnormalities considered to be the result of damage to the areas of the brain subserving motor activity. The manifestations of the damage depend upon the location and extent of the lesion. Paralysis, weakness, uncoordination, and other aberrant motor functions are the primary behaviors displayed. Sometimes the nonfocal effects of the damage are observed before the focal effects. This is particularly the case in less severe forms or in early infancy. As we will see in the case of Art, his atypical behaviors in nonmotor functions were attributed to other causes before cerebral palsy was finally diagnosed.

ART

They say colic lasts only three months. Perhaps this wasn't colic, thought Jane Black. Her little Arty was in his sixth month and still kept her up most of the night. Neighbors said he'd grow out of it; some said she should relax since infants are sensitive to high-strung mothers. While she was willing to accept herself as an inept mother, perhaps even accept responsibility for Art's uneasiness, her husband, Bob, was not ready to let her take this responsibility. He felt something was basically wrong with Art. Art had always been an exceptionally alert and attractive baby, but why didn't he sleep? Both he and Jane were exhausted from staying up with him night after night.

The pediatrician felt that Art just needed less sleep than other children. Neither parent could agree with this opinion. Some children require less sleep, yes, but Art hardly slept at all, and when he did, it was excessively light and characterized by inordinate movement and irregularity. When placed in his crib he would cry until taken out and held.

Resolved to ignore his crying, the Blacks would lie in their bed each night listening to Art cry. When the crying reached almost hysterical proportions, Jane couldn't stand it any longer and would pick Art up and comfort him. Bob critized Jane for her weakness, and they fought over their difference of opinion. Bob, who originally was convinced that something was wrong with Art, now was confused and bewildered by the whole situation. Out of frustration, he would lash out at Jane for not following their plan, even though neither really believed its basic premise.

Consulting baby and child care manuals was no help. They labeled babies who behaved like Art as hypertonic (Spock, 1957), a term used to describe babies whose immature nervous and digestive systems have difficulty adjusting to the external environment. The manuals recommended ignoring crying at night.

Jane and Bob decided to take turns staying up with Art and not to expect him to sleep much. With time, perhaps he would grow out of it. At least they wouldn't be fighting with each other.

Art had started to drool excessively at about 3 months. Jane and Bob anxiously awaited his first tooth. At least something was going right. At 6 months, no tooth had arrived. The pediatrician said not to worry, since many children drool, bite, and have periods of fretfulness for sometimes four months until the first tooth actually arrives.

At about 9 months, Art's parents noticed that he fatigued easily. After creeping vigorously for several minutes, he would become irritable and require rest. Nevertheless, he wouldn't sleep for very long, even when extremely fatigued. Jane would put him down for a nap and within ten minutes he'd be up and shaking the crib. His motor development seemed slower than that observed in neighbor's children. Again the pediatrician's opinion was that, although Art may be a little slow to develop, there was no cause for alarm; different children have different patterns of development. Developmental charts reflect only averages; not every child can be expected to fall exactly at the average.

Both parents feared that Art might be mentally retarded, but neither would say so for fear that somehow their words might make it true. His alert and attractive features, however, seemed to contradict this suspicion.

One night Bob noticed that Art favored his right hand. Closer observation revealed that he grasped objects almost exclusively with this hand. The child care manuals stated that some children establish a preferred hand early but most use both hands interchangeably during infancy. Jane noticed that the right knee of Art's overalls was always more dirty and worn than the left. Close inspection of Art's motor activities revealed that he placed most of his weight on his right side when creeping. His grasp with his left hand was poor and his thumb seemed to turn in. The Blacks discussed these observations with the pediatrician. He recommended they take Art to a pediatric neurologist associated with the Child Development Center at the Children's Hospital.

Art's evaluation

Art went to the hospital on several occasions for an evaluation that included the gathering of detailed historical material, a developmental assessment, and a neurological examination. The evaluation revealed brain damage to the right cerebral hemisphere. The technical diagnosis was given as cerebral palsy with mild spastic hemiplegia, or incomplete paralysis of the left side. Art favored his right leg and right hand because his left side functioned poorly.

Since Art's motor involvement was primarily on the left side, the damage was located somewhere in the motor region of the right cerebral cortex. As we know, there is a crossing over, or decussation, of most of the neurons of the corticospinal tract as they pass from the brain stem into the spinal cord. For this reason, the muscles on one side of the body are controlled by the cortex of the opposite side. Let us examine more closely how the neurologist arrived at his decision.

The neurologist's examination Unless a child is grossly damaged, neurological evaluations are perhaps more an art than an exact science, particularly when performed in early childhood. At present, a diagnosis is reached by piecing together information gathered from historical material, observation, and some thirty specific assessment procedures. Should the neurologist suspect that abnormalities revealed by these procedures are the result of a tumor or intracerebral hemorrhage (bleeding within the brain), he would employ more complex diagnostic procedures. Many of the procedures employed in Art's neurological evaluation also are used when evaluating older children suspected of having minor brain injury (see Chapter 8).

The first procedure undertaken was developmental assessment. To avoid Art's becoming bored or irritable, assessment was carried out before the history was taken. The neurologist placed a 1-inch cube on the table in front of Art. Immediately Art grabbed the cube with his right hand. While Art was still holding the first cube, the neurologist handed him another. The neurologist noted that Art did not use his thumb when grasping with his left hand. Instead, he held the block in his palm rather than between his thumb and forefinger, as he did with his right hand. Also noted was that he did not transfer cubes from one hand to another. When he had a cube in each hand, however, he would bring them together for comparison. Next, a small pellet was placed on the table, and Art touched it with his finger. Both an index finger approach to a pellet and block comparison dates development of manipulation at about 9 months. Both hands were then observed for presence of spasticity or ataxia (irregular movement). Jane was instructed to ask Art to hand her a cube. Art was able to comply with this request.

Art was then undressed and his sitting stability, position in the prone, ability to crawl or creep, and weight-bearing were assessed. His muscle tone (the state of tension in resting muscle necessary to maintain posture) in all limbs was assessed by palpitating the muscles, putting the joints through passive movements, and testing the degree of movements of joints, especially the hips and ankles. His reflexes were then tested, particularly the knee jerks, since the area over which a tendon jerk is obtained increases in spastic forms of cerebral palsy. Finally, Art's head circumference was measured and his urine tested for biochemical abnormalities.

In addition to formal assessment, the neurologist observed Art's postural activities during his stay in the center. Close attention was paid to their quality, quantity, and symmetry. Art's appointment was scheduled so that the neurologist could join the family for lunch and observe Art eating.

Following lunch, historical information was gathered. The chief importance of the history lies in the determination of the previous rate of development, or developmental history, and in the elicitation of factors which might have influenced development. The Blacks were asked whether any genetic conditions had ever existed in the family, such as degenerative diseases of the nervous system, mental deficiency, or hydrocephalus. Jane was asked about her health during pregnancy, the mode of delivery, and Art's condition at birth and thereafter. Regarding Art's development, Jane was asked questions about his feeding habits, alertness, sleep patterns, and motor functioning.

The neurologist knew the average age at which certain skills are acquired and compared Jane's description of Art's development with these norms. Jane and Bob could not remember exactly when Art first performed all of the activities the neurologist inquired about, but had recorded some of these events in his baby book. Although parental recall is not always accurate (Wenar & Coulter, 1962), the neurologist still considered such questioning helpful.

The psychologist's involvement On a second visit to the hospital, Art's performance on the Cattell Infant Intelligence Scale (Cattell, 1947) was compared with national norms. The Cattell scale is considered a downward extension of the Stanford-Binet scale discussed in Chapter 1. The test items are grouped at age levels, as they are on the Binet, with groupings provided at each month, from 2 months through 12, and at two-month intervals in the second year. At 10 months, Art's age, a child should be able to uncover a toy, put a cube inside a cup, attempt to take a third cube when holding two, hit a cup with a spoon, and poke his finger into the holes of a form board. If he does all these functions successfully, then he scores at a 10-month level. Like the Stanford-Binet, the Cattell scale obtains a basal age, adds the credits obtained at higher levels to obtain a mental age, and from that obtains a ratio IQ. Art's IQ was within the average range.

Most intellectual measurement taken in infancy fails to correlate substantially with measurement taken at a later date, primarily because later measures include tasks requiring verbal mediation, analysis, and synthesis, while early measures are primarily those of state of alertness and physical health. Until language develops, prediction of the child's ultimate intellectual handicap is difficult.

Clinical findings and interpretation Art's assessment was performed at a favorable age because of the readily available milestones of manipulation, motor development, imitation, and beginning speech. Art's pediatrician had performed developmental assessments as part of his routine check-ups, but he had performed them at an earlier and more difficult age (Illingworth, 1962) and was not a specialist in neurology trained to notice minor deviations in development. While neurological evaluation of the neonate (newborn) is possible, minor abnormalities are difficult to assess at that age. In addition, both individual variability and the slow temporal sequence of developmental stages make diagnosis difficult (Paine, 1960a).

The pediatrician first saw Art in a more or less amorphous state shortly after birth. He developed certain attitudes about Art's parents, viewing the mother as high-strung and the father as solicitous toward his wife. His later examinations of Art were influenced by his earlier perceptions of both Art and his parents. Since his later percepts were related to the first by recall, they were subject to distortion.

In contrast, the neurologist had greater experience with cerebral palsied children, and he was not influenced by earlier opinion. In addition, he performed the evaluation prior to taking a history and therefore prior to forming an opinion about the family.

The cardinal alerting signs were that Art held his left arm against his body, had an immature grasp, and dragged his left leg when tired. In addition, his left hand would contract spontaneously after mild stimulation, and the range of movement of his left extremities was limited. Behavioral signs were Art's abnormal sleep patterns, his excessive crying, his delayed teething, and his delayed motor development; the last sign is a specific effect, while the other signs are the general effects. Many of the same nonfocal effects are observed in other brain-damaged children as well as in children with suspected damage who display learning disorders but no other obvious signs of dysfunction.

What the neurologist ruled out   A loss of muscle tone can be a sign of neuromuscular disease (Chapter 6) or of a progressive disorder. These disorders are usually accompanied by an absence or low intensity of reflex. The neurologist could rule out both these disorders since Art had exaggerated responses and increased muscle tone. Increased tone could result from a heart disorder, such as rheumatoid arthritis (Chapter 6), but other signs were present that were not associated with heart disorder. Normal head size, absence of intracranial pressure, and absence of symptoms such as vomiting and excess drowsiness ruled out brain tumor. Normal cranial nerve functioning ruled out disorders of the brain stem.

Reevaluation for the assessment of related disorders   Art's condition was considered mild because the motor abnormalities were not marked. Psychological evaluation as well as informal observation suggested that the impairment was confined largely to motor functioning. Art's alertness, interest in his surroundings, responsiveness, and powers of concentration were considered normal. Consequently, his prognosis was favorable.

Nevertheless, Art would need continual reevaluation, since many of the sensory and cognitive deficits that often accompany cerebral palsy are difficult to assess at younger ages. Approximately 50 percent of palsied children have speech and perceptual disorders as well as sensation losses (Paine, 1960b). Over 50 percent have intelligence quotients in the mentally retarded range (Rutter, Graham, & Yule, 1970). The cerebral palsied child may also have one or more of the following difficulties: impaired vision, defective hearing, convulsions, orthopedic defects, dental anomalies, perceptual difficulties, and emotional problems (Cardwell, 1965; Cass, 1966; Cruickshank, 1966; Daley, 1965; Levin, 1965; Love, 1970; McDonald & Chance, 1964).

More specifically, a child like Art, who has right-side hemiplegia, may have right hemianopia (loss of vision of the right side of the visual field) which makes it difficult to follow a line of print (see Figures 2.2 and 2.3). He may also be unable to deal with spatial relationships and have disturbances in body image as a result of some parietal lobe damage. Retarded speech development and dysphasia (inability to discriminate sounds) are common. Behavioral and emotional disorders are frequent,

Figure 2.2 *Demonstration of a right visual field defect in a 10-month old infant with a congenital lesion of the left cerebral hemisphere. A, she failed to turn to the toy hatchet when it was presented on the right side. B, she turned to hatchet in the left visual field. Note also the attitude of the hemiparetic right hand. (From P. R. Dodge. Neurologic history and examination. In T. W. Farmer (Ed.), Pediatric neurology, p. 25. New York: Harper & Row, 1964.)*

A   B

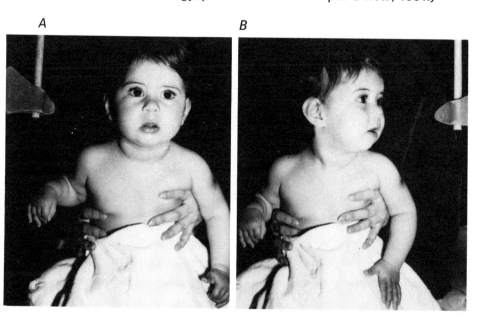

Figure 2.3 *Testing of nystagmus (involuntary eye movement) by moving a printed cloth across the field of vision. The patient also had a right hemianopia and a supranuclear facial weakness, which is visible in the photograph. The deformed knees are the result of recurrent joint disease. (From P. R. Dodge. Neurologic history and examination. In T. W. Farmer (Ed.), Pediatric neurology, p. 220. New York: Harper & Row, 1964.)*

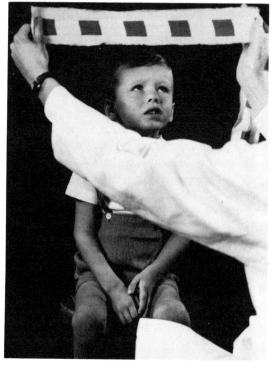

but they are related more to family factors than to the degree of motor or perceptual deficit present (Skatvedt, 1960).

Assessment for these disorders usually is not possible until early childhood. Prognosis depends upon the kind of environment in which the child is raised and how his parents react to him. If he suffers from emotional deprivation, he may achieve less than his developmental potential would indicate. We will discuss disorders associated with cerebral palsy in more detail in later sections.

Even Art's motor functioning would be easier to evaluate at a later date because reactions of muscle tone are more pronounced when the child attempts activities beyond those under his control. Although Art may creep or crawl in a relatively normal way, he may become stiff and show signs of spasticity when trying to stand and walk. If he attempts to move quickly or fears loss of balance, he may become spastic. Increase in tone also can appear when he attempts to speak.

Art would be reevaluated in six months. In the meantime, his parents were instructed in procedures that would assist Art to develop as normally as possible.

Art's treatment

"How can we help him now?" was the first question Art's parents asked. Treatment of Art's problem would aim primarily at producing a more normal state of muscle tone to prepare for movement.

Muscles work in groups and the brain responds by making groups of muscles work in particular patterns. The muscles of the cerebral palsied child also work in groups, but their patterns are abnormal. For example, in spastic paralysis, the child may want to extend his arm but instead it involuntarily contracts; when he reaches for an object, instead of contracting his fingers extend.

The Bobaths (Semans, 1967) have observed that abnormal muscle activity can be changed by changing the relationship of parts of the body to each other and thereby changing output patterns. Special handling is believed to accomplish these changes. Art will be handled in such a way that abnormal patterns are blocked. By changing pattern, muscle tone is changed. The Bobaths theorize that by such handling synaptic connections can be broken by blocking the visible muscular reaction, thus preventing aberrant impulses from being channeled into abnormal reflexes. It then becomes possible to redirect impulses into the desired responses being stimulated at the same time. The child's reaction to handling is carefully observed for changes in postural tone, and the handling is adjusted to these changes.

The Bobaths have pointed out that spasticity affects parts of the body other than those directly related to the brain damage. The sound side of the body becomes involved in the disability by attempting to compensate. The compensation movements are often different from normal patterns of muscular coordination. Consequently, the child can develop into a one-sided youngster, with decreased chances of recovery and of coordinated action between the two sides of the body. In treating Art, the entire left side would be included, starting with proximal parts. The abnormal compensatory activity of the sound side would be retrained to facilitate whatever responses are available on the involved side.

The family was scheduled to see the physical therapist at the child development clinic associated with the local hospital. Jane and Bob were taught to handle Art very much as would the physical therapist, facilitating normal reactions while stopping the abnormal, and giving help only when Art needed to control abnormal postures. The therapist identified each important step as goals and gave tips on how to assist Art toward these goals in his everyday handling and play. Emphasis was placed on the desired responses from Art, and Jane was encouraged to use her own common sense and ingenuity. Although Jane was given several specific suggestions, the clinic staff felt it improper to instill a faith in some system or ritual of exercises as a kind of magic pill. Teaching a list of exercises, the significance of which a parent might not understand, often has adverse effects (Semans, 1966). Jane would have a better chance than the therapist to seize the moment of readiness and encourage a desired response. Consequently, she learned the steps in development that could be expected and ways of handling and playing with Art that would elicit a wide variety of movement responses at each step.

The Blacks were told that physical improvement would be slow and not to become discouraged or to blame themselves if Art's progress was not as rapid as they might hope. The affected arm and leg would never become perfect no matter how much they improved. The leg usually tends to do better than the arm. Most hemiplegic children manage to use the affected leg well enough to be able to walk, primarily because they could not walk without it.

The affected hand and arm are not as important, since the child can do a great deal with his good hand without the assistance of the other. The ability to use the affected hand depends on many things beside the stiffness and weakness of the arm. For example, if the sense of touch is affected, the child may be unable to recognize objects by touch, shape, size, and texture when they are placed in his affected hand. If blindfolded, he may be unable to distinguish objects from one another using only the affected hand. Since he is clumsier using this hand, he comes to rely more and more on his good hand; the affected hand becomes a nuisance to him (Culloty, 1964).

The Blacks were told to encourage Art to use the affected hand, not only to make it useful but to prevent deformity as he grows older (Semans, 1966). Since the hand will never become normal, Art was to use it as a helping hand, but not instead of the good hand. Several suggestions were made, such as encouraging his play with objects or containers requiring the use of two hands and helping him to learn to support his weight on both hands and to crawl properly. Correct crawling was facilitated by placing a sling under his chest and supporting his weight while he was on his hands and knees.

The effects of treatment Although proponents of various physical therapies attribute favorable outcome to their methods, no adequately controlled studies appear in the literature. Using the subject as his own control is not a satisfactory procedure because children have been known to show improved motor functioning without any intervening treatment (Illingworth, 1960).

How can spontaneous recovery occur when nerve tissue does not have the capacity to repair itself? Other tissues can do so through the division of adjacent cells, a process not available to central nerve tissue. At birth a child's brain has practically all the neurons that it will ever have. Damage to any of the cells means they cannot be replaced. How then can a child spontaneously improve his functioning if his brain cells cannot be replaced through mitosis (cell division) of adjacent cells? Studies by Isaacson (1970) and his collegues help answer this question.

In animals with brains damaged as adults, supportive cells and connective tissues fill in the cite of the lesion. In infancy many of the supportive cells have not had time to form in the brain. Instead, nerve cells that appear normal are found in the originally damaged area. How does this happen? In infants most of the nerve cells are fully formed and have migrated to their final destinations in the brain. Nerve cells are not produced in equal amounts along all ventricular surfaces; cells from more active areas migrate considerable distances to their final position. Isaacson theorizes that when areas of active production are not damaged they will continue to function and new cells will continue to move to their target areas. Finding these areas damaged, they reach other areas, form novel connections, and operate in a somewhat different manner than would be expected. Some operate as if they were in the area for which they were originally intended. In mature brains lesions destroy completely developed nerve cells and there are no new cells being formed. The wound, then, cannot receive new cells. Instead, supportive cells mix with blood vessel tissue linings to form a cover for the wounded area.

In order to assess the effects of a therapeutic program, children matched according to disability need to be assigned to a treatment and nontreatment condition. Only then can the effects of a treatment be determined. No one, however, is willing to assign a child to a nontreatment condition when he really believes in the treatment. Perhaps advocates of different approaches could match children on relevant variables and then compare the results of their different procedures. At present, however, no such study exists. For such a study to be performed, some adequate form of classification would have to be developed and much more learned about the course of the disorder. The natural history of cerebral palsy has not yet been precisely chronicled. Consequently, classification accurate enough to predict outcome is difficult. Many factors contribute to this difficulty. First, a wide range of variation exists, both between children and within the same child from one day to the next. Second, certain signs become manifest only at certain stages of maturation. Third, the disorders are labile, dependent in kind and degree upon environmental circumstances. Fourth, no agreed terminology exists for signs nor is there a satisfactory system of classification. Fifth, different clinicians are more adept at perceiving different cues in the same array of signs. Consequently, the experience and data of different clinicians often cannot be pooled for comparison (Abercrombie, 1960a).

Although abnormal patterns may be changed, the handling techniques themselves may not produce the changes in the manner hypothesized. Luria's (1966) research has demonstrated that motor disorders can be compensated for by strengthening the intellectual organization of the movement, bringing into play higher cortical levels of control over the motor act. For example, a patient who could not voluntarily unclench his fist when instructed to do so could unclench it when instructed to point to the window with his finger. The instruction to perform a new motor task abolished the perseverance of the previous action (clenched fist), and the transfer of the movement to the complex cortical level overcame the elementary automatism.

The infant with cerebral palsy has not developed control over complex motor acts, so that such a shift in control of simple acts to higher cortical centers cannot take place. The Bobaths' handling techniques, however, may facilitate greater cortical control over motor acts, and it is perhaps such shifts in control that produce the changes they note, rather than a redirection of impulses into desired responses. Further research may shed some light on this topic.

TYPES OF CEREBRAL PALSY

Because Art's prognosis was considered favorable, the reader may wonder why his case is included in a section devoted to incapacitating disorders. There are three reasons for selecting Art to represent the cerebral palsied. First, as we will see later, the degree of incapacitation is not always directly correlated with the extent of disability. Society tends to reject the physically disabled as social companions, so that many children with less severe forms of cerebral palsy find themselves social outcasts and unable to compete successfully in our society. Second, cerebral palsy can exist in a variety of forms without accompanying intellectual retardation; Art serves to emphasize this fact. Third, Art displayed many of the same behaviors displayed by children with brain injury varying from mild to severe: irregular sleep, poor mastication of food, and excessive drooling. With advanced age, they display other behaviors, such as short attention span, excessive variation in mood, and impaired concentration ability. Many never show the degree of motor involvement that leads to early referral for neurological evaluation. The signs they show are often subtle and until recently were thought the result of emotional difficulties, motivational factors, or mild mental retardation (see Chapter 8). Of those with major motor involvement, involvement easily identified at birth or within the first year, the majority are not as fortunate as Art.

A child whose brain injury results in paralysis, weaknesses, incoordination, or other aberration of motor function is labeled as cerebral palsied. This term is employed to categorize a heterogeneous group of brain-injured children who have palsy (lack of muscular control) as a result of damage to the motor centers of the brain (motor cortex, cerebellum, or basal ganglia). As we have seen, damage is rarely confined solely to motor centers, and damaged children usually have associated difficulties.

Classification systems

Although the symptoms and signs of cerebral palsy are variable, cases can be roughly divided into three groups, according to whether the damage is to the motor cortex, basal ganglia, or cerebellum. On this basis they are classified as spastic, athetoid, or ataxic. In 1954 the Nomenclature Committee of the American Academy for Cerebral Palsy adopted a classification system derived from observable symptoms. The six classes represent some attempt to correlate the neuromuscular disorder with the site of the lesion.

Spastic paralysis is the most frequent form and results from lesions in the pyramidal tract of the motor cortex and in other areas at the base of the brain. Spasticity is an exaggerated contraction of muscles when they are stretched; when suddenly elongated, the muscles contract, the degree of contraction depending upon the degree of spasticity. When Art pressed his arm against his body, with his forearm bent and his fingers flexed, and dragged his involved leg, he displayed two classic signs of spastic paralysis.

Athetosis usually results from lesions to the extrapyramidal motor tracts (structures outside of, or extra to, the pyramidal system) and is characterized by involuntary, incoordinate motion in various parts of the body. The child displays uncontrollable, jerky, irregular twisting movements of the extremities.

A small number of children who display disturbances in balance and posture are classified as *ataxic*. Lesions in the middle lobe of the cerebellum usually cause this disorder. Children who have extremely flaccid muscles and unusually deep tendon reflexes (abnormally strong muscle contraction when a tendon deep within the muscle is stimulated) are classified as *atonic*. While the exact anatomical basis of this disorder is unclear, lesions somewhere in the cerebellum are partially responsible for its occurrence. Those children who show fine involuntary muscular movements that are rhythmic in character are classified as *tremor*. Lesions in the midbrain and cerebellum are responsible for tremor. Children are labeled *rigid* who display a functional noncoordination of extensor and flexor muscles that results in rigidly held limbs that resist movement. Lesions in the midbrain near the pons are most often responsible for this disorder (Cardwell, 1965).

There is usually no clear-cut dividing line between the types of cases, and admixtures are the rule rather than the exception. The incidence of cerebral palsy is somewhere between 2 and 3 per 1000 of population (Rutter et al., 1970). Approximately 50 percent are spastic, 25 percent athetoid, 13 percent rigid, and the remainder divided among the various other types.

Some investigators question the usefulness of classifying patients into these various categories as they believe them to be artificial categories based on unphysiological tenets. They suggest more careful study of the physiological basis for motor reactions in both normal and abnormal children.

Twitchell (1965) presents the view that there is no clear-cut dividing line between normal and abnormal behavior and that motor development is no exception. Many of the abnormal motor reactions of the cerebral palsied are identical in nature to similar reactions of the normal infant. There also are children whose motor development proceeds through the same sequence as does the normal infant's but is stretched out over a five- to six-year period. At 3, these children reveal features of spasticity, increased reflexes, inability to stand without assistance, a "scissor gait," and overextension of ankles when assisted in walking. Several years later a number of these children can walk and function reasonably well. Although clumsy, they show no spasticity or reflex changes, and they walk without the overaddation characteristic of the scissor gait of the palsied. Twitchell (1965) considers the patient with cerebral palsy to represent the most advanced form of physiological defect in sensory-motor maturation.

Another system of classification is based on the clinical criterion of the topography (location) of the handicap. *Paraplegia* is the classification used when only the legs are involved, *hemiplegia* when half the body is involved, and *quadriplegia* when all four extremities are involved. Less prevalent are *monoplegia* when only one limb is involved, and *triplegia* when three extremities are involved (Cruickshank, 1966). Approximately one-third of cerebral palsied children are hemiplegic and about one-half are quadriplegic in varying degrees of severity (Rutter et al., 1970).

What causes the injury that results in cerebral palsy?

Although we know that brain injury causes the various motor disorders subsumed under the label cerebral palsy, we have yet to discover exactly what causes brain injury. There is considerable disagreement concerning the relative importance of prenatal and perinatal factors. In a great many cases the relative importance of these factors cannot be determined. Current evidence indicates that many cases originate at or near the time of birth, anoxia or asphyxia (diminished oxygen in the blood) being a chief cause. Allen (1964, p. 211) states: "Although considered a likely cause of congenital spastic paralyses for over a century, the causative role of asphyxia has been exceedingly difficult to prove, particularly due to the equivocal nature of obstetric histories and the usual lack of physiological data."

ASSOCIATED IMPAIRMENTS

Art's prognosis was considered favorable because of the apparent absence cf associated disorders. He was fortunate to have a normal IQ, since only 30 percent of all cerebral palsied children have an intelligence quotient above 90. Approximately 50 percent have IQs below 50 (Cardwell, 1965; Cruickshank, 1966; Rutter et al., 1970). Monoplegic and hemiplegic children are more likely to have IQs closer to the normal range (Rutter et al., 1970), because there is less diffuse damage in these conditions than in triplegia or quadriplegia.

Intelligence is affected not only by damage to areas of the brain governing higher thought processes but also by damage to visual-perceptual sensory and language centers, basic processes through which the child learns about his environment. About 50 percent of spastics have some type of visual problem, usually some form of strabismus (squinting). Figure-ground discrimination, stereognosis (inability to recognize objects by touch), and two-point discrimination can be impaired, particularly in spastics. Defective speech is common. Dysarthria, an articulation defect caused by poor motor control, delayed speech, voice disorders, stuttering, and various forms of aphasia can be present.

Language problems are more common in those with severe intellectual retardation than in those with normal or borderline intelligence. Very few cerebral palsied children who attend school are severely retarded in language, although approximately one-half have articulation defects (Rutter et al., 1970). In contrast, 80 percent of those not in school have little or no useful language.

There are several possible causes of the speech and language problems of cerebral palsied children. Intellectual retardation is probably the most important factor. Hearing difficulties are a factor in some children, but deafness is rarely the main cause, except in children with athetosis. Aphasia resulting from cortical damage is sometimes important (Cohen & Hannigan, 1954). (Children whose primary problem is aphasia will be discussed in a later section of this chapter.) Partial paralysis or incoordination of the articulatory organs can cause dysarthria. Nevertheless, many of the articulation problems displayed by the palsied child are developmental ones since they resemble those of normal children just learning to speak.

Strabismus, refraction errors, and other visual defects are present in the majority of cerebral palsied children studied (Breakey, Wilson, & Wilson, 1974). Forty percent of those excluded from school and 26 percent of those attending school have strabismus (Rutter, Graham, & Yule, 1970). Hemianopia (blindness for half the field of vision in one or both eyes) occurs in 10 to 25 percent of hemiplegics, but good compensation is usual so that this disorder is not a major handicap (Ingram, 1964). Degenerative myopia (nearsightedness) is common, particularly in those born prematurely. Spastic children show qualitatively and quantitatively more defects than athetoid children (Breakey, Wilson, & Wilson, 1974).

Epileptic fits occur in 30 to 40 percent (Rutter et al., 1970). The rate of epilepsy is about two and one-half times higher in those excluded from school. Frequent medical complications, dental abnormalities, specific learning disorders, emotional problems, and family strife are common.

About 6 percent of cerebral palsied children are deaf (Nakano, 1966), with larger percentages having milder hearing impairments, the rate varying with the type of cerebral palsy (Gerber, 1966; Shore, 1960). Approximately 23 percent of athetoids have hearing losses, particularly in high frequencies (Ingram, 1964).

Vernon's (1970) study of deaf cerebral palsied children revealed the extent of associated impairments in such children. Table 2.1 summarizes Vernon's findings. The presence of aphasia in over half of the sample indicates that, while deafness and somewhat lower IQ could account for problems in expressive and receptive language, many of the problems are due to associated neuropathology.

Assessment of intellectual deficits

When Art grows older, his parents will undoubtedly have his intellectual functioning evaluated by a psychologist. As discussed previously, IQ scores obtained in infancy correlate poorly with those obtained at later dates. Most cerebral palsied youngsters are not evaluated in early infancy because the tests available are primarily tests of motor development, and motor impairment is the child's most apparent deficit. Most parents begin to wonder about their child's intelligence when they notice other abnormalities, such as slow speech development.

Although evaluating Art may not be difficult, other children present

Table 2.1 **MULTIPLE DISABILITIES OF 47 DEAF CEREBRAL PALSIED CHILDREN**

Etiology	Vision		Seizures		Orthopedic		Heart		Aphasia		Mental retardation		Emotionally disturbed	
	No.	%	No.	%	No.	%	No.	%	No.	%	No.	%	No.	%
Rh factor	6	33.3	4	22.2			1	5.5	7	43.7	1	4.7	4	23.5
Prematurity	12				1	8.3			10	71.4			5	31.2
Meningitis	3	50.0			4	80.0			2	33.3	5	50.0	5	16.6
Rubella	2	66.6			2	8.3			2	66.6			1	50.0
Unknown	4								3	75.0	3	30.0	2	25.0
Total	27	57.4	4	8.5	7	16.0	1	2.1	24	54.5	9	22.2	17	36.0

From M. Vernon. Clinical phenomenon of cerebral palsy and deafness. *Exceptional Children*, 1970, **36**, 743–751. Reprinted with permission of The Council for Exceptional Children.

complications. How can a child who cannot speak intelligibly define a word or repeat a number? How can a child with visual or hearing difficulties respond to objects, pictures, or sounds presented to him? How can the examiner obtain responses if the child cannot control the movements of his arms to point to parts of objects or manipulate them adequately? Although a standardized test can be used, Taylor (1959) feels that no one test is sufficient for adequate evaluation. Consequently, she has selected items from tests which measure a variety of abilities. Each test item has been given to children at different ages, and the percentage of children passing the item at each age has been determined.

Taylor describes the evaluation of Bobby, a boy with severe athetosis and dysarthria. Bobby was unable to use his hands and was barely able to talk. His development had been extremely slow. At 6 months of age, his fists were tightly clenched and he made no effort to grasp objects. He was unable to hold up his head at 15 months and did not sit, but lay on his back, his head turned to one side. He was unable to roll over and rarely used his hands. He did not chew food, often did not swallow, and frequently regurgitated food. He was fed five or six times a day because light feedings were less fatiguing. When wet or soiled, he would cry until his mother picked him up.

When brought for evaluation at 15 months, Bobby lay passively in the examining crib. His face was expressionless, but his eyes followed his mother as long as she stayed in sight. When she went beyond his field of vision, he looked perturbed and agitated his arms and head in jerky, uncoordinated movements.

A red ring was moved in front of him across his line of vision. He was unable to approach the ring with either hand, but followed it with his eyes without turning his head. The ring was then moved toward a screen, made to disappear behind it, and then to come out the other end. After two repetitions of this action, Bobby ignored the spot where the ring disappeared and quickly shifted his gaze to the other side where he had learned to expect the ring to reappear. Infants under 12 months typically fixate on the spot where the ring disappears and eventually lose interest.

When a set of jingle bells was placed under a cloth, Bobby stared at the cloth and expressed pleasure each time the bells were uncovered, covered, and recovered again. The bells were then moved to another spot and covered with another cloth. Bobby quickly switched his gaze to the second spot. Infants under 12 months typically expect the bells to appear in the first position.

Given a picture book and asked "Where is the doggy?" Bobby fixated on the correct page. When the page was turned and he was asked the same question, he looked about the page without finding a point to fixate, seemed frustrated, and smiled when the page was turned back for him. Several other measures of visual search and motor manipulation were administered.

The evaluation revealed that Bobby was more alert and observant than he appeared at first glance. His comprehension of objects and motions was nearly adequate for his age and he seemed to comprehend some language. The evaluation revealed that most of his retardation was due to motor impairment rather than intellectual inability. However, lack of effective manipulation, locomotion, lip movements, and sound locomotion would limit the scope of his activity and consequently his interests, and his inability to develop independence and initiative would restrict him in learning to deal effectively with his environment.

Bobby was evaluated again at 4 years of age, at 7, and at 12. On each occasion test results revealed better intellect than expected. At 4, his comprehension and reasoning abilities were within normal limits. At 7, though competent and able to learn, he demonstrated enough variations from normal mental functioning to warrant a cautiously planned educational program. (His language contained remnants of primitive syncretic qualities usually abandoned by children of his mental level.) In early examinations Bobby needed defending from those who thought him defective; later, he needed protection from overly optimistic persons who dismissed his deviations from normal as resulting from motor deficiencies and lack of experience (parental attitudes and expectations are discussed in Chapter 3).

Taylor's (1959) detailed descriptions of evaluations and the signs that led to her conclusions in each case are unparalled in the literature. Not only does Taylor present extremely useful techniques of evaluation, but she also helps the reader to understand parental attitudes and expectations based upon their own appraisal of their child's intelligence. Frequently, parents magnify their child's assets to try to compensate for perceived weaknesses. Frequently, they forget to allow for fatigue in their pressures for better achievement. The harder the children try, the more praise and encouragement they may receive from parents, teachers, and relatives. Consequently, they are under constant pressure to achieve goals which are beyond them. Unable to judge for themselves how much they can achieve, they accept assignments more conscientiously than most normal children, thriving on the approval they get for effort, not for results. The psychologist's role in these situations is to clarify actual strengths and weaknesses in an effort to modify such pressure.

Reliability of intellectual evaluations Since evaluation of the severely impaired cerebral palsied child relies more on informal procedures, to what extent are the psychologist's judgments valid? We saw in Bobby's case that the examiner's predictions were accurate. The judgment at 15 months that his intellect was within the normal range was supported by later evaluations. Was this a chance occurrence or can such predictions be made with a high degree of confidence? Since we know that IQ scores of normal infants correlate poorly with those obtained later, we would expect an even poorer correlation based on informal procedures. Before answering this question, however, the more basic question of whether the test scores are reliable needs to be answered.

Whether the psychologist uses a test score alone or whether he combines it with other sources of information, he is involved in a process of measurement; he is assigning individuals to a place on a scale of scores or to a place on a subjective scale which he formulates as a clinical judgment. How consistent is he when evaluating children with motor and language disabilities? Would he assign the same score or make the same judgment if he evaluated the same child on two occasions? Would two psychologists arrive at the same opinion if they evaluated a child independently? Successful prediction cannot be expected if the measures on which the predictions are based do not consistently discriminate between individuals who differ in ability.

When severely handicapped youngsters are assessed, there are two questions that are asked about reliability. First, are the test instruments reliable, that is, are consistent scores obtained by the same individuals on two occasions or with equivalent tests? Second, how reliable is the psychologist's judgment concerning a child's problem solving ability (Doris, 1963)? If the psychologist relies entirely on the test score to form a judgment, then the second question need not be asked. Dependence on the actual score, however, is rare. More typical is the combination of test score with observations of how the score was achieved. Attention span, attitudes toward testing, distractibility, perseverance, motivation, and emotionality are all considered. The tester then considers material from the patient's history, parental interviews, school reports, and pediatric examinations. His final clinical judgment about the child results from a combination of all this diverse information.

When used by an experienced tester, the Binet has been found to be a reliable instrument for use with cerebral palsied children, even where the tester varies from standard administration and scoring to make allowances for the child's handicaps (Doris, 1963; Sattler & Anderson, 1974). Some individuals do show marked changes in IQ scores from test to retest, but the number doing so is only a small proportion of the total tested. If the time interval involved between test and retest is a long one, there is the possibility that marked changes in scores reflect actual changes in the child's functioning rather than an error of the test instrument or its user. When considerably long intervals occur between test and retest, such a study should be considered one of IQ constancy rather than reliability of measurement. Let's look at the results of such studies. Knowing how stable an IQ score is allows one to place more confidence in predictions about a child's performance (validity).

Taylor (1959) retested 214 cerebral palsied cases from 3 to 12 years following their initial evaluations, the majority of which took place before the child was 6 years old. In 57 cases the child had been judged to have average or above-average intelligence. In all 57 cases the second testing verified the earlier judgment. Consequently Taylor had correctly assured the parents before the child was of school age that he was of normal intelligence. In 9 cases Taylor had correctly predicted superior intelligence. In 107 cases she had believed the child was mentally retarded. The second testing verified this opinion in 91 (85 percent) of the cases. Fifty cases were initially considered to be of borderline intelligence (between retarded and normal, or IQs between 70 and 90). Of these 50, 6 had better intellect on the second examination, 18 were more defective, and 26 remained in the borderline category.

Looking at the data from a slightly different viewpoint reveals that, of the 214 cases, 157 (73 percent) fell into the same category on both examinations, 33 (15 percent) were in a lower category on reevaluation, and 24 (11 percent) fell into a higher category. Examination of the reasons for disagreement between first and second categorization reveals several findings. In some cases physical deterioration accompanied mental decline and in others physical development accompanied mental improvement. These differences reflect changes in the child rather than errors of measurement. In many cases, however, errors in prediction occurred when the first examiner placed undue emphasis on language skill rather than on other signs of comprehension. The most flagrant disagreements were found in those children having pure extrapyramidal involvement (involuntary movements). Of 11 cases originally considered retarded (IQ below 70), but who turned out to be borderline (6) or average (5), 5 were subsequently found deaf or hard-of-hearing. The remainder had serious speech delays due to dysarthria. Speech delay was also responsible for errors in classification among other diagnostic groups. Errors in the opposite direction occurred because the examiner placed undue emphasis on early speech development. Early high ratings because of verbal ability masked errors of reasoning and judgment apparent on later reevaluation (Taylor, 1959).

Taylor's results are summarized clinical impressions rather than detailed presentations of predictions and outcomes. Perhaps psychologists should attempt to distinguish between the reliability or stability of ratings obtained from test instruments alone and those obtained from test scores combined with clinical judgments. Making this distinction could result in determining which of the factors involved in clinical judgment can result in a greater degree of reliability than the test score alone (Doris, 1963). Perhaps these factors can be isolated and standardized so that better test instruments themselves can be developed. As a result, there would be less dependency upon clinicians with unusual skill. Obvious from Taylor's book was the vast experience she brought to bear in the evaluation of each child. The average psychologist could not hope to duplicate this experience and would rely more on formal test procedures.

A study by Klapper and Birch (1967) provides better information about estimates of intelligence made solely from scores on standardized tests administered without making allowances for an individual's handicap (that is, with no variations from standard administration). The intelligence test scores received by a group of 51 cerebral palsied individuals on two occasions were studied to determine the stability of IQ score. The first test was administered prior to age 6 in all 51 cases, and an average interval of 14 years occurred between the two testings. Table 2.2 presents shifts from the initial IQ score to the follow-up IQ score. The greatest stability occurred in individuals with initial IQs below 50 and above 90. The least stable individual scores were obtained when the initial IQ was between 50 and 89, and most particularly in the range from 75 to 89. The changes that occurred in this group were largely in the direction of improved IQ. Seventeen individuals showed an IQ change of 15 points or more, with 14 showing a gain and 3 a decline. The total group tended to have a higher IQ in adulthood.

Two reasons could account for these changes. First, intellectual functions of cerebral palsied children may be transiently depressed as a consequence of early restriction of sensory and motor experiences. Second, the higher scores obtained in adulthood may result from accelerated development of verbal skills as a compensatory reaction to motor and perceptual-motor disturbances. Because adult IQ tests permit greater reflection of verbal skills than do tests in early childhood, the scores would tend to be higher (Klapper & Birch, 1967).

The validity of the IQ score   Klapper and Birch (1966, 1967) related IQ scores obtained in childhood to adjustment in adulthood of cerebral palsied subjects. Their results showed that the initial IQ as a predictor of educational achievement or occupational level is valid only in certain IQ ranges. In their study no child with an initial IQ under 50 went

Table 2.2   IQ-LEVEL SHIFTS FROM INITIAL TEST SCORE TO FOLLOW-UP TEST SCORE, N = 51[1]

Initial IQ score	Correlation with follow-up IQ score	Follow-up IQ score (percentage of individuals)			
		0–49	50–74	75–89	90+
0–49	—	100	—	—	—
50–74	.62†	6	47	18	29
75–89	.31 n.s.	—	7	40	53
90+	.54*	—	7	7	86

[1] Includes PPVT scores except those of the three patients who were initially untestable.
   * $p < .05$.
   † $p < .01$.
   From Z. S. Klapper & H. G. Birch. A fourteen-year follow-up study of cerebral palsy: intellectual change and stability. *American Journal of Orthopsychiatry*, 1967, **37**, 540–547. Copyright © 1967, the American Orthopsychiatric Association, Inc. Reproduced by permission.

beyond the sixth grade; every child with an IQ above 110 went at least as far as high school and some went further. No individual with an early IQ under 50 was economically independent or even contributing to his economic maintainence; of the 22 with IQs about 110, 13 were earning a small income. The value of IQ as a social predictive measure was relatively low in children with IQs between 50 and 89. In these children, neither school attendance nor specific levels of education or work achieved related to early IQ.

Studies of individuals without cerebral palsy also indicate that the predictive validity of IQ scores within the range of 50 to 89 is poor (see Chapters 3 and 11). We can say, therefore, that predictions from standardized IQ test scores are as valid for those with cerebral palsy as they are for nonpalsied children.

THE EMOTIONAL ADJUSTMENT OF THE CEREBRAL PALSIED CHILD

Perhaps the most important question of all is "How does the cerebral palsied child experience himself?" At present there is no clear answer to this question. Investigators have paid relatively little attention to how the child feels about his disorder. Several studies of self-concept, attitudes, and emotional and social adjustment of children with physical handicaps have included cerebral palsied subjects among their samples. They did not, however, examine these variables separately within cerebral palsied groups. Studies of emotional difficulties of intellectually retarded children appear in the literature, but they do not analyze separately the data on children with accompanying motor disorders.

While there is an absence of research to support many of the statements made regarding the feelings of cerebral palsied children, clinicians generally agree that the seriously impaired gradually realize they are living in social isolation. They see their siblings performing in ways that they cannot. Each activity in which they cannot participate drives them further into social isolation. Some eventually accept their isolation, giving up hope of normal social contact. But others become determined not to accept it, striving to equal peers, and with great exertion strain their already weakened stamina. Eventually, they may gain social acceptance, but they are never certain whether the acceptance is genuine or the result of charitable motives of tolerance and sympathy. They may come to distrust friends and even family. Development under these conditions must have an effect on personality characteristics. The exact nature, however, remains to be determined. Some Russian research (Kirichenko & Trifonov, 1969) indicates a high prevalence of neurotic disorders among cerebral palsied groups, but the research failed to employ proper control groups for comparison.

The Graham, Chir, and Rutter (1968) survey revealed that children with organic brain dysfunction display five times more psychiatric disorder than found in the general population and three times more than found in children with chronic physical handicaps not involving the nervous system. Because of the unfavorable comparison of the organic group with those having chronic physical handicaps, the authors concluded that psychiatric disturbances are the general effects of organic damage rather than a reaction to disability. However, since only 30 percent ($n = 35$) of Graham's sample were cerebral palsied, we can't say for certain that these results can be generalized to cerebral palsied groups.

Several studies have appeared that seem to support the notions of Bender (1934) and Bender and Silver (1948) that brain-injured children suffer a disturbance in body image. They believe that the attention focused upon particular body parts by the disease itself and by the attention of others at early stages of development results in attributing increased psychological value to those parts and thus produces a disturbed body image.

Machover (1949) studied the projection into figure drawings of unconscious determinants related to body image. Klapper and Weiner (1950) and Machover (1949) present findings that individuals project important features of their reaction to their disability into their drawings of a person. These projections usually take the form of illustrations of the specific bodily impairments which correspond to their own disability, for example, relatively useless or indefinite limbs, hidden hands, etc. In other cases the drawings are primitive or bizarre, drawings thought to reflect a disordered body image.

Abercrombie and Tyson (1966) question whether the drawing of a man really allows for the perception of body image, pointing out that some cerebral palsied children have difficulties drawing other things also. Consequently, their failure to draw a person may be a reflection of their general weakness in drawing rather than weakness in body image. Figure 2.4 presents the drawings of six children which could be interpreted as showing signs of physical impairments. Actually these drawings were made by normal children.

Silverstein and Robinson (1956) found no significant differences between normal and physically handicapped children in signs of impairment on human figure drawings. The mental ages of cerebral palsied children, as estimated by the Goodenough Draw-a-Man Test, are similar to those estimated from the Bender Visual Motor Gestalt Test (Abercrombie & Tyson, 1966). These findings suggest that many of the drawings of "impairment" made by cerebral palsied children may be similar to drawings of normal children of similar mental age. "It is as meaningful, and no more meaningful, to say these children have a body image disorder as it is to say that they have a diamond image disorder" (Abercrombie & Tyson, 1966, p. 12).

Figure 2.4 *Drawings of a man by normal 6-year old schoolchildren. The drawings might be thought to show signs of physical impairment if they had been drawn by handicapped children. (From M. J. L. Abercrombie & M. C. Tyson. Body image and Draw-a-Man test in cerebral palsy.* Mental Medicine and Child Neurology, *1966,* **8,** *9-15. Redrawn by permission.)*

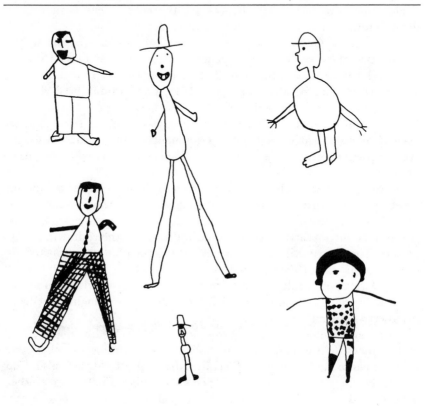

This author has observed normal preschool children whose drawings of human figures were distorted but who could construct well-proportioned figures from clay. Perhaps brain-injured children might perform similarly.

THE PALSIED CHILD'S FAMILY

Parental reactions to the atypical child

The birth of an atypical child is considered a crisis situation for a family. Parents can react to the birth of such a child with a variety of conflicting feelings and thoughts. The almost universal parental reaction is one of shock, followed by grief and disappointment. Frequently, guilt and anger accompany great anxiety, bewilderment, and confusion. Many reactions are responses not only to reality problems but to real or imagined feelings, thoughts, or actions. If the parents did not really want the pregnancy, they may feel they were punished for this feeling. Some may believe their own sinful thoughts were somehow visited upon the child. Mothers who attempt abortion and then give birth to an abnormal child display strong guilt reactions. Mothers with poor self-concepts may feel they have given birth to a "bad" part of themselves for all to see (Kohut, 1966).

The shock, the sorrow, and the related feelings of guilt or resentment severely test a family's capacity to maintain emotional balance. These feelings are not only present at the time of crisis but also emerge as the child develops and faces crises himself. Various professionals have described parental reactions as evolving through three stages. The initial period is one of emotional disorganization; such disorganization can be so severe as to disrupt normal ways of coping with stress. During the second stage reintegration takes place, usually by the adoption of defense mechanisms, such as denial of the reality of their predicament. In the third stage, mature adaptation, the handicap is accepted and constructive attitudes are adopted. Some parents achieve the third stage spontaneously, others need help to do so, and some never reach this stage. One measure of the family's health is its capacity to achieve each stage (Kohut, 1966).

What is a natural response in the second stage of adaptation may develop into a neurotic reaction, if the family is unable to progress to the third stage. For example, denial is a natural defense mechanism, the parents' way to assuage overwhelming feelings of chronic sorrow. However, when it extends beyond a reasonable period, it becomes a neurotic response, with negative consequences for the child, because such parents usually place undue pressure on the child to achieve beyond his capabilities.

Kohut (1966, p. 161) describes several families whose behavior is representative of each of the three stages of adaptation. The family described below serves as an example of a family threatened with disintegration (Stage 1) following the birth of their second child who was brain-injured:

Mr. B. was an anxious immature man with good intellectual endowment. Mrs. B. was a Viennese refugee who had spent time in a concentration camp. She had a realistic appreciation of her husband's strengths and limitations and accepted her marriage for the security it offered her after her years of suffering and deprivation. Both Mr. and Mrs. B. had an inordinate concern about financial security and lived frugally to accumulate savings.

Mrs. B. was less attracted to parenthood than her husband and was satisfied with the birth of her first child who was a normal, healthy little boy. To Mr. B., on the other hand, having children strengthened his weak male identification. Horrified at fathering a defective child, he needed to project all of his feelings onto his wife, refused to permit her to see the child, and kept restating his fears that she would become mentally ill if she were in any way involved in planning for the child.

Several studies have related family variables to the child's emotional adjustment. Parents have been classified into three groups: (1) parents who overstimulate and put great pressure to achieve on the child, creating in the child a sense of rejection if he fails to achieve up to their expectations; (2) parents who grossly overprotect their child, leaving him little opportunity for independent achievement; (3) parents who come to terms with their child's handicap and who accept him realistically. Using Piaget-type tests and object-sort tasks, Williams (1960) found that differences in conceptual reasoning among cerebral palsied children roughly matched on IQ were related to parental attitudes. Children whose parents fell into group 3 displayed conceptual reasoning that was closer to normal than did children in the other two groups. Children whose parents fell into group 1 were more impaired conceptually than children in the other groups.

A parent's positive regard for a child is an essential element in the child's development of a concept of himself as a worthwhile person. Without love and acceptance in the early stages of infancy, the child is grossly impaired, even though he may be stimulated by those around him, as is the case with parents in group 1. Intense anxiety, resentment, and guilt are experienced by most parents of cerebral palsied children. Coming to grips with these feelings occurs at a time in the child's development when the need for secure and accepting parents is crucial. Severe depression in the mother during a child's first year of life correlates highly with the child's emotional maladjustment in later childhood (Williams, 1960). The crippled child is not just a neurological case; he is the object of long expectations, dreams, and fantasies. If the mother feels her child will never be normal, she may become deeply depressed. To cope with these feelings, families need the continued support and assistance of professional personnel.

Supportive roles of professional personnel

When the parents of a handicapped child first meet the clinician, they are likely to be in a confused and disoriented state. Something terrible has happened to them; their child is not normal. Some frightening decision may have to be made, such as sending him away. They endow the clinician with some of the properties of a parental figure who is wiser and more powerful than they. They try to get not only medical help, but also information that will help them deal with their mental distress, to rebuild their world. When they ask "What caused it?" they want answers not in etiological terms, but in terms related to their often unasked questions, "Was it my fault?" or "Was it her fault?" or "Will it happen next time?" They try to make some sense out of the misfortune that has befallen them. But it has to be sense to them in terms of their feelings and that is not necessarily medical sense. Consequently, they find it difficult to bring up problems that they recognize are not medical problems. They do not expect their child's doctor to help them handle their feelings (Abercrombie, 1960b).

Not too much information is given to parents after their child's first evaluation. Information is usually better accepted by parents if given a little at a time. Initial interviews with parents have a special importance. Once told that their baby is somehow defective, the child turns into a question mark and is seen only in terms of the handicap. Until the parents have been given some kind of answer, the baby remains this "awful thing" you don't talk to or play with, but just look at in anxious despair (Mac Keith, 1960).

The early interviews are particularly crucial with families whose children are severely impaired. Mothers who "shop" for a better prognosis may be those who at the first interview were bluntly told about their child's sad future. If clinicians spent three instead of one interview to convey in stages that a child is defective or handicapped, the mother might accept the condition more readily and listen to useful advice (Mac Keith, 1960). Mothers want to know that their child has a second chance. Clinicians should emphasize that, although treatment will begin immediately, the diagnosis may change at a later time. It is important to stress the idea of joint work with parents; "We know something about many children, you know all about this child, and we shall work together."

Interviews are spaced not only to enable the parents to ask more questions, but also to give clinic staff the opportunity to find out more about the parent's anxieties. Mothers in particular feel responsible for the child's handicap and need assistance in expressing and working through guilt and shame. Fathers also can feel guilty, particularly if they have experienced an illness they feel might have influenced their physiological functioning. Tizard (discussion in Gibbs, 1960) surveyed 250 parents regarding their attitudes about having more children. About 50 percent were worried, but only 5 percent had spoken to their doctors about this concern. Frequently, successive interviews bring out anxieties which parents may be unable to reveal without encouragement.

The nurse is often a more important person than the doctor when the handicap is revealed at birth. Since she usually has more time to spend with parents, her reaction to a disabled child can foster or hinder the parent's acceptance of the youngster. Perhaps the most a physician can do is to provide the parents with information about what is best for their impaired child and how it can be obtained. He can reassure parents about their role in the cause of the disorder and can be readily accessible to help them feel they are not traveling a lonely road (Holt, 1960).

As the child matures, the psychologist's role becomes more important.

When the child becomes old enough for psychological appraisal, parental anxieties loom large again. "He is quite normal, isn't he?" or "You're not saying he's retarded, are you?" are frequent questions. If the child cannot speak, the parent may say, "He understands everything you say." A typical statement is "He has an excellent memory." If the parents witness the examination, as they do in the young child, and the child does poorly, the questions turn against the test, "We have not taught him to do that yet" and "You people don't know him like we do. You should see him at home."

The psychologist needs to work out a schedule of spaced assessments, not necessarily for better evaluation of the child, but to help parents gradually accept their child's limitations. The psychologist can suggest that between visits the parents teach their child certain conceptual tasks. Frequently the parents discover for themselves that the child is not as bright as they thought. Such a change in attitude may make it easier to show them the child's limitations. The psychologist should reassure parents that a permanent label will not be placed on their child and that the child will be given every chance to reveal his true potential. Many parents want basic information about their child's learning ability. They also need to come back to discuss or refute the psychologist's results. Joint planning for observing various strengths and weaknesses helps the parents to accept the child's limitations and to assist him to develop his strengths. When parent questions are directed at masking or denying the handicap, the outlook is grim, no matter what the measured intelligence (Gibbs, 1960).

EDUCATION AND TRAINING

Habilitation of the child with cerebral palsy depends largely upon the severity of the disorder. If the child's disability is primarily motor, treatment is confined to physical therapy and supportive guidance. Many methods of physical therapy have been proposed. As we mentioned previously, the strongest supporters of each method of therapy are the method's originators, their students, and those parents who feel their child has been helped by the method. Nevertheless, scant evidence is available to demonstrate the superiority of one method over another nor have current treatments been adequately tested through carefully controlled studies (McDonald & Chance, 1964).

The child with multiple handicaps requires more services. Some communities are fortunate to have a multidisciplinary child development center where physical, occupational, and speech therapists work in cooperation with teachers, psychologists, social workers, and medical specialists. In such a setting a program can be tailored to meet the exact needs of each child. The most important member of the team is the child himself, with each team member coordinating his activities to help the child reveal his abilities and minimize his disabilities.

Education of the child with motor abnormalities is made more difficult when other associated disorders are present. As we have seen, a large percentage of palsied children have one or more additional disabilities. In addition to associated difficulties that may result from diffuse brain damage, there are the nonfocal effects of the lesions. Remember from our general discussion of brain lesions that a local lesion affects those functional systems that include the damaged link in their composition. We also stated that brain injury can have different consequences at different ages. Because complex motor activities develop from a basis of precisely differentiated motor functions, a deficit in simple motor behavior significantly impairs the acquisition of more complex motor behaviors.

Not only does development proceed from the simple to the complex, but once complex acts are acquired they, in turn, modify the work of the elementary behavioral processes and change the form of their organization. The organizing influence of the higher forms of behavioral processes on their elementary forms has been well studied by Soviet psychologists (Leont'ev, 1959; Luria, 1958; Vygotsky, 1960). For example, after practice in externally aided memorizing, the structure of unaided memory is modified and converted into a complex, internally organized logical process. The young child memorizes material by repeating it aloud, while the older child memorizes the same material by resorting to logical methods of organizing the material. In other words, in early stages of development the intellect looks for help from memory processes, while in later stages memory itself is compensated by the organizing role of the intellect (Luria, 1966). The same may be said of motor behavior.

Motor behavior and perceptual development

Precise relationships between simple motor and higher order perceptual-motor behavior have not been clearly delineated, but the work of some investigators implies that impaired motor behavior will result in impaired perceptions.

Piaget (1953) describes the infant's visual inspection of grasping objects, his assimilation of visual schemata to manual schemata, and the resulting reciprocal assimilation of visual and motor schemata. He also regards successful assimilation as rewarding. Similarly, development of intersensory analytic, synthetic, and discriminatory ability proceeds from the initial independence of the various forms of perception, or ability to use a single sensory modality, to intermodal interaction dominated by vision (Birch & Lefford, 1963).

The child who cannot walk well, who cannot physically manipulate objects, and whose peripheral sensory system is not intact will be hindered in perceptual development (Isom, 1966). In Piaget's (1953) terms, if schemata are not extended, modified, and coordinated through exploratory behavior with physical objects, intelligence is adversely affected. For Piaget, the development of intelligence is attributed to experience resulting from a child's own activities. The learning pattern possible at one developmental stage determines the type of behavior pattern at the next stage. Adaptive behavior and the acquisition of new schemata result only when a child is capable of successful assimilation of and accommodation to stimuli. When the child cannot readily assimilate stimuli, he is less motivated to deal with that stimuli when it is presented again.

Other investigators state, almost unequivocally, that motor deficiency leads to perceptual deficiency. Kephart's (1964, 1970) perceptual-motor theory stresses the importance of movement and perceptual-motor skill as the foundation upon which all other learning is based, including the symbolic and conceptual activities of the classroom. A child must learn to change his posture in space readily and his balance and posture must be flexible to permit movement and awareness of positions of body parts. Consistent and efficient movement patterns permit perceptual data to be systematized and compared with motor systems. Through such activities, the perceptual and behavioral worlds come to coincide, providing an organized system of symbolic and conceptual material. Learning difficulties are considered the result of a breakdown in the perceptual development of the child.

Unfortunately, very little empirical evidence exists to support the notion that movement underlies all learning nor have relationships been established between movement, perception, and academic training (Mordock & DeHaven, 1969). The degree to which severe motor handicaps limit perceptual and conceptual development also is not clear (Webb, 1971). Some patients with severe athetosis have almost no motor control except for the eyes, and yet develop considerable intellectual capacity (Semans, 1970).

Support for these assumptions could be derived from studies demonstrating changes in learning proficiency resulting from perceptual-motor education. Adaptive physical education has improved balance, gross motor skill, and fine motor skill of brain-injured children, but has had no appreciable effect on other behavior or academic functioning (DeHaven, Bruce, & Bryan, 1971). Other investigations have showed that perceptual training increases perceptual ability, but there is no evidence to support even the assumption that perceptual motor training on specific tasks increases the ability to perform related perceptual motor skills.

If remediation has a beneficial effect on perceptual motor behavior, most likely that effect is possible because tasks may be performed by several different methods based on different combinations of active brain units. Remediation enables a system that has become dysfunctional because of a damaged link to become functional again through the aid of new, intact links (Luria, 1966). More knowledge about the functional links between the motor region of the brain and other analyzers is necessary before one can say that a particular remedial procedure will improve particular behaviors.

Let us examine how a link may or may not be involved in a particular function. For example, it has been demonstrated that athetoid children are inferior to spastic children in speech intelligibility and speech articulation (Rutherford, 1944; Hammill, Myers, & Irwin, 1968). Because this inferiority stems from an inability to control the speech musculature adequately, it is a motor inability. If motor efficiency is necessary for the development of other speech-related behaviors, then athetoids should show an inability in more advanced language skills. This is not the case. There are no differences between spastics and athetoids on measures of sound discrimination, vocabulary, and abstraction (Irwin & Hammill, 1964, 1965; Hammill et al., 1968), indicating that control of speech musculature is not a critical link in these other functions. These findings also suggest that when auditory material is presented to cerebral palsied children, there is no need to modify the material simply because the athetoid group has more difficulty making themselves understood.

Eye movements and perceptual development In addition to poor motor control over the extremities, cerebral palsied children frequently display disordered eye movements, both of version (abnormal eye position) and of vergence (a horizontal or vertical turning of one eye with reference to the other). These disorders may contribute to some of the perceptual dysfunctions that accompany cerebral palsy and which make learning difficult (Abercrombie, 1964; Bortner & Birch, 1962; Cruickshank, 1968; Simpson, 1967). Cerebral palsied children may be retarded in attaining full control of eye movements and this retardation may be related to delayed development of perceptual skills.

A study by Abercrombie, Davis, and Shackel (1963) is worth reporting in some detail not only because of the unusual techniques employed but also because the procedure can be adapted for use in the study of those reading disorders presented in Chapter 8. The study was inspired by Piaget and Inhelder (1956) and by Hebb (1949), who speculated that the infant's scanning movements of the eyes around the contours of different shapes assisted him to make discriminations between the shapes. The aim of the study was to establish that eye movements differed between non-brain-impaired and cerebral palsied children.

Each child was wired for recording. Four electrodes, attached with rubber suction cups, recorded both vertical and horizontal eye movements. Two tasks were employed, one involving saccadic (rapid visual fixations) and one involving pursuit movement. The eye movements involved in the saccadic task were considered analogous to those involved in reading. The child sat at a table on which the visual target was presented at eye level. The task required the child to move his eyes from one spot to another when the experimenter said "now the next one" at approximately 2-second intervals and moved her finger to the next spot. When the child got to the end of the row of spots, he went back to the beginning and repeated the process.

The records obtained from normal children revealed that the eyes fixated on each of the seven spots with a fairly steady position in the vertical plane. In contrast, the palsied child's movements were characterized by unsteady fixation and irregular movement from one dot to the next.

In the pursuit task the child was to follow an electric train which moved out of a tunnel in a straight line and into another tunnel. The train traveled both backward and forward. A good performance on this task showed smooth movements from left to right and steady fixation on the tunnel. A poor performance showed erratic following of the train and unsteady fixation on the tunnel, with many movements away from the tunnel, considerable time spent off it, and many vertical movements.

Both of these tasks were extremely simple, requiring little thinking or interpretation. Nevertheless, the performance of the 15 cerebral palsied children whose records were scorable was approximately 50 percent worse than physically handicapped youngsters without brain disorder and normals (15 other palsied children had unscorable records because of eye squint, body movements, or distractibility). Performance tended to be related to chronological age, but was significantly related to mental age. The correlation with mental age is consistent with the views on the importance of eye movements in perceptual development (Hebb, 1949; Piaget & Inhelder, 1956). The more accurately a child can direct his eyes to a target and the longer he can maintain fixation when required, the less time irrelevant images occupy the retina and the quicker he learns to perceive. In contrast, a child with disorderly eye movements is slowed down in learning because of the greater proportion of irrelevant images occupying the retina and being relayed to the visual cortex.

Some educators have suggested that training eye movements may benefit those with disordered movements. Both Getman (1966) and Kephart (1970) describe methods they have developed for training eye movements. At present, however, there is scant evidence that training improves disordered movements or that such training improves other perceptual activities.

HOW DO THEY FARE?

In the sculptured monuments of Egypt there are figures of individuals who appear to have been cerebral palsied. In the Holy Scriptures there are references to individuals crippled since birth. Many early medical works make reference to the paralyses and deformities of crippled children. Early in the nineteenth century physicians began to suspect that some of the crippling conditions were caused by brain lesions (McDonald & Chance, 1964), but until the late 1950s and early 1960s relatively little information was available regarding the life course of these children (Crothers & Paine, 1959; Ingram, 1964; Taylor, 1959). Crothers and Paine related physical status and extent of orthopedic handicap in adult life to early diagnostic category. But this work, as well as that of Ingram and Taylor, provides only limited information on the predictive worth of diagnostic evaluation, primarily because the earlier psychological characteristics of the patients selected for follow-up were not systematically defined.

Both European (Dunsdon, 1952; Hansen, 1960; Ingram, Jameson, Errington, & Mitchell, 1964; Stephen, 1961) and American (Machek & Collins, 1961) studies of the vocational functioning of the cerebral palsied suggests that they have a difficult time integrating themselves into the job market. The difficulties occur in spite of organized attempts to improve their vocational and social adjustment. These findings agree with those of Crothers and Paine who found only 25 percent of adults with cerebral palsey to be suitable for nonsheltered employment.

Although clinical experience suggests that the degree of physical handicap and of intellectual retardation in childhood obviously affects outcome in later life, little information exists regarding the childhood characteristics of the adults studied.

In spite of Twitchell's (1965) belief that existing diagnostic categories are artificial, initial diagnosis had prognostic significance. Spastic groups tend to have higher IQs, achieve a higher level of schooling, and tend to function more independently both socially and economically than do athetoid, ataxic, and mixed groups. In fact, it is only in spastic groups that individuals can be found who have obtained an education beyond the high school level. Among athetoids, only 30 percent complete an elementary education (Klapper & Birch, 1967).

Achievement in school for those bright enough to attend is more a function of self-care than of intellectual ability. Of those with an initial diagnosis of mixed cerebral palsy, none is found to be independent in self-care. Of those with athetosis, approximately 50 percent are completely independent, but display abnormal gait or other stigmata. Poor self-care rather than low IQ is considered responsible for the poor educational attainment of many with athetosis and ataxia, since often their IQ scores are similar to those of spastics who achieve at higher levels.

Adequate self-care is also a prerequisite for functional social interaction. About 50 percent of those who become independent have no significant social involvement, with 20 percent being complete isolates. Less than 20 percent are actively involved with friends and social groups. Of these, very few have any major physical stigmata.

The majority of cerebral palsied studied to date have been from lower middle class families who probably could not afford the special costs required to enable their child to participate more fully in society. Findings with a more affluent sample may be different.

Follow-up data of those who are not mentally retarded can be summarized as follows: the palsied achieve a high level of self-care and ambulatory independence, but the stigmatic remnants of childhood cerebral palsy interferes with maximal social and economic achievement. Only those completely free from physical stigmata and awkwardness in gait or speech integrate socially into society. The remainder, despite progress in self-care and physical functioning, accompanied by substantial educational achievement, are socially isolated. Unfortunately, the progress they make in motor functioning is not accompanied by corresponding progress in social integration. "The typical individual at follow-up, therefore, was a young adult with a high school education, a menial job, financially dependent, unmarried, living at home with his family and minimally involved in community activities and interpersonal relationships" (Klapper & Birch, 1967, p. 654).

Aphasia: a language disorder

We have seen how lesions in areas of the cortex involved in motor behavior have both a specific (motor abnormalities) and general (associated disorders) effect. We do not always know, however, to what degree the associated disorders observed in a child are the nonfocal results of a focal lesion; some may be due to diffuse brain damage. While sophisticated neurological and psychoneurological procedures can sometimes make this distinction, most of the time we are uncertain. In this section we discuss children whose brain damage affects the ability to use or comprehend language symbols. The deficit, called *aphasia*, is considered the result of a defect in the central nervous system rather than the result of hearing loss, muscular paralysis, mental retardation, or severe emotional disturbance (Agranowitz, 1964; Kleffner, 1959; Weisenburg & McBride, 1964). Children with such a disorder are labeled aphasic.

The aphasic child usually manifests perceptual dysfunction in one or more sensory modalities, but both his auditory and intellectual inefficiency are worse than would be predicted from his scores on quantitative tests. Linguistically, the aphasic child demonstrates severe retardation for both the reception (comprehension) and production of language, although he is generally able to understand more than he is able to verbalize. What language the child does achieve is usually characterized by an absence of conventional grammar, a smaller vocabulary size, and shorter sentence length. As he matures, he is not likely to reveal the expected increments in language and the ordered pattern that characterize the language achievement of normal youngsters (Eisenson, 1968).

Children with these characteristics give the impression of being severely hard-of-hearing or deaf. In fact, many do have mild or moderate hearing loss. Nevertheless, the hearing disability tends to vary with conditions not directly related to the intensity or frequency range of the auditory events to which the child is exposed. While they may have difficulty in the physical reception of sound (Chapter 5), the greater handicap is the functional and practical difficulty in dealing with the sounds, the streams of utterance, that are received (Eisenson, 1968).

TYPES OF APHASIA

Expressive and receptive aphasia

Two main types of aphasia are reported among children, *expressive*, or *motor*, aphasia and *receptive*, or *sensory*, aphasia. Expressive aphasia is characterized by: (1) lack of expressive speech and language; (2) adequate understanding of speech and language; (3) limited one- or two-syllable patterns of vocalization; (4) partial or complete inability to imitate tongue, lip, and jaw actions, sounds, or words; (5) absence of muscular paralysis; and (6) adequate intelligence for speech. The expressive aphasic child can understand speech, but cannot reproduce sound patterns or sequences. Whenever the child attempts verbal communication, a limited pattern of one or two syllables is all that is repeated (Wilson, 1965).

Receptive aphasia is characterized by: (1) lack of understanding of speech; (2) lack of expressive speech; (3) discrepancy between intelligence and understanding of language; and (4) discrepancy between hearing and understanding of language. McGinnis (1963) describes four types of receptive aphasics: silent, echolalic, jumbled speech sounds, and jumbled speech with some meaningful phrases.

Developmental aphasia

Osgood and Miron (1964) believe that symptoms of aphasia differ according to the age of onset. They distinguish between aphasia present at birth (developmental aphasia) and aphasia occurring after language had been acquired in the normal manner (childhood aphasia or adult aphasia). Although this may be a useful distinction, little data is available which compares age of onset of aphasia with behavioral symptoms. We do know from Halstead and Rennick's (1966) work that damage in infancy is often associated with severe impairment of culturally acquired skills, while acquired skills may be retained when damage is imposed upon the mature brain.

Acquired aphasia

Most children diagnosed as aphasic have failed to acquire normal speech and language use. A small number, however, acquire the ability to use language in an apparently normal fashion and subsequently lose it. Landau and Kleffner (1957) present six such cases. In each of the cases the children developed aphasia for periods ranging from a day to several months. The symptoms then persisted from two weeks to several years. In all the children a variety of convulsive manifestations were present. In three of the six cases various professionals at one time considered the child emotionally disturbed. Landau and Kleffner found that when language deficit was an island of behavioral deficit, the distinction of acquired aphasia from a primary psychotic disorder was obvious. Nevertheless, when the child developed a regressive reaction to the loss of communication, differential diagnosis was difficult.

DIFFICULTIES IN DIAGNOSIS

One drawback of employing labels to subsume a constellation of interrelated symptoms is that individuals not trained in language disorders tend to use the labels inappropriately. Such misuse of labels occurs not only with aphasia but also with other conditions discussed throughout this book. Any child who does not perform according to the teacher's or the psychologist's expectations is likely to have a label pinned on him. Many parents of children with hearing impairments report that their child's teacher said he was not only deaf but also aphasic (Rosenberg, 1964). When they asked what the teacher meant by "aphasic," the reply was "He isn't doing average work in the classroom, which means he's aphasic."

Chappell (1970) describes the patterns of language behavior in developmental aphasics and provides a diagnostic and prognostic key, but even with such aids diagnosing aphasia is no simple matter. To diagnose motor aphasia requires formal test results and informal observation of the child's basic skills. To evaluate the ability to control the tongue, the child is asked to imitate lip and tongue actions. When the child has cerebral palsy, the diagnosis is more difficult. In the classroom the motor aphasic demonstrates difficulties in writing. Reversals or distortions in copies of letters or in their recall are typical. After progress in language is made, there may be reversals in word order within sentences, both written and oral, as well as letter omissions. The child does not use meaningful speech sounds for appropriate communication, but uses repetitive speech patterns such as bu-bu-bu, du-du-du, or la-la-la with appropriate voice inflections (Wilson, 1965).

Classifying a child as sensory aphasic is a more difficult process. A hearing loss often is present, but not severe enough to account for the language deficit. Intellectually, the sensory aphasic may range from superior to retarded, but below dull-normal the classification aphasia is thought inappropriate because intellectual retardation is actually the predominant handicap. If retarded, the prognosis is less favorable.

As in cerebral palsy, most cases present multiple handicaps in varying degrees (Doehring, 1960; Goldstein, Landau, & Kleffner, 1960; Rosenstein, 1957; Weinstein, 1964; Wilson, Doehring, & Hirsh, 1960). Associated deficits include sensory and motor defects, inadequate body schema, inability to locate embedded geometrical figures (figure-ground confusion), poor performance in complex visual problem solving tasks, and poor spatial orientation, all deficits which are also associated with cerebral palsy.

Differentiation from delayed language development

All children with delayed language development are not aphasic. Language difficulties can result from a number of causes, and accurate diagnosis depends upon careful observation of the particular symptoms associated with aphasia, not just the presence of the general symptom of language retardation. For example, McGinnis (1963) describes a pattern of language retardation in 4- to 5-year-olds where they hear well but do not talk and are indifferent to encouragement. In contrast to aphasic children, they seldom vocalize or gesture; occasionally they may say a word, but appear startled by having said it. Sometimes they respond to suggestions, obey commands, or act on cue words in parental conversations. Their social behavior does not differ greatly from other children their age, except for more frequent temper tantrums and obstinate behavior. Descriptively, they might be referred to as "late bloomers" or as cases with a familial pattern of delayed speech because eventually they develop normal speech (Beagley & Wrenn, 1970).

Differentiation from mental retardation

Differentiating intellectual retardation from aphasia is not always a simple task. There are, however, some characteristic differences. The articulation growth pattern of 350 mentally retarded children has been compared with the developmental sequence of consonant sounds established in normal children (Blanchard, 1964). Only one child in ten achieved acceptable adult speech. Only five out of seven reached the 4-year level of articulatory competence, though chronological ages ranged from 8 to 15 and IQs from 27 to 68. Those with retardation resulting from postnatal head trauma and those without evidence of neurological disorder (familial retarded) had the most normal speech patterns and were more likely to reach adult standards of articulation. Those with mongolism, mechanical birth injury, and prenatal infection were the most retarded in verbal communication. Nearly 60 percent had articulation patterns considered peculiar to the mentally retarded, such as omission of word parts and bizarre substitutions for unknown consonants. These articulation patterns are important in distinguishing mental retardation from aphasia, for they are behaviors not normally seen in aphasics.

Differentiation from hearing disorders

Hearing is also difficult to evaluate in the young child. Very little is known about the hearing process or about its relation to neurological processes in general. Consequently, while discrete measurement of auditory functioning may be possible, there is no certainty about the relation of what is measured to the total hearing process.

Many things can interfere with the auditory signal sent to the central nervous system (see Chapter 5). If the signal is imperfect, the central nervous system experiences difficulty in handling the auditory information. More distorted signals are probably sent to the brain of hearing-impaired children than to that of normals. Therefore, faulty interpretation of auditory signals may be the result of a distorted signal, rather than of brain damage (Goldstein, 1965).

Goldstein makes references to cases where auditory capacity deteriorates over time. When hearing deteriorates, understanding of speech is well below what is anticipated from hearing loss alone. "The patient seems to have auditory sensitivity, but no understanding; he seems to have psychic stability, the intellectual capacity, a satisfactory home life and total environment, and yet he neither perceives nor learns from the sounds he hears" (Goldstein, 1965, p. 21). This description would certainly fit aphasia. Nevertheless, current evidence suggests that when hearing deteriorates the signal is not transmitted normally. Hence, even though the signal can be perceived adequately from the standpoint of loudness, it cannot be encoded. Peripheral rather than central nervous system factors, therefore, are responsible for the picture which resembles aphasia (Goldstein, 1965).

Differentiation from emotional problems

Emotional factors also complicate differential diagnosis. If a child fails to respond to maternal overtures because of a peripheral deficit, the parents may withdraw their interest and affection or place undue pressures on the child to perform. The child reacts to their behavior and a vicious cycle of interaction may result. Delayed speech, therefore, may result from this abnormal parent-child relationship rather than from brain dysfunction.

The case of Hank below serves to highlight the difficulties involved in diagnosing aphasia.

HANK

Hank's teacher in the day care center initially thought him to be extremely shy. Like many children from disadvantaged families, Hank said very little in school (see Chapter 9). He preferred to run about, handle objects, throw things, and make a general nuisance of himself.

Most of the children in the center, unlike those from advantaged families, were poor monitors of their own behavior, relying almost exclusively on the teacher to calm them down and to set limits for them. After about six months in the center, most were fairly well behaved and used verbal rather than motoric means of expression. Rather than pulling their teacher to the window and pointing, they could say to her "Mrs. Green, it's snowing!" "See the big black dog!" The shy ones usually were less withdrawn and the loud ones more subdued.

Hank had remained the same, shy and withdrawn and without speech. Mrs. Green didn't think him retarded because he seemed to comprehend events that went on around him, but she wasn't sure. Perhaps, he was deaf; yet sometimes he heard her. Mrs. Green remembered reading that certain children could hear within the normal range but responded to sound inconsistently, while others had hearing losses only within certain restricted ranges. Since federal funds were available for audiometric evaluation, she arranged for Hank to be seen at the speech and hearing clinic associated with the local hospital.

Hank's evaluation

Hank's audiometric evaluation revealed consistent responses to low but not to high tones. Unless the sound stimulus was very close to his ear, responses to environmental noises were inconsistent. Hank was given a hearing aid and the clinic agreed to provide speech therapy. The therapist reported that Hank understood no words or phrases and his response to sound with or without amplification was still inconsistent. He could respond to both soft and loud sounds but often ignored them. Although he made vocal sounds and occasionally imitated the therapist, no meaningful, spontaneous speech occurred during the sessions.

Hank's mother was extremely vague about his early history, but did recall that he had "bad blood." She could not elaborate on this statement but gave the name of the hospital where Hank was born so they could write for more information. The hospital report revealed that Hank developed a blood disease at birth due to Rh incompatibility. He had two exchange transfusions, one at 8 hours and another at 45 hours. His mother was told to watch him carefully for signs of jaundice (yellowing of the skin), but since he never returned to the hospital no further entries appeared on his record.

The clinic then requested a psychological evaluation. The evaluation revealed that performances on various nonverbal tasks were within the

4-year level, while perceptual-motor functioning was one year below normal. The total evaluation revealed borderline intellectual functioning, but suggested at least low normal potential.

The clinic staff held a conference devoted to discussing Hank's disabilities. Mrs. Green attended and reported on Hank's current behavior in the day care center. Her report read as follows:

Hank still has extreme difficulty monitoring his behavior. When given a crayon and pencil, he does not wait for instructions like the other children. Instead he begins scribbling and it's very hard to get him to stop. If you tell the children that something special will take place later in the day, Hank will be pleased and excited and will tug and pester you until the special event takes place. On the playground, he runs until he loses control of himself, laughing and giggling almost compulsively.

Considering this report along with the other information available, the clinic staff considered Hank to be an aphasic child who had more difficulty in expressing words than in understanding them.

Originally, Hank's hearing loss together with his deprived environment and absence of verbal stimulation at home were considered responsible for his language deficit. After a program of language stimulation failed to bring about noticeable improvement, the staff began to suspect a more severe deficiency. In school Hank was not progressing in other sensory modalities, failing to understand language symbols visually or motorically. If his deficiencies were simply the result of an auditory problem, he should have been able to handle language symbols when presented in other sensory modalities. Indications of strength in other areas ruled out intellectual retardation as a prime factor. The decision to proceed as if he were aphasic was actually arrived at by a process of elimination.

Hank's treatment

Classification and education Although we can identify criteria for different types of aphasia, children classified as aphasic demonstrate a great variation of language problems. Kleffner (1964, p. 10) now believes we should exclude reference to deficits in the child's nervous system: "In everyday clinical life the practical application of the term aphasia is not based upon observations of the nervous system." He prefers an operational rather than a neurological classification, applying the term aphasic to one who "presents a greater deficiency in speech and language than we would expect on the basis of our observations of his hearing, intelligence, social behavior, and (if he has had any) his schooling" (p. 11).

For Kleffner, the real question is not whether the language difficulty is due to hearing loss or aphasia, but whether the child shows the type of difficulty that prevents him from learning from ordinary methods. The aphasic's inability to learn language results from inability to retain and recall symbols and to transfer what is learned in one situation to another. Classifying a child as aphasic means only that he will be taught in a certain manner. Children classified as deaf, psychotic, or intellectually retarded would receive a different teaching approach (Wilson, 1966). The system believed to be most effective with children classified as aphasic is called the *association method* (McGinnis, 1963).

The association method of speech and language instruction   Hank was removed from the day care center and placed in a special class operated by the hospital. There were six other children in this class, all of whom were bused from various parts of the county in cooperation with the local public schools who helped support the program. For approximately eight weeks, Hank's daily schedule consisted of a set routine that emphasized early establishment of a given order for daily lessons and the ability to imitate the teacher's actions. During this introductory period, Hank made name tags and stick figures, which later he used to relate actions with words. Imitation of actions, board games, puzzles, art, guided play, and some formal speech training predominated during this period. Change in programming was made gradually, until eventually Hank's program included more language training.

The teaching method chosen to provide a basic foundation for Hank's speech and language was the association method developed by McGinnis (1963). The major principles of this method are summarized below:

1. A phonetic or elemental approach to learning words.
2. Emphasis on the precise articulatory position for each sound.
3. Careful association of each articulatory position and sound with the appropriate letter symbol(s) of cursive script.
4. Use of expression as the foundation or starting point in building language.
5. Systematic sensory-motor association.

The basic units used in building words are individual sounds. Hank was taught to produce each sound and to associate the sound with its written letter symbol. The sounds were taught one at a time and precise articulatory production was required. Before Hank could combine the individual sounds into a connected articulation of a complete word, he first learned to produce each individual sound in the word in the proper order until certain of their sequence. Initially, Hank's words were articulated in a stilted and abrupt manner. Teaching smooth articulation was delayed until Hank knew words well enough to attempt smooth articulation without losses in accuracy.

Cursive script, rather than manuscript or printing, was used because it emphasized the continuity and grouping of letters and because the transition from reading cursive print to reading printed letters was considered easier. Hank was not expected to understand any word he heard until he could pronounce the word himself. Production of words, therefore, preceded attempts to establish recognition of the meanings of words.

The association method is based upon systematic association of motor skills and sensory abilities. The seven steps used in teaching nouns best illustrates the method.

1. The child produces in sequence from the written form the sounds composing a noun.
2. He matches the picture of the object denoted by this word to the written form of the word.
3. He copies the word and articulates each sound as he writes the letter(s) for it.
4. He repeats the word aloud after watching the teacher say it and matches the object or picture to the written form of the word.
5. He says the name of the object from memory.
6. He writes the word for the object from memory, articulating each letter sound as he writes it.
7. He repeats the word spoken into his ear and matches the picture to the written form of the word. The child does not watch the teacher, as in step 4, and thereby receives only the auditory pattern (McGinnis, Kleffner, & Goldstein, 1956).

These specific procedures constitute only the initial phase of the program. Once the child has gained some skill in language use, he develops increasing ability to learn without formal instruction. The essence of the total approach is building simple speech acts and then combining these acts into more complex expression and understanding. This method takes about three years to complete and even then the children are still behind equal-age peers.

In order to profit from such instruction, the child must be fairly attentive. Typically, however, aphasic children have secondary emotional difficulties as a result of limitations imposed by the handicap or their parents' reactions to it. Initially, the aphasic child may be inaccessible to the teacher's efforts. The teacher who cannot relate adequately to the child and make him feel he is valued will be relatively unsuccessful. Many of the teaching techniques discussed in Chapter 12 are applicable to the aphasic child since his needs and his response to need-frustration differ only in degree from that of the normal child. Patience, tolerance, understanding, and interest pay off with these children as with any other. The aphasic, like any handicapped child, is first a child, and second a child with a specific disability. Significant people in the child's environment must provide a human basis for human language usage.

WHAT ARE THE APHASIC'S DEFICITS?

In this section we will review some of the speculations concerning the nature of the specific deficits associated with aphasia. The first hypothesis to be considered postulates that the child's storage system for speech signals is defective (Eisenson, 1968). If a child cannot store auditory-linguistic events, even for a brief time, he can appear deaf as well as mute. If he can store them briefly, he still will not be able to speak, but he may be able to imitate speech immediately following a word's presentation, although not after a delay. This hypothesis suggests that the characteristics of auditory events which constitute speech require different control and storage than do other auditory events (Lieberman, Cooper, Shankwelier, & Studdert-Kennedy, 1967).

The second hypothesis postulates impairment of discrimination and perception of phonemes in context (Eisenson, 1968). The child can usually discriminate between isolated letter sounds, but cannot make the discriminations when the sounds are incorporated into words. Sounds may be stored as discrete entities rather than generalized into phoneme categories.

The third hypothesis postulates difficulty in receiving and processing auditory signals at the rate at which such signals are normally processed. In essence, this hypothesis states that the aphasic child cannot listen as fast as normals. He cannot make rapid matchings between on-going auditory events and images of the events. A correlated disorder may be difficulty in determining the order in which events occur.

To test this hypothesis requires comparing normals and aphasics on the minimum time intervals necessary for awareness of succession of stimuli (is it one or two events?). Surveys of studies in this area indicate that successiveness may be perceived within a range of from 2–10 msec (Fay, 1966; Hirsh, 1967). A longer interval is required to decide the order of a sequence of stimuli, an interval of 20 msec to report correctly 75 percent of the time (Hirsh & Sherrick, 1961). When subjects have not been previously exposed to the stimuli, the interval is considerably longer (Broadbent & Ladefoged, 1959; Hirsh & Fraisse, 1964).

For normal adults approximately 50–60 msec are required for correct judgment of the order of two 10-msec sound pulses differing in frequency. Aphasic subjects, however, require as much as a full second interval between the two sound pulses before they can make a correct judgment (Edwards & Auger, 1965; Efron, 1963; Lowe & Campbell, 1965).

The ability to recognize the serial order of sound pulses or noises may not be the same as the ability to sequence speech sounds. Nevertheless, it has been firmly established that aphasics, as a group, display a marked defect in auditory sequencing. Clinical observations and psychoeducational test findings support this statement (Stark, 1967). Tests which measure sequencing differentiate aphasic children from those who are deaf or retarded and aid substantially in differential diagnosis.

The aphasic also has delayed reaction times to auditory signals (Brookshire, 1971). Of interest is that improved reaction times to an auditory word comprehension test has been related to recovery, a finding that suggests that initial reaction time intervals may be related to prognosis (Croskey & Adams, 1970).

How much of this data applies to motor or expressive aphasics? Unless there is clear evidence to suspect dysarthria or oral apraxia, expressive difficulties are considered by some to be simply another aspect of auditory or sensory aphasia (Eisenson, 1968). If sounds are not correctly, reliably, and consistently recorded, the child cannot adequately store units of language for retrieval and production. His expressive difficulties are simply the result of faulty reception of sound; what is "heard" incorrectly cannot be reproduced correctly. On the other hand, Weiner (1972) feels that production difficulties are more common among aphasic children. He notes their inadequacy in using oral structures in nonspeech activities and their difficulty in making repetitive tongue movements. Obviously, more research needs to be done before the two categories of aphasia can be considered to denote discrete behavioral differences.

Where does the damage occur?

While references to the central nervous system can be removed from definitions of aphasia, considerable data does exist regarding the behavioral effects of lesions in different parts of the brain.

If auditory aphasia is assumed to be a breakdown in the ability to analyze the flow of spoken utterance, then some general statements can be made about the location of brain damage. Luria (1966) reports that the functions involved in phonemic analysis are carried on by the secondary divisions of the auditory cortex of the left cerebral hemisphere. Numerous studies have demonstrated that patients with right hemisphere damage perform poorly in perceptual-motor tasks, while those with left hemisphere damage perform poorly on verbal tasks (Vega & Parsons, 1969). Both Reitan (1962) and Luria (1966) provide an extensive review of this literature. However, even though the left hemisphere is considered the "speech dominant" hemisphere, findings are not always consistent. Some patients whose left cerebral hemisphere was completely removed were reported to show little or no change in speech or hearing (Goldstein, 1965; Hodgson, 1967). Other research has demonstrated aphasia to result from damage to the right cerebral hemisphere (Goodglass & Quadfasel, 1954; Humphrey & Zangwill, 1952). In addition, clinicopathological studies of children with congenital aphasia (Benton, 1964; Landau, Goldstein, & Kleffner, 1960) sometimes reveal bilateral damage as well as severe degeneration in the speech centers. Nevertheless, the children acquired considerable useful language following special instruction. Language function, therefore, can be subserved by pathways other than the primary auditory center.

Because of the preceding studies, most investigators agree that anatomical speculations are not a legitimate basis for making decisions concerning the education and rehabilitation of aphasics (Davis, 1962; Goldstein, 1965; Kleffner, 1964). The congenitally aphasic child probably has bilateral or global damage. The fact that a child is labeled aphasic simply means that the language dysfunction manifests itself more strongly than other dysfunctions; language disorder is the primary symptom. Like cerebral palsy, where motor disorders are the primary symptom, many other deficiencies accompany aphasia. Consequently, the question of whether aphasia is the direct result of a cerebral insult or a secondary consequence of some other forms of impairment, awaits further research into its functional relationships.

HOW DO THEY FARE?

McGinnis, Kleffner, and Goldstein (1956) summarized the educational progress of 141 children initially diagnosed as aphasic by the staff of the Central Institute for the Deaf in St. Louis. Of these 141, 26 were referred to schools for the retarded after mental deficiency was found to be the principal impediment to learning speech and language; 115 were promoted to other schools. Seventy-one of those promoted were tested prior to discharge. The average grade equivalent was 3.6 and the average age 10.5 at testing. This data indicates approximately two and one-half years academic retardation for the average tested graduate. The authors note that these figures are an underestimation of the total group functioning because the 44 children who left without testing were, in general, those who had progressed rapidly and reevaluation was considered unnecessary.

Considering that the majority of the 141 children did not begin their training at Central Institute until they were past 6 years of age, and some not until 8 or 9, and that they initially had almost no language, the progress reported is substantial in spite of the two-year lag. Nevertheless, no subsequent reports have been published about this sample nor have any long-term follow-up reports of aphasic children appeared in the literature.

CONCLUDING REMARKS

Both Art and Hank had central nervous system impairment, but each had a different disorder. Art's was primarily motor, while Hank's was primarily verbal. The prognosis for Art was better than that for Hank because Art's disability would minimally affect his response to educational programs. Hank needed special educational techniques in order to learn, techniques which required his removal from the main stream of education and resulted in his isolation from normal peers.

The exact cause of each boy's disorder remains unknown. Even if the brain of each was actually damaged, as opposed to structurally malformed, the amount of damage does not always correlate with the amount of behavioral deficit. Art might actually have had more actual tissue damage than Hank, but in a less critical area of the brain. In both cases, however, the impairment was not substantial enough to affect adversely other perceptual, conceptual, and intellectual functions. Both were fortunate since most cerebral palsied and aphasic children have associated impairments. Many suffer more diffuse damage and are intellectually retarded. If so, they are better classified as retarded. The next chapter discusses children who fall into this classification.

References

Abercrombie, M. L. J. Can we improve the perceptual skills of the clinical examiner? In M. C. O. Bax, E. Clayton-Jones, & R. C. Mac Keith (Eds.), *Child neurology and cerebral palsy*. (Little Club Clinics No. 2) London: Spastics Society, Heinemann, 1960a.

Abercrombie, M. L. J. Comments of a participant observer. In M. C. O. Bax, E. Clayton-Jones, & R. C. Mac Keith (Eds.), *Child neurology and cerebral palsy*. (Little Club Clinics No. 2) London: Spastics Society, Heinemann, 1960b.

Abercrombie, M. L. J. *Perceptual and visuomotor disorders in cerebral palsy*. (Little Club Clinics No. 11) London: Spastics Society, Heinemann, 1964.

Abercrombie, M. L. J., Davis, J. R., & Shackel, B. Pilot study of version movements of eyes in cerebral palsied and other children. *Vision Research*, 1963, **3**, 135–153.

Abercrombie, M. L. J., & Tyson, M. C. Body image and Draw-a-Man test in cerebral palsy. *Developmental Medicine and Child Neurology*, 1966, **8**, 9–15.

Agranowitz, A. *Aphasia handbook*. Springfield, Ill.: C. C Thomas, 1964.

Allen, N. Developmental and degenerative diseases of the brain. In T. W. Farmer (Ed.), *Pediatric neurology*. New York: Medical Department of Harper & Row, 1964.

Beagley, H. A., & Wrenn, M. Clinical follow-up of 192 normally hearing children with delayed speech. *Journal of Laryngology and Otology*, 1970, **84**, 1001–1011.

Bender, L. Psychoses associated with somatic diseases that distort the body structure. *Archives of Neurology and Psychiatry*, 1934, **32**, 1000–1024.

Bender, L., & Silver, A. Body image problems of the brain injured child. *The Journal of Social Issues*, 1948, **4**, 84–89.

Benton, A. L. Developmental aphasia (DA) and brain damage. *Cortex*, 1964, **1**, 40–52.

Birch, H. G., & Lefford, A. Intersensory development in children. *Monographs of the Society for Research in Child Development*, 1963, **28** (5, Whole No. 89).

Blake, F. G., & Wright, F. H. *Essentials of pediatric nursing*. Philadelphia: Lippincott, 1963.

Blanchard, I. Speech pattern and etiology in mental retardation. *American Journal of Mental Deficiency*, 1964, **68**, 612–617.

Bortner, M., & Birch, H. G. Perceptual and perceptual-motor dissociation in cerebral palsied children. *Journal of Nervous and Mental Disease*, 1962, **134**, 103–108.

Breakey, A. S., Wilson, J. J., & Wilson, B. C. Sensory and perceptual functions in the cerebral palsied. III. Some visual and perceptual relationships. *Journal of Nervous and Mental Disease*, 1974, **158**, 70–77.

Broadbent, P. E., & Ladefoged, P. Auditory perception of temporal order. *Journal of the Acoustical Society of America*, 1959, **31**, 1539.

Brookshire, R. H. Effects of trial time and inter-trial interval on naming by aphasic subjects. *Journal of Communication Disorders*, 1971, **3**, 289–301.

Cardwell, V. E. *Cerebral palsy: advances in understanding and care.* New York: Ronald, 1965.

Cass, M. T. *Speech habilitation in cerebral palsy.* New York: Hafner, 1966.

Cattell, P. *The measurement of intelligence in infants and young children.* New York: Psychological Corporation, 1947.

Chappell, G. E. Developmental aphasia revisited. *Journal of Communication Disorders*, 1970, **3**, 181–187.

Cohen, P., & Hannigan, H. M. "Aphasia" in cerebral palsy. In H. D. Bauman (Ed.), *Proceedings of the Annual Meeting of the American Academy of Cerebral Palsy.* Springfield, Ill.: C. C Thomas, 1954.

Croskey, C. S., & Adams, M. R. The experimental analysis of certain aspects of an aphasic's recovery. *Journal of Communication Disorders*, 1970, **2**, 177–180.

Crothers, B., & Paine, R. *The natural history of cerebral palsy.* London: Oxford University Press, 1959.

Cruickshank, W. M. *Cerebral palsy: its individual and community problems.* Syracuse, N.Y.: Syracuse University Press, 1966.

Cruickshank, W. M. Perception and cerebral palsy, studies in figure-background relationship. *Research in Education*, 1968, **3**, 40. (Abstract)

Culloty, V. *The hemiplegic child: suggestions for home training.* (Parents Handbook No. 5) London: Spastics Society, Heinemann, 1964.

Daley, W. T. (Ed.) *Speech and language therapy with the cerebral palsied child.* Washington, D.C.: Catholic University of America Press, 1965.

Davis, H. Occam's razor and congenital aphasia. *Psychosomatic Medicine*, 1962, **24**, 81–84.

DeHaven, G. E., Bruce, J. D., & Bryan, D. B. Remediation of coordination deficits in youth with minimal cerebral dysfunction. (Final Report, Research Grant 15-P-55120/3-02.) Devon, Pa.: Social and Rehabilitation Service and the Devereax Foundation Institute for Research and Training, 1971.

Doehring, D. G. Visual spatial memory in aphasic children. *Journal of Speech and Hearing Research*, 1960, **3**, 138–149.

Doris, J. The evaluation of the intellect of the brain-damaged child: historical development and present status. In A. J. Solnit & S. A. Provence (Eds.), *Modern perspectives in child development.* New York: International Universities Press, 1963.

Dunsdon, M. J. *The educability of cerebral palsy children.* London: Newnes, 1952.

Edwards, A. E., & Auger, R. The effect of aphasia on the perception of precedence. *Proceedings of the 73rd Annual Convention of the American Psychological Association*, 1965, **1**, 207–208.

Efron, R. Temporal perception, aphasia, and déjà vu. *Brain*, 1963, **86**, 403–424.

Eisenson, J. Developmental aphasia: a speculative view with therapeutic implications. *Journal of Speech and Hearing Disorders*, 1968, **33**, 3–13.

Fay, W. H. *Temporal sequence in the perception of speech.* Amsterdam: Mouton, 1966.

Gerber, S. E. Cerebral palsy and hearing loss. *Cerebral Palsy Journal*, 1966, **27**, 6–7.

Getman, G. N. The role of the visuomotor complex in the acquisition of learning skills. In S. R. Rappaport (Ed.), *Childhood aphasia and brain damage.* Vol. 3. *Habilitation.* Narberth, Pa.: Livingston, 1966.

Gibbs, N. Questions parents ask. In M. C. O. Bax, E. Clayton-Jones, & R. C. Mac Keith (Eds.), *Child neurology and cerebral palsy*. (Little Club Clinics No. 2) London: Spastics Society, Heinemann, 1960.

Goldstein, R. Discussion of aphasia by panelists. In S. R. Rappaport (Ed.), *Childhood aphasia and brain damage*. Vol. 2. Differential diagnosis. Narberth, Pa.: Livingston, 1965.

Goldstein, R., Landau, W. M., & Kleffner, F. R. Neurologic observations on a population of deaf and aphasic children. *Annals of Otology, Rhinology and Laryngology*, 1960, **69**, 756–767.

Goodglass, H., & Quadfasel, F. A. Language laterality in left-handed aphasics. *Brain*, 1954, **77**, 521–548.

Graham, P. U., Chir, B., & Rutter, M. Organic brain dysfunction and child psychiatric disorder. *British Medical Journal*, 1968, **3**, 695–700.

Halstead, W. C., & Rennick, P. M. Perceptual-cognitive disorders in children. In A. H. Kidd & J. L. Rivoire (Eds.), *Perceptual development in children*. New York: International Universities Press, 1966.

Hammill, D. D., Myers, P. J., & Irwin, O. C. Certain speech and linguistic abilities in subclasses of cerebral palsy. *Perceptual and Motor Skills*, 1968, **26**, 511–514.

Hansen, E. *Cerebral palsy in Denmark*. Copenhagen: Munksgaard, 1960.

Hebb, D. O. *The organization of behavior*. New York: Wiley, 1949.

Hirsh, I. J. Information processing in input channels for speech and language: the significance of serial order of stimuli. In A. H. Millikan & F. L. Darley (Eds.), *Brain mechanisms underlying speech and language*. New York: Grune & Stratton, 1967.

Hirsch, I. J., & Fraisse, P. [untitled] Periodic Progress Reports, Central Institute for the Deaf. 1964, **8**, 20.

Hirsh, I. J., & Sherrick, E. E. Perceived order in different sense modalities. *Journal of Experimental Psychology*, 1961, **62**, 423–432.

Hodgson, W. R. Audiological report of a patient with left hemispherectomy. *Journal of Speech and Hearing Disorders*, 1967, **32**, 39–45.

Holt, K. S. What parents want from doctors. In M. C. O. Bax, E. Clayton-Jones, & R. C. Mac Keith (Eds.), *Child neurology and cerebral palsy*. (Little Club Clinics No. 2) London: Spastics Society, Heinemann, 1960.

Humphrey, M. E., & Zangwill, O. L. Dysphasia in left-handed aphasics. *Journal of Neurology and Neurosurgery in Psychiatry*, 1952, **15**, 184–193.

Illingworth, R. S. Difficulties in developmental prediction. In M. C. O. Bax, E. Clayton-Jones, & R. C. Mac Keith (Eds.), *Child neurology and cerebral palsy*. (Little Club Clinics No. 2) London: Spastics Society, Heinemann, 1960.

Illingworth, R. S. *An introduction to developmental assessment in the first year*. (Little Club Clinics No. 4) London: Spastics Society, Heinemann, 1962.

Ingram, T. T. S. *Paediatric aspects of cerebral palsy*. Edinburgh: Livingston, 1964.

Ingram, T. T. S., Jameson, S., Errington, J., & Mitchell, R. G. *Living with cerebral palsy*. London: Heinemann, 1964.

Irwin, O. C., & Hammill, D. D. Some results with an abstraction test with cerebral palsied children. *Cerebral Palsy Review*, 1964, **25**, 10–11.

Irwin, O. C., & Hammill, D. D. Effects of types, extent, and degree of cerebral palsy on three measures of language. *Cerebral Palsy Journal*, 1965, **26**, 7–9.

Isaacson, R. L. When brains are damaged. *Psychology Today*, 1970, **3**, 38–42.

Isom, J. B. Perceptual development: visual and kinesthetic. *Physical Therapy*, 1966, **46**, 734–740.

Kephart, N. C. Perceptual-motor aspects of learning disabilities. *Exceptional Children*, 1964, **31**, 201–206.

Kephart, N. C. *The slow learner in the classroom.* (2nd ed.) Columbus, Ohio: Merrill, 1970.

Kirichenko, E. I., & Trifonov, O. A. On the pathological formation of personality in children and adolescents with cerebral palsy. *Zhurnal Nevropatologii i Psikhiatrii,* 1969, **69,** 1553–1556.

Klapper, Z. S., & Birch, H. G. The relation of childhood characteristics to outcome in young adults with cerebral palsy. *Developmental Medicine and Child Neurology,* 1966, **8,** 645–656.

Klapper, Z. S., & Birch, H. G. A fourteen-year follow-up study of cerebral palsy: intellectual change and stability. *American Journal of Orthopsychiatry,* 1967, **37,** 540–547.

Klapper, Z. S., & Weiner, H. Developmental deviations in brain-injured (cerebral palsied) members of pairs of identical twins. *Quarterly Journal of Child Behavior,* 1950, **2,** 288–313.

Kleffner, F. R. Teaching aphasic children. *Education,* 1959, **79,** 413–418.

Kleffner, F. R. Discussion of aphasia by panelists. In S. R. Rappaport (Ed.), *Childhood aphasia and brain damage: a definition.* Narberth, Pa.: Livingston, 1964.

Kohut, S. A. The abnormal child: his impact on the family. *Physical Therapy,* 1966, **46,** 160–167.

Landau, W. M., Goldstein, R., & Kleffner, F. R. Congenital aphasia, a clinico-pathological study. *Neurology,* 1960, **10,** 915–921.

Landau, W. M., & Kleffner, F. R. Syndrome of acquired aphasia with convulsive disorder in children. *Neurology,* 1957, **7,** 523–530.

Lashley, K. S. *Brain mechanisms and intelligence.* Chicago: University of Chicago Press, 1929.

Lashley, K. S. *The neuropsychology of Lashley: selected papers.* New York: McGraw-Hill, 1960.

Leont'ev, A. N. *Problems in mental development.* Moscow: RSFSR Academy of Pedagogic Sciences Press, 1959.

Levin, A. K. *Cerebral palsy.* Baltimore: Williams & Wilkins, 1965.

Lieberman, A. M., Cooper, F. S., Shankweiler, D. P., & Studdert-Kennedy, M. Perception of the speech code. *Psychological Review,* 1967, **7,** 431–461.

Love, N. W., Jr. The relative occurrence of secondary disabilities in children with cerebral palsy and other primary physical handicaps. *Exceptional Children,* 1970, **36,** 301–302.

Lowe, A. D., & Campbell, R. A. Temporal discrimination in aphasoid and normal children. *Journal of Speech and Hearing Research,* 1965, **8,** 313–314.

Luria, A. R. *The human brain and psychological processes.* New York: Harper & Row, 1966.

Luria, A. R. (Ed.) *Problems of the higher nervous activity of the normal and abnormal child.* Vol. 2. Moscow: RSFSR Academy of Pedagogic Sciences Press, 1958.

Machek, O., & Collins, H. A. Second year review of evaluating and classifying the vocational potentials of the cerebral palsied. *Archives of Physical Medicine and Rehabilitation,* 1961, **42,** 106–108.

Machover, K. *Personality projection in the drawing of the human figure.* Springfield, Ill.: C. C Thomas, 1949.

Mac Keith, R. C. Improving one's technique. In M. C. O. Bax, E. Clayton-Jones, & R. C. Mac Keith (Eds.), *Child neurology and cerebral palsy.* (Little Club Clinics No. 2) London: Spastics Society, Heinemann, 1960.

Magoun, H. W. *The working brain.* Springfield, Ill.: C. C Thomas, 1958.

McDonald, E. T., & Chance, B., Jr. *Cerebral palsy.* Englewood Cliffs, N.J.: Prentice-Hall, 1964.

McGinnis, M. A. *Aphasic children: identification and education by the association method.* Washington, D.C.: Volta, 1963.

McGinnis, M. A., Kleffner, F. R., & Goldstein, R. Teaching aphasic children. *Volta Review,* 1956, **58,** 239–244.

Mordock, J. B., & DeHaven, G. E. Movement skills of children with minimal cerebral dysfunction: the role of the physical therapist. *Rehabilitation Literature,* 1969, **30,** 2–8.

Nakano, T. Research on hearing impairment in cerebral palsied school children. *International Audiology,* 1966, **5,** 159–161.

Osgood, C. E., & Miron, M. S. *Approaches to the study of aphasia.* Urbana: University of Illinois Press, 1964.

Paine, R. S. The immediate value of the neonatal neurological evaluation. In M. C. O. Bax, E. Clayton-Jones, & R. C. Mac Keith (Eds.), *Child neurology and cerebral palsy.* (Little Club Clinics No. 2) London: Spastics Society, Heinemann, 1960a.

Paine, R. S. Disturbances of sensation in cerebral palsy. In M. C. O. Bax, E. Clayton-Jones, & R. C. Mac Keith (Eds.), *Child neurology and cerebral palsy.* (Little Club Clinics No. 2) London: Spastics Society, Heinemann, 1960b.

Piaget, J. *The origins of intelligence in the child.* Translated by M. Cook. London: Routledge, 1953.

Piaget, J., & Inhelder, B. *The child's conception of space.* Translated by F. J. Langdon & J. L. Lunzer. London: Routledge, 1956.

Reitan, R. M. Psychological deficit. *Annual Review of Psychology,* 1962, **13,** 415–444.

Rosenberg, P. E. Discussion of aphasia by panelists. In S. R. Rappaport (Ed.), *Childhood aphasia and brain damage: a definition.* Narberth, Pa.: Livingston, 1964.

Rosenstein, J. Tactile perception of rhythmic patterns by normal, blind, deaf, and aphasic children. *American Annals of the Deaf,* 1957, **102,** 339–403.

Rutter, M., Graham, P., & Yule, W. *A neuropsychiatric study in childhood.* (Clinics in Developmental Medicine Nos. 35–36) London: Spastics International Medical Publications, Heinemann, 1970.

Rutherford, B. A comprehensive study of loudness, pitch, rate, rhythm, and quality of children handicapped by cerebral palsy. *Journal of Speech and Hearing Disorders,* 1944, **9,** 263–271.

Sattler, J. M., & Anderson, N. E. The Peabody Picture Vocabulary Test, Stanford-Binet, and the Modified Stanford-Binet with normal and cerebral palsied children. *Journal of Special Education,* 1974, **7,** 119–123.

Semans, S. Principles of treatment in cerebral palsy. *Physical Therapy,* 1966, **46,** 715–720.

Semans, S. The Bobath concept in treatment of neurological disorders. *American Journal of Physical Medicine,* 1967, **46,** 732–785.

Semans, S. Comments by discussant. *Physical Therapy,* 1970, **50,** 342–343.

Shore, M. O. The cerebral palsied child with a hearing loss. *Volta Review,* 1960, **62,** 438–441.

Silverstein, A. B., & Robinson, H. A. The representation of orthopedic disability in children's figure drawings. *Journal of Consulting Psychology,* 1956, **20,** 333–341.

Simpson, S. Perceptual functions in cerebral palsied children. *Dissertation Abstracts,* 1967, **28,** 508-A.

Skatvedt, M. Sensory, perceptual and other non-motor defects in cerebral palsy. In M. C. O. Bax, E. Clayton-Jones, & R. C. Mac Keith (Eds.), *Child neurology and cerebral palsy.* (Little Club Clinics No. 2) London: Spastics Society, Heinemann, 1960.

Spock, B. *Baby and child care.* New York: Pocket Books, 1957.

Stark, J. A. A comparison of the performance of aphasic children on three sequencing tests. *Journal of Communication Disorders,* 1967, **1,** 31–34.

Stephen, E. Assessment, training and employment of adolescents and young adults with cerebral palsy. I. An introductory review. *Cerebral Palsy Bulletin,* 1961, **3,** 127–134.

Taylor, E. M. *Psychological appraisal of children with cerebral defects.* Cambridge: Harvard University Press, 1959.

Twitchell, T. E. Variations and abnormalities of motor development. *Physical Therapy,* 1965, **45,** 424–430.

Vega, A., & Parsons, O. A. Relationship between sensory-motor deficits and WAIS verbal and performance scores in unilateral brain damage. *Cortex,* 1969, **5,** 229–241.

Vernon, M. Clinical phenomenon of cerebral palsy and deafness. *Exceptional Children,* 1970, **36,** 743–751.

Vygotsky, L. S. *Development of higher mental functions.* Moscow: RSFSR Academy of Pedagogic Sciences Press, 1960.

Webb, R. C. Is movement necessary in the development of cognition? *Mental Retardation,* 1971, **9,** (4) 16–18.

Weiner, P. S. The perceptual level functioning of dysphasic children: a follow-up study. *Journal of Speech and Hearing Research,* 1972, **15,** 423–438.

Weinstein, S. Deficits concomitant with aphasia or lesions of either cerebral hemisphere. *Cortex,* 1964, **1,** 154–169.

Weisenburg, T., & McBride, K. *Aphasia: a clinical and psychological study.* New York: Hafner, 1964.

Wenar, C., & Coulter, J. B. A reliability study of developmental histories. *Child Development,* 1962, **33,** 453–462.

Williams, J. The effect of emotional factors on perception and concept formation in cerebral palsied children. In M. C. O. Bax, E. Clayton-Jones, & R. C. Mac Keith (Eds.), *Child neurology and cerebral palsy.* (Little Club Clinics No. 2) London: Spastics Society, Heinemann, 1960, pp. 123–132.

Wilson, L. F. Assessment of congenital aphasia. In S. R. Rappaport (Ed.), *Childhood aphasia and brain damage.* Vol. 2. *Differential diagnosis.* Narberth, Pa.: Livingston, 1965.

Wilson, L. F. The language of living. In S. R. Rappaport (Ed.), *Childhood aphasia and brain damage.* Vol. 3. *Habilitation.* Narberth, Pa.: Livingston, 1966.

Wilson, L. F., Doehring, D. G., & Hirsh, I. J. Auditory discrimination learning by aphasic and nonaphasic children. *Journal of Speech and Hearing Research,* 1960, **3,** 138–149.

That mentally deficient children realize their incapacity is well known to those who have experience in teaching them. One of the problems connected with dealing with them is to give their minds relief from the paralyzing sense of inferiority.

—John Madison Fletcher

3
Brain disorder
and mental retardation

Binet first developed his intelligence test in order to predict who would do well in school. Eventually, children scoring below certain levels were placed in a slower-moving class or excluded from school altogether. In this chapter we present Nick, a boy who is intellectually limited and whose IQ score is between 45 and 55. Hank, the aphasic child presented in Chapter 2, also had a verbal IQ in the retarded range, but his performance functioning was close to average. Hank's retardation resulted from a specific language deficiency, and if his communication skills improved, his verbal IQ would increase. Nick, unlike Hank, is limited in all areas of functioning and, even with special educational techniques, is expected to function throughout his life like an 8- to 10-year-old.

Like Hank's language deficiency, Nick's intellectual deficiency resulted from central nervous system pathology. Autopsy studies have revealed that almost all individuals who had had an IQ below 50 had brain pathology (Crome, 1960; Zigler, 1967). How does this information square with the typical textbook presentation of a plot of intelligence test scores which looks like the normal, bell-shaped curve?

The normal curve hypothesis implies that intelligence is distributed like height and weight. Except for physiological disorders (thyroid or pituitary deficiencies) or genetic abnormalities (dwarfs and pygmies), the distribution of height or weight begins in adult groups at some base level considerably higher than zero (say 4 ft. 10 in. or 80 lbs). The same is true for intelligence. The normal distribution probably starts somewhere around 60–70. Individuals with lower IQs are analogous to those with physiological or genetic abnormalities that result in small height or low weight. A low IQ can result from cerebral trauma, infection, and toxic agents, all of which destroy brain tissue, or from chromosomal abnormalities, gene peculiarities, or Rh incompatibility. These diverse etiologies all result in cerebral pathology or abnormal physiological processes (Zigler, 1967). Consequently, individuals with a cerebral pathology that lowers intellectual functioning should be considered abnormal. Their intelligence scores should be excluded from distributions of those without physiological defects, because including them results in a skewed distribution.

Research reveals that there is an overabundance of individuals at the very low IQ levels (Penrose, 1963)—what we would expect when abnormal and normal subjects are combined in a distribution of scores. Consequently, Zigler (1967) proposes a two-group approach toward classifying mental retardation. The first group includes only individuals with known physiological defects. An IQ distribution for this group would have a mean near 35 and a standard deviation of approximately 12.

The second group includes normal individuals, that is, the bulk of the population. The IQ curve for this group would be a normal distribution with a mean of 100 and a standard deviation of approximately 16, with lower and upper limits of 50 and 150 respectively. A number of individuals in the normal group would still have an IQ below 75. They would be considered mentally retarded, but retarded as a result of normal manifestations of the genetic pool in our population, rather than as the result of physiological abnormality. While less intelligent than other children, they are as integral a part of the normal distribution as are the small percentage of children viewed as superior.

Figure 3.1 illustrates the two-group approach. Note that because there are a small number of individuals with known defects throughout the IQ continuum (see Chapter 8), the population encompassed by the smaller curve extends beyond the 70 IQ point—the arbitrary cut-off point below which individuals are considered retarded. The larger curve represents the polygenic distribution of intelligence; the smaller represents the distribution for all those whose intellectual functioning reflects factors other than normal polygenic expression, that is, those retardates having an identifiable physiological defect. This chapter will discuss mental retardation resulting from physiological defects, while Chapter 11 will discuss those at the lower end of the polygenic distribution of intelligence.

Nick is a member of the first group, the child whose retardation results from brain dysfunction. Nick's dysfunction had a marked effect on his intellectual functioning, but left his motor and language functioning relatively unimpaired.

Figure 3.1 *The two-group approach to classification of intelligence. The shaded curve represents the IQ distribution for individuals with known physiological defects; the unshaded curve is the IQ distribution for normal individuals.*

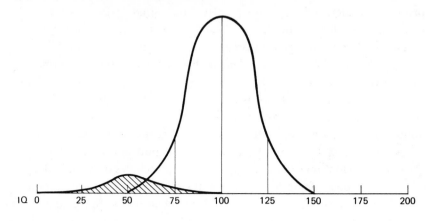

NICK

Nick's social development, vocalization, interest in his surroundings, alertness, social responsiveness, and powers of concentration were all retarded. In addition, slight microcephaly was present. Recall from Chapter 2 that serial measurements of Art's skull were part of his developmental evaluations. His measurements were recorded on a graph which showed the average rate of increase for normal children. Each successive measurement indicated adequate head size in relation to body size. In Nick's case head size was small in relation to body size. Some investigators have reported that head size at 1 year of age is a valid predictor of measured IQ at 4 years of age (Nelson & Deutschberger, 1970).

Nick's evaluation

Nick's developmental history disclosed excessive sleepiness and drowsiness. His mother described him as a "very good baby" who slept the greater part of the day. As he got older, however, the mother became concerned about both his vision and hearing, primarily because he failed to follow movements with his eyes or to respond adequately to sound. Hand regard (fascination with hand movement) persisted for some time after 2 years of age, and he was late to chew properly, frequently spitting up and sometimes vomiting. Formal evaluation revealed that Nick was retarded in many areas of development, although his motor development was close to normal. Because of his adequate motor skills, his parents had not suspected retardation until after 2 years of age. The pediatrician, however, had been aware of Nick's retardation from a much earlier period. Let's retrace the steps which led to the pediatrician's awareness and to Nick's eventual evaluation.

The pediatrician's decision   Complications at Nick's birth had resulted in neonatal asphyxia, and although relations between asphyxia and retardation are not clear, the obstetrician recommended that the pediatrician follow Nick's development closely. The pediatrician did not immediately inform Nick's parents of these suspicions. While he believed in early identification, his bias was against identification which took place "too early." He preferred to allow mothers to become as attached to their retarded infants as they would to any other. If informed immediately following birth, the parents might reject the child or request his early institutionalization. Such rejection prevents the establishment of an affectional bond between mother and child. Without this bond, the child's condition could deteriorate rather than improve.

Institutions have long waiting lists. If, while awaiting admittance, the mother merely looks after the child's physical needs and neglects his needs for affection and stimulation, the child's chances of improving within the institution could decrease considerably. The doctor knew of parents who could not relate to their child once they were told he was retarded. They would not play with him and would keep him confined to his crib. Such confinement, and the resulting lack of stimulation, could result in the development of repetitive and stereotyped behavior which would interfere with later development (Warren & Burns, 1970). Stereotyped behavior (rocking, sucking, object hitting, rubbing and scratching, body manipulation, complex hand movement, head banging, and even self-destructive behavior) has been related to a lack of sensory stimulation (Berkson & Mason, 1963, 1964; Guess, 1966). Confining a child to a crib and avoiding contact with him may make him more retarded. In addition, infant depression, delayed speech, and severe ego deficits have been traced to maternal deprivation (Philips, 1967).

Numerous investigators have emphasized the importance of affection as well as tactile stimulation during the first six months of life. Nick's pediatrician felt that too many children had been institutionalized because of the physician's insensitivity to the feelings of parents and their own needs as doctors to avoid the unpleasant experience of doctoring a "defective" child. Because of their own ignorance about retardation, they support, if not subtly encourage, early institutionalization. When the child fails to prosper in the institution, their belief is supported, "I'm glad we recommended institutionalization. What a burden that child would have been!"

Institutional living also can contribute to increased deficits because of the inadequate stimulation often present in such settings (Provence & Lipton, 1962). The physician's prophecy, then, becomes self-fulfilling. He recommends early institutionalization, thereby preventing the parents' attachment to their child; without a strong parental bond, the child's emotional and intellectual growth suffers; the child is then institutionalized when a vacancy occurs; the institutional environment fails to stimulate the child; the child fails to thrive; and the pediatrician observes the final result without knowledge of the intervening variables and concludes that he was wise to recommend institutionalization. Nick's pediatrician tried to avoid this cycle of events.

During his second year, Nick's parents began to realize that he was slow in social development. During this same period, the pediatrician was more convinced that Nick was retarded. He expressed his suspicions and helped the parents to both discover and accept Nick's retardation as he tried to prepare them for its consequences.

While Nick's pediatrician chose to delay presenting Nick's young parents with his suspicions, there is no widespread agreement regarding this practice. The practice of withholding information from parents has been criticized. Some feel that such a practice is based on an a priori decision by the professional that he knows how much "truth" a parent can take for his own future good and that the professional who takes this approach may not have resolved his own feelings about retardation. "Since a professional has, by his own life pattern, indicated that he values intellectual accomplishment, he may assume that a diagnosis of even mild retardation will be a devastating blow to any parent. This may or may not be the case" (Anderson, 1971, p. 4).

Nick's pediatrician, who had known both parents since their childhood, preferred to withhold his opinion until he could maneuver the parents into arriving at their own diagnosis of retardation. By that time, a mother-child bond would be established. He would continue, however, to evaluate whether the mother's developing concerns interfered with the mother-child relationship.

A diagnostic team decision In Art's case careful evaluation over a period of years failed to disclose intellectual deficit, a fortunate occurrence for Art since the majority of cerebral palsied children are intellectually retarded. In Nick's case, in spite of relatively normal motor and manipulative development, intellectual deficit accompanied neurological deficiency. Once Art and Nick reached 2 years of age, the presence or absence of intellectual retardation was easier to establish. Diagnosis of retardation can be complicated by other conditions, for example, by aphasia, as in Hank's case, or by behavioral syndromes which resemble retardation (several of these will be presented in Chapter 4). Deaf children and those with delayed maturation also can appear retarded.

Nick's pediatrician's various developmental assessments supported his initial impression of intellectual retardation. He was not, however, an expert in retardation, and when Nick reached 3, he referred the family to the diagnostic center affiliated with an institution for the retarded. He put off the decision for some time because of the center's location on the grounds of an institution, an institution that conveyed a gloomy outlook to parents who took their child there for evaluation. He remembered the negative reactions of many young people who worked as volunteers in this facility. "Will he have to go there?" was a question that hurt him deeply. He wished there was a child development center in the community so that Art could be evaluated in more favorable surroundings.

Nevertheless, the center staff were better equipped than he to make an etiologic and pathologic diagnosis and to determine the effect of the retardation on intellectual, emotional, and social growth. They were better trained to evaluate the adjustment of the family to Nick's presence, to discuss and counsel the parents regarding his prognosis, and to suggest techniques for present and future management of his behavior.

At the center Nick was given the Vineland Social Maturity Scale, the Stanford-Binet Intelligence Scale, a speech and hearing evaluation, and a neurological evaluation. The results indicated mild diffuse brain damage, and intelligence quotient of 48, and a social quotient of 51 (an SQ of 100 represents a social age equivalent to chronological age). The social worker felt that the parents had made a favorable adjustment to Nick, but would need help in specific methods of training.

Nick's speech and communication skills were markedly deficient. Center staff said he could be trained to talk and to communicate with gestures. He also could be trained in elementary health habits and would profit from systematic habit training (what is meant by the term *trainable*).

PSYCHOLOGICAL EVALUATION:
CLARENCE, AGE 28

Present test results. Weschler Adult Intelligence Scale (WAIS): verbal IQ 48, performance IQ 44, full scale IQ 43; Stanford-Binet (Form L–M): MA approximation 4-6; Goodenough Draw-a-Man: 4 years.

General observations. One can tell from Clarence's general behavior that he is functioning well below his age level since even his pidgin English is characteristic of a preschooler. He was at ease during testing but never spoke spontaneously or called attention to objects in the room. He was quick to respond and was rather persistent in his efforts to master certain tasks, while he gave up quickly on others.

Test interpretation. The examiner first obtained a measure of mental age using the Stanford-Binet. The ceiling level was reached at 7 years, where he failed all items. His MA was 6 years, although his drawing of a man placed him somewhat lower than that level. The Draw-a-Man score was deflated because of poor perceptual-motor functioning. Clarence could not integrate what his eye could see with what his hand could do. His perceptual functioning was adequate; he got 5 out of 6 correct on the Binet pictorial similarities subtest and 9 out of 10 correct on the discrimination of forms subtest (the subtest requires that the testee select from among a number of geometric shapes the one that looks like the sample). Clarence also could state that his drawing of a diamond (completed adequately by most 7-year-olds) looked more like a circle and his square more like a triangle.

Clarence's functioning on the WAIS digit span subtest was at a moderately retarded level. He could repeat up to 4 digits forward but could not repeat any digits backward. Several examples were given of what was meant by the word "backward," but Clarence continued to give his answers forward. Such perseveration and/or rigidity is often noted in brain damaged individuals. All efforts to get Clarence to give digits backward were unsuccessful. He seemed confused and unable to understand the instructions.

On the WAIS digit symbol subtest, Clarence could not duplicate the figures which went with each number. For example, if an 8 ($\times$) was given, he would give an 8 (=); if a 7 ($\wedge$) was given, his $\wedge$ would not look like the symbol. When asked whether his drawings looked like the examples, his answers were inconsistent. He missed the first two designs of the WAIS block design subtest, did the third correctly, but missed the remainder. On those he missed, the examiner asked him if his looked like the model. Again, he gave affirmative answers on some occasions but not on others. If the examiner placed a correct and incorrect block arrangement before him, however, he could select the correct one as the best match (adequate perceptual ability). On the WAIS picture arrangement test, he got the first two correct but could not explain why he selected the order he did.

On both the WAIS picture arrangement and WAIS object assembly subtests, the examiner sought to determine if Clarence could learn with repeated practice. On the picture arrangement subtest, the reason for each order was given, and Clarence was asked to put them in the order corresponding to the story he had just heard. Clarence did not benefit from this type of practice. On the object assembly subtest, Clarence tried to assemble the manikin five times and no improvement was noted. The examiner had demonstrated how to assemble the manikin, had told him which were the arms, legs, etc., but on the fifth attempt, he still tried to put the arms in the leg slots.

Summary and recommendations. Although Clarence is functioning at a 6-year-old level, considerable patience will be needed to teach him those things which a 6-year-old can master. He is eager to learn, however, as he spontaneously wrote the word *man* over his drawing of a man and the word *vot* under his drawing of a foot. With his positive attitude toward learning and his pride in his accomplishments, it should be rewarding to see him make whatever progress is possible; but the goals should not be set too high, since his ability to learn with practice is quite limited.

A controversial treatment for Nick—patterning

Over the next five years the gap widened between Nick's development and that of other children. A second child was born, leaving the parents with less time to devote to Nick. He could not attend school with the neighborhood children because he did not qualify for the educable classes in the public school setting. He had been attending the trainable classes at the state institution for a year, but the long bus ride to this setting seemed to negate progress. In addition, Nick had never been accepted by the neighborhood children. While similar to his normal peers in size, he lacked the alertness to compete with them. When other children moved from parallel to cooperative play, he was still engaged in parallel play. When ready for cooperative play, he had outgrown those younger children with whom he could now play. Neighbors would not allow their children to play with him because of their ignorance about retardation. The lack of playmates and the teasing which eventually followed his rejection intensified Nick's feelings of inferiority. Eventually, he isolated himself from others and inhibited his attempts to solve new problems.

Nick's parents became increasingly worried about his emotional well-being. Frustrated by his lack of progress and desirous of avoiding institutionalization, they wanted to do something more for him, to see more rapid improvement. Nick's father had read of a controversial treatment designed to help children with brain injury. He did not fully understand the theory but was impressed by the articles he had read and the number of professional persons listed as associated with the development of the theory and its therapeutic application. Consequently, he arranged for Nick's evaluation at a nearby center which employed this approach to treatment.

The theoretical basis of patterning The treatment is derived from a theory of neurological development which postulates that ontogeny (the process of individual development) recapitulates phylogeny (the process of species development). Physical abilities are theorized to proceed through four main stages of development governed at four levels of the brain (Delacato, 1959, 1963, 1966). The simplest movements are governed at the level of the medulla and spinal cord. Crawling comes with the development of the pons. With the development of the midbrain comes creeping on all fours. Finally, as the cortex matures, the child learns walking, talking, and the full range of motor skills. With the cortex's development also comes dominance of one side of the brain. This dominance is considered necessary for normal functioning.

The child's development of mobility, manual competence, tactile competence, vision, audition, and language is functionally related to and parallels anatomical development. Delacato and other members of the Institutes for the Achievement of Human Potential, a center established to treat children according to the premises of this theory, assert that the neurological development of a child must proceed through the normal sequence of stages. If this does not occur, either because of brain damage or improper stimulation, the child will exhibit difficulties in mobility, speech, and cognition. Delacato asserts that most learning difficulties stem from the poor neurological organization that results from a failure of the child's nervous system to develop phylogenetically. To correct these difficulties, it is first necessary to determine the exact stage at which neurological growth halted or, at best, was incomplete. Determining the stage of arrest identifies the area of the brain damaged.

The theory holds that insufficient practice at one stage of development retards the entire process of future development. Remediation involves retraining the child to perform movements characteristic of the stage where arrestation took place and then moving him from that point through the higher stages until proper neurological organization is reached. Delacato claims that such retraining enables undamaged nerve cells to be activated and to take over functions impeded by dead or atrophied cells. In order to determine the appropriate treatment in each case, the Doman-Delacato Developmental Profile (Doman, Delacato, & Doman, 1964) is used to profile precisely the developmental levels reached in various motor activities.

Neurological organization is assessed at the highest cortical level by observing whether the child has established clear unilateral dominance in activities involving the feet, hands, and eyes. Mixed laterality (for example, a combination of right-eyed, left-handed, right-footed) is considered evidence of poor neurological organization.

Neurological organization at the second highest cortical level is evaluated by observing whether the child walks in a cross-pattern manner, i.e., extending the right arm with the left leg, in a well-coordinated manner. Smooth movements of the eyes during visual pursuit also are considered evidence of satisfactory organization at this level.

At the level of the midbrain, good neurological organization is revealed in smooth, rhythmic, cross-patterned creeping and smooth eye movements during visual pursuit of an object held in the child's hand.

At the level of the pons, good neurological organization is evidenced by a sleeping position appropriate to the child's laterality, crawling in the prone position culminating in cross-pattern crawling, and smooth visual pursuit with each eye while the other eye is occluded.

The lowest level at which a child fails a subtest determines the level at which training is initiated. Training consists of teaching the child to perform those activities the profile reveals as deficient. Typically, the following activities are included: patterning (reproduction of normal activities that the brain would have controlled had it not been injured), assisted crawling and creeping on the floor, eye exercises, tactile exercises with different materials, drawing, and reading. Patterning is usually recommended four time a day, five minutes at a time, seven days a week. In more severe cases patterns of passive movement are imposed. Several adults manipulate repeatedly the child's head and extremities into positions dictated by the theory. Additional procedures may include: rebreathing of expired air into a plastic face mask for 30 to 60 seconds once each waking hour (alleged to increase vital capacity and stimulate cerebral blood flow); a special diet low in salt and sugar content combined with restricted liquid intake (alleged to decrease cerebrospinal fluid production and the consequent build-up of pressure in the brain); establishment of cortical hemispheric dominance through restrictions on hand or eye use; sleep and rest positioning; and visual and gait training.

Proponents of the approach also believe that enhancement of one function will result in improvement in other areas. For example, improvement in coordination may, without special attention to speech, lead to improvement in expressive language (Institutes for the Achievement of Human Potential, undated). Improvements in areas not specifically treated are believed to stem from improved brain functioning. The Domans and Delacato state they are not treating the visible results of brain injury but the injured brain itself.

In the normal child each successful attempt at crawling and creeping sends sensory nerve messages to the area of the brain that governs these movements. Repeated successes build up movement-controlling circuits within the brain and thereby establish reflex patterns that permit the child to make coordinated movements without conscious planning. Since most brain injuries do not damage all the cells in the injured area, advocates of patterning believe that repeated patterning through limb manipulations may eventually send sensory messages which activate those undamaged cells in the injured area; such activation results in the ability to carry out those movement patterns the child previously could not perform. This stimulation of the brain is believed to facilitate the return of other functions, including cognition, as the brain approaches its full functional achievement.

Nick's response to treatment Nick's parents went to the patterning center near them for an evaluation of Nick's condition and instruction in the theory and therapeutic practices involved. Nick was put through a series of tests adopted from the Doman-Delacato Profile. The testing took approximately two days. Following this evaluation, two days were devoted to explaining the basic theory and one day to explaining how to carry out the treatment program.

Nick's parents were told that the success or failure of treatment depended largely on their unswerving efforts. Every day lost in making Nick better would make him worse, because he would lose another day in the race with his peer group. In order to maximize treatment opportunities, Nick was removed from the trainable class he was attending and kept at home.

The family began the treatment hoping that the result of their efforts would be a completely normal child. The prognosis they had received following the evaluation at the state institution was temporarily forgotten as they forged ahead with treatment. Almost immediately, they began to feel the strain caused by the total family's involvement in Nick's treatment; they began to feel that their efforts were never enough. Told never to miss a day of treatment, their daily lives revolved around patterning, crawling, breathing exercises, dietary restrictions, flashing lights, bedtime positions, and other treatments which took up most of the day. Family friends and helpful neighbors became involved in assisting the family to carry out the daily program when mother needed to shop or care for other members of the family.

After three months of treatment, Nick was reevaluated at the center. Nick showed considerable gain on the Doman-Delacato Profile, some gain in measured intelligence, increased awareness and ability to understand a sequence of commands, and some gain in vocabulary. The family was told to continue the same treatment and to return again in three months.

After three more months of the demanding routine, the second reevaluation also showed gains on the profile, but gains in other areas were minimal. Gradually, Nick's parents lowered their expectations for him. Like the parents of many brain-injured and retarded children, they began to realize that, while their child might improve in some areas, it was unfair both to the child and to themselves to expect too much. Many parents actually learn to resent the child who never fulfills their image of what he should be. Many are eager to mislead themselves about how normal their child will become under any treatment.

Nick's parents eventually felt that the program kept Nick from participating in other activities which they now realized were important for his development. Conversations with other parents who were using the approach revealed the same degree of involvement (parental devotion to patterning is discussed by Melton [1968]). Nick had little time to spend with other children and to develop social skills. For these and other reasons, the family discontinued Doman-Delacato treatments. Although they felt Nick had made some progress because of the program, they suspected the change resulted from the tremendous care and attention they had given him rather than from the specific treatment. More realistic in their view of Nick, they reenrolled him in the trainable class and arranged for social gatherings between Nick and the other retarded children in his classroom.

If the diagnostic center had not been attached to an institution and had been closer to home, if a local chapter of the National Association for Retarded Children had existed in Nick's community, if comprehensive services had been available, and if the classes for the trainable had not been attached to an institution an hour away from their home, perhaps Nick's parents would not have involved themselves in a controversial treatment. Perhaps their motivation resulted more from fears of eventual institutionalization should Nick fail to progress than from an inability to accept his limitations.

In Chapter 1 we described the facilities needed within each community to serve the retarded effectively. We also presented Wolfensberger's twenty predictions about the future of services for the retarded. But until these hopeful predictions are put into effect, families like Nick's must continue to search wherever they can for the services they need.

Professional opinions of patterning   But what about other children who remain longer in such a treatment program? Do they improve? Informal surveys of parents reveal divided opinion (National Association for Retarded Children, 1968). Some professionals have expressed rather strong objections to the patterning approach (Brown, 1964; Cole, 1964; Hudspeth, 1964; Wepman, 1964). Freeman (1967) has summarized these objections as follows.

1. The approach tends to ignore the natural clinical course of some children with brain injuries. Physicians have observed children who recover spontaneously without having received any treatment whatsoever. To attribute beneficial changes to specific methods without the proper experimental design to control for nontreatment effects is scientifically gratuitous.

2. Doman-Delacato followers assume that their methods treat the brain itself, while other methods treat only symptoms. However, there is no solid evidence that stimulation can raise the functioning capacity of functionally depressed cells. There is also no agreement as to what constitutes a "pattern" or whether passive movements have a specific central effect.

3. The treatment assumes that because the full potential of the brain is not known, it can be concluded that each child not "genetically defective" may have above average intellectual potential. Such an assumption can raise false hopes. The diagnosis of mental retardation is a major disappointment to all parents. Many never accept the condition and continually seek a different viewpoint or a treatment which will return the child to "normal." Since advocates of the patterning approach assume that most mental retardation is the result of brain injury, they convey the impression that the child can return to normal if given the proper treatment (*Institutes for the Achievement of Human Potential Bulletin*, 1965).

4. The treatment program makes parents the therapists. Placing the burden on parents can change the nature of parent-child relationships and result in the neglect of other important aspects of family life. Making

the parents the therapists also places the burden of possible failure on their shoulders. Should failure occur, it could add to the feelings of guilt and inadequacy that already exist in most parents of handicapped children.

5. The child under treatment is frequently prevented from performing certain self-motivated activities. If he begins to sit or walk before the profile indicates he has properly mastered the preceding stages of mobility, he is prevented from doing so by a variety of devices. The long-term effects of such procedures are not known, and the parents may become the target of the child's anger and frustration.

6. The Institutes' statements may increase parental anxiety. Freeman cites three examples. (a) The threat of death: the Institutes imply, according to Freeman, that delay in treatment may create complicating illnesses that could eventuate in death. (b) The possibility of damage to a child's potential by a variety of almost universal child-rearing practices. Freeman cites Doman and Delacato's (1965) article in *McCall's* which had the following title and subtitles: "Train Your Baby to Be a Genius! Is your baby in a playpen? Are his clothes snug? Is his crib near a wall? Then you may be inhibiting his mental development." The article implied that many common practices were detrimental to a child's intellectual growth. (c) The need for rigid performance of patterning to obtain successful results: parents are encouraged to carry out the routine without deviation and are led to feel they may be interfering with their child's progress should they permit any deviation.

7. The Institutes assume that improvements are the result of their specific treatments. However, the treatment program involves changes in family life, perhaps eliciting hope where there was none and sometimes generating interest and support from the community. These factors must be considered when analyzing reasons for improvement. It is precisely these factors, however, that are the most difficult to control in evaluative studies.

8. The Doman-Delacato Profile is purported to permit simple and conclusive diagnosis of brain damage and other developmental problems that most other professionals have found to be quite complex and most difficult to assess. The Institutes state that "the cause in the vast majority of individuals with behavioral problems is brain injury" (Institutes for the Achievement of Human Potential, undated). This opinion is not shared by most other workers in the area of behavioral disorders. Most professionals question the assumptions behind the profile and the failure to report studies that adequately relate it to any standard methods of assessing development.

9. The studies Delacato cites in support of his theory suffer from statistical defects. A critique of the studies in three published works by Delacato (1959, 1963, 1966) found them "exemplary only for their faults" (Glass & Robbins, 1967). The majority were naively designed and clumsily

analyzed, performed in "ignorance of the fundamental principles of comparative experimental design which have been known to researchers for thirty years." The results in the majority of studies were vitiated by the use of matched groups instead of random assignment to groups and failure to take into account regression toward the mean (groups of individuals selected because of extreme scores on a variable will tend to have less extreme scores when tested again on the same or related variables).

Regarding Freeman's second point, Delacato's followers are not alone in their belief that stimulation of parts of the central nervous system may increase the probability of that part's system reaching its full potential. For example, optimal visual stimulation is thought to maximize structural and functional growth of the visual system. The "optimal period" hypothesis, however, would predict that optimal stimulation needs to take place during a particular stage in development and that stimulation from that point forward would have a decreasing effect.

Regarding Freeman's third point, we will see later in the chapter that very few severely or moderately retarded children, regardless of the type of treatment, reach normal levels of functioning. Some do, however, perhaps because of early errors in diagnosis and a prognosis that limited treatment. When prognostic errors are followed by improvement under treatment, the specific therapeutic regimen frequently receives credit.

Concerning his fifth point, some parents sampled by *Children's Limited* (National Association for Retarded Children, 1968) claimed that their children were adversely affected by the demanding routine since it limited their contact with others their own age at school or at play. Those parents who were critical of the Doman-Delacato treatments said this isolation impeded their child's development.

What does the research say? At present, there are no carefully designed research studies that support the theory of neurological organization. Robbins (1966) concluded from his review of the literature that the various treatments dictated by the theory have not achieved favorable results. Children in Katzen's study (cited by the National Association for Retarded Children, 1968), sponsored by the United Cerebral Palsy Association and the Rockland County Center for the Physically Handicapped in New York, showed no appreciable difference in IQ or physical condition after one year of patterning, while the Doman-Delacato Profile indicated more than an average year's growth in two of the five cases. Similarly, Taylor (1968) reported that among 335 brain-damaged children, only gross muscle tone—1 out of 155 items on a case history form —was related to improvement on the Doman-Delacato Profile.

Kershner (1968) found that a patterning program improved the creeping and crawling as well as the motor proficiency of retarded children, but that similar improvement in motor proficiency was displayed by a group given general physical exercise. Using 149 children under different treatment conditions, Robbins (1967) reported no relationship between reading improvement and a treatment program similar to that employed at the Institutes. Similarily, O'Donnell and Eisenson (1969) found no differences between treated and untreated groups in reading.

The search for the miracle cure   The reader may question why so much space was devoted to presentation and discussion of a program which has not been supported by research. In all fairness to the Institutes, the more traditional treatment approaches also have not been adequately evaluated. The Bobaths's treatment, presented in the last chapter, while accepted by many professionals, has never been adequately tested. The difference between the programs of the Institutes and those of others lies in the publicity given to the one and not to the others.

The mass media bestowed much favorable publicity on the work of the Institutes (*Chicago Tribune Magazine,* September 13 and 27, 1964, both articles reprinted for wider distribution; *Good Housekeeping,* September 1962; *Life,* August 23, 1963; *Reader's Digest,* October 1964, November 1966; *Saturday Evening Post,* July 29, 1967). Reprints of the 1964 *Reader's Digest* article have accompanied mailings from the Institutes during fund-raising drives and have been sent to individuals inquiring about the Institutes' programs. It is tragic that such outstanding claims have been made in lay literature when so little support for the program exists. To the uninformed reader, the approach seems to make good sense. Bits of truth from other well-established theories are included in the theory and their inclusion gives the theory an air of credibility, although some have stated that the theory of neurological organization is based on eighteenth-century neurology. Until adequate research supports the theory's postulates, the statements of its proponents must be accepted with caution.

Patterning is certainly not the first miracle cure. At one time, a diet of foods high in glutamic acid was felt to have a significant influence on intellectual development. Currently, the use of megavitamins appears to fall into the same category (Cott, 1972).

In the late 1940s a number of articles appeared in popular magazines which stated that at long last a scientist had produced an educational procedure that would change children from the status of "feeblemindedness" to that of "normalcy" in intellectual, social, and personality traits ("They Are Feebleminded No Longer," *Reader's Digest,* September 1947; "Feebleminded Children Can Be Cured," *Women's Home Companion,* September 1947). These articles referred to a study by Schmidt (1946) which claimed to demonstrate that children classified as feebleminded (mean IQ of 52.1) increased nearly 20 IQ points in intelligence following completion of three years of special training. This training took place under Schmidt's supervision of several special classes for the retarded in Chicago. At the completion of five years of post-school experience, the

IQs had increased nearly 40 points and approached average (mean IQ of 89.3).

Kirk (1948) doubted the credibility of these findings and reexamined portions of the original data. He concluded that the majority of children probably had IQs between 50 and 79 rather than 50 and below. In fact, he estimated that approximately 50 percent of the children enrolled in special classes in Chicago during the period covered in Schmidt's investigation had IQs between 70 and 79. This is not surprising since public school classes for the trainable did not exist in Chicago in that era. Kirk could not determine the IQs of the actual children in Schmidt's sample because she refused to provide him with their names, stating that spotlight scrutiny would hinder the present adjustment of the subjects.

Schmidt (1948) replied to Kirk's criticisms with some of her own regarding his reanalysis. They were not convincing. In light of recent knowledge regarding IQ and social class, we know that many of Schmidt's subjects may not have been retarded but were, rather, from disadvantaged backgrounds. Some, therefore, could have improved in intellectual functioning following special schooling. Recall from Chapter 2 that cerebral palsied children with IQs below 50 faired poorly on follow-up. Those having IQs between 50 and 89, however, were less predictable. The majority, however, had IQs within 10 points of their original score. Follow-up studies presented later in this chapter also indicate that over two-thirds of those retested have IQs within 10 points of their original score. Although Schmidt called for replication of her study in her reply to Kirk, no such replication was ever published by her.

Glutamic acid, patterning, and megavitamins will not be the last of the miracle cures. More will come in the future, raising the hopes of parents of retarded and brain-injured children, hopes that will be short-lived. Some may even achieve the status of patterning (expenses related to patterning are deductible as medical expenses according to the Office of Internal Revenue's Publication 502, "Deductions for Medical and Dental Expenses"). Even treatments that have research support often turn out to be of benefit to only a portion of the group for which they were originally intended. As we will see in our discussion of phenylketonuria later in this chapter, diet treatment, originally predicted to cure this disorder, is effective with only a portion of those afflicted.

Many families, like Nick's, will try the miracle cures. In some cases their child will improve and they will attribute the improvement to the specific treatment followed. Others will not be so fortunate and, like Nick's parents, may come to realize that their child will remain less than what they had hoped. Some, out of frustration and anger, will send their retarded child to residential centers and divert their attention to their normal offspring.

In any case, no one has proved that unusual treatments harm children. Perhaps future research should be directed to this topic. So-called traditional cures, such as institutionalization or expensive private residential treatment, may be no more beneficial than remaining at home and being given unconventional treatment. Any form of residential treatment isolates the child from his family and community, eliminating benefits that might be derived from remaining at home.

Also needed is research on the exact nature of the population affected by special treatments. Patterning, for example, has been used to treat children varying widely in IQ and social behavior. Within a restricted range of IQ or with a particular type or degree of brain injury the treatment may prove beneficial. Cause and effect relationships must also be studied carefully so that the pragmatic observation of effect in treatment is not confused with understanding the mechanisms of the brain or the cause of the condition treated. Should the Institutes' treatments help certain youngsters, this does not necessarily support the theory on which the treatments are based. Certain drugs have been helpful in controlling convulsive disorders in children, yet we would not assume that convulsions are due to a lack of these drugs in childhood.

We have seen how Nick's family dealt with his retardation and have discussed how parents with retarded children hope for some treatment that will return their child to normal. This hope is not unlike that of the early pioneers in mental retardation who envisioned a "cure" for this disorder. These pioneers were unaware of the causes of retardation. Had they had such awareness, they would have set more realistic goals for themselves. Since their time, we have accumulated more knowledge about what causes retardation. This knowledge will now be presented.

PSYCHOLOGICAL EVALUATION: SANDRA, AGE 6

Reason for referral. Plans to place Sandra in a special classroom require contemporary information. Sandra has been under the care of a neurologist for three years. He has diagnosed her as suffering from a "developmental aphasia, with receptive and expressive elements." Yearly checkups have resulted in judgments of increasingly effective communication functions.

Sandra was examined a year ago and received a WISC verbal IQ of 60, performance IQ of 54, and full scale IQ of 53. Special class placement was recommended. Sandra has received specialized speech therapy from the child development center. They reported an IQ of "approximately 67" and added that "she does not possess intelligence above the upper limits of the retarded range." Placement in as small a class as possible was recommended at that time, but her parents refused to cooperate.

Sandra is currently repeating kindergarten. During her first year in school, she aggressed other children and could not respond to regular classroom routine and expectations. In her second year in school, Sandra's aggressiveness and occasional inappropriate behaviors diminished and all but disappeared. At first, Sandra spent part of her school day in a first grade classroom and the rest in a kindergarten classroom. The first grade teacher did not respond to inappropriate dependency gestures and felt important progress was being made in developing age-appropriate behaviors. Nevertheless, her parents intervened, believing too much stress was being generated, and since then she has spent all her time in a kindergarten class. Her current teacher reports that she has been unhappy over those events. She reports that Sandra does not have strong relationships with her peers, remaining on the periphery of play and work groups and attending events without participating. Lately, she has developed a strong liaison with another child who also has obvious intellectual and maturational deficits.

Behavioral observations. In the classroom Sandra drifted silently and slowly from one on-going group to another. Peers seemed oblivious to her presence. When she noticed my presence, Sandra came directly to me, curious and unafraid. She stood inches from my face and looked at me for a few minutes. She did not initiate conversation and only smiled softly when I spoke her name. She was tall for her age, well developed, and well groomed, but her gait was unsteady. A slight "hitch" to her walking resulted from her right leg being placed askance, and her right shoulder drooped.

During psychological examination, Sandra was gay and cooperative. Sometimes she became foolish, apparently a defense against anxiety and a strategy to lead the examiner and herself away from areas of threat. Attention span was moderate. As avoidance increased during a task, commands to continue were sufficient to return her to appropriate behavior. Midway through examination a rest period was needed, and we played with a soft ball. Sandra delighted in our play together. Her large muscle performance was very good during this activity. Her ball throwing, however, became progressively assertive, until she was throwing the ball to hit me.

Tests administered. Wechsler Intelligence Scale for Children (WISC), Bender-Gestalt, House—Tree—Person technique.

Test results. On the WISC Sandra earned a verbal IQ of 58, a performance IQ of 44, and a full scale IQ of 47. As noted above, threat and anxiety intruded upon her performance. Frequently, she was loquacious but unintelligible. She did not comprehend some of the tasks presented to her, particularly those requiring psychomotor processing of information. Without constant attention and direction, she was unable to persist in a coding task for two minutes.

Perceptual-motor performance was severely impaired. On the Bender-Gestalt test Sandra apprehended only a few simple designs and was unable to reproduce satisfactorily even the simplest. Projective testing (House—Tree—Person technique) revealed the same primitive, unconsidered expression found in psychomotor evaluation. Concepts were perseverated and hastily judged when produced.

Sandra's expressive difficulties were paramount. Asked to name her school, she said "kin-gar school." She described herself as 5 years old and a boy. She was in grade "four-day."

At the completion of structured testing, I attempted to interview her about her feelings toward her classroom and peer experiences. She became immediately upset and anxious. Pulling her knees up onto the desk, she began to rock in her seat. She laughed loudly, but fear was obvious in her eyes. She presented one of the most clear messages she ever produced, "No, no, oh good by, I go now."

Summary and recommendations. Sandra is functioning in the retarded range of intelligence, ranging from trainable to educable levels. Perceptual-motor deficit is severe. While her social skills have improved, she remains distant from her peers, unable to use the resources of modeling and imitation, and she is overly dependent upon a one-to-one teaching arrangement. The emotional side effects arising from her psychosocial and intellectual developmental problems are becoming more obvious. She is learning she is different and inadequate, and she tries to suppress her pain and confusion. She can relate to adults and is able to adjust her social behaviors to accepted norms, suggesting untapped potentials for further development of peer relations. Communication problems persist and must be cared for by specialists in that area. It is recommended that Sandra be placed in a special classroom.

Sandra's parents need counseling, since their interventions in programs that serve Sandra's needs hinders her progress. At the same time, as they overprotect and infantilize her, they deny her mental retardation. The term aphasia is evidently more palatable to them. Actually, the primary diagnosis should be mental retardation. It is not even clear whether Sandra's deficiencies are due to aphasia, since her speech problems resemble those often displayed by cerebral palsied children.

CAUSES OF RETARDATION

In Chapter 2 some of the causes of brain dysfunction were briefly mentioned: Rh incompatibility, rubella (German measles) in the mother, premature birth, damage to nervous tissue during delivery, infections, toxicity, or high fever. These factors can cause nervous tissue damage resulting in a variety of disorders: cerebral palsy with or without associated defects, aphasia, mental retardation, or any combination of these and related disorders and in any degree of severity. Why this is so remains to be determined. Limited knowledge is available regarding the specific factors that give rise to developmental defects. Even where there is knowledge, it is limited to what causes the disorder rather than to how the particular disorder comes about. High fever, for example, can result in retardation in one case, cerebral palsy in another, and aphasia in a third. This discussion, then, could just as easily appear in the previous chapter. Mental retardation, however, has a greater incidence than either cerebral palsy or aphasia without accompanying retardation. The disorders presented in Chapter 8 also are thought to result from mild brain dysfunction, but the extent to which actual brain damage is a factor is still unclear. For these reasons, the causes of brain dysfunction are presented at this time.

Severe intellectual retardation (IQ < 50) occurs in about 3.4 per 1000 individuals (Kushlick, 1964; Rutter, Graham, & Yule, 1970). The prevalence rate of children with developmental language disorders of a severe nature is slightly less than 1 per 1000 and that of cerebral palsy without accompanying severe retardation is about 2 per 1000. Among those with severe retardation where etiology is known, about a third have Down's syndrome (0.8 per 1000 in general population) and about a third have cerebral palsy (0.8 per 1000 in general population). The remainder includes those with ill-defined conditions. A very small percentage have lesions below the brain stem—muscular dystrophy and muscular atrophy (Chapter 5). Over 5 percent of institutionalized retardates are those whose retardation is due to unknown prenatal influences and structural defects from unknown causes (Payne, Johnson, & Abelson, 1969).

No effort will be made to catalogue the different types of structural defects leading to mental retardation or to present a comprehensive coverage of their various causes. Instead, several of the more puzzling types will be presented in detail. The reader interested in other types, some of which are listed in Table 3.1 but not described in the text, is referred to the standard texts on pediatric neurology or mental retardation (Ford, 1966; Sarason, 1969).

Structural malformation during fetal development

Four principles that apply to human fetal development are: (1) the kind of fetal effect an agent produces is dependent upon the time of its

Table 3.1 TYPES OF MENTAL RETARDATION

Chromosomal defects
1. Cri du chat (deletion of short arm of chromosome 5)
2. Trisomy 13–15
3. Trisomy 17–18
4. Down's syndrome (Trisomy 21)
5. Familial hydrocephalus (defective recessive gene?)
6. Female retardates with an additional X chromosome

Inborn errors of metabolism (associated with retardation)
1. Overflow aminoacidurias
   a. Phenylketonuria
   b. Maple syrup urine disease
2. Disturbances of lipid metabolism
   a. Cerebroretinal degenerations (e.g., amaurotic family idiocy)
   b. Niemann-Pick disease
   c. Heller's disease
3. Disturbances in carbohydrate metabolism
4. Gargoylism
5. Congenital ectodermosis
6. Miscellaneous
   a. Demyelinating disease
   b. Cretinism (thyroid deficiency)
   c. Lowe's disease

action during development; (2) a fetus can be greatly malformed by an agent that produces little or no effect on the mother; (3) the time of action of an agent may long postdate the time of its administration; and (4) the unborn child, particularly in the earliest phases of development, should not be considered as beyond the possibility of damage even within the safety of his mother's womb (Goldman, 1965). Keep these four principles in mind during the following discussion.

Chromosomal defects   Before considering genetic factors which lead to malformation, some basic genetics as well as the periods of neonatal development will be reviewed. *Meiosis* is the process of chromosomal division which occurs only in the development of egg or sperm. The number of chromosomes in every egg or sperm is reduced in two consecutive divisions from 46 to 23 with restoration to 46 following the union of sperm and egg in fertilization. All other chromosomal divisions during the entire life span of an individual are *mitotic* (the number 46 is reduplicated for each new cell formed).

During female fetal development, following development of the ovaries, eggs contained within the ovum start the first chromosomal division of meiosis and stop midway through the process. Nothing further happens until the woman is mature and ready to conceive. At that time, the egg is shed from the ovary to a fallopian tube. Ovulation then stimulates the egg to continue its first meiotic division where it left off many years earlier when the mother herself was a fetus. After such a long delay, abnormalities in this chromosomal division would not be surprising. Twenty-four to twenty-six hours after ovulation a father's sperm may fertilize the egg, whereupon the second meiotic division is completed. All further chromosomal divisions in the embryo and fetus are mitotic. The multicellular egg then makes its way down the fallopian tube and implants itself in the uterus. The implanting takes place around the ninth day of pregnancy. Differentiation of the embryo proceeds in this site until about the eighth or ninth week of pregnancy, at which time almost all central nervous system structures and other body organs are fully formed. From this period forward, the embryo simply grows.

Down's syndrome   While most genetic defects are lethal for the embryo, some chromosomal defects, such as an extra chromosome, result in central nervous system defects in a surviving infant. Mongolism (Down's syndrome) is one such defect. The usual form of mongolism, a trisomy of the twenty-first chromosome, occurs most frequently in older mothers and does not run in families. In some mongoloids of this type, the child has some cells containing an extra chromosome while the remainder have the normal number. This second kind is called a chromosomal mosaic (Richards, 1969).

The extra chromosome in the usual trisomy occurs during the second meiotic division in the fallopian tube between ovulation and fertilization.

This type of defective chromosomal division is not likely to occur more than once in any mother. It occurs more frequently in older mothers, where the tendency for abnormal division is greater in more aged eggs. The mosaic defect undoubtedly occurs within the first few mitotic divisions of early cleavage in the tube and within 24 to 48 hours after fertilization, since any chromosomal defect occurring during meiosis would be transmitted to all daughter cells. The highest correlation between maternal age and mongolism occurs with mosaic mongoloids.

A rare type of mongolism occurs when a part of or a whole extra twenty-first chromosome becomes attached to another chromosome so that the total number is still 46. This type, called chromosomal translocation, can occur in two or more children in the same family and is not correlated with age. The translocation defect is thought to occur during the first meiotic division when either the mother or grandmother of the mongoloid child is still a fetus. If formed in the grandmother, the translocated chromosome is passed to her offspring, half of whom would be normal with 46 chromosomes, while the other half would be carriers of the translocated chromosome. If a second error occurred during meiosis of these children, the following could happen: the normal, separate twenty-first chromosome could pass to the egg or sperm along with the twenty-first chromosome that is attached to the translocated chromosome, and a 21 trisomy would result upon fertilization. The other egg or sperm missing the twenty-first chromosome presumably would not survive following fertilization. Since the mother or father is the carrier of the translocated chromosome, a mongoloid child could occur more than once in the family. Because the defect occurs in the mother or grandmother's fetal life, the syndrome occurs independently of maternal age.

What causes these chromosomal abnormalities? We know that errors in mitosis occur more frequently in older women; perhaps the ovum, either through its own aging process or through some extraovarian bodily process, becomes more susceptible to virus attacks (Penrose & Smith, 1966). Extensive X-ray treatments, diseases such as hepatitis, and drugs such as LSD are suspected causes in some cases.

Because translocation defects occur in only 2 percent of all mongoloids, less is known about this phenomenon. The probability that a mother who is a carrier of the chromosomal translocation will have a second mongoloid child is about one in four. Fortunately, this condition can be diagnosed in the fetus through the use of amniocentesis of the mother's amniotic fluid, a process by which the amniotic fluid is placed in a centrifuge, the liquid part discarded, and the remaining pellet placed in a culture to grow. If this culture shows the translocation characteristic of mongolism, an abortion can be performed upon the mother's request.

CHARACTERISTICS OF CHILDREN WITH DOWN'S SYNDROME. The term mongoloid was first used over a hundred years ago by a physician named John L. H. Down. He erroneously labeled retarded children as mongoloids because certain characteristic physical features reminded him of the Mongoloid race. He felt their deficiency reflected regression to a primitive level of life, a level at which he considered the Mongol people. (Japanese physicians feel that patients with Down's syndrome resemble Caucasians, and Russians have always preferred the term Down's syndrome.)

There are eight striking features characteristic of children with Down's syndrome: (1) the back of the head is flattened, (2) the eyes have epicanthic folds (the skin at the inner corner of the eye forms a fold, making the eye look somewhat slanted), (3) the tongue is furrowed or fissured, (4) the neck is broad and short, (5) the iris of the eye is speckled (e.g., blue eyes with brown spots), (6) the hands are short and broad, with deep creases running straight across the palms, and the little fingers are curved, (7) the big toe and the second toe are separated by a relatively large gap, and (8) the bridge of the nose looks flat and the nostrils are noticeably tilted upward. Some of these stigmata can be seen in Figure 3.2. The three types of Down's syndrome (trisomy of the twenty-first syndrome, mosaicism, translocation) do not differ in the number or kind of stigmata (Payne et al., 1969), and only a few mongoloids possess all the characteristics. These stigmata are not unique to mongoloids. Other brain-disordered children often show some of these features. Their presence in children, therefore, can be diagnostic of central nervous system dysfunction.

The mongoloid child goes through a fairly normal development during early fetal growth. About the fifth to seventh week of pregnancy, developmental deceleration takes place, and anomalies of the brain, heart, bones, and eyes become apparent. After birth, development also is slow. The child will not walk until approximately 3 years, will not learn simple speech until 4, and will not be fully toilet trained until 5. One mongoloid in four will have a heart defect and approximately half will die before the age of 5. Most do not live to the age of 50. Early death is associated with higher incidence of leukemia, respiratory disease, heart lesions, and congenital duodenal disorders (Kirman, 1970).

The intellectual functioning of most mongoloids is quite limited. In an institutionalized sample of over 2500 cases, the mean IQ was 28.6 (Payne et al., 1969). Even the brightest do not score much above an IQ of 60. Rosecrans (1968) suggested that those with comparatively high ability are more often cases of mosaicism. However, another study found translocations to be the highest, trisomies intermediate, and mosaics the lowest in intellectual ability (Payne et al., 1969). The discrepancies in the findings have been ascribed to sample bias and variability. Previous research dealt, for the most part, with individuals whose comparatively high ability caused them to be selected for karyotyping (typing of chromosomal abnormality). "It may be that mosaics show a high amount

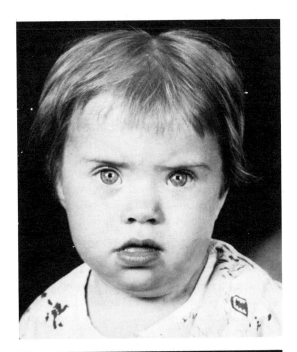

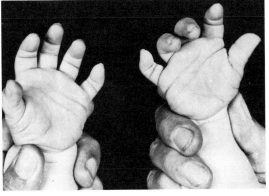

Figure 3.2
Characteristic features of mongolism: slanting eyelid fissures, epicanthal folds, protruding tongue, short head, prominent transverse palmar creases, small incurved fifth digits. (From N. Allen. Developmental and degenerative diseases of the brain. In T. W. Farmer (Ed.), Pediatric neurology. *New York: Harper & Row, 1964.)*

of variation in ability so that if, for example, one were testing the brightest 1 percent of Down's cases, one would find many of them to be mosaics, despite the fact that the mean for all mosaics is below that of the other two types of Down's cases" (Payne et al., 1969, p. 67). Some support for this interpretation was found in a sample of 296 karyotyped cases. Mosaics comprised only 6 percent of the sample, yet of the five cases with IQs above 60, one was a mosaic.

The finding that translocations had higher IQs supports Rosecrans's (: `l) hypothesis that the degree of excessive chromosomal material (which would be less in partial translocations) is related to the degree of physical and mental deficits. Rosecrans presented a child with partial translocation whose verbal IQ (86) was considerably higher than the majority of Down's cases. This child's behavior was overactive, aggressive, disruptive, and negativistic, in contrast to the bland and docile friendliness typically associated with Down's syndrome.

PSYCHOLOGICAL ADJUSTMENT OF DOWN'S CASES. Individuals with Down's syndrome are better adjusted and less aggressive than children of a similar age with other kinds of retardation (Moore, Thuline, & Capes, 1968; Johnson & Abelson, 1969). Mongoloids show significantly less maladaptive behavior and greater social competence than other retarded children of the same age despite their being slightly less intelligent. The differences in favor of Down's cases are largest in the area of self-help. Down's cases, however, are strikingly deficient in communicating to others understandably (Spreen, 1965).

Nevertheless, ward attendants in state schools for the retarded report that while most cases are happy, somewhat passive, and affectionate, some are active and aggressive. Johnson and Abelson (1969), therefore, examined their data for differences between the three types. They did find translocations to be more active and aggressive than the other two groups, but only a small proportion displayed problem behaviors. Of the five who did display aggressivity-activity, all were translocations. Rosecrans's case also displayed aggressive behaviors. Evidently, mongoloids with higher IQs are more aggressive. Strange, that the most abnormal possess those traits we'd like most for humanity—increased affection and decreased aggression.

Hydrocephalus Hydrocephalus is a condition in which the normal circulation of spinal fluid is impeded, resulting in increased intercranial pressure and progressive enlargement of the head. For various reasons, the absorption-reabsorption cycle of spinal fluid is irregular, causing progressive accumulation of unabsorbed fluids that distend the ventricles and cause the head to enlarge and the brain cortex to thin. With continued enlargement of the head, the skull sutures separate and the infant becomes progressively more helpless, first, because of inability to support the large head and later, because of accompanying damage to the brain.

Although hydrocephalus is usually a sporadic disorder that rarely recurs in the same family, there is a rare variety which is hereditary. Bickers and Adams (1949) were the first to propose that one form of hydrocephalus is inherited. Since then other investigators have reported family histories that reveal hereditary factors in hydrocephalus (Price & Horne, 1968). The disorder is probably due to a defective recessive gene on an X chromosome, since female carriers are unaffected while their male offspring can be affected. Around 5 percent of male hydrocephalies may be due to this hereditary factor.

Inborn errors of metabolism—phenylketonuria   The metabolism of various biochemicals (amino acids, fats, carbohydrates, etc.) is necessary for adequate brain tissue functioning. A disturbance of the metabolic process can result in brain dysfunction. A list of disorders resulting from inborn errors of metabolism appears in Table 3.3. We will discuss only one type of one form of disorder—phenylketonuria, an overflow disorder.

The overflow aminoacidurias are disorders characterized by elevated concentrations of one or more amino acids in the blood or urine. The metabolic defect results from an absence of the appropriate enzyme system to mediate the conversion of a particular amino acid to its end product. Excessive amounts of the unmetabolized amino acid accumulate in the body and are excreted in the urine. For this reason the disorders are referred to as overflow disorders.

Phenylketonuria (PKU) is a hereditarily transmissible defect in the metabolism of one of the amino acids—phenylalanine. The accumulation of the products of the incomplete metabolism of this acid are believed to lead to progressive damage of brain tissue and to eventual mental retardation. Fortunately, the incomplete metabolism leads to the excretion of an abnormal substance in the urine, which can be detected by a simple chemical test. When the urine test is positive, the defect can be partially controlled by a diet low in phenylalanine (Knox, 1960; O'Flynn, 1967). The extent to which diet can preserve mental functioning is currently being evaluated. Since most well-baby clinics now routinely screen for this disorder, a great deal more should soon be known about PKU.

Although the urine test is a relatively successful diagnostic technique, it was found that many cases of the disorder still went undetected. Affected infants frequently do not show a positive test until 4 to 6 weeks of age (Hsia, Berman, & Slatis, 1964), and by then the majority of children are discharged from the newborn nursery. Fortunately, a blood screening method has been developed which can be employed just prior to the child's discharge. Perfection of this technique has resulted in a method that combines a high probability of detecting affected infants with a small frequency of false positives.

PKU was first described by a veterinarian, Fölling, in 1934, and had it not been for the errors of others the discovery might have been delayed. Fölling was a relative of a Norwegian woman who had been unsuccessfully treated by a psychiatrist for an "obsession"; she had insisted that her child had a strange odor. When she persisted in this obsession, she was referred to a New York psychiatrist. After his "failure" to cure her of the obsession, she returned to Oslo and consulted her cousin Fölling. He accepted her obsession as real and proceeded to work out the nature of the metabolic defect (Jervis, 1953).

An infant suffering from PKU may appear normal for the first few weeks of life. Within six months, however, motor retardation becomes obvious. The child is usually unable to sit by 1 year and, like the mongoloid, may not walk until 3 or 4 years of age. A variety of eczema resistant to the usual forms of treatment may accompany the disorder, and skin and hair pigmentation may be lighter than the child's ancestry suggests.

Severe behavior problems with hypermobility, tantrums, and convulsions accompany the retardation, PKU groups being markedly more active and aggressive than other retarded children (Johnson, 1969). Mental retardation is usually severe in untreated children, the majority having IQs below 50 and usually below 20.

Although their numbers are small, intellectually normal children and adults have been found whose phenylalanine levels are above 20 mg per 100 ml, the classic PKU level (Hansen, 1970; Fisch, Doeden, Larshy, & Anderson, 1969). Other cases show mild hyperphenylalaninemia (levels above 4 mg per 100 ml) without adverse effects on their intelligence (Hansen, 1970). Of interest is that PKUs with normal intellectual ability do not show aggressive behavior (Siegel, Balow, Fisch, & Anderson, 1968).

Children with this disorder represent approximately 1 percent of all institutionalized retardates (Payne et al., 1969). The incidence calculated from those institutionalized was 1 in 25,000, but more recent surveys from screening of newborns places the incidence at a much higher rate, varying from 1 in 6800 (Ashley, 1970) to 1 in 14,000 (Hanley, Partington, Rathbun, Amies, Webb, & Moore, 1969; Levy, 1969). Levy's survey is perhaps the largest reported. Out of 517,206 newborns screened, 73 were considered hyperphenylalaninemics. Of these, 34 were classical PKUs, 11 were atypical cases, and 28 were cases in which phenylalanine tolerance later became normal. In Israel routine screening of 178,174 children revealed 7 cases of classic PKU (1 in 25,000) (Szeinberg, Cohen, Golan, Peled, Lavi, & Crispin, 1969). Perhaps Israelites are less prone to develop this disorder. Two disorders that occur almost exclusively in Jews are amaurotic family idiocy and Niemann-Pick disease. Both lead to rapid mental deterioration and early death (2 to 3 years of age). If true, low incidence of PKU among Jews would certainly be a blessing to them.

Control through diet PKU was only of academic interest until 1953 when Bickel (Bickel, Gerrard, & Hackmans, 1954) described considerable improvement in the behavior of a 2-year-old PKU child who was fed a diet low in phenylalanine. Based on the belief that phenylalanine was toxic to the brain, Bickel fed the child an artificial diet with a greatly reduced phenylalanine content. As the blood phenylalanine level fell, the girl's behavior improved and she became more manageable. A commercially produced diet was developed and has been available since about 1957.

Early research seemed to demonstrate that the sooner the child was started on the diet, the more favorable the results. One of the first studies of diets was that of Paine (1957). He presented data on children treated before 2 months, after 2 months, and those who were untreated. The mean IQs of the three groups were 85, 56, and 17 respectively. The mean IQ of unaffected siblings, however, was 109, suggesting that dietary restriction was not the entire solution to treatment.

Initially, clinicians assumed that the most effective dietary treatment would involve bringing blood phenylalanine levels to the same levels as found in normals. Early treatment attempts, therefore, tried to maintain blood phenylalanine levels at 1 to 2 mg per 100 ml, the reported norm. However, about a third of children with PKU failed to improve on the diet and another third made only moderate improvement (Fuller & Shuman, 1969). Some studies have shown no improvement in any subjects (Birch & Tizard, 1967). Some PKU children show malnutrition when blood serum phenylalanine levels are maintained at the norm (Sutherland, Berry, & Umbarger, 1970). Reports on the most effective phenylalanine level are in conflict. Some maintain that levels close to normal are more effective and others believe optimal levels should be higher.

In one study children under 18 months whose blood phenylalanine levels were kept below 5 mg per 100 ml through dietary regimens declined in intelligence, while those with diet regimens producing higher levels showed no IQ decrease (Fuller & Shuman, 1971). These results suggest that the phenylalanine need of younger PKU children is greater than that of normal infants. The level of serum phenylalanine does decrease with age (Pitt, 1969). Perhaps this natural decrease indicates less need for phenylalanine after the period of the body's most rapid growth. Dietary differences after a certain interval, therefore, would have less effect.

The finding that phenylalanine levels decrease with age explains why studies using institutionalized populations placed the incidence figure too low; with advancing age the serum level in many PKUs returns to normal. Blood tests, therefore, would fail to identify them as retarded due to PKU.

Another problem involved in dietary treatment of PKU children is determining when to discontinue the diet. A number of children have been taken off the diet before the age of 5, the age at which the brain has reached 90 percent of its adult size. Several early (pre-1965) follow-ups of children taken off the diet between 3 and 4 years of age revealed no deterioration (Horner & Streamer, 1959; Vandeman, 1963). O'Flynn (1967) discontinued the diets of eight children at approximately 5 years of age and reported no adverse effects. None of the children in the study displayed the behavior problems (hypermobility, aggressiveness, tantrums) noted in untreated children. She felt that children should be taken off the diet at about age 5, picking this age because there seemed to be no ill effects from such an action and because dietary maintenance places a strain on the family. Although there was less information available about dietary effects when she reached this conclusion, the reasons cited may still be valid.

1. As long as the infant can eat only exactly what his parents give him, there are few problems in diet maintenance. Once the child can walk, however, he becomes strongly motivated for regular foods and will go to great lengths to obtain forbidden goods. As he gets older and plays with other children, he will eat his friend's food. Extra-mealtime stealing, therefore, may render the diet ineffective. Consequently, after the first 12 to 18 months the ability to maintain good dietary control becomes increasingly more difficult.

2. Family problems are precipitated by the situation just described. Because the parents realize the importance of dietary restriction, the child's stealing results in problems between them and the child.

3. Poor response to the diet may be an indication to discontinue. A child whose improvement is minimal after a reasonable time on the diet may do better without the diet, since the family can relax its pressure on the child.

4. Although most states provide the diet free to affected persons, prior to state aid it was a financial burden to most families to keep a child on the diet.

The treatment model assumes that excess phenylalanine is toxic to the developing brain and that early termination, when the brain is less developed, should result in decreased functioning. Later termination should have less effect. Paradoxically, however, some children whose treatment is discontinued early (Fuller & Shuman, 1971) respond more favorably than those whose treatment is discontinued later. Perhaps this paradoxical effect is due to decreases in blood serum levels of phenylalanine with increases in age or to nutritional deficiencies in the artificial diet.

Fuller and Shuman's (1971) research showed that dietary discontinuation produced a decrease in IQ. The age at which diet was stopped, however, was not a factor. The significant factor was the degree of dietary control in the year prior to discontinuation. Of those on loose dietary control (9+ mg per 100 ml) the average loss was 3.9 IQ points; for those on a strict dietary control (2 to 9 mg per 100 ml) the average loss was 10.9 IQ points. These results suggest the use of less rigid dietary controls. When to terminate the diet, however, is still unclear. Termination, regardless of timing, resulted in a decrease in IQ, although the decrease was less for those on a loose diet during the preceding year. Since the brain does not reach its full growth until early adolescence, why not maintain the special diet until that time—why take chances?

Sex differences in PKU Some surveys report that the sexes are equally represented among institutionalized PKUs; others report that significantly more males make up younger PKU groups. This suggests that more male PKUs are born but that the total frequency for each of the sexes is equal because of a higher death rate among males (Payne et al., 1969). A second possibility, although no evidence exists for its support, is that testing for PKU may yield more false negatives for males than for females and that the undetected and thus untreated males become more severely handicapped and are, therefore, more likely to be institutionalized. This situation is unlikely for two reasons: first, screening tests miss females more often than males (Hsia & Dobson, 1970); second, studies of diet therapy show no sex differences (Baumeister, 1967). A third hypothesis is that institutional screening misses more younger females because of some yet undiscovered sex difference in fluctuations in blood phenylalanine levels.

The children of PKU children   We stated that PKU is hereditarily transmissible. Studies are now being made to check the effect of PKU on eventual pregnancies and births. A number of PKU children who have become mothers have given birth to children who were retarded but not necessarily PKU. Mothers with PKU undiagnosed in childhood also have given birth to retarded children as have those with hyperphenylalaninemia. Two sisters of near normal IQ and undiagnosed PKU had a total of 28 pregnancies; 16 terminated in spontaneous abortions and 12 resulted in microcephalic and mentally retarded live borns (Huntley & Stevenson, 1969). One PKU woman of normal IQ gave birth to 6 non-PKU but retarded children and had one spontaneous abortion (Fisch et al., 1969).

PKU screening usually is recommended as a part of an obstetric workup, and PKU women, if pregnant, are advised to avoid high protein diets and restrict phenylalanine intake, particularily if any previous pregnancies resulted in retarded offspring. Some physicians recommend tubal ligations or avoiding pregnancy, since the effects of dietary restrictions are unpredictable.

Examinations of those mothers with high phenylalanine levels indicated that mental retardation in their offspring was more closely associated with subnormal intelligence of the mother, low birth weight, and microcephaly of the child (Hansen, 1970). The biochemical disturbance was more likely to affect the child if it also had affected the mother's mental development.

A simplistic disease and treatment model   All these findings question the simplistic disease and treatment model originally proposed for children with PKU. The model states that the mental retardation in those with excess phenylalanine in the blood is caused by this excess, and the treatment for the disorder is simply the prevention of this excess. Obviously, investigators have barely scratched the surface in their efforts to uncover knowledge about this disorder. Most likely, differences among PKU cases will eventually be attributed to differences in development yet undiscovered.

Noxious agents and disease   Recall the principle that the kind of effect an agent produces on the fetus is dependent upon the time of the agent's action during development. The earliest period is the maturation of the egg in the mother. We have considered some of the influences on egg formation in our discussion of Down's syndrome. The earliest period during which an agent could affect sperm is when sperm is manufactured, a process which occurs in two to four week cycles. Several reports have described defective children whose fathers have taken thalidomide before conception. This phenomenon has been demonstrated in animals. Malformed rabbit fetuses have been born following thalidomide intake in fathers prior to conception (Goldman, 1965).

A second period in development occurs during the week following conception when the egg travels down the tube. Malformed infants have been born following the administration of several drugs during this period.

A third period is the period of embryonic differentiation that occurs between one and eight or nine weeks of pregnancy. This period is perhaps the most critical. At this time, metabolic influences, such as radiation, viral infection by German measles, hormones, drugs, or chemical agents, can produce malformed infants. Most studies show that German measles during the first two months of pregnancy can result in cardiac defects and cataracts that produce blindness. During the second to fourth months, it may produce central nervous system damage with or without deafness (Goldman, 1965). The damage at the later stage would be attributed to tissue injury rather than to structural malformation, and the symptoms displayed would resemble those resulting from postnatal encephalitis.

Drugs can produce infant malformation during the period of embryonic differentiation. Those taken by the mother for anticancer treatment prior to planned abortions are known to produce malformation. Others are considered harmful because malformation occurred in children whose mothers took the drug during this period. Drugs also produce malformations when taken by the mother during the fourth period of development, the period of fetal growth.

Malnutrition and maternal disease (e.g., respiratory infections, maternal diabetes, etc.) can cause brain disorders in offspring. The ancient beliefs that fright, shock, or stress could cause retardation were largely discounted during this century. Nevertheless, several studies have appeared that relate anomalies in animals to maternal immobilization, crowding, or isolation (Goldman, 1965). These findings could result in renewed interest in this topic.

Geography and season of the year also are related to the incidence of retardation. Knoblock and Pasamanick's (1958) work is perhaps the most significant piece of research in this area to have been performed prior to 1961. These two investigators reported a heightened incidence of retardation among children born in the winter and a lowered incidence among those born in the summer. They also showed an increased frequency of retarded children born in years when the summer was particularly warm. Consequently, they postulated that mothers who are exposed to high temperatures during the eighth to twelfth weeks of gestation are more likely to produce retarded offspring.

This finding contrasts with the knowledge that the maternal diseases that affect fetal development occur more frequently in the winter months. As a consequence, a greater percentage of retarded children should be conceived in late fall and winter and born in the summer. Payne, Johnson, and Abelson (1969) analyzed the birth records of 2666 institutionalized individuals retarded as a result of known prenatal causes. Those conceived in the period from October through March showed a significantly higher proportion of retardation resulting from prenatal influences. These investigators explain Knoblock and Pasamanick's contrasting findings as due to sampling error. Knoblock and Pasamanick simply examined the birth records of all individuals admitted to a state school. Many of the subjects in their study could have been retarded as a result of damage at birth or thereafter. Payne, Johnson, and Abelson examined only those with prenatal causes (10 percent of most institutionalized populations are retardates due to prenatal causes).

Prematurity Premature birth has been related to both intellectual and neurological impairment. Premature birth, itself, however, is probably not the causal factor in retardation (Drillien, 1954). Most likely, the mental and neurological abnormalities associated with prematurity result from defects originating early in fetal life that also cause premature birth. Research shows that complications of pregnancy or of delivery usually are not the primary causes of gross defect. If cerebral damage does occur because of these complications, prenatal conditions often are the predisposing causes of these occurrences.

Low birth weight, which usually accompanies prematurity, is related to lowered intellectual functioning. A preponderance of low birth weight children (below 4.4 lbs.) has been found among dull, retarded, and defective school age children (Drillien, 1954). Low birth weight, regardless of gestation period, has also been associated with mild and moderate mental retardation (Drillien, 1970). The incidence of low birth weight neonates and infants with a variety of developmental malformations is high among mothers with a history of infertility. In addition, low birth weight occurs more often among children from impoverished and deprived environments.

Relatively minor undernutrition during a time of relatively rapid brain growth can result in decreased weight and brain size (Davies & Davis, 1970). Rectal and axillary temperatures are higher in underweight children during their first week of life. If these conditions prevailed prenatally, perhaps energy derived from food was being diverted to heat production instead of being available for growth.

In any case, the majority of children born prematurely do not show major handicaps. In a follow-up study of 60 prematures, the IQ scores ranged from 64 to 111 with the majority falling in the range 70 to 100. IQ scores, however, were not predictive of achievement since many with high IQs showed underachievement. Underachievement may have resulted from the attentional deficiencies and extreme fatigability frequently found in such children (Boy, Lafont, & Villemin-Glog, 1969). The correlation of birth weight with IQ was not calculated in this study. In general, other studies have demonstrated that in infants below 4.5 lbs. there is a direct relation between intellectual functioning and birth weight (Wiener, 1970). Both very low and very high birth weight is associated with higher probability of subsequent mental retardation (Babson, Henderson, & Clark, 1969).

Functional deficits

Functional deficits in cognitive development may occur in cases where there are no detectable signs of prenatal structural malformation due to chromosomal defects, metabolic imbalance, or noxious agents. We do know that metabolic factors may produce subtle defects, and research with animals has explored some possible relationships between a variety of prenatal factors and functional difficulties.

Several studies have demonstrated that X-irradiation of pregnant rats results in offspring who appear normal but who perform more poorly than other rats on maze problems (Hicks, 1958). Rats exposed to tranquilizers during pregnancy (Werboff & Havlena, 1962), as well as to crowded living conditions (Keeley, 1962), also showed variations in behavior, most notably decreased activity and depressed exploratory behavior. In humans, however, the relationship between maternal psychoactive medication and later cognitive development has not been determined (Desmond, Rudolph, Hill, Clashorn, & Wreesen, 1969).

Hopefully, future research will ascertain the relationships between prenatal factors and functional difficulties. The interested reader is referred to Joffe (1969) for an in-depth presentation of this topic.

Tissue damage

Jack was only 5 months old when he underwent an operation for a hernia. He was a bright and cheerful baby, a joy to parents and grandparents alike. The operation was expected to be uneventful and while his parents were certainly anxious, they had been told not to worry. Nevertheless, during the operation Jack's heart stopped for a full five minutes before cardiac massage could restore its functioning. Five minutes! An interval of time which passes unnoticed in most lives. For Jack it meant profound retardation!

Evaluation revealed an undisclosed muscle atony (lack of muscle tone), and with the stress of anesthesia the heart muscle had relaxed completely.

Consequently, no blood was pumped to the brain. Since blood carries oxygen to the tissues, the brain tissue experienced profound lack of oxygen and, therefore, suffered irreversible tissue damage.

Of course, Jack's case is an unusual occurrence. In fact, in full-term infants the relationship between asphyxiation and neurological damage is still unclear. Careful follow-up studies of full-term infants with varying degrees of asphyxiation at birth have failed to reveal clear-cut relationships (Bakwin & Bakwin, 1966). Probably between 1 and 2 percent of retardation can be traced to anoxic damage at birth (Payne et al., 1969).

Damage to brain tissue can occur during the birth process or following any number of conditions to which the brain is exposed. Reitan (personal communication) feels that falls from bicycles, while rarely causing major retardation, do result in many minor neurological disorders.

Table 3.2 below lists those causes of retardation that may occur during or following birth. Surveys of institutional populations reveal that infectious diseases account for between 8 and 9 percent of the retarded children and physical trauma for approximately 12 and 13 percent. These figures are probably an underestimation considering that about 18 percent of institutional populations are diagnosed as retarded due to defects of an unknown origin and twice that number are considered hereditarily dull (Payne et al., 1969). The interested reader will find detailed presentations of these causes in most standard texts on mental retardation, the most recent edited by Koch and Dobson (1972) or in the annual review edited by Wortis (1972).

TRAINING AND EDUCATION

Mentally retarded children usually have sensory, perceptual, motor, and language defects accompanying their intellectual retardation. Abstracts of studies related to these defects appear in *Mental Retardation Abstracts*, a quarterly publication of the Division of Mental Retardation, Rehabilitation Services, U.S. Department of Health, Education, and Wel-

Table 3.2 POSTNATAL CAUSES OF RETARDATION

Perinatal
1. Anoxic damage to brain tissue
2. Birth trauma, i.e., hematoma, laceration
3. Hyperbilirubinemia (kernicterus)

Postnatal
1. Infections, e.g., meningitis, encephalitis, pertussis
2. Trauma, i.e., hematoma, laceration
3. Hypoglycemia
4. Spontaneous cerebrovascular accidents
5. Anoxic damage following drownings, shock, operations, etc.

fare, *Child Development Abstracts and Bibliography* published by the Society for Research in Child Development, and *Psychological Abstracts* published by the American Psychological Association. Reviews of these studies appear in *The Handbook of Mental Deficiency* (Ellis, 1963) and in the *International Review of Research in Mental Retardation* (Ellis, 1972).

The training and education of the retarded with brain impairment should proceed only after thorough assessment of the strengths and weaknesses of each child. Formerly, the large majority of these children received their training as residents of large state institutions. More recently, many are trained in public school classes for the trainable mentally retarded or in child development centers.

Remaining in the community is usually advantageous for the retarded child since institutionalization retards the development of many trainable children. For example, mongoloid children reared at home for at least the first two years of life are intellectually superior to mongoloids who are institutionalized at birth (Meindl, Barday, Lamp, & Yater, 1971; Cornwell & Birch, 1969; Shipe & Shotwell, 1965). There is some debate as to the nature of this superiority. Shipe and Shotwell (1965) found that home-reared children maintained their superior intellectual development for three years after being placed in an institution. Some investigators feel that these are short-lived differences, stating that noninstitutionalized mongoloids simply reach ceiling levels of intellectual development earlier than those reared in institutions (Barclay & Goulet, 1965). Still other studies suggest that the home-reared mongoloids maintain their higher functioning (Cornwell & Birch, 1969).

Kershner's (1970) study is one of the few indicating that institutionalization has a positive affect on some children. Community families, that is, families in which a retarded child is kept at home, showed decreases in functioning over the years in all measures taken, whereas institutional families, that is, families which institutionalize their retarded child, tended to improve in functioning. The continued presence of the retarded child interfered with the functioning of both the child and his family; separation of the child from his family resulted in improved family functioning. Nevertheless, intellectual functioning decreased in both home and institutionally reared children. Family functioning as well as the child's social and intellectual ability were both related to a family's decision to institutionalize their child. The significantly higher social than intellectual functioning among community-reared children may reflect a concerned family's efforts to help their child, while the higher intellectual than social functioning in the institutionalized children may be symptomatic of a stressful family situation that led to institutionalization.

The specific components of institutional and home environments need to be analyzed before one can articulate the question of institutionalization versus community as a series of meaningful and researchable hypotheses (Kershner; 1970; Tizard, Cooperman, Joseph, & Tizard, 1972). Investigators are just beginning to identify variables common to both home and institutional environments and to examine the reciprocal relationships between these variables and the development of retarded children. For example, an acceleration in verbal development has been observed when the social milieu in an institution is reorganized to resemble a family-type residential unit (Lyle, 1960). We will now discuss changes in institutional structure and organization that may lead to the improved functioning of residents.

PSYCHOLOGICAL EVALUATION: EDWARD, AGE 11-4

Reason for referral. Edward was referred for psychological evaluation in an effort to determine a meaningful treatment program for his difficulties. His family was completely disorganized, either because of his presence or because of their own interpersonal problems.

Behavioral observations. Edward was neatly dressed and very cooperative. He comprehended instructions and was responsive to the examiner. When complying to requests, Edward would fidget, squirm, and shift positions frequently, displaying considerable restlessness and attention to irrelevant detail. He often demonstrated difficulty in articulation; his rate of speech was uneven, with verbal perseveration, circumlocution, and flight of ideas. Eddy expressed his apprehension through excessive questioning and a careful check of the office. During testing, he displayed impulsive, careless behavior by responding quickly to problems without autocriticality.

Tests administered. Wechsler Intelligence Scale for Children, Rorschach, Kinetic Family drawings, Bender-Gestalt.

Results. Current intellectual functioning, as measured by the WISC, is at a moderately retarded level (verbal IQ 58, performance IQ 58, full scale IQ 54) and is consistent with results from previous testing (IQ 51). In spite of Edward's absence from school, he has managed to maintain his relative ranking within his age group and has even gained slightly. Nevertheless, analysis of the total picture indicates serious impediments to anything but minimal achievement functioning; vocabulary and general fund of information are at moderately retarded levels, while attention and concentration are at severely retarded levels. He functions at somewhat higher levels if materials are pictorial and anchored more to real-life situations requiring minimal conceptual ability. He can proceed as instructed on highly structured tasks, such as matching of symbols to numbers, but he is so slow and careful that his resulting performance is deficient.

Edward's best performance is on tasks calling for the assembling of objects that require anticipation of final products and appropriate motor manipulations; his functioning on these tasks is at mildly retarded levels and would be a place to start in efforts at remediation of academic deficits through use of strengths.

Edward's speaking vocabulary and expressive manner indicate potential for better functioning. Such discrepancy between test results and behavior, together with uneven intellectual functioning, points to the presence of interfering factors which could vitiate reaching this potential. Given the proper environment, Edward would function more adequately, but, at best, expectations would not exceed moderately retarded levels.

An analysis of projective data indicate weak, rather feeble defenses against expression of aggressive impulses in response to fears of aggression from others. It is apparent that hostile interchange is the rule in his home, interchange that colors his perception of external events. Such perception and limited conceptual understanding disrupt his appraisal of interpersonal situations and thereby prevent him from adequately coping with them. When feeling comfortable, however, he does demonstrate better ability to organize and integrate experiences, is less hyperactive, and is more attentive.

Edward has incorporated the view that he is crazy and inadequate, a view continually reinforced by the presence in the home of more competent siblings. In an effort to compensate for these inadequacies, he has taken to disrupting the family and being disrespectful; manipulation of his parents and siblings is reinforcing in spite of the punishing consequences, since it is his only way of exerting his influence and, thereby, feeling important. His father is viewed as more demanding, but there is little other differentiation between his parents, as if both are at times fused into one, and perhaps they are in their efforts to control him.

In spite of his difficulties, Edward is eager to relate to adults and this eagerness, coupled with his appealing qualities, forecasts an ability to profit from a more therapeutic environment.

Summary and recommendations. Edward is a moderately retarded youngster with an emotional overlay resulting from mismanagement. It is suggested that placement in an institution for the retarded would not only benefit Edward, but would also allow his parents to concentrate on solidifying other family relationships, which appear strained. It must be trying for all family members, including Edward, to have him continually at home. In another setting, rivalry with siblings would be reduced and manipulative behavior would become less necessary. Freed from managing Edward's behavior, his parents might develop a more positive relationship with him during visits and vacation periods.

Modifying the architecture

In Chapter 1 we discussed new service models, particularly small residential units employing live-in house parents, family subsidy, and day care. However, most states lack these facilities. Large institutions still flourish and new ones continue to be built. Because many severely retarded children will continue to live in institutional settings, we will give examples of how institutions can modify their physical structure in order to facilitate the application of new training techniques for developing self-care, perception, and socialization.

Redesigning a living unit Most modern institutions are composed of separate residential units of approximately 18 to 20 children. These units may be separate cottages or wings of a larger building. Figure 3.3 presents a fairly typical floor plan of such a unit. The unit is a single, large room with an adjacent bath. A 5-foot-high lattice room divider separates the bed area from the day area. An attendant station is located in a hallway outside the unit, with a "dutch door" between the unit and the hallway. Furnishings in the day hall consist only of a built-in bench and a wall-mounted television set. The bath contains two bathtubs, three toilet bowls, a wall-type sink, a service sink, and a wooden bench where the children are placed when their diapers are changed.

Children placed in such a unit are usually of the same sex and approximately the same age and IQ. These units house the severely retarded and could be described as medical-nursing units since little else can be provided for children who live in them. Occupants who cannot dress or feed themselves or care for their personal hygiene are not uncommon. The residents often lie on the floor for long periods and display behavior such as self-destructive biting, head banging, rocking, hair pulling, smear-

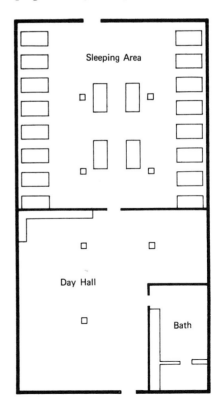

Figure 3.3 *Plan of residential living unit before architectural modification. (From C. E. Gorton & J. H. Hollis. Redesigning a cottage unit for better programming and research for the severely retarded.* Mental Retardation, *1965,* **3,** *16-21.*

ing of feces, masturbation, or preoccupation with minutia; the younger are often victimized by the more aggressive. Ward attendants provide only minimal protection since they cannot anticipate the aggressive behavior in time to intercede nor can they separate the children. Play materials are limited to paper or soft plastic objects so as to curtail injuries that can result from inappropriate use of more sturdy toys.

In such a unit, contact between attendants and children is limited; consequently, interaction that would stimulate learning of social skills is absent. Staff attend only to those children in imminent danger from self-destructive acts or from the aggression of others, those who soil themselves, or those who tear or attempt to destroy their clothing.

Teaching children to eat, dress, bathe, and care for their personal hygiene in such a facility can be more difficult than simply doing these things for them. The role of attendants, therefore, is frequently restricted to administering to physical needs, housekeeping, and paper work, a role which many find distasteful (Platt, Mordock, & Dorgan, 1969).

Gorton and Hollis (1965) demonstrate how architectural modification of the unit described can change its whole character. The unit was redesigned to satisfy two main requirements; the need to control and to facilitate acceptable interaction between the children and the need to delimit environmental space.

As depicted in Figure 3.4, the system consists of seven areas. The aide or attendant station is centrally located to provide closer contact between aides and children; windows in the various internal walls facilitate visual supervision. Bathing and toileting facilities were designed so as to be more conducive to training in self-care. A group play area accommodates children who can play together appropriately. The larger day hall, the operant area, was originally equipped with partitioned units to provide individual play spaces, but this system was later abandoned because one aide could not monitor children in all the units adequately. The units were replaced by three large tables. Two have flat surfaces for drawing, puzzles, or games. The third table has six recessed boxes with transparent lids, each box containing candy that children could obtain by operating various types of latches.

Staff assigned to this redesigned unit are trained to observe children more objectively, to use reinforcement procedures to increase desirable and to extinguish undesirable behavior, and to group children in ways that ease management problems. The following procedures are incorporated into daily care: (1) immediate positive reinforcement following a desirable behavior, (2) frequent reinforcements at first and then a gradual reduction of frequency after the desired behavior is established, (3) reinforcement of small improvements and building toward a more complicated, larger chain of responses, and (4) ignoring undesirable behavior (Gorton & Hollins, 1965).

Procedures were developed to encourage independent eating habits

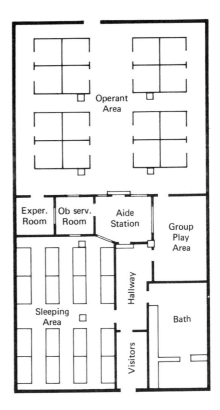

Figure 3.4 *Plan of residential unit after architectural modification. (From C. E. Gorton & J. H. Hollis. Redesigning a cottage unit for better programming and research for the severely retarded.* Mental Retardation, *1965,* **3,** *16-21.*

for nonfeeders. The instructor takes the child's hand and secures it to a spoon filled with food. He moves the child's hand and the spoon to his lips several times and then stops the spoon about half an inch from the child's lips. Eventually, the child moves the spoon the remaining distance. The instructor then releases the hand at increasing distances from the child's lips. In this fashion, the child eventually learns to feed himself.

This procedure can be applied to most behavioral acts. The child is first taken through all the steps that comprise a specific act. Then he is required to perform the final step, then the last two steps, until, by completing successively more of the sequence, he is able to perform the entire act by himself. A manual for child care workers prepared by the Southern Regional Educational Board (Bensberg, 1965) gives more examples of this procedure.

Redesigning the institution Procedures such as these can be employed more effectively in units architecturally designed for such purposes. Another example of how an institution can modify its architecture to suit its training approach is the Children's Habilitation Unit at Wassaic State School in Dutchess County, New York. The Habilitation Unit within the larger institution is divided into four wards to suit children at varying levels of ability. The wards are labeled P-1, P-2, P-3, and P-4. P-4 receives severely retarded children who need extensive training in basic self-care practices, particularly toilet training. P-3 receives patient-residents who are physically handicapped in addition to retardation and who require an intensive physical therapy program. P-2 functions as an extension of P-4 and receives children from P-4 who are approximately 70 percent toilet trained. P-2 is concerned with completing toilet training and beginning perceptual and socialization training. P-1 receives children promoted from P-2 and is concerned with developing greater social and perceptual abilities. In this ward emphasis is placed upon the child's developing responsibility for managing his own behavior. Most of the children in P-1 simultaneously attend trainable classes in the school associated with the institution. Within each ward children are cared for in small groups (4–6), the members of whom engage in activities suited to their developmental level.

The Children's Habilitation Unit uses an operant approach to developing behaviors and also employs game-like training aids to encourage perceptual development, sequential thought, and socialization. On the day-room floor separating P-1 from P-2 are colored designs. The first design, the coordination figure eight, is laid out in bright red in the shape of the figure eight. Design 1 has a path width of 32 inches. The child, under supervision and according to ability, negotiates the course by using a walker, walking, or riding a bike; the idea is to stay on the path. Reward follows each successful approximation of the desired performance. Improved coordination, orientation of body in space, directionality, and ability to function within definite limits are the goals of participation in this activity. Improving these skills is thought to increase the child's ability to adapt to new situations, to avoid simple hazards in the environment, and to develop confidence in the control of his own body.

Design 2, the 180 degree switchback, is painted bright yellow and used to impart the concept of angular navigation in order to improve the child's ability to negotiate sidewalks, hallways, and other situations requiring abrupt turns. The design is an extension of the first, since the severely retarded has more difficulty negotiating sharp turns in rapid succession than negotiating slow winding turns.

Designs 1 and 2 are the first in a series of figures, each designed to increase judgment, planning ahead, and sequential thought. Each can be adapted for many games, games that increase attention while avoiding monotonous routine.

Goals of training

Goals for trainable youngsters include the development of self-help skills; physical coordination and manual dexterity; communication skills, including a protective vocabulary; limited proficiency in selected academic areas, including acceptable work habits; and adjustment to change and challenge. This last goal is particularly important in order to avoid the development of the "institutional personality," so often mentioned as a feature of long-term residential placement.

Repetition is essential with these youngsters, but healthy repetition rather than extended classroom drill. Varied experiences free the child from monotonous, routine learning. The aide or child care worker, as a part of the child's day-to-day living situation, can offer this varied exposure, having at her disposal more tools and opportunities than does the classroom teacher.

Certainly, the classroom teacher has a variety of educational materials available to her, but as materials they are one step removed from life, often only representations of real objects. As representations, the materials are abstract. Retarded youngsters have difficulty with abstract and symbolic material. No amount of formal instruction about the weather, for instance, will substitute for the multisensory experience of being exposed to changes accompanying the rapid onset of a rainstorm, nor can a lesson in geography adequately substitute for the child's "map" of his immediate personal surroundings.

PSYCHOLOGICAL EVALUATION: BARBARA, AGE 3-6

Reason for referral. To determine the extent of her mental functioning.

Previous testing. None.

Tests administered. Stanford-Binet Form L–M (IQ indeterminable).

Test interpretation. Although Barbara sat still for testing, she moved her head constantly and her eyes did not fixate on objects. Stimulation for head movement did not seem to be a function of the external environment. When objects were placed in front of her, she rarely looked at them. The examiner had to hold the objects in front of her eyes, move them back and forth or tap them on the table to elicit her attention. It could not be determined if the tapping was heard, as this method of eliciting attention was not always effective. She made no effort to put blocks into a formboard or to look for a kitty hidden under a cup. She would not imitate the examiner's actions when he played with toys, but she was stimulated by candy.

Summary and recommendations. Barbara's mother states that she is just beginning to play with toys. Possibly testing at a later date, when her play has become more frequent, might show some change from the present administration. At present, she is considered a severely retarded youngster.

The child care worker should ask himself three basic questions about each child in his care: What can he do with what we present to him? What does it mean to him? What could it lead to later on? An outline of general methods to be employed by workers in the residence is presented in Table 3.3.

Table 3.3 SENSORY TRAINING IN THE HOME: METHODS AND TECHNIQUES

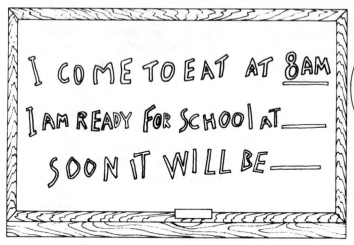

I. Concept formation

A. Direction, location, motion
1. Up-down—stairs
2. Left-right—shoes, parts of the body, locations in the residence
3. Top-middle-bottom—dressers, ranking progress, etc.
4. First-last—group formations, games, etc.
5. Slow-fast (motion)—walking to class, dining hall, activity areas

B. Size, weight, height
1. Big-small—comparisons among peers
2. Tall-short—people, objects, buildings, etc.
3. Light-heavy—objects in their environment

C. Amount
1. Few-many-some—(during snacks)
2. All-none—(trips)
3. Pair—shoes, socks, etc.
4. Numbers—counting by 1's, 2's, etc.

D. Time
1. Morning-afternoon-evening
2. Sequence of days, months, and year
3. Calendar
4. Four seasons
5. Telling time
    a. Wrist watch
    b. Room clock, school clock
    "I come to eat at _____."
    "I get ready for school at _____."
    "Soon it will be _____."

E. Temperature (thermometer)
1. Hot-cold—while washing and showering, touch window pane, while eating (tea, soups, etc.)
2. Warm-cool—room temperature, outside temperature changes
3. Changes in weather
    a. Rain, snow, cloudy, mild, etc.
    b. Proper dress for weather conditions

II. Arithmetic

A. Use of numbers
1. Home and school addresses
2. Telephone numbers and telephone directories
3. Important holidays, birthdays, etc.
4. Counting objects
   a. Laundry—"6 sheets in laundry bag," etc.
   b. Evening "treat"—"1 candy bar each, 2 cookies," etc.
   c. Money concepts—35 cents for admission to roller rink, 25 cents for candy and cokes, $1.00 bus fare, school lunches, savings, earnings for a job well done

III. Language arts

A. Speaking
1. Relating incidents—personal or general nature
2. General information
   a. Name and address (repetition)
   b. Telephone number
   c. Birthdate, etc.
3. Telephoning
4. Ability to arrange events in sequence
5. Expressing opinions
6. Making oral reports
7. Vocabulary development
8. Good speech habits
   a. Reproducing songs or short poems
   b. Memory and recall
   c. Speaking clearly
B. Listening—to home requests and commands
C. Handwriting—letter writing, laundry slips, etc.
D. Spelling—general communications
E. Reading—magazines, library books, home letters, etc.
F. Geography
1. Personal geography of immediate environment
2. Directions—"How do you get to the bathroom?"

IV. Social competencies

A. General expression—"good morning," "good afternoon," "good evening"; "thank you," "you are welcome," "OK"; "excuse me," "I beg your pardon," "pardon me"; "may I _____?"
1. School
   a. Upon arrival and departure
   b. Asking for school materials and supplies
   c. Small group formations
   d. Asking for privileges
   e. Recreation and play period (others)
2. Residential setting
   a. Upon arising and retiring
   b. General everyday information
   c. Permission and assistance requests
   d. During meals
   e. School functions—parties, dances, etc.
B. Other social skills
1. School
   a. Getting along with teacher and classmates
   b. Obedience to school rules and regulations
   c. Sharing with others in school
2. Residential setting
   a. Getting along with roommates and house parents
   b. Obedience to home rules and regulations
   c. Sharing with others in residence

From J. B. Mordock & V. J. Selvaggio. The child care worker and sensory training. *Devereux Schools Forum*, 1969, **5**, 25–32.

Very few trainable youngsters can play together. Child care workers often comment on this inability and fail to understand why it exists. A closer examination of what constitutes play will clarify this situation. To play, a child has to interpret a situation and recreate it in some manner in a meaningful fashion. If a child cannot understand the daily symbols to which he is exposed, he certainly cannot use these symbols to recreate anything meaningfully. These youngsters exploit objects only for their sensory qualities, since to use them in any other fashion requires abstract abilities that they do not possess. They therefore have to be taught to play, and the child-care worker is in an excellent position to provide such teaching.

Many retarded children become impatient when anticipating events because they think such events should happen immediately (Mallison, 1968). Time should not be taught in hours or minutes, but as large and meaningful divisions of the child's day. Only when the child has time concepts involving sequences of events, can he be helped to anticipate what is going to happen next. Again, such instruction is within the province of the child care worker or aide. As such understanding develops, tantrum behavior often decreases since many outbursts result from a lack of real understanding of what to do, causing anxiety, frustration, and loss of behavior control.

Retarded children lose control more easily when in groups. A child withheld from participation in group activities is not being deprived if these activities cause disorganization. Often birthday parties and family visits are disappointing, since the child cannot handle the change in routine and becomes upset. Until he gains security in his abilities, can communicate better, and can understand what is involved and what he is expected to do, these events will only precipitate tantrums, disruptive behavior, and acting out.

Mallison (1968) suggests rehearsal of special events. For example, when a birthday party is to occur, the child should invite only one or perhaps two friends, he should rehearse beforehand the games he will play, and the party should last only a short time. Rehearsal of trips and visits home or to the hospital can help prepare the child for a change in routine. He can make a picture-storybook about the coming event to itemize some of the things that will occur, and he can take it with him as a reference should he become confused. Having him make his own book is better than reading or telling him what to expect since he can "read" it over and over until he develops security in the knowledge of what is expected. This procedure can be modified to include the development of social understanding. The child care worker, through the medium of a play or show, can, in a pretend fashion, reshape the pattern of usual conflicts that occur between children. Questions can be asked such as "What could they do instead?" Various alternative courses of action can be tried in the safety of a show.

Mallison also states that many retarded youngsters are confused by television viewing. They see actors behaving in ways not acceptable in real life. They lack the sophistication to interpret such observed actions as untrue and often do not comprehend the language that accompanies such actions. Since they tend to imitate what they see, their conceptual inadequacies get them into trouble. The procedure of reenacting interpersonal conflicts can be employed to clarify television shows. Restricted viewing is necessary, however, as many shows cannot be reenacted.

Turning to more specific individualized techniques, an example will be given from a program developed for a 6-year-old neurologically impaired child who communicated in single words only, appeared "willful," either taking what he wanted or pointing with others' hands, and displayed frequent temper tantrums. No one could determine how much he understood.

The child care worker participated in programming in the following manner. Although handedness was not established, the child seemed to prefer his left hand, and so the child care worker attempted to promote the child's left hand as dominant. The worker was not to tell the child to switch hands when he played by himself, but was to hand things to his left side or place things in his left hand. Simple toys that the child could assemble, such as graded rings and boxes, were used to introduce the concept that he not only had to assemble toys but also had to wait for a verbal command, for instance, "Take it out," before being handed a desired item. The child was handed nothing unless told its name and unless he looked directly at the speaker. He was also forced to look directly at people when he returned an object, since many children with similar disabilities often expect someone or something to be there to receive what they return, a level of conceptual development characteristic of the very young infant. The child must be forced to realize that other people exist separately from him and his whims. Many times the youngster's hand had to be moved around to facilitate his looking at the worker.

Simple manipulative toys were used to teach colors, sizes, and counting. Concepts such as *big* and *little* were introduced and later combined with color concepts, e.g., *big red, little red*. Everything to which the child was exposed was given a name, starting with nouns that could be used as a basis for later communicative skills. The noun *apple* was learned and then the verb which went with it—"Eat apple." Articles of clothing were treated in the same way, for instance, *hat*—"Put on hat." "Put on hat" is considered a better phrase than "wear your hat" because the child can later substitute only two words and ask "Can I put on hat?" Since imitation is so common in these youngsters, we should use it to our advantage. To promote abstract abilities, pictures of common objects were placed on the wall of his room rather than remote objects that he probably would never see.

Language development

Perhaps more important than any other skill is skill in communication. The delayed speech and language deficits of retarded children constitute a major impediment to their social, emotional, and vocational adjustment. Five levels of normal speech development have been detailed. The first level, *reflex activity*, is the production of isolated sound and syllabic chain utterances without apparent auditory awareness. The second level, *babbling*, emerges in the second month. The child amuses himself by producing phonemes and gurgles ranging from soft to loud. The third stage, *lalling*, occurs when the child uses more frequently sounds that influence others. At about 10 months, the child becomes aware of the sounds of others and imitates these sounds (Goda, 1960; Rigrodsky & Goda, 1961). The latter stage is called *echolalia*. The final stage of speech development, the stage of *language*, is the acquisition of one or several meaningful words. The retarded child may not be able to progress unaided through these levels or may make only extremely slow progress. Goda (1969) presents specific procedures to develop speech in children at each of the different levels. For example, if the child makes sounds for kinesthetic pleasure only, without auditory awareness, the program would seek to involve the child in hearing his own sounds. If the child is at the lalling stage, an instructor would repeat the utterance of the child and reinforce him for repeating it back. Through such a procedure, a speech response is developed between the child and another individual.

Goda stresses that language should be associated with activities the child finds pleasurable. Initial language training should involve words that are important to the functioning of the particular child receiving the language stimulation. In this vein, Goda (1969, p. 24) relates his experiences with one youngster.

The writer related language naturally to toy trains and cars which one non-speaking retarded youngster of four years always carried in his pockets. He would remove them, place them randomly on the floor, and then put them back in his pocket. His play activities were enlarged to include holding of the toys in the air, putting them on various surfaces, and placing them in the four corners of the room. The speech associated with the activity was "car," "see the car," "see the car now," "here is the car," "see the train," "here is the train," "I have the train," etc. The parts of the toys were examined. The wheels were manipulated. There was finally a collision between the train and car. The first word imitated by the youngster emerged from the collision. The word "crash" was spoken. The child enjoyed the activity and imitated the word. There were many "crashes" following the initial one. Each happening resulted in the word and gales of laughter. From these initial episodes we were able to "talk" about cars and trains. This youngster liked chocolate candy and he selected a piece whenever he desired from a metal box decorated with animals, a favorite toy of his brought from his home.

Goda is a highly trained speech pathologist, but language-based curricula can be implemented by nonprofessionals (Hallet, Sype, & Gates, 1971). Child care workers and psychiatric aides have been successfully trained as language developmentalists under the supervision of speech pathologists (Guess, Rutherford, Smith, & Ensminger, 1970). In addition, operant conditioning techniques have been successfully used with severely retarded children (Bricker & Bricker, 1970; MacCubrey, 1971). These techniques can be implemented by child care staff or attendants or perhaps by volunteers. For example, children given intimate personal contact with a foster grandparent, a person age 60 or over, during the first few weeks of institutionalization, were judged to be better adjusted than those without such contact (Friedsam & Dick, 1968). Perhaps such contact could also be used to increase verbal skills.

What are educational programs like today?

While we are hopeful that institutions for the retarded will change their institutional design so as to make better use of their staff, surveys of institutions reveal that architectural modifications such as we have presented are still the exception rather than the rule. This handicap and a shortage of personnel make it difficult to institute the kind of remediation we have just been discussing.

Each year newspapers and television stations run feature editorials describing the deplorable conditions that exist in many institutions. In 1966 Blatt and Kaplan (1966) published *Christmas in Purgatory*, a pictorial essay of the back wards of hospitals for the retarded in five eastern states. In 1969 Philadelphia television stations did a feature on Pennhurst State School for the Retarded, which they considered a public disgrace. In 1972 conditions at Willowbrook State School in Staten Island were exposed to the public. As a result of such exposure, congressional investigations are called for, institutional personnel ask for more money, politicians make promises to parent groups, and token amounts of money are made available. Since the parents of retarded children represent a small minority, politicians rarely formulate platforms designed to capture their votes. Usually change comes about because influential people take a personal interest, President Kennedy because of his retarded sister or Vice-President Humphrey because of his mongoloid grandson.

The National Association for Retarded Children and its state and regional chapters, along with the American Association for Mental Deficiency and the Council for Exceptional Children, have been successful in obtaining legislation on behalf of the retarded. In order to support change, however, people need to know what change to bring about.

HOW DO THEY FARE?

Like cerebral palsied individuals with IQs of less than 50, the majority of severely retarded individuals remain dependent upon others throughout their life. Most remain within institutional settings, and their IQ score is the best predictor of the degree of independent functioning they display (Johnson, 1970). Many children decline in intelligence and social competence after placement in institutions and as a result are less competent as adults (Mitchell & Smeriglio, 1970; Provence & Lipton, 1962; Vogel, Kun, & Meshorer, 1967). The average IQ of the institutionalized adult mongoloid was found to be 24 (Sternlicht & Wanderer, 1962), a figure less than would have been expected had they remained in the community.

We have already mentioned that decline in cognitive functioning can be avoided and that the institutional environment can perhaps be as adequate as a home environment, provided that daily learning experiences beyond simple attendant care are present. Nevertheless, atypical patterns of social competence and intellectual functioning, together with language retardation, still occur in children exposed to relatively stimulating environmental regimens (Mann, 1967). Consequently, while improvement within the institution is possible, most severely retarded children will remain institutionalized.

A small percentage of those with IQs between 50 and 60 do leave the institution and make a satisfactory adjustment. If a prevocational and vocational training program exists on the grounds of the institution or a sheltered workshop is provided within the community, many more can return to community settings following vocational training. Some can leave the institution to work in the community during the day and return to the institution at night.

The largest number of retarded individuals are employed in occupations such as cleaning, food service, and maid service. But even as our institutions are developing better job training programs, our society has less need for unskilled labor. The severely retarded lack the stamina for physical labor, the coordination for key punch or stenographic work, and sometimes the attentional skill for many assembly line tasks. While the outlook for residential care looks brighter, the outlook for employment looks dimmer. Shoe repair, book binding, and other trades previously open to the retarded have all but disappeared.

Wolfson (1970) examined the status of a group of retarded adults twenty years after their return to the community. The majority of the retarded in this study, however, were in the mildly retarded range and probably would be considered as falling within the familial group of retardates discussed in Chapter 11, rather than the brain-disordered group discussed in this chapter. The sample also included 66 males and 97 females who were expected to become self-supporting. Among the 66 males, 38 (57.5 percent) had been steadily employed for a number of years. Employment levels varied from holding positions with some responsibility, such as railroad work, factory work, or practical nursing, to farming, dishwashing, or working in bowling alleys. Ten were dependent and worked in a sheltered workshop or remained at home; 7 had led a vagabond existence, 1 of whom died in a prison; 10 developed psychoses and of these 8 were in state hospitals, 1 died, and 1 returned to the institution and died while in residence; the status of the last of the 66 was unknown.

The status of the 97 female patients was as follows: 49 (50 percent) were married, 39 living on a modest but adequate socioeconomic level and 10 living on a marginal socioeconomic level; 15 were single, widowed, or separated, but working steadily; 6 who were admitted as adults because of failure to cope with family were back in the community and adjusting satisfactorily; 8 were dependent; 9 were making a poor adjustment; 6 had developed psychoses and were hospitalized; and 4 had returned to the institution and remained there. Evidently, a greater number of women make a more favorable adjustment to the community than men, perhaps because marriage demands less from them than the responsibilities of employment.

The IQ scores of the individuals studied were compared with those obtained during their institutionalization some twenty years earlier. While IQ scores are fairly stable, one-third of retested retardates achieve scores that vary from their original scores by more than 10 points, usually in the direction of higher scores; variations in scores are more common in males than in females (80 percent of females score within 10 points of their school IQs). In addition, there are ethnic differences in the frequency of discrepant scores. More than 50 percent of Puerto Rican males and 40 percent of black males achieve retest scores 10 points or more higher than their original scores (Tobias, 1970).

Most likely, only a few children classified in the category of retardation discussed in this chapter are included among those released from institutions; the majority released have IQs in the mild and borderline retarded category, and they represent only 14 to 15 percent of most institutional populations. Approximately 70 percent of institutionalized retardates need help in grooming, nearly 60 percent need help in dressing, and over 40 percent need help in toilet use; about 65 percent have impaired speech and are on drug medication (Payne et al., 1969). Obviously, the large majority of brain-disordered retardates remain in institutions throughout their life. Arnold is such a case.

ARNOLD, AGE 34

Minutes of the team meeting in 1966, when Arnold was 30, described him as a problem student who had difficulty with self-control. During June of 1966, Arnold was transferred to Unit 6 where it was felt that he might profit by being with others of a similar age who had developed some responsibilities.

Arnold was enrolled in the vocational program but failed to meet the unit's work standards. He was effective doing routine and repetitive tasks, but his performance was not predictable. His behavior, however, did change substantially. He became more cooperative, related well to both students and staff, and his attitude was regarded as excellent.

The parents applied for social security benefits for Arnold in late 1969, but the claim was denied after he was examined and considered able to obtained some kind of substantial, gainful work. The case was reexamined and, in the light of reports sent from the institution, the decision not to give benefits was reversed.

During August, 1970, Arnold was transferred to Unit 5. Staff indicated that he had again presented problems of impulse control. At Unit 5 Arnold was a helper, doing necessary chores to assist the aides. He had an avid interest in watching television and reading about sporting or current events. At this time his functioning was described as follows.

Arnold had limited ability to handle many elements of his environment simultaneously. He could not discriminate accurately and wasn't equipped for decision making. His solutions to problems were unrealistic and, because he preferred to act on the impulse of the moment, his effectiveness in coping with his environment was reduced to a bare minimum. Arnold's attitude was pollyannaish and his grasp of reality immature. Never having taken much responsibility for his own actions nor having achieved much through his own efforts, his characteristic attempt to master situations was to hope for the best. Wish-thinking was, therefore, omnipresent as a palliative.

In a very general way, Arnold was aware of his limitations. On the one hand, he outwardly expressed wishes to support himself and to make his family proud of him, while on the other hand, he feared that he would never leave the institution. Because he had no idea as to the procedures he should take toward realizing his goals, he turned to accomplishment through wishing. He had no real sense of self and no understanding of what is meant by self-determined behavior. He acted as if all he had to do was to wait and things would work out for the best. Self-initiative was, therefore, foreign to his thinking. He had no idea of behaviors and their meaning nor did he understand the consequences of social actions. His life was reduced to the simplest interactions and most of what went on around him was not fully appreciated nor understood.

Primitive religious concepts pervaded his life. He proclaimed that if one had faith enough, things would work out for the best. Life was dichotomized into the good and the bad, and if one was good, he would be taken care of. Religion was the controlling force in his life. In kind of a magical way problems would be solved by the deity. Thus his super-ego was primitive. If he did wrong, he feared punishment from external sources rather than from his own conscience. Internal standards for conduct were, therefore, minimal.

Arnold was extremely dependent upon support from his environment. His reactions to these dependent needs were mixed. He projected the responsibility for his own actions onto others and rationalized his failures by denying their importance. He also became very hostile when his impulses were not immediately gratified, and in anxiety-arousing situations he would deny the existence of affect. He showed ambivalence when discussing his goals by first saying he wished he were a responsible person and then saying he would like to retreat from responsibilities and just sleep. He was concerned that his parents would die and that there would be no one to care for him. Unconscious hostility was directed toward his parents, for he believed they had rejected him. His defense against these feelings was to deny them and adamantly profess love for his parents. Further, by denying the existence of hostile feelings toward all people, he attempted to convey the impression that he was never aggressive or assertive.

On a standard test of social maturity, given to him when he was 34, Arnold attained a social age of 13-6 years. He was reported to be interested in reading and keeping up with current events, particularly those of the sporting world. He could communicate by letter and handle the purchase of minor articles, but inconsistently performed responsible routine chores. He no longer participated in those social activities he enjoyed in the past. Although he was never one for dances and social gatherings, he had been involved in the sports program. Due to his age, he now limited himself even further by no longer participating in athletics. Evidently, he had not developed age-appropriate interests in athletic activities of an individual nature. He did not play table games nor did he have any hobbies with which to occupy his time. He spent most of his leisure time watching television or socializing around the unit.

Although Arnold's intelligence as measured by the Wechsler was at marginal levels, when confronted with problem solving situations, he produced oversimplified and inaccurate solutions. His thinking was at very immature levels, as he could not deal with any sort of complex situations. Even when coaxed to try harder, he had no procedure to follow to arrive at any sort of solution. When he did not know an answer, he gave up rather than struggle with even trial-and-error methods.

Comparison of most recent to prior evaluations indicates that Arnold has consistently functioned within the marginal range of intellectual ability. It appears unlikely, therefore, that future testing will reveal any hidden abilities. Further, certain vocational outlets will be unavailable to him, since he displays the perceptual-motor dysfunction often characteristic of brain-damaged retardates.

Arnold's inability to maintain himself in a heterosexual environment and his state of nonstriving point to a very guarded prognosis. The outlook is for life-care, in a supervised and controlled environment.

Factors impeding adjustment

More of the moderately retarded like Arnold could return to the community after residential placement or perhaps avoid institutionalization altogether. We have stressed that inadequate training programs and community facilities limit the retarded's potential for adjustment. Over 60 percent of the retarded in Payne, Johnson, and Abelson's (1969) survey never went home to visit, 30 percent never had visitors, and 28 percent never received mail. This isolation from family and community makes community adjustment all the more difficult.

Another impediment to satisfactory community adjustment is the attitude of community members about the retarded. People with extremely low intelligence tend to be the least popular members within the community social framework and those who are considered retarded are often avoided (Dentler & Mackler, 1962). Guskin (1963) summarized the research related to attitudes held about mental retardation as follows: (1) associations to the term mentally retarded include abnormality, inadequacy, and helplessness; (2) the term is seen as similar to mentally ill and emotionally disturbed, as somewhat related to delinquent, and very different from average; (3) these associations are widely held, particularly by unsophisticated people.

Guskin also formed the following hypotheses about interaction between the retarded and other members of the community. (1) Adults who believe that a child is defective will be more likely to give him easier tasks, to assist him more in play, and to be less critical of his performance. (2) A retarded individual will do less well on tasks when others present are concerned with his needs for protection and assistance than when others are not so concerned. (3) If a subnormal and normal person work together on a task defined as requiring ability and the subnormal individual is labeled retarded, (a) the normal person will tend to help the retarded person with his task in addition to doing his own, (b) the retarded individual will not learn the task as well, but (c) he will be judged favorably by the normal person. (4) If subcultures or communities hold particular views regarding the retarded, the behaviors displayed by the retarded in these communities will tend to conform to these views. For example, retarded individuals living in groups that expect childlike behavior from them will show less adult behavior, and those living in groups that expect delinquent behavior will be more delinquent. (5) Parents or parent surrogates who react to all children in terms of protectiveness, authoritarian control, and fostering of dependency would adapt more readily to having a retarded child than parents who foster independent functioning in children. However, retarded children reared by the latter may show more adult behavior, in spite of the parents' initial adjustment problem.

Still another factor that prevents favorable adjustment and which is related to attitudes of community members is the attitude of the retarded toward himself. A series of studies at the Laurelton State School and Hospital in Pennsylvania demonstrated the relationship between self-attitudes and effectiveness of performance (Guthrie, Gorlow, & Butler, 1967). Although the majority of adolescents in this institution were retarded because of cultural or familial etiology, the findings probably apply to the brain-impaired retardate as well.

Problems in handling hostility and resentment emerged in almost every study. Hostility was the outstanding factor differentiating those who were in the institution from those in the community. Some institutionalized retardates organized their views of themselves around negative themes of being hateful and angry, useless, shy, weak, and unloved. The angry, aversive behavior often accompanying retardation can be a defensive method of dealing with or avoiding feelings of hopelessness, helplessness, and low self-esteem. Other retarded individuals denied their hostility as well as their difficulties, emphasized conformity and compliance, and insisted they were as good as the next person. The latter group, those denying and suppressing their hostility, made more favorable adjustments upon return to the community.

What leads some retardeds to adopt defensive attitudes leading to better community adjustment? Psychotherapy while in the institution does not seem to be a significant factor. Traditional group psychotherapy has failed to produce greater self-acceptance in those with poor self-concepts. Jackson and Butler (1963) found that the variables related to better community adjustment are age, with the older doing better, high verbal intelligence, residence with parents for at least the first five years of life, and living in a rural environment. Since IQ is relatively stable by age 5, and since other research demonstrates a decline in IQ following early institutionalization, the higher IQs in Jackson and Butler's successful subjects may be accounted for by their longer stay at home prior to institutionalization. Similarly, Bloom's (1964) research indicates that personality and self-attitudes are formulated at an early age and remain relatively stable. The finding that retardates who are separated from their parents at an early age express more negative attitudes is consistent with Bloom's findings and serves to further emphasize the negative consequences of early institutionalization. Those retardates avoiding institutionalization placement have the most positive attitudes about themselves.

Compliance and submission to adults are higher in those institutionalized after age 5 and are related to subsequent community adjustment. Why is this so? Would it not be predicted that those subjected early to the regimentation of institutional living would be more submissive than those subjected to such a regime at a later date? Apparently not. Perhaps compliance to institutional regimentation is only superficial and that actual compliance is an internalized attitude that occurs only in the early atmosphere of a mother-child relationship. According to the stages of development outlined in Harvey, Hunt, and Schroder (1961), a child reaches the stage of mutuality only after successful advancement through the stage of negativism. If negative behavior is actively punished or disallowed, the child's development is arrested at this stage. Perhaps such arrest is characteristic of children separated from their mothers at an early age and subjected to an institutional environment. Similar self-attitudes also characterize many dependent and neglected children of average IQ who are placed in child care institutions at early ages.

CONCLUDING REMARKS

With genetic counseling, therapeutic abortion, better prenatal care, and improved standard of living, there should be fewer severely retarded children in the future. Nevertheless, there will always be retarded children who will need care. Rather than hiding them in large institutions away from society, hopefully, we will help them to achieve their fullest potential within their own community. Shapiro (1973) and Spencer (1973) report successful group home placement of retarded individuals. Unfortunately, most states are far from reaching this goal. New institutions continue to be built; some are smaller than usual (250 children as the upper limit), but they are institutions none the less.

Since institutions will be around for some time, conditions must be improved within them; they must be humanized. New funds must be made available to attract well-trained staff members to improve the programs and management of the institutions and to provide other services such as parent guidance groups, family counseling, emergency placements, and extended visiting. If these services are not provided, families will be forced to do without essential help or to seek help where they think they can find it. Unconventional treatments offer some hope where there is only despair and, in this fashion, may even perform a service for the wealthy parent. For the disadvantaged parent, however, there is only despair.

References

Anderson, K. A. The "shopping" behavior of parents of mentally retarded children: the professional person's role. *Mental Retardation*, 1971, **9**, (4) 3–5.
Ashley, C. G. Evaluation of Oregon's PKU program. *Oregon Health*, 1970, **48**, 1–8.

Babson, S. G., Henderson, N., & Clark, W. M. The preschool intelligence of over-sized newborns. *Pediatrics*, 1969, 44, 536–538.

Bakwin, H., & Bakwin, R. M. *Behavior disorders in children*. Philadelphia: Saunders, 1966.

Barclay, A., & Goulet, L. R., Short-term changes in intellectual and social maturity of young non-institutionalized retardates. *American Journal of Mental Deficiency*, 1965, 70, 257–261.

Baumeister, A. A. The effects of dietary control of intelligence in phenylketonuria. *American Journal of Mental Deficiency*, 1967, 71, 840–847.

Bensberg, G. *Teaching the mentally retarded, a handbook for ward personnel.* Atlanta, Ga.: Southern Regional Education Board, 1965.

Berkson, G., & Mason, W. A. Stereotyped movements of mental defectives: III. Situation effects. *American Journal of Mental Deficiency*, 1963, 68, 409–412.

Berkson, G., & Mason, W. A. Stereotyped movements of mental defectives: IV. The effects of toys and the character of acts. *American Journal of Mental Deficiency*, 1964, 68, 511–524.

Bickel, H., Gerrard, J., & Hackmans, E. M. The influence of phenylalanine intake on chemistry and behavior of a phenylketonuric child. *Acta Paediatrica*, 1954, 46, 64–71.

Bickers, D. S., & Adams, R. D. Hereditary stenosis of the aqueduct of Sylvius as a cause of congenital hydrocephalus. *Brain*, 1949, 72, 246–262.

Birch, H. G., & Tizard, J. The dietary treatment of phenylketonuria: not proven. *Developmental Medicine and Child Neurology*, 1967, 9, 9–12.

Blatt, B., & Kaplan, F. *Christmas in purgatory*. Rockleigh, N.J.: Allyn & Bacon, 1966.

Bloom, B. S. *Stability and change in human characteristics*. New York: Wiley, 1964.

Boy, J. L., Lafont, C., & Villemin-Glog, L. The weight, stature and psycho-motor future of premature children: results of a survey of former premature children. *Revue d'Hygiene et de Medecine Sociale*, 1969, 16, 753–783.

Bricker, W. A., & Bricker, D. D. Development of receptive vocabulary in severely retarded children. *American Journal of Mental Deficiency*, 1970, 74, 599–607.

Brown, J. R. Review of C. H. Delacato, *The diagnosis and treatment of speech and reading problems. Neurology*, 1964, 14, 599–600.

Cole, E. M. Review of C. H. Delacato, *The diagnosis and treatment of speech and reading problems. Harvard Educational Review*, 1964, 34, 351–354.

Cornwell, A. C., & Birch, H. G. Psychological and social development in home-reared children with Down's syndrome (mongolism). *American Journal of Mental Deficiency*, 1969, 74, 341–350.

Cott, A. Megavitamins: the orthomolecular approach to behavioral disorders and learning disabilities. *Academic Therapy Quarterly*, 1972, 7, 245–258.

Crome, L. The brain and mental retardation. *British Medical Journal*, 1960, 1 (5117), 897–904.

Davies, P. A., & Davis, J. P. Very low birth-weight and subsequent head growth. *Lancet*, 1970, 2(7685), 1216–1219.

Delacato, C. H. *The treatment and prevention of reading problems: the neuropsychological approach*. Springfield, Ill.: C. C Thomas, 1959.

Delacato, C. H. *The diagnosis and treatment of speech and reading problems.* Springfield, Ill.: C. C Thomas, 1963.

Delacato, C. H. *Neurological organization and reading*. Springfield, Ill.: C. C Thomas, 1966.

Dentler, R. A., & Mackler, B. Ability and sociometric status among normal and retarded children: a review of the literature. *Psychological Bulletin,* 1962, **59,** 273–283.

Desmond, M. M., Rudolph, A. J., Hill, R. M., Claghorn, J. L., Dreesen, P. R., & Burgdorff, I. Behavioral alterations in infants born to mothers on psychoactive medication during pregnancy. In G. Farell (Ed.), *Congenital mental retardation.* Austin: University of Texas Press, 1969.

Doman, G. J., & Delacato, C. H. Train your baby to be a genius. *McCalls,* March 1965.

Doman, G. J., Delacato, C. H., & Doman, R. J. *The Doman-Delacato Developmental Profile.* Philadelphia: Institutes for the Achievement of Human Potential, 1964.

Drillien, C. M. *The growth and development of the prematurely born infant.* Baltimore: Williams & Wilkins, 1954.

Drillien, C. M. Complications of pregnancy and delivery. In J. Wortis (Ed.), *Mental retardation: an annual review.* Vol. 1. New York: Grune & Stratton, 1970.

Ellis, N. R. (Ed.) *Handbook of mental deficiency.* New York: McGraw-Hill, 1963.

Ellis, N. R. (Ed.) *International review of research in mental retardation.* Vol. 5. New York: Academic Press, 1972.

Fisch, R. O., Doeden, D., Lansky, L. L., & Anderson, J. A. Maternal phenylketonuria: detrimental effects on embryo genesis and fetal development. *American Journal of Diseases of Children,* 1969, **118,** 847–858.

Ford, F. R. *Diseases of the nervous system in infancy, childhood and adolescence.* (5th ed.) Springfield, Ill.: C. C Thomas, 1966.

Freeman, R. D. Controversy over "patterning" as a treatment for brain damage in children. *Journal of the American Medical Association,* 1967, **202,** 385–388.

Friedsam, H. J., & Dick, H. R. A note on the facilitation of early institutional adjustment of retarded children. *Mental Retardation,* 1968, **6,** 15–18.

Fuller, R. N., & Shuman, J. B. Phenylketonuria and intelligence: trimodal response to dietary treatment. *Nature,* 1969, **221,** 639–642.

Fuller, R. N., & Shuman, J. B. Treated phenylketonuria: intelligence and blood phenylalanine levels. *American Journal of Mental Deficiency,* 1971, **75,** 539–545.

Glass, G. V., & Robbins, M. A critique of experiments on the role of neurological organization in reading performance. *Reading Research Quarterly,* 1967, **3,** 5–51.

Goda, S. Vocal utterances of young moderately and severely retarded non-speaking children. *American Journal of Mental Deficiency,* 1960, **65,** 269–273.

Goda, S. Language therapy for the non-speaking retarded child. *Mental Retardation,* 1969, **7** (4), 22–25.

Goldman, A. S. Predisposing genetic and metabolic factors to developmental defects of the central nervous system. *Physical Therapy,* 1965, **45,** 345–356.

Gorton, C. E., & Hollis, J. H. Redesigning a cottage unit for better programming and research for the severely retarded. *Mental Retardation,* 1965, **3** (3), 16–21.

Guess, D. The influence of visual and ambulation restrictions on stereotyped behavior. *American Journal of Mental Deficiency,* 1966, **70,** 542–547.

Guess, D., Rutherford, G., Smith, J. O., & Ensminger, E. Utilization of subprofessional personnel in teaching language skills to mentally retarded children: an interim report. *Mental Retardation,* 1970, **8** (2), 17–23.

Guskin, S. Social psychologies of mental deficiencies. In N. R. Ellis (Ed.), *Handbook of mental deficiency.* New York: McGraw-Hill, 1963.

Guthrie, G. M., Gorlow, L., & Butler, A. J. The attitude of the retarded toward herself: a summary of research at Laurelton State School and Hospital. *Pennsylvania Psychiatric Quarterly*, 1967, **7**, 24–34.

Hallet, P., Sype, S. M., & Gates, J. K. A language-based curriculum for the mentally retarded. *Mental Retardation*, 1971, **9** (6), 9–12.

Hanley, W. B., Partington, M. W., Rathbun, J. C., Amies, C. R., Webb, J. F., & Moore, J. E. The newborn phenylketonuria screening program in Ontario. *Canadian Medical Association Journal*, 1969, **101**, 185–190.

Hansen, H. Epidemiological considerations on maternal hyperphenylalaninemia. *American Journal of Mental Deficiency*, 1970, **75**, 22–26.

Harvey, O. J., Hunt, D. E., & Schroder, H. M. *Conceptual systems and personality organization*. New York: Wiley, 1961.

Hicks, S. P. Radiation as an experimental tool in mammalian developmental neurology. *Physiological Review*, 1958, **38**, 337–356.

Horner, F. A., & Streamer, C. W. Phenylketonuria treated from earliest infancy; report of three cases. *American Journal of Diseases of Children*, 1959, **97**, 345–347.

Hsia, D. Y. Y., Berman, J. L., & Slatis, H. M. Screening newborn infants for phenylketonuria. *Journal of the American Medical Association*, 1964, **188**, 203–206.

Hsia, D. Y. Y., & Dobson, J. Altered sex ratio among phenylketonuric infants ascertained by screening the newborn. *Lancet*, 1970, **1** (7653), 905–908.

Hudspeth, J. W. The neurobehavioral implausibility of the Delacato theory. In M. P. Douglas (Ed.), *Claremont Reading Conference Yearbook*. Claremont, Calif.: Claremont Reading Conference, 1964.

Huntley, C. C., & Stevenson, R. E. Maternal phenylketonuria. *Obstetrics and Gynecology*, 1969, **34**, 694–700.

Jackson, S. K., & Butler, A. J. Prediction of successful community placement of institutionalized retardates. *American Journal of Mental Deficiency*, 1963, **68**, 211–217.

Jervis, G. A. Phenylpyruvic oligophrenia deficiency of phenylalanine oxidizing system. *Proceedings of the Society of Experimental Biology and Medicine*, 1953, **82**, 514–515.

Joffe, J. M. Prenatal determinants of behavior. In *International series of monographs on experimental psychology*. Vol. 7. New York: Pergamon, 1969.

Johnson, R. C. Behavioral characteristics of phenylketonurics and matched controls. *American Journal of Mental Deficiency*, 1969, **74**, 17–19.

Johnson, R. C. Prediction of independent functioning and of problem behavior from measures of IQ and SQ. *American Journal of Mental Deficiency*, 1970, **74**, 591–593.

Johnson, R. C., & Abelson, R. B. Intellectual, behavioral and physical characteristics associated with trisomy, translocation, and mosaic types of Down's syndrome. *American Journal of Mental Deficiency*, 1969, **73**, 852–855.

Institutes for the Achievement of Human Potential Bulletin, 1965, **10**, 46.

Institutes for the Achievement of Human Potential. *A summary of concepts, procedures and organization*. Philadelphia, undated.

Keeley, K. Prenatal influence on behavior of offspring of crowded mice. *Science*, 1962, **135**, 44–47.

Kershner, J. R. Doman-Delacato's theory of neurological organization applied with retarded children. *Exceptional Children*, 1968, **34**, 441–450.

Kershner, J. R. Intellectual and social development in relation to family functioning: a longitudinal comparison of home vs. institutional effects. *American Journal of Mental Deficiency*, 1970, **75**, 276–284.

Kirk, S. A. An evaluation of the study by Bernardine G. Schmidt entitled: "Changes in personal, social, and intellectual behavior of children originally classified as feebleminded." *Psychological Bulletin,* 1948, **45,** 321–333.

Kirman, B. H. *Down's syndrome.* In J. Wortis (Ed.), *Mental retardation: an annual review.* Vol. 1. New York: Grune & Stratton, 1970.

Knoblock, H., & Pasamanick, B. Seasonal variations in the births of the mentally deficient. *American Journal of Public Health and the Nation's Health,* 1958, **48,** 1201–1208.

Knox, W. E. Evaluation of treatment of phenylketonuria with diets low in phenylalanine. *Pediatrics,* 1960, **26,** 1–11.

Koch, R., & Dobson, J. C. *The mentally retarded child and his family.* New York: Brunner-Mazel, 1972.

Kushlick, A. The prevalence of recognized mental subnormality of IQ under 50 among children in the South of England. *Proceedings of the International Conference on the Scientific Study of Mental Retardation.* Copenhagen: Statens & Andssvage-forsorg, 1964.

Levy, H. L. Large-scale studies in Massachusetts. In G. Farrell (Ed.), *Congenital mental retardation.* Austin: University of Texas Press, 1969.

Lyle, J. G. The effect of an institution environment upon the verbal development of imbecile children: II. *Journal of Mental Deficiency Research,* 1960, **4,** 14–23.

MacCubrey, J. Verbal operant conditioning with young institutionalized Down's syndrome children. *American Journal of Mental Deficiency,* 1971, **75,** 696–701.

Mallison, R. *Education as therapy—suggestions for work with neurologically impaired children.* Seattle: Special Child Publications, 1968.

Mann, E. T. The symbolic process of recidivist and non-recidivist children as assessed by the Kahn Test of Symbol Arrangement. *Journal of Projective Techniques and Personality Assessment,* 1967, **31,** 40–46.

Meindl, J. L., Barday, A. G., Lamp, R. E., & Yater, A. C. Mental growth in non-institutionalized mongoloid children. *Proceedings of the 79th Annual Convention of the American Psychological Association,* 1971, **6,** 621–622.

Melton, D. *Todd.* Englewood Cliffs, N.J.: Prentice-Hall, 1968.

Mitchell, A. C., & Smeriglio, V. Growth in social competence in institutionalized mentally retarded children. *American Journal of Mental Deficiency,* 1970, **74,** 666–673.

Moore, B. C., Thuline, H. C., & Capes, L. Mongoloid and non-mongoloid retardates: a behavioral comparison. *American Journal of Mental Deficiency,* 1968, **23,** 433–436.

National Association for Retarded Children. *Childrens Limited,* 1968, **17,** (2).

Nelson, K. B., & Deutschberger, J. Head size at one year as a predictor of four-year IQ. *Developmental and Child Neurology,* 1970, **12,** 487–495.

O'Donnell, P. A., & Eisenson, J. Delacato training for reading achievement and visual-motor integration. *Journal of Learning Disabilities,* 1969, **2,** 441–447.

O'Flynn, M. E. Diet therapy in phenylketonuria. *American Journal of Nursing,* 1967, **67,** 1658–1660.

Paine, R. S. The variability in manifestations of untreated patients with phenylketonuria (phenylpyruvicaciduria). *Pediatrics,* 1957, **20,** 290–302.

Payne, D., Johnson, R. C., & Abelson, R. B. A comprehensive description of institutional retardates in the western United States. Boulder, Colo.: Western Interstate Commission for Higher Education, 1969.

Penrose, L. S. *The biology of mental defect.* London: Sidgwick & Jackson, 1963.

Penrose, L. S., & Smith, G. F. *Down's anomaly.* London: Churchill, 1966.

Philips, I. Psychopathology and mental retardation. *American Journal of Psychiatry,* 1967, **124,** 29–35.

Pitt, D. B. Variations in the level of serum phenylalanine with age. *Australian Paediatric Journal,* 1969, **5,** 234–236.

Platt, H., Mordock, J., & Dorgan, N. B. *Multidisciplinary training program for houseparents: final report.* (Grant No. 4 TI MH 8108) Devon, Pa.: National Institute of Mental Health and The Devereux Foundation Institute for Research and Training, 1969.

Price, J. R., Jr., & Horne, B. M. Family history indicating hereditary factors in hydrocephalus. *Mental Retardation,* 1968, **6,** (5) 40–91.

Provence, S., & Lipton, R. *Infants in institutions.* New York: International Universities Press, 1962.

Richards, B. W. Mosaic mongolism. *Journal of Mental Deficiency Research,* 1969, **13,** 66–83.

Rigrodsky, S., & Goda, S. Language behavior of a group of non-speaking mentally retarded children. *Training School Bulletin,* 1961, **58,** 52–59.

Robbins, M. P. The Delacato interpretation of neurological organization. *Reading Research Quarterly,* 1966a, **1,** 57–78.

Robbins, M. P. A study of the validity of Delacato's theory of neurological organization. *Exceptional Children,* 1966b, **32,** 517–523.

Robbins, M. P. Test of the Doman-Delacato rationale with retarded readers. *Journal of the American Medical Association,* 1967, **202,** 389–393.

Rosecrans, C. F. The relationship of normal 121 trisomy mosaicism and intellectual development. *American Journal of Mental Deficiency,* 1968, **72,** 562–565.

Rosecrans, C. J. A longitudinal study of exceptional cognitive development in a partial translocation Down's syndrome child. *American Journal of Mental Deficiency,* 1971, **76,** 290–294.

Rutter, M., Graham, P., & Yule, W. A. *A neuropsychiatric study of childhood.* (Clinics in Developmental Medicine, No. 35/36) London: Spastics International Medical Publications, Heinemann, 1970.

Sarason, S. *Psychological problems in mental deficiency.* (4th ed.) New York: Harper & Row, 1969.

Schmidt, B. G. Changes in personal, social, and intellectual behavior of children originally classified as feebleminded. *Psychological Monographs,* 1946, **60** (Whole No. 5).

Schmidt, B. G. A reply. *Psychological Bulletin,* 1948, **45,** 334–343.

Shapiro, H. Circle of homes. *Mental Retardation,* 1973, **11**(3), 19–21.

Shipe, D., & Shotwell, A. M. Effects of out-of-home care on mongoloid children: a continuation study. *American Journal of Mental Deficiency,* 1965, **69,** 649–652.

Siegel, F. S., Balow, B., Fisch, R. O., & Anderson, V. E. School behavior profile ratings of phenylketonuric children. *American Journal of Mental Deficiency,* 1968, **72,** 937–943.

Spencer, B. G. Utah community group homes. *Mental Retardation,* 1973, **11**(3), 13.

Spreen, O. Language functions in mental retardation: a review. I. Language development, types of retardation, and intelligence level. *American Journal of Mental Deficiency,* 1965, **69,** 482–494.

Sternlicht, M., & Wanderer, Z. W. Nature of institutionalized adult mongoloid intelligence. *American Journal of Mental Deficiency,* 1962, **67,** 301–302.

Sutherland, B. S., Berry, H. K., & Umbarger, B. Growth and nutrition in treated phenylketonuric patients. *Journal of the American Medical Association,* 1970, **211,** 270–276.

Szeinberg, A., Cohen, B. E., Golan, R., Peled, I., Lavi, U., & Crispin, M. Persistent mild hyperphenylalaninemia in various ethnic groups in Israel. *American Journal of Diseases of Children,* 1969, **118,** 559–564.

Taylor, R. G. Identification of variables useful in prognosis for brain-injured children. *Perceptual and Motor Skills,* 1968, **27,** 606–607.

Tizard, B., Cooperman, O., Joseph, A., & Tizard, J. Environmental effects on language development: a study of young children in long-stay residential nurseries. *Child Development,* 1972, **43,** 337–358.

Tobias, J. Vocational adjustment of young retarded adults. *Mental Retardation,* 1970, 8(3), 13–17.

Vandeman, P. R. Termination of dietary treatment for phenylketonuria. *American Journal of Diseases of Children,* 1963, **106,** 492–495.

Vogel, W., Kun, K., & Meshorer, E. Effects of environmental enrichment and environmental deprivation on cognitive functioning in institutionalized retardates. *Journal of Consulting Psychology,* 1967, **31,** 570–576.

Warren, S. A., & Burns, N. R. Crib confinement as a factor in repetitive and stereotyped behavior in retardates. *Mental Retardation,* 1970, 8(3), 25–28.

Wepman, J. M. Review of C. H. Delacato, *The diagnosis and treatment of speech and reading problems. Contemporary Psychology,* 1964, **9,** 351–352.

Werboff, J., & Havlena, J. Postnatal behavioral effects of tranquilizers administered to the gravid rat. *Experimental Neurology,* 1962, **6,** 263–269.

Wiener, G. The relationship of birth weight and length of gestation to intellectual development at ages 8 to 10 years. *Journal of Pediatrics,* 1970, **76,** 694–699.

Wolfson, I. N. Adjustment of institutionalized mildly retarded patients twenty years after return to the community. *Mental Retardation,* 1970, 8(4), 20–23.

Wortis, J. (Ed.) *Mental retardation: an annual review.* Vol. 3. New York: Grune & Stratton, 1972.

Zigler, E. Familial mental retardation: a continuing dilemma. *Science,* 1967, **155,** 292–298.

Sometimes the crisis of unreality supervened on the street. Everything looked dead, lifeless, stony, ridiculous and in the stillness a baby's cry would arouse me and rewaken the fear.

—"Renee"

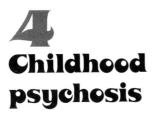

Childhood psychosis

In Chapters 2 and 3 we showed some of the ways in which both brain injury and structural malformations of the brain can affect the developing child. We also mentioned that psychiatric disorders among brain-disordered children are five times that found in the general population. We assumed, however, that the psychiatric disorder is a nonspecific rather than specific effect of the brain dysfunction. In this chapter we will present children whose disturbances in interpersonal relations have been attributed by some investigators to brain dysfunction. These children have been labeled psychotic or childhood schizophrenic.

Although psychotic children display a variety of behaviors, perhaps the feature that sets them apart from others is their bizarreness; they often engage in activities which appear meaningless to the observer. Specific behaviors that accompany their bizarre actions include alternating periods of overactivity and inactivity; extreme anxiety expressed in excessive fears; purposeless, repetitious, and unexpressive behavior; sexual preoccupation; self-destructive attempts; and aggression. The child is often detached and pressures to socialize him lead only to negativism.

Bright children with the disorder frequently display an unusual degree of interest in abstract notions. For example, one 12-year-old psychotic devoted considerable time to the study of mythology but experienced auditory and visual hallucinations of Greek heroes rescuing her from her enemies.

A group of British clinicians (Creak, 1961) listed nine observable clinical signs and behaviors which characterize the childhood psychotic: (1) gross impairment of emotional relations with people, (2) apparent unawareness of personal identity, (3) pathological preoccupation with objects or particular attributes of them, (4) sustained resistance to change in the environment, (5) abnormal perceptual experience, (6) acute, excessive, and seemingly irrational anxiety, (7) speech arrested at levels characteristic of an earlier age or absent altogether, (8) distorted mobility patterns, and (9) considerably uneven intellectual development.

A review of 52 published reports which featured diagnostic symptomatology in childhood psychosis substantiated that all the behaviors described as characteristic of the children studied could be embodied in the above nine points (Goldfarb, 1970a).

No single symptom is diagnostic nor do all the symptoms need to be present before a child can be diagnosed as psychotic. Each of the nine symptoms can be found in children with other disorders, such as children with brain injury without the schizophrenic syndrome and children with severe neurotic disorders (see Chapter 7).

Although the childhood psychoses can occur at any age, there are three main periods when the disorders appear. *Infantile psychosis* or *infantile autism* begins in early infancy but occasionally occurs as late as the second or even third year of life. In *regressive psychosis* or *childhood schizophrenia* the child apparently develops normally in the first few years and then shows disintegration of behavior and a regression in speech and other functions. *Adolescent schizophrenia* begins in early adolescence and appears indistinguishable from schizophrenia as it occurs in adults, that is, the diagnostic symptoms of childhood schizophrenia, such as pathological preoccupation with objects, speech abnormalities, and resistance to change, are not characteristic features.

The case of Bill serves as an example of blatent childhood schizophrenia.

Schizophrenia

BILL *Boucher*

Bill, a frail Oriental boy of 7, was referred for psychological evaluation because of hyperactive and disruptive behavior in his classroom. His teacher reported that he hit other children, took things from their desks, and continually talked without permission. He was preoccupied with girls, looked up their skirts, and went into their bathroom. On the playground, he was aggressive and oblivious to danger, and he spent considerable time lying atop the jungle gym. He wove elaborate fantasies about a nonexistent sister. During the previous year he had been fixated to the color red.

Observations by the psychological assistant added the following. During reading, Bill was in constant motion. He fidgeted continually, turned around in his chair numerous times, and twice fell from it onto the floor. Although he did try to read occasionally, most of the time he was in a world of fantasy, smiling to himself in a peculiar, secretive manner. Without provocation, he pinched in the rear the girl who sat next to him. Data from an observation schedule revealed that he was on-task only 10 percent of the classroom period.

In music class he was completely disruptive, stimulating others to the point where little music resulted. He talked out constantly, saying repeatedly to other boys, "You should marry Miss Brown," and "Pull down Miss Brown's underwear." While the other children sang the song assigned, Bill sang, "Take off your underwear," and then laughed hysterically. When reprimanded, he could desist only momentarily.

The aide concluded that most of Bill's behavior was unrelated either to that of the teacher or to the other children; more likely it resulted from his response to internal promptings. Several other children derived pleasure from egging him on, getting him to do things they would like to do but were fearful of doing, but, in general, Bill was his own stimulator. Consequently, he received a great deal of teacher attention, attention which he seemed to relish even though it included scolding and punishment.

The school psychologist described Bill as a boy of average intelligence whose current functioning was hampered by thought disorder and anxiety provoking fantasies. Foremost among his worries was extreme fear of animals. Preoccupation with ways of avoiding fantasied dangers consumed much of his time and energy; an abnormal interest in airplanes probably reflected his effort to escape imagined threats.

Bill's intellectual efficiency was seriously hampered by the intrusion of these fantasies into his responses to questions. For example, when asked, "What do we do to make water boil?" Bill said, "To the sink, hot water, some sleeping tablets." In response to "How are paper and coal alike?" he replied, "White paper with poison. You can draw pictures on them. Could kill you. Some bug foods are poison, some bees bite. If you eat them, you could get sick 'cause they are poison."

The psychologist recommended Bill's removal from the regular classroom. Until this was accomplished, school staff were advised to restrict his attendance to highly structured classes, avoiding music, art, and gym. Specific recommendations regarding his instruction were deferred until school placement was decided. The next step was to hold a parent conference.

Bill's father came to the parent conference about fifteen minutes before his wife, but saw no reason to wait for her before beginning the discussion. He described his typical day with Bill, but omitted behavioral descriptions. He gave some brief background information, but mostly about a younger son who was institutionalized as a mental retardate. After Bill's mother arrived, his teacher described his school behavior. At first the parents seemed surprised, but gradually opened up and admitted having difficulty with Bill at home. The father described outbursts of anger where Bill bit, pinched, and destroyed things. He said that Bill was stubborn and disobedient and would obey only when threatened with punishment, punishment that included the threat of sending him to the institution where his brother was or hitting him with a big stick. The mother reported that Bill had nightmares every night and refused to sleep unless threatened with the stick.

The parents were told that Bill's problems were of sufficient magnitude to require therapeutic intervention, and they were referred to the local child guidance center. At the same time, Bill was placed in a special class for emotionally disturbed children. School personnel suggested that the parents spend more time playing with Bill, decrease their pressures for school performance, stop threatening him, and be more supportive. Staff stressed that Bill did not always misbehave on purpose but found self-control extremely difficult. Bill's parents left the impression of two rather inadequate people floundering in a tenuous relationship with a very difficult child.

Decisions made about Bill

While referral and evaluation proceeded smoothly, a number of critical decisions were made during the process, decisions based on the data gathered by the various professionals involved and on their particular viewpoint about schizophrenia. Questions were posed, alternatives considered and rejected, and recommendations decided upon. First, the teacher decided she could not handle Bill without professional advice. Second, based on both test results and the aide's observations, the psychologist did not attempt behavior modification in the normal class. Instead, he recommended removal from less structured classrooms, referral to the clinic, and special class placement. Third, school staff rejected the idea of tutoring, psychoeducational counseling, or use of the resource room. Instead, they placed him in a special class for the emotionally disturbed. Fourth, clinic staff considered therapeutic alternatives. They could see Bill in individual therapy, refer him to a residential center or psychiatric hospital, see his parents as a couple or assign them to a couple's group. The staff selected family therapy as the treatment modality.

The psychologist's decision Psychological evaluation of Bill was not actually necessary because classroom functioning was so bizarre. In more withdrawn cases test results can add significantly to decision making, but Bill was tested essentially to substantiate classroom impressions.

FRANK

Frank arrived on time, asked clearly if he was in the right place and if the examiner was the right person, and, after being introduced to another boy who was in the office at the time, took the seat offered to him. Because of this initial favorable impression, the examiner was surprised by what followed. After the other boy left, Frank began hitting the keys of the examiner's typewriter. He hit only one key over and over and would not answer questions unless he was allowed to continue this activity. He rambled, asked incomprehensible questions, and showed inappropriate affect. At certain times, he would clutch his arms to his chest, grimace, and squeal loudly. Then, suddenly, he would return to the task before him and calmly answer a question. In general, he refused to do anything, but with persistent coaxing he directed his attention to some tasks.

Although he engaged in fantasy throughout testing, all efforts to get him to reveal their nature were fruitless. He would not tell stories or divulge his wishes. He went to the bathroom several times during testing, where he could be heard squealing and talking to himself. When presented with a pair of scissors, he mumbled that he would kill the examiner. He was quite hostile when he refused to cooperate and eventually formal testing was discontinued.

His feelings of helplessness in the face of the anxieties generated by testing were prominent. He responded to these feelings by simply refusing to cope with tasks presented. Further, responses to affect-laden situations were delayed, making it difficult to determine whether his behavior was due to the memory of some previous events or to the current source of frustration.

After the testing materials were put away, the examiner asked if there was something else he would like to do in the time remaining. Frank replied that he did not want to play, that he never played, but only watched television. He stood by the doorway, mumbled about playing kickball, said something about "really giving it a good kick," and asked if he could go.

The impression was clearly that of a psychotic child. In addition, his psychotic behavioral reactions increased whenever he was challenged. When these behaviors did not work (i.e., questioning persisted) he would withdraw entirely from the challenge by physically removing himself from it (i.e., going to the bathroom, standing by the door, and requesting removal).

Although no one test pattern is characteristic of childhood psychosis, several signs indicate this diagnosis (Des Lauriers & Halpern, 1947). Intellectual functioning is quite uneven. Unexpected failures occur irregularly in a series of successes, perhaps resulting from sudden preoccupation with unessential details. Responses sometimes seem illogical and associations unusual. Drawings of human figures show confusion and disorganization. Responses to projective tests (Rorschach or Thematic Apperception Test) reveal a poor match between the child's perceptions and the stimulus presented, for example, the child sees a horse when the shape is that of a bat. Sometimes the match is correct but the child's elaborations are bizarre, for example, he sees the bat about to devour a little girl (Myer & Caruth, 1967).

The school's decision   The decision to refer Bill to a special class rather than to attempt behavior modification in his regular class was based on the relative ineffectiveness of this procedure with psychotic children. Extremely disturbed and disruptive children negatively influence other children in the regular classroom. Efforts to control this influence consume time needed to give proper education to the remaining children. In the smaller special class a total class approach can be employed (O'Leary & Becker, 1967) and individualized programs can be more efficiently arranged (Lovaas, 1967; Sailor, Guess, Rutherford, & Baer, 1968).

The resource room was rejected because Bill needed environmental programming of the whole day (Hewett, Taylor, & Artuso, 1969). Psychoeducational therapy was rejected because short-term therapy would not bring rapid diminution of inappropriate classroom behavior. In addition, individual psychotherapy with psychotic children requires a unique set of skills and therapist availability beyond that of limited contact (Ekstein & Wallerstein, 1954).

The teacher of the special class where Bill was placed followed the approach described by Douglas (1961). Her initial goal was to gain Bill's trust by establishing firm limits. Firmness would give Bill the security that he would not hurt others or himself. The classroom was highly structured, so that Bill could learn what was expected of him hour by hour and could be prepared well in advance for any changes that would occur in his daily routine. The teacher felt that imposition of external control and organization helped the psychotic child to develop internal organization. Short work periods, lowered achievement demands, and remedial work designed to improve self-esteem were the chief characteristics of classroom organization. When Bill developed better control over his behavior, she would increase her demands for achievement commensurate with his intellectual capacity. Her most difficult job would be limiting Bill's aggressive outbursts without being punitive.

The clinic's decision   Several investigators have trained parents to modify their psychotic child's behavior (Walder, Breiter, Cohen, Daston, Forbes, & McIntire, 1966), but the extent of parental pathology was not ascertained in these studies nor was adequate follow-up presented. The clinic staff, therefore, rejected this approach. They also ruled out individual and group therapy, not only because the staff believed these procedures to be relatively ineffective with children like Bill, but also because pathology was clearly evident in other family members. The family, rather than Bill alone, was identified as the "patient," and improvement of family functioning was the chief objective.

The outcome of these decisions

For approximately four months, the family came regularly to the clinic. Although the parents tried to hide their weaknesses, it became apparent that Bill's mother was quite disturbed; historical material brought up in the sessions revealed her peculiar functioning since early childhood.

This disclosure was not surprising since psychiatric disorders are common in the parents of schizophrenics (Rosenthal, 1971). As a child, Bill's mother showed a lack of frustration tolerance, lack of social adaptation, emotional immaturity, and a variety of obsessive-compulsive behaviors. Most of the time she could function normally, but when alone or frustrated, she withdrew into fantasy or vented severe temper outbursts against siblings.

Ekstein (1966) and Geleerd (1958) refer to children who display such behavior as "borderline psychotics." Such children who show psychotic symptoms when under stress, but for the most part remain mildly eccentric. They appear arrested at a stage of development where their sense of security is dependent upon their mother's approval. As they grow older, they need an adult's approval to feel secure, but have difficulty sharing the loved object with another person. As long as they can control the caretaker, they function more or less adequately.

Bill's mother became attached to one therapist and looked to him for support during the family interviews, support which didn't come from her husband except in their mutual agreement that Bill was the sick one. The father's cold, detached manner, while predictable, failed to provide the security the mother needed to function. Children were her rivals for the limited affection available. Unfortunately, the therapist went on vacation. Upon his return, Bill's mother vented tremendous anger toward him and refused further treatment. The father, evidently seeing the therapist as a rival, went along with this decision.

Following this setback in treatment, Bill was given medication during school hours. Chemotherapy was designed to modify certain target symptoms in order to facilitate other aspects of treatment (Fish, 1968). In Bill's case medication was employed to help relieve his tremendous anxiety. It was hoped that the medication would also reduce his hyperactivity, since hyperactivity is sometimes a response to anxiety. If Bill became less hyperactive, he could participate more fully in the educational program. Numerous studies have demonstrated the disruptive effects of anxiety on attention, perception, and cognition. Diminishing anxiety restores functioning in these areas and also assists the loosely organized to function more coherently.

Bill remained in the special class, but was being considered for placement in a specialized day care program for seriously disturbed youngsters. This program was being developed by the county community mental health center. Had the family continued in treatment, perhaps Bill could have remained in the special education class. His behavior had improved, but he was still considerably more disturbed than the majority of youngsters in the class. Day care staff hoped to involve the parents again, but were not optimistic. Should Bill fail to improve in the multidisciplinary day care program, commitment to the children's center of the state hospital would be likely. While removal from the home imposes new adults, new peers, new school situations, and new group living on a child who already suffers severely, communities cannot always tolerate such a disruptive member; removal becomes the only alternative.

THE CAUSES OF SCHIZOPHRENIA

Childhood schizophrenia, or regressive psychosis, is frequently, but not always, associated with mental retardation and organic disease (Goldfarb, 1961). Many investigators have attributed the disorder to organic factors because a similar picture of regression often occurs after a known brain disease, such as encephalitis. This belief in organic causation is strengthened by the frequent association of schizophrenia with known neurological abnormalities. Some of these are abnormal sighting and postural responses, disturbances of body schema, abnormal muscle tone, epileptic seizures, pathological reflexes, motor abnormalities, and language disorders (Eaton & Menolascino, 1966; Gittelman & Birch, 1967; Goldfarb, 1961; Rutter, 1965). Even after eliminating children with obvious localizing signs and those with abnormal reflexes and sensory-motor dysfunction, Goldfarb (1970b) found over 60 percent of the remainder to show subtle signs of neurological impairment. Similarly, approximately 50 percent of schizophrenic children have abnormal EEGs which are qualitatively and quantitatively similar to each other (Stevens & Milstein, 1970; White, DeMyer, & DeMyer, 1964).

The fact that many psychotic children are free from these associated disorders has led some investigators to postulate two types of regressive childhood schizophrenia, organic and nonorganic. However, the major differences reported between organic and nonorganic groups are primarily quantitative rather than qualitative. Organic groups have significantly lower IQs and display greater inability on a variety of perceptual and psychomotor functions. In many cases where there is no overt brain disorder, the subsequent course of development often reveals a degenerative condition of the brain (Bender, 1947; Creak, 1963).

One group of investigators feels that different disorders are incorrectly subsumed under the label schizophrenia. In Chapter 3 we emphasized that originally all retarded children were grouped together; the common symptoms of their disorders made them look identical. Eventually, different syndromes were identified, and this identification led to different lines of research on prevention, diagnosis, and treatment. Similarly, many physical diseases have common features, for example, high fever, vomiting, and pallor, but the etiology and treatment of the diseases are considerably different. Consequently, this group of researchers expresses the need for precise behavioral diagnosis in order to study causative factors in schizophrenia (Eisenberg, 1966). At the present time differential diagnosis into agreed upon categories is not widespread. In one study (Rimland, 1971) 445 psychotic children were each seen by two different diagnosticians; only 55 were assigned the same diagnosis twice (see Table 4.1). This data suggests that more work is necessary before subclassifications of psychosis can be reliably employed.

Another group views schizophrenia as a relatively endogenous disorder, a disorder that can appear at any time in life and that varies among individuals quantitatively rather than qualitatively (Bender, 1971). Those who hold this position make no distinction between infantile autism, childhood schizophrenia, or schizophrenia in adolescents or adults. They regard separation into syndromes based on clinical symptoms or age of onset as wasted effort. They attribute the differences observed at different ages to developmental factors. In other words, the developing child is more adversely affected by the disorder than is the adult. This same group of investigators holds the view that certain individuals are predisposed to develop schizophrenia and that the disorder occurs at different ages because of different precipitating events. They attribute schizophrenia to an interaction between genetic and environmental factors.

The genetics of schizophrenia

Research has not been able to establish the exact roles of genetic and behavioral factors in schizophrenia. Several studies have revealed significant relationships between the disease and possible causative factors, but none is conclusive.

The likelihood of a person being schizophrenic increases as a function of his biological relationship to a schizophrenic(s). In approximately 45 percent of the cases, the identical twin of a diagnosed schizophrenic is also schizophrenic or schizoid, regardless of whether he was reared apart from or with his twin (Allen, Cohen, & Pollins, 1972; Buss, 1966; Heston, 1970; Shields & Gottesman, 1972). About 45 percent of the relatives of a schizophrenic are schizophrenic or schizoid (Heston, 1970). The term *schizoid* is used to describe behaviors consistent with the schizophrenic syndrome but displayed only to a mild degree. Heston feels that the labels schizoid and schizophrenic refer only to the degree of pathology. He believes that the same genetic defect accounts for the genetic contribution to both schizoid and schizophrenic disease.

Several investigators have used studies of adopted children who became schizophrenic to tease apart hereditary and environmental factors in the genesis of schizophrenia. If schizophrenic disorders are transmitted be-

Table 4.1 AGREEMENT BETWEEN PAIRS OF DIAGNOSTICIANS ON THE DIAGNOSES ASSIGNED TO 445 CHILDREN SHOWING SEVERE BEHAVIOR DISORDERS

First diagnosis	Second diagnosis								
	Autistic	Infantile autism or early infantile autism	Childhood schizophrenia	Emotionally disturbed or mentally ill	Brain damaged or neurologically damaged	Retarded	Psychotic (symbiotic psychosis), etc.	Deaf or partly deaf	Total
Autistic	33	5	53	18	23	51	10	7	200
Infantile autism or early infantile autism	1	10	6	—	4	6	—	2	29
Childhood schizophrenia	17	3	1	2	8	1	—	—	32
Emotionally disturbed or mentally ill	12	2	4	2	9	13	3	—	45
Brain damaged or neurologically damaged	14	3	2	5	4	15	—	1	44
Retarded	21	2	6	18	16	5	2	2	72
Psychotic (symbiotic psychosis), etc.	4	—	1	1	2	2	—	—	10
Deaf or partly deaf	4	1	—	2	—	5	1	—	13
	106	26	73	48	66	98	16	12	445

Reprinted from B. Rimland. The differentiation of childhood psychosis: an analysis of checklists for 2218 psychotic children. *Journal of Autism and Childhood Schizophrenia*, 1971, **1**, 161–174. With the permission of V. H. Winston & Sons, Publishers.

haviorally, then a greater incidence of schizophrenia should be found among the adoptive relatives of schizophrenics than among the biological relatives. The studies revealed that the degree of psychopathology in adoptive parents is significantly less than that of the biological parents of schizophrenics (Rosenthal, 1971).

Studies of twins have been extremely helpful in investigating schizophrenia. The classic design (Kallman, 1946) is based on comparisons of monozygotic (one-egg) twins, who have the same heredity, with dizygotic (two-egg) twins, who have only about half their genes in common. The finding that there is a greater incidence of concordance for schizophrenia among monozygotic twins (both have schizophrenia) than among dizygotic twins, suggests a genetic contribution to this disorder. The findings from these twin studies are not conclusive, however, since monozygotic twins could both have the disorder as a result of a similar response to noxious environmental conditions. If the twins have been reared apart, the evidence for the genetic position is stronger, except that both could have responded similarly to noxious events before separation, such as faulty interuterine development or damage at birth (Birch & Hertzig, 1967). The likelihood of this latter possibility is remote, however, since other evidence suggests that childhood schizophrenia is not caused by anoxia or non-mechanical injury at birth (Terris, Lapouse, & Monk, 1964).

Genetic determination of stress-response mechanisms At the present time we are uncertain about the type of genetic disorder that predisposes one to schizophrenia, but evidence is accumulating that points to a deficiency in the brain systems that regulate responses to stress. Building on the work of Eysenck (1947), who attempts to anchor major personality dimensions to physiological substrata, Claridge (1972) has theorized that schizophrenic behaviors represent exaggerated form of behaviors distributed among the general population. The predisposition to display these behaviors has a discoverable physiological basis in the form of particular kinds of nervous typological organization (Pavlov originated the idea of different nervous typologies some 50 years ago). Each typology differs in anxiety-proneness as a result of variations in central nervous system activity or arousability. From this viewpoint, those with the typology prone to greater autonomic arousal would be likely to act psychotic when they are extremely anxious.

Support for this position comes from the work of two groups of researchers. The first group followed the development of 207 children of schizophrenic mothers. During the interval covered (6 years), 20 of the 207 children developed psychoses. Matching these children with both those who did not develop psychoses and those who had normal mothers revealed that certain electrodermal responses appeared in the psychotic group almost exclusively. In general, they displayed hyperlabile and hypersensitive autonomic nervous system functioning. In addition, 53 percent of the mothers of the children who became psychotic suffered from serious pregnancy or birth complications. This percentage was much higher than in the other two groups, 15 and 28 percent respectively (Mednick & Schulsinger, 1970). Mednick (1971) postulates that complications during pregnancy or at birth impair the child's ability to regulate his body's stress-response mechanisms. These complications apparently trigger or exacerbate an already vulnerable nervous system.

A second group of investigators have suggested that biochemical abnormalities may be responsible for the deficient functioning of the stress-response mechanisms. Pollin and Stabenau (1968) have noted the high rate of a particular group of organic compounds (catecholamines) in the urine of both schizophrenics and their nonschizophrenic twin. Some of these compounds carry messages to different parts of the brain, and all of them play an essential role in the body's efforts to cope with stress. In the past the presence of these catecholamines in the urine was attributed to the patient's anxiety. Stress usually produces an elevation of other compounds as well (adrenal steroids, for example). These compounds were found in the schizophrenic twin. The nonschizophrenic twin, however, showed no parallel rise in the latter compounds, suggesting that the high amount of catecholamines in the schizophrenic twin was not solely a response to stress (Pollin & Stabenau, 1968; Stabenau, Pollin & Mosher, 1969). Further studies by Pollin's group determined that the amount of catecholamines in both twins was under genetic control. Perhaps hypersecretion of catecholamines impedes the ability to cope with stress and thus leads to schizophrenia.

If the causes of serious psychopathology are rooted in the systems that respond to stress, then a pathological spiral could develop in the following fashion. If a child has biochemical abnormalities that diminish his ability to react appropriately to stress, he may overreact in increasingly nonproductive ways. These reactions reduce the child's ability to cope with stress. As the ability to cope with stress decreases, external threats loom larger, leading to a greater overreaction, and finally to a pathological spiral that eventuates in schizophrenia.

Identification of the preschizophrenic child

From our discussion of genetics and the stress-response systems, we might postulate that childhood and adolescent schizophrenia, or even adult schizophrenia, are the same disorder, the only difference being the age of onset. Different behavioral manifestations occur at different ages because the disorder occurs at different stages of development. A child who has developed to a stage where he can think logically and then has a schizophrenic breakdown is bound to differ from a child only at the level of animistic thinking when he becomes schizophrenic. The adolescent schizophrenic is considered to be an individual who has been exposed to increasing increments of stress over time. When this stress is added to the stress of adolescence and its accompanying bodily changes, the combination is too much to handle and a schizophrenic reaction is activated.

According to this view the childhood histories of adolescent schizophrenics should differ from those of nonschizophrenics, and the differences should become more pronounced with advancing age. Current information suggests that this is the case. Through contacts with parents, family members, teachers, friends, school reports, and clinic records, the childhoods of schizophrenic adults and adolescents have been reconstructed.

While retrospective studies have increased our knowledge about schizophrenia, they have a number of weaknesses. (1) It is not known how many other children with childhood symptoms similar to the schizophrenic group grew up to be normal. (2) Facts may be altered or distorted with the passage of time. (3) Informants may be influenced by what they have heard about mental illness, what they think the interviewer wants to know, and their possible knowledge that the person in question is under psychiatric care. (4) The original life history, clinic, or school records may be unreliable. (5) Informants, particularly teachers, often form impressions from scant information (halo effect). (For example, if the child did good work in a subject, he may be remembered more favorably than one who did poor work.) Keeping these shortcomings in mind, we will examine the results of retrospective studies.

In general, children destined to be schizophrenic adults behave differently in school than other children. Nevertheless, not all preschizophrenic children are distinguishable in early childhood; deviation becomes clear by adolescence in about half of them. The type of deviation found depends upon how far back in time the study goes.

Ricks and Berry's (1970) retrospective studies suggest that the child headed for schizophrenia knows he is vulnerable and makes various efforts to defend himself. They describe three stages of retreat into schizophrenia: protest, despair, and apathy. In the first stage, *protest*, the adolescent whose past was a series of continual failures eventually attempts to deal with his world by angry confrontation. He demands special attention and privileges, throws temper tantrums, or displays provocativeness that tests the limits to which he can violate norms and still be loved. If this protest is successful, or if he can find some route into a low-pressure life style, then stabilization as an impulsive or schizoid character, or even recovery, may take place.

The second stage, *despair*, is characterized by hopelessness, withdrawal, and depression. The person who stabilizes at this stage may be diagnosed as depressed or as acute schizophrenic but will usually be discharged from the hospital.

"THEY TELL YOU"

They tell you, "One out of two hospital beds in the country is filled with mental patients."

And, "Mental illness strikes one out of every three families."

And, "Boys are especially prone to this, boys in their teens."

And you go on shopping, working, playing bridge with your friends, and pay no attention. All this can happen to other people, you think. But to you? Don't be ridiculous.

Then your own son turns sixteen.

Sixteen, a difficult age at best. Boys are all rebels then, moody, easily angered, given to criticizing their families. It's hell on parents, sure, but you'll live through it, and so will he. Remember, they're going through a change of life themselves, these kids. Be firm, but be patient and understanding in your firmness . . . and hang on.

Unfortunately, the dividing line between adolescent cussedness and emotional illness is thin. And they don't run pressure gauges to warn you where natural behavior leaves off and the danger point begins.

Gradually, so gradually it is impossible to say just when it started, we had become aware of a change in Ken. From the friendly, tractable, energetic boy we had known he was changing into someone disagreeable, often sullen, quick to flare into fits of temper for no apparent reason. He was bitterly critical of us, our home, the food we served, even his friends. He sought them out less and less, and when he did play it was as if some demon were driving him. He let his homework slide, studied little, and although he didn't miss any appreciable time from school, his marks began to decline.

Alarmed, his father and I consulted his teachers. Perhaps they, too, had felt the brunt of his distemper and could advise us what to do? To our relief and surprise, they assured us his deportment at school was above reproach. "Don't worry; they always act worse at home. Just see that he studies more," they said.

And so we relaxed, lulled into false security for a time. But as Ken's defiance grew worse, we became uneasy once again, then irritated, then outright angry. There was simply no rhyme nor reason for his attacks and tirades. To curb them, we tried withholding his allowance, restricting his activities. In our poverty of understanding, we did not realize that his perversity was the poison spurting from some deep, unsuspected sore of wretchedness . . . an anguish so dark, so mysterious, that he was totally unable to recognize or to cope with it.

When discipline failed, we tried the other end of the measure, excessive kindness. Surely this had something to do with that adolescent change of life we'd heard about, the precarious balance of boy striving for manhood. We wanted desperately to help, to understand, and in our desperation we explored ourselves, searching our lives and our very souls for mistakes, baffled, guilt-driven, actually hoping to find in our own behavior some clue. And although we are far from the perfect family (if such an entity exists) we could not, in all honesty, find ourselves sufficiently wanting in decency, harmony, and humanity to produce this state.

Why, then? Why? Why?

In the third stage, *detachment and apathy*, periodic protests no longer occur and depressive feelings and self-blame give way to apathetic unconcern. Energy directed at restitutional efforts, efforts sometimes helpful at the two earlier stages, is channeled into creating an imaginary world.

What leads to protest, despair, and apathy? Ricks and Berry propose that the immediate impetus to psychotic retreat is a set of intolerable feelings. Retrospective reports indicate that the schizophrenic's early years were marked by insecurity and uncertainty. During these years he was preoccupied, self-conscious, insecure, tense, or worried and had feelings of being overcome with anxiety. He felt unloved and unable to communicate with others (Fleming & Ricks, 1970).

Life from early childhood was a series of defeats and failures. Efforts to make sense out of his dismal situation led to unusual interpretations and helped create feelings of unreality. The psychological vacuum that resulted when the child started to isolate himself from others was filled with compensatory fantasies and magical hopes. These fantasies, never tested out in reality, increased already existing feelings of bodily detachment, for the person who only lives in "his head" has little sense of wholeness and realness. While finding some safety in this inner world, it is never totally satisfactory. This untenable and intolerable position eventually leads to some form of protest or despair.

Whether the process moves through to the final stage of apathy depends more on neurological integrity, intelligence, and social skill than upon intensity of feeling. If the individual can be active, effective, and successful in a reasonably receptive environment, his chances of recovery are greater (Ricks & Berry, 1970).

In struggling with their disorders, boys and girls tend to display different behaviors. Boys are more likely to be irritable, aggressive, negativistic, gloomy, and unhappy; girls appear extroverted and emotionally immature in grade school and then become more cooperative, shy, and less involved in groups by adolescence. Some children, however, do display the behaviors regarded as characteristic of the opposite sex; boys may be overinhibited and girls unsocialized aggressive.

Family background and parental social class are sometimes related to the pattern of maladjustment. A background of parental repression may contribute to the overinhibited pattern (see Chapter 7), whereas a disorganized or hostile background may lead to the unsocialized aggressive pattern (see Chapter 9; Watt, Stolorow, Lubensky, & McClelland, 1970).

The finding that many schizophrenics are antisocial as children (O'Neal & Robins, 1958; Watt, 1972) is at odds with the generally held belief that the majority of schizophrenics are introverted in childhood. A retrospective study of 606 males seen at a child guidance clinic 26 years earlier revealed that children originally classified as introverts, that is, shy and withdrawn, were not those who developed severe mental disorders in adult life (Michael, Morris, & Soroker, 1954). This study also suggested that when withdrawal did occur in schizophrenics, it was most prevalent just prior to the onset of psychosis.

Because the onset of schizophrenia proceeds through several stages, results of retrospective reports will differ depending upon the stage the child was in when the informants knew him or when he was referred to a clinic. Consequently, there are no distinct traits that could identify the preschizophrenic child from his peers at any given period in his life prior to his protest reaction. Radical changes of mood from extreme rebelliousness to extreme withdrawal and preoccupation may be a signal that a child should be referred for evaluation, but many adolescents go through similar personality changes as part of normal development. Should evaluation reveal illogical thought processes or distorted body imagery as well, the likelihood increases that the child may later show more serious difficulties.

Stress response and family influences

Differential responsiveness of family members How can we explain identical twins who are discordant for schizophrenia? It is true that the nonpsychotic twin often is considered peculiar; only about 13 percent are regarded as normal or nearly normal and the remainder are often diagnosed as schizoid. Nevertheless, some reason has to be advanced in order to explain why one twin becomes overtly psychotic while the other does not. Before we examine this question, reference to another genetic disorder will help us to understand the possible transmission of schizophrenia.

Congenital dislocation of the hip clearly has a genetic as well as an environmental etiology. It runs in families, with identical twins concordant for it in 40 percent of the cases. Certain aspects of the anatomy of the hip joint are controlled by heredity. Visualizing the hip joint as a modified ball and socket, the shape of the socket and size of the ball, both determined by heredity, can determine the relative ease with which the head of the thigh bone (the ball) can pop out of the socket. The finding that dislocation of the hip is considerably more frequent in girls than in boys is explained as resulting from a generalized laxness in all joints of the girl, a laxness that results from a release of hormones just before birth that temporarily loosens connective tissue.

Perinatal and postnatal conditions also affect the disorder. Dislocation is more common among children born by breech presentation, a position where the legs are bent and the thigh bone is likely to pop out. The custom of swaddling has similar effects because of the misdirected pressure on the baby's legs. Consequently, there is a higher rate of dislocations among certain American Indian tribes. In contrast, dislocation among Chinese children is rare because mothers carry their infants on their backs, a position that pushes the ball back further into the socket.

When twins are discordant for hip dislocation, it often turns out that one twin was a girl or was subjected to conditions that would increase the likelihood of dislocation, e.g., breech birth or swaddling.

Returning to schizophrenia, we can now ask if the schizophrenic twin was somehow different from the other in spite of identical genetic structure or if he was exposed to different rearing conditions. We do know that there is often a lower birth weight and a higher number of neonatal difficulties in the twin with schizophrenia. The schizophrenic twin also appears to identify with the psychologically less healthy, cognitively less clear-thinking parent (Mosher, Pollin, & Stabenau, 1971). Perhaps this identification is a result of the weaker physical condition. Perhaps the parent focuses on constitutional differences to select one twin as "needing her more." Although this process may be related to a real need in the smaller twin, it may lead to the parent's projecting onto the smaller twin behaviors that may not characterize the child. Similarly, particular physical and behavioral characteristics of the preschizophrenic child that set him apart from his sibling often lead the parents to attribute to him unacceptable elements of their own personalities. These repudiated aspects of the parent's own psyche are constantly drawn to the child's attention and subtly encouraged to become enduring, though negative, qualities of his personality. Later, the parents react to these qualities by punishing the child for having them (Stabenau & Pollin, 1970). Bill's mother called him a hateful monster who needed to be watched continually lest he harm his sister. In reality, Bill was not a hostile child. One of his assets was his genuine concern for other children when they were hurt. It was his mother who harbored the hate and who took to beating Bill with a stick.

In contrast, the positive aspects of the parent's personality are projected onto the healthy sibling. Consequently, the healthy sibling develops a clearer and more positive sense of self, traits that lead him to develop greater competence in social and interpersonal situations (Stabenau & Pollin, 1970).

Whatever the reason, parents seem to concentrate their efforts on the small twin. Once established, this pattern persists as the twins grow up. The smaller twin is praised for things taken for granted in the larger, and he is babied and overprotected. As a consequence, the smaller twin performs less successfully and is perceived as the less competent of the two. From age 6 until adolescence, the weaker twin becomes increasingly dependent on his healthier co-twin, who simultaneously expands his friendships. As the healthier one moves further out into society, the weaker becomes isolated from others, and his stress mounts as he grows up (Stabenau & Pollin, 1970).

If family members respond differently to identical twins, they obviously respond differently to the different children in their family. This differential responsiveness may explain why only a particular child in a family becomes schizophrenic. In addition, some families provide an environment where stress is kept to a minimum, while others expose their children to severe stress. If a child is brain-damaged or unintelligent, he also is less able than other siblings to cope with stress. Let's examine the interpersonal factors that may lead to reduced ability to handle stress.

Stress arousing family structures Reviews of the literature (Kantor & Winder, 1961; Roff, 1970) suggest that the early home environment of many schizophrenics is characterized by excessive emotional turmoil. This turmoil can result from the early death of the mother, a psychotic or severely neurotic parent, severe marital discord, rejection of the child, a dominant, overprotecting, or cold mother, or an ineffectual and passive father. Alcoholism, neuroticism, psychosomatic ailments, psychopathic personalities, and schizophrenia occur frequently among the family members of the schizophrenic.

A study of family histories reveals that many families of schizophrenics experienced periods of major crisis when the schizophrenic was between 6 months and 3 years of age, being at their peak when the child was 18 months old. Also, this was frequently a time of periods of depression in the mother, precipitated by the crises or by the birth of another child within two years after the birth of the preschizophrenic child. Maternal depression has a profound effect on the subsequent development of a child and in some way determines the child's style of response to stress later in life. Reiser (1966) found a relation between prolonged depression in mothers after childbirth and infantile psychosis.

Many of the family difficulties that exist in schizophrenic families also occur in families whose children later become delinquent or show other emotional maladjustment. Some years ago schizophrenia was considered a response to family disorganization. But, because disorganization is found in families without schizophrenic children, it is now considered only one of several factors that can precipitate schizophrenia in children already predisposed to develop this disorder.

What may be unique about the family of the schizophrenic is a particular style of family structure that leads to continual arousal of stress. To the casual observer, many families with a schizophrenic member seem no different from other families. Nevertheless, a considerable number display what Lidz and his colleagues call *marital schisms* and *marital skews* (Lidz, Fleck, & Cornelison, 1966). A marital schism exists when the marriage is always in a state of chronic disequilibrium and discord, a condition that aggravates the personality troubles of each parent and constantly threatens the marriage. In a marital skew the marriage is secure as long as the more normal parent allows the psychopathology of the other to dominate the home and thus distort the child's development.

An example given of a schismatic marriage was one where the wife was Catholic and the husband bitterly anti-Catholic. The husband had informed her shortly after their marriage that they would never quarrel about the children's religion because there would be no children. When a daughter was born, he refused to let her be baptized. Conflicts such as this occurred throughout the daughter's childhood, and in late adolescence she became schizophrenic. Looking back, she could remember no period when her parents were not threatening to separate. Her mother overprotected her when she was young and intruded into her life when she was older. Her father was chronically irritable, extremely suspicious, and offered no emotional support to his unusually insecure wife.

An example of a skewed marriage was one where the mother was quite disturbed but got along well with her husband because he was grateful for her attention. When their first child was born, the father bathed him because the mother feared she might accidently drown him. This child and his younger sister were isolated from other children until they went to school. The mother continually pestered the children's teacher to recognize the special abilities that each possessed. When the two children quarreled with their mother in later years, the father advised them to do as he did and never oppose her. The boy became psychotic in late adolescence.

Some of the deficiencies found in families with a schizophrenic child are considered deficiencies in the structure or organization of the family. Others are disturbances in the way parents communicate to their children, particularly to the child who is schizophrenic.

Deficiencies in structure When a marriage works properly, each parent supports the other in the primary roles assigned to each. Their mutual support and fulfillment of roles are basic factors in the development of the child.

In schizophrenic families the parents often fail to form a coalition; the coalition is formed instead between one parent and the schizophrenic child. The parents' lack of mutual support encourages the child to develop a manipulative technique of further dividing them to get what he wants or needs. These findings are revealed through the use of various experimental strategies that assess how families arrive at decisions. One common strategy is to have each family member respond individually and privately to a questionnaire, attitude survey, or projective test. The family members then come together and are asked to discuss the items on which they privately disagreed and to reach agreement on an answer for each item that would best represent the family's decision. Families with and without a schizophrenic member participate and the patterns of each are observed. In comparison to normal families, schizophrenic families manifest less spontaneous agreement and are impaired in their ability to reach a group decision. The parents of a schizophrenic child are unable to form working coalitions, and all family members share equally the number of decisions "won" and the amount of support received. They spend more time in silence, express more negative affect toward each other, are less expressive, and lack role differentiation in decision making (Ferreira & Winter, 1965; Mishler & Waxler, 1968; Schuham, 1970, 1972).

Parents in schizophrenic families often fail to maintain the essential boundaries between the generations (Lidz et al., 1966). In families with a schizophrenic son, there is often a reversal of generational roles between father and son; the boy and his mother take relatively high power positions and tend to defer to each other in decision making, while the father exerts little influence. In families with a schizophrenic daughter, the mother exhibits the high power position, but the daughter is isolated and little attention or respect is given to her (Mishler & Waxler, 1968). These patterns of role differentiation do not provide suitable identification models for either sons or daughters.

These patterns lead to efforts by one parent, and sometimes both, to use the child to satisfy emotional needs that are not met by the other parent. For example, one father whose wife would remain aloof after a quarrel would become excessively attentive to his daughter, until their relationship bordered on the incestual. Sometimes a mother lives through her child, unable to differentiate between her own needs and anxieties and those of the child. She may constantly supervise the child, fight all his battles, and constantly intrude into his life. One mother, when she needed a laxative, also gave her twin sons a laxative; when the doctor prescribed a sedative for her, she gave it to the boys as well (Lidz et al., 1966).

When generational boundaries are confused, energies that the child should be directing toward his own development are directed toward providing emotional support to a parent, struggling with a rivalry imposed by a parent, or simply trying to survive.

The parents of schizophrenics also fail to maintain the sexual roles appropriate to them. Rather than being warm, expressive, and helpful, the mothers of schizophrenic girls are often distant and cool toward their daughters. The fathers of schizophrenic boys tend to be weak and ineffective as husbands and parents, although they often are successful in their occupations.

Distorted communication Communication within many schizophrenic families is fragmented, amorphous, and undifferentiated (Mosher et al., 1971). A vague and rambling mother who is schizoid or schizophrenic exposes her child to blurrings and inconsistencies of meanings. A father who seems somewhat rigid and overbearing to his business associates dominates the behavior and thinking of his family with his paranoid distrust.

Training in irrationality predominates (Lidz et al., 1966). Many families, even those without an outright delusional member, distort reality to meet their own emotional needs. A father pretends to be successful when he is not; a mother denies a characteristic that is obvious to others. The result is that the child comes to distrust his own perceptions and becomes confused about the meaning of words. In addition, to be accepted by the parent, the child has to accept the role of being the one who is wrong, who perhaps is even "crazy."

Goldfarb describes mothers of schizophrenics as being bewildered or bland in the face of the bizarre behavior displayed by their child. They show passivity, marked uncertainty, lack of spontaneity, absence of empathy for the child, and frequent failure to recognize or acknowledge their child's feelings and meanings (Goldfarb, Levy, & Mayers, 1966). For example, a mother might ask her child what he had for lunch, ignore his reply, and repeat her question.

Bateson and his colleagues (Bateson, Jackson, Haley, & Weakland, 1956; Weakland, 1960) observed what they call the "double-bind" pattern of communication in families of schizophrenics. The essential feature of the double bind is that the child is caught in a situation where someone intimately involved with him communicates two messages to him and one of these denies the other. He is not allowed, however, to comment on the messages being expressed. Bateson describes the reaction of a mother to her son's attempted embrace—she stiffens, pulls away from him, and says, "Don't you love me anymore?" Verbally she implies love but behaviorally she is rejecting him. Because of the child's dependent relationship with her, he is unable to respond to the double-binding situation; he cannot make explicit what he implicitly feels. Eventually, the child learns reciprocal patterns of communication, such as giving incongruent messages of his own.

Olson (1972) examined studies investigating communication in schizophrenic families and concludes that, although the double-bind concept has generated considerable interest, the concept is still being defined and refined and that more valid measures of the concept are needed. He asks whether double binds are necessarily pathogenic. Perhaps schizophrenic patients are not as well prepared as others to integrate paradoxical experiences.

The effects of rearing conditions Children reared under conditions such as those just described are likely to lack the skills necessary to cope with challenging experiences. Unable to cope, they experience considerable anxiety when challenged. We have seen how many schizophrenics suffer from strong feelings of insecurity and live with constant anxiety. Should a deficiency exist in their stress reducing neural mechanisms, they are likely to display an exaggeration of those characteristics they learn from their parents—delusions, unreal communication, and irrational and illogical thought. If the neural transmission of messages within the brain also is faulty, these behaviors could be more pronounced.

Do not forget, however, that not all families of schizophrenic children show dysfunctional relationships and distorted communication patterns. Other stresses, such as prolonged failure due to minimal cerebral dysfunction, low intelligence, illness, or the bodily changes at adolescence, can bring about schizophrenia in those predisposed (Pollack, Levenstein, & Klein, 1968; Pollack, Woener, & Klein, 1970).

If prolonged stress helps produce schizophrenia, then children of schizophrenic parents who are reared under conditions of differing stress should show different rates of schizophrenia. One might assume that being reared by a nonschizophrenic mother would be less stressful. Studies of the fate of offspring of schizophrenic parents who are reared adoptively produce inconsistent findings. Wender (1969) reports that one-third of such a group display psychiatric disorders of a schizophrenic character. This figure may be somewhat high, since Mednick (1971) reports that only 10 to 15 percent of children reared by their schizophrenic mothers become schizophrenic before age 6. There are investigators who report similar rates of psychiatric disorder for children reared by their schizophrenic mothers and for those reared adoptively (Heston, 1966; Higgins, 1966).

In contrast, other studies suggest that adoptive rearing conditions can reduce the severity of the disorder and perhaps even its expression (Mednick & Schulsinger, 1964; Rosenthal, 1971). While this research will need replication, other research supports the position that adoptive rearing conditions can have a beneficial effect. For example, children of schizophrenic parents are more often neglected and subjected to beatings than are children of normal parents and, therefore, display a higher incidence of emotional disturbance than would be expected on purely a genetic basis (Landau, Harth, Othnay, & Sharfhertz, 1972). Similarly, Rosenthal's (1971) studies of children of normal parents who were adopted by parents who became schizophrenic revealed that these children were subjected to considerable stress, stress which eventually resulted in emotional disorders. Waxler's (1974) study demonstrated that schizophrenic adolescents who display a cognitive deficit show significant improvement after working on the cognitive task with normal parents. We also know that the number of critical comments made by key relatives of adult schizophrenic patients is strongly associated with the patients' relapses; following improvement, patients whose relatives show marked warmth without expressing criticism or overinvolvement have a better outcome (Brown, Birley, & Wing, 1972).

The highest incidence of psychopathology in Landau's study was displayed by children who comprised the third generation of mentally ill parents (61 of 70 children). While this data offers strong support for the genetic theory of transmission of mental illness, it also implies that the more ingrained the psychopathology of a family, the greater the chances that a child will have an emotional disorder.

The child living with a psychotic parent, particularly the mother, has to cope daily with bizarre behavior and illogical thinking. In addition, he has no clear parental image with whom to identify. Grace, mentioned in Chapters 9 and 12, lived with her psychotic mother until she was placed in a residential treatment center. Her extreme anxiety and depression resulted from having lived with this delusional mother, a mother who attacked a neighbor with a meat cleaver and who attributed qualities to Grace that she did not possess.

One distraught girl who lived with her paranoid mother remarked, "Mother always tells me that the neighbors put poison in our water pipes and through the doors. I don't believe it. I know my mother is sick, but still maybe mother knows something; probably the neighbors hate us, so I don't go out and play with children" (Landau et al., 1972, p. 43).

Before we conclude this section, we should note that Goldfarb (1961) reported that the children with severe pathology, his organic group, had better adjusted parents than those with mild pathology. Several other investigators also report fewer differences between families of schizophrenics and normals when the schizophrenic member is severely impaired (Caputo, 1963; Farina, 1960; Mishler & Waxler, 1968). Goldfarb suggested, therefore, that schizophrenia could result from both organic and psychogenic causes. Considering the role of stress in schizophrenia, another explanation is plausible.

Parents of a severely schizophrenic child may learn to ignore his behavior so as to minimize disruption and disturbance in the family (Mishler & Waxler, 1968). The parents accept that their child was "born that way" and that his behavior is largely beyond their control. In contrast, parents of the less disturbed youngster, a youngster with no apparent organic abnormalities on which to focus the blame, may come to disagree violently on how the child should be handled, blame each other for the child's difficulties, or be burdened with guilt. The increased incidence of psychosis in the mothers of the nonorganic children may result from the family's disharmony—the stress of marital discord activating the mother's disorder.

We can best conclude this section by summarizing Bender's (1968a) position regarding schizophrenia. She holds that individuals have a constitutional predisposition to develop schizophrenia, but an environmental stimulus is necessary to activate it. The etiological factor activating the predisposition is a physiological crisis, such as anoxia at birth, severe illness or accident, or prepubertal and pubertal crisis. Social and psychological factors determine the pattern of the psychosis. Because the child is unable to perceive reality correctly, he experiences considerable anxiety. The final clinical picture is influenced by the type of defenses the child develops to handle this anxiety.

Bender's position regarding stress as an activator of schizophrenia can be expanded to include psychological as well as physiological stress. Heston (1970) remarks, "The importance of genetic factors in the development of schizophrenia has been established beyond reasonable dispute, although it is clear that environment too plays its etiological role." We shall add that social class is not an important factor (McDermott, Harrison, Schrager, Lindy, & Killins, 1967), except perhaps in determining behavioral expression. Nevertheless, not all investigators accept the genetic hypothesis (Bettelheim, 1967). Bender (1971) has remarked that genetic factors have been disregarded more because of a wish to disbelieve than for valid reasons.

EDUCATION OF THE SCHIZOPHRENIC: BEHAVIORS THAT MAKE IT DIFFICULT

Intelligence, language, and logic

While large variations in measured IQ occur within groups of children diagnosed as schizophrenic, the majority score below an IQ of 90. Gittelman and Birch (1967) reported that only 18 percent of a group of 97 psychotic children scored above 90, 26 percent scored between 70 and 90, and 56 percent scored below 69. Nevertheless, intelligence quotients as high as 169 have been reported (Bender, 1969).

In addition to low measured intelligence, the majority of psychotic children display deficiencies in visual and auditory discrimination and in language use. Their speech is infantile, and they display a lack of questioning, infrequent use of personal pronouns, greater use of imperatives, decreased verbal output, and more frequent idiosyncratic uses of words (Hingtgen & Bryson, 1972).

The psychotic child with considerable intellectual, perceptual, and language deficiency would be educated similarly to the retarded child discussed in the last chapter. In the discussion of infantile autism later in this chapter we will describe some specialized educational procedures which also have been employed with severely impaired psychotic children. The psychotic child whose intellect approaches or exceeds the average range would be educated similarly to normal children. However, his extreme anxiety, hyperactivity, and confused ideation make his instruction difficult, particularly if attempted in regular class settings.

The first step in educating a boy like Bill is to help him develop control over his own behavior and to provide him with an atmosphere where his anxiety can decrease. The next step is to help him improve his language ability. Let's examine more closely Bill's manner of communication.

Bill's language had meaning only to himself. Its meaning was not shared by others around him. Sullivan (1944) believed the language peculiarity of the schizophrenic results from the need to maintain personal security. Being convinced that needs will remain unsatisfied, the schizophrenic uses language to pursue security; verbally, he manipulates events magically in a fruitless effort at self-satisfaction.

Language not only is a means of relating but also expresses thoughts. For most people, thought processes are based on some form of logic. Bill's responses to the Rorschach ink-blot test revealed his lack of normal logic (see Table 4.2). For example, on card 9 he saw a clown. When asked what makes it look that way, he replied "clown animal." This response represents a very primitive form of logic. To him, the nose looked more animal than human. Instead of rejecting the clown response for one incorporating the nose into the percept, he dealt with both images simultaneously by perceiving a "clown animal." This form of logic is characteristic of schizophrenic adults. Schizophrenics also seem to accept identity based upon identical predicates rather than identical subjects (Arieti, 1959). For example, if presented with "Jack is a member of the class and Jack is mean," Bill might draw the conclusion that since he was a class member, he must also be mean. A number of investigators have related the schizophrenic's inability to formulate abstract concepts to overpersonalized thinking and to associations that lead to overinclusiveness in concept making (Harrow, Himmelhoch, Tucker, Hirsh, & Quinlan, 1972; Payne & Sloan, 1968; Shimkunas, Gynther, & Smith, 1967). Feldman and Mordock (1969) noted *pars pro toto* thinking (a part is taken to be the whole), dysfunction in evaluative operations, and observable intrusions of personal and highly emotional ideas into "ordinary thinking." Concepts of self, future, and time also are distorted (Farnham-Diggory, 1966).

Overinclusive thinking is displayed when unessential elements are in-

Table 4.2 SELECTED RORSCHACH RESPONSES OF BILL, AGE 6–11

Card 3—cat	Has teeth; some cats bite and ran from you; doesn't have any bones, just eats branches and that takes out their bones
Card 5—a moustache, a bug, a bug moustache	Go on your nose and bite, stings and hurts; it's a bug like an alligator, it bites things and alligators like to eat bug moustaches; [why look like] cause its made of soft things and comes in water
Card 6—looks like a fox, has four legs	It could come and look at you, follow you, and chase you, eat you up, you come down to their stomach; if play with their skins you can get out, if you punch and break their skins; then someone could come and take them; you have to go some place else—in a airplane in the sky cause they can't reach up there
Card 9—clown too	His face; nose is like an animal, mouth is like a clown; has red lips; it's a clown animal
Card 10—looks like a face	A flower face, has a moustache, has eyes; it has bugs, bees could eat them to make honey, they sting you; [face or flower?] a flower face, looks like eyes and moustache

cluded in concepts; there is an inability to separate the relevant from the irrelevant. For example, if a normal child is given an array of objects and asked to put together those that are alike, he might group objects by size, shape, color, use, or category, such as "These are tools." The psychotic child might group together a spoon, a candle, and a pair of pliers and say "They are all roundish" or "They can all be washed in a sink." In the first response the child has focused on only one aspect of one item, the round part of the candle, and overgeneralized this aspect so that his resulting concept is inaccurate or diffuse. In the second response he has focused on the spoon, which he has seen washed in a sink, and relates the remaining two objects to the spoon on this irrelevant dimension. *Pars pro toto* thinking, a variety of overinclusiveness, would be displayed in a response such as "You can eat with them all." Sometimes an overinclusive response is highly idiosyncratic, such as "They all hurt you"; perhaps the child has been burned by a candle or pinched by pliers and overgeneralizes this idiosyncratic response to other "harmless" items like the spoon.

In Chapter 7 we describe the illogical thinking of an obsessive-compulsive child who said a thimble, a whistle, and a bottle of mercurochrome were all metal because mercury comes from mercurochrome. Since this child was exceptionally bright, he would not be expected to show such confusion. This response suggests that obsessive-compulsive disorders may sometimes mask a schizophrenic process. Bender (1955) would classify such children as pseudoneurotic schizophrenics, those whose neurotic defenses against anxiety are actually defenses against the profound anxiety and disorientation that accompanies schizophrenia.

Schizophrenic children and adults respond in affective terms to many stimuli and are unable to separate their affective reactions from more neutral reactions (Quinlan, Harrow, Tucker, & Carlson, 1972). They are likely to become emotionally aroused by objects presented to them and group them in a category such as "They are all bad" (Wahl & Wishner, 1972). One schizophrenic adolescent said that three objects were alike because they all "were painful." Her chain of associations elicited after this response was as follows. One object was a lipstick tube. She said the lipstick reminded her of blood, the blood of her menstrual period, and her period of pain. Hence the objects were "painful" objects. This response was immediate, the lipstick generating associations rarely made by normal adolescents, even when they are instructed to make unusual associations. Bill's response to questions also showed highly idiosyncratic associations.

Bill was unable to relate appropriately to other children. One interpretation of the bizarre thought processes of older schizophrenics is that they result from severely disturbed interpersonal relationships (Cameron, 1938; Haley, 1963; Jourard, 1964; Sullivan, 1944). The schizophrenic's interpersonal experiences are presumed to have been so noxious that he has chosen a life style that negates interpersonal relationships via his use of nonconsensual, autistic language. This position has been supported by findings that reveal that schizophrenics become more bizarre when requested to establish fairly intense personal relationships (Shimkunas, 1972), perform more poorly on motor and conceptual tasks when the experimenter behaves in a "warm" as opposed to an "aloof" manner (Berkowitz, 1964; Brenner, 1967), and perform more efficiently when the experimenter's absence is contingent on good performance (Gelburd & Anker, 1970).

Evidently, the schizophrenic tries to avoid interacting with people when he can and suffers when he is reminded of people and human interaction. When he cannot escape from relationships, he verbalizes distorted beliefs and autistic associations, suggesting that his symptoms function as covert messages aimed at controlling social interaction in a devious manner so as to avoid self-disclosure. Mednick and Schulsinger (1970) explain this phenomenon as a learned disorder of thought. The thought disorder consists of a set of conditioned avoidance responses that enable the schizophrenic to control his autonomic hyperresponsivity. The avoidance responses are learned on those occasions when the preschizophrenic escapes from an arousal producing stimulus by switching to a thought interrupting this arousal stimulus; the intruding association enables the individual to avoid the arousal stimulus. By such avoidance, anxiety is reduced and the association reinforced between the arousal stimulus and the avoidant thought. When these avoidance responses become automatic, they seriously interfere with sustained thinking and, therefore, hamper the child's learning.

Overinclusive thinking may be the result of interference by affective stimuli, intrusion of irrelevant associations, failure to maintain set, conditioned avoidance reactions, temporary disruptions in attention, or some other factor. Whatever the reason, such thinking makes difficult the teaching of children like Bill. The teacher's lesson deals with one topic, but the child's unusual associations to it or to unessential parts of it take him far afield from the topic.

Arieti (1965) has asserted that thought disorders in schizophrenia can be reversed. He urges early identification, stating that in the early stages of schizophrenia manifestations are evident primarily in relation to the individual's own inner anxieties. Consequently, they are more amenable to treatment than when generalized to impersonal domains. At present, there is no evidence to support this supposition. Instruments are available, however, to test this hypothesis, as well as to assist in educational planning (Feldman & Mordock, 1969; Mordock & Feldman, 1969; Wahl & Wishner, 1972).

Limited understanding of cause and effect

Like so many psychotic children, Bill had limited understanding of cause and effect, thought and action. One afternoon he was stung by a bee. After medical treatment, his chief concern was "Why would the bee want to sting me?" According to Fraiberg (1959), a boy of 5 understands that human intelligence is different from animal intelligence. Bill, at 7, had not clearly grasped this concept. Not only did he believe that the bee had desires analogous to humans, but that the bee had actually singled him out to sting. Ideas such as these (called *ideas of reference*) caused him to mistrust others because he believed they intended to harm him. When a tent set up outside school fell down on Friday, Bill believed his pulling the tent ropes on Thursday caused the tent's collapse. He probably wished the tent would collapse, for his pulling on the ropes clearly had a destructive intent. To Bill, the mere wish to pull down the tent was sufficient to make it happen. Fraiberg (1959, p. 183) tells of a boy of 5 who came into therapy with the news that two boys set fire to a house being built across the street from his house. He said soberly, "You know, I think those boys have worser problems than I have! . . . Cause if you only think about doing something like that, it can't hurt anyone. But if you do it, then you can really hurt someone." In some respects, Bill had not learned what this 5-year-old had learned—that thoughts and actions are not identical, that thoughts cannot magically produce effects. One reason for Bill's difficulty was his acting-out behavior. Thought and action were not distinct from each other because Bill's thoughts usually were translated into action. He had no controls to enable destructive thoughts to remain thoughts; he usually performed them. This inability to control himself contributed to his difficulty in understanding that thoughts themselves do not produce events. His teacher believed that firm imposition of external control would help clarify the relation for him.

Lost in fantasy

Many psychotic children are difficult to teach because they are preoccupied with their fantasies. Recently, investigators have studied the meaning of these fantasies. Chethik and Fast (1970) speculate that fantasy provides a realm of pleasure largely divorced from reality, reflects terrors being denied, and changes in response to events in the child's life.

Freud (1925) described a stage of development where the child divides experience into the pleasurable and the painful. Only the pleasurable is accepted as real, while the unpleasant and painful is denied and excluded from conscious experience. Such behavior is evident in the fantasies of Sandra, described by Chethik and Fast (1970, p. 758).

Sandra, a 9-year-old patient, developed her Cinderella story. In her therapy sessions, her "doctor" was given the role of fairy godmother. In the game, Cinderella and her protector were inseparable. When Cinderella went to bed, her fairy godmother tucked her in and sang to her. Each night as the Cinderella-child slept, her companion remained awake, never once shutting her eyes—scrubbing floors, sorting laundry, and drying dishes. Toward the early part of the morning, fairy godmother began to bake. As Cinderella awakened at dawn, she was immediately greeted by her godmother who hugged and kissed her and asked, "How many cookies do you want for breakfast?" Sandra at times reversed the roles in the repetitive games with the therapist, but the format of the story—the separation in sleep, the godmother's nighttime activity and chores, the gentle reunion upon awakening—had to be repeated along exactly prescribed lines. Interventions, comments, attempts to understand by the therapist were met with fury, or treated as no more than annoying intrusions to be overcome. Actual internal or external tension in Sandra's daily life had its immediate effect on the Cinderella story, binding godmother and daughter even more closely together in the fantasy. During a period when Sandra was suffering from nightmares (dreams containing monsters and earthquakes), the Cinderella story intensified. Cinderella became younger and younger, requiring more and more care. Finally, in one session, she was a tiny baby, just two days old. She was fed by a bottle in the game, sucked and fell asleep satiated, the bottle still in her mouth. On other anxiety producing occasions (vacation of therapist, change of appointment time, sharing therapist with another ward patient) when Sandra felt her union with the therapist was threatened, the Cinderella story became more rigid and the roles for the elaboration of the story theme became more controlled by Sandra. *(Copyright 1970, the American Orthopsychiatric Association, Inc. Reproduced by permission.)*

Sandra's Cinderella world was exhilarating and totally pleasurable; Cinderella was endlessly fed and protected. Eventually, if she is to improve, Sandra must recognize the external world as independent of herself and make a commitment to give up fantasied gratifications. Reality must be felt as real whether pleasurable or not, and pleasurable fantasies recognized as unreal if they cannot come true. The result is an integration without disorganization of both pleasure and pain into experience (Freud, 1925).

In psychotic and borderline children this transition is extremely difficult. For many psychotic children failure experiences are so painful they are denied and avoided. Avoiding work by staying in fantasy means safety from anxiety. Consequently, learning tasks should be structured for maximal success until the child gets bored and asks for more challenging work, work which he must also do significantly well. Bill's teacher combined a highly structured organization with low achievement demands to reduce anxiety and improve self-esteem, the framework suggested by Douglas (1961). Other teachers employ a variety of methods. Many advocate permissive and unstructured approaches, allowing the child freedom to work or not to work, permitting him to play out unconscious fantasies and to engage in regressed behavior. Bill's teacher felt that the theoretical basis underlying her approach was more consistent with her readings, experience, and personality makeup, and more important, it worked better for her than other approaches. Although some evidence suggests that structured approaches are more appropriate (Ney, Palvesky, & Markely, 1971), research supporting the various theories of instruction is lacking. These methods are reviewed by Haring and Phillips (1962).

"THE DICTATOR"

The satisfaction Paul derived from just thinking that he could order us about may have helped him to behave less wildly. In any event, while his "wild critter" and "crazy man" episodes had been accompanied by a marked lack of control over his body, when he was the "Great Dictator," he exercised stringent control, marching about rigidly, Nazi style. He was still hitting out at the world, but he also ordered others to do his fighting and killing, which in turn meant that he had less need to be violent himself. This also represented some progress over the "wild critter." "I'm the Great Dictator," he would announce. "All kids do what I tell. They've (to do) what I want."

As he strutted about, stiff as a robot or mechanical toy, he would laugh uproariously. But as the act wound up, he would relapse into making infantile sucking noises. Finally, when he calmed down, he would profess to be hungry and devour any food we offered him—quietly.

What lurked behind these delusions of being a dictator? Was it a desire to wield such great power that he need never again go hungry? His hunger reactions as his act subsided seemed to justify this interpretation. In any case, both the "wild critter" and the "Great Dictator" characterized Paul at his least controlled. And as these episodes became less frequent, he at last embarked on the long, laborious process of acquiring mastery over himself.

From B. Bettelheim. *Paul and Mary.* New York: Doubleday, 1960, p. 98–99.

Early infantile autism

John was an exceptionally healthy and attractive 2-year-old whose sparkling blue eyes made him look quite intelligent. Nevertheless, his family as well as his pediatrician had been worried about him almost since birth. He would sit for hours staring into space, with no one able to distract him. His disinterest in his mother troubled her greatly. But then John always had been more interested in objects than in people; he was an unusual infant, disinterested in his surroundings and extremely fearful of strangers. He insisted his toys remain in certain arrangements, and he engaged in highly repetitive play. Fantasy was absent. Speech, which, to the delight of his parents, he had acquired early, now seemed peculiar and noncommunicative. Desires were expressed by leading his mother by the hand to what he wanted.

John was referred to the child guidance clinic for evaluation. Staff opinion was that he displayed infantile psychosis, more specifically, that he was autistic.

This unusual behavioral disturbance was first described by Kanner (1943). He found the major features to be: early preference for being alone, failure to relate to parental figures, abnormal speech development, desire for sameness, and extreme anxiety when confronted with change. Kanner felt that early infantile autism is distinguished from severe mental retardation by the autistic child's normal motor development, thoughtful facial expression, rote memory (his concern for sameness implies recall of previous arrangements), and spatial ability (frequently he does well on jigsaw puzzles). Table 4.3 presents the symptoms of four autistic children.

Kanner's research led to a series of investigations into infantile autism and an effort to distinguish this syndrome from childhood schizophrenia. In 1964 Rimland, the scientist-father of an autistic child, published a comprehensive review of the literature on infantile autism that reiterated many of Kanner's original findings. Rimland also added some criteria of his own: low incidence of psychosis among the child's ancestors, lack of clinically detectable hallucinations or delusions, fetishlike preoccupation with mechanical objects, extremely well-developed spatial memory, and musical ability.

Lotter (1966, 1967) surveyed all the children in Middlesex County who were between the ages of 8 to 10 during the period of his study (with 97 percent coverage of 78,000 children). His research included a well-constructed screening questionnaire, clinical interviews by Lotter of all 135 possible cases of autism, testing of children and families, and complete medical histories. Final identification of two groups of autism, nuclear and less severely psychotic, were made by comparing all information against 24 items (Table 4.4) considered characteristic of autism.

Lotter's criteria are not completely consistent with those of Rimland and Kanner. Not included in Lotter's list were several of Rimland's criteria. For example, Lotter does not include excellent motor ability, physical attractiveness, or musical ability, since these traits were not confirmed by other experimenters (Goldfarb, 1970a). In addition, Lotter's survey included children who developed the disorder between 2 and 5 years and those who manifested gross organic features, criteria clearly at odds with Kanner, who emphasized that autism differed from other cases of childhood psychosis because of its manifestation in early infancy.

CAUSES OF INFANTILE AUTISM

If infantile autism is an early version of schizophrenia, then we have already discussed current thinking regarding its etiology. Those who hold the view that the disorder differs from the schizophrenias postulate various causes. Kanner (1943) felt the disorder was due to an inborn disturbance of affective contact. Later, he placed greater emphasis on the emotional coldness seen in the parents of the children. While he still considered the defect inborn, he felt psychogenic factors were also contributory. Still

Table 4.3 CLINICAL NOTES ON DISTURBANCES OF PERCEPTION, MOTILITY, RELATEDNESS, AND LANGUAGE IN FOUR AUTISTIC PATIENTS

Patient			Symptoms			
Name	Age	Perception	Motility	Relatedness	Language	
John	13	At times, failed to respond to spoken command or loud noise. Devoted considerable time to smelling, tasting, and feeling the texture of objects. Intermittently stared at people and objects. Marked textural food preferences. Refused to eat for several days.	Hand-flapping, persistent finger-wiggling, total body-rocking, darting and lunging movements alternated with periods of prolonged immobility.	Failed to imitate, avoided eye contact, "looked through" people. Could not form a meaningful relationship with psychotherapist, teachers, or familiar staff personnel.	Predominantly echolalia and delayed echolalia. Occasional spontaneous verbalizations of realistic demands and bizarre fantasies.	
Richard	9	Regarded objects and hands in a stereotyped manner. Rubbed surfaces and objects to sense their texture. Spun himself and objects and stared at spinning objects. At times, unresponsive to soft and hypersensitive to loud as well as soft sounds. Frequently failed to respond with appropriately painful affect to bumps and falls.	Persistent toe-walking, hand-flapping, finger-flicking. At times, darting and lunging movements alternating with posturing.	Failed to imitate and avoided eye contact. Had no social smile or anticipatory response to being picked up. Used others as an extension of himself and inappropriately climbed onto a lap as if it were a chair.	Mute except for crying and screaming when severely upset.	
Pedro	4	Intermittent staring, regarding of hands and objects, and finger movements. At times, unresponsive to sounds. Frequently tasted objects and showed food preferences based on textures.	Oscillated objects such as pencils with his fingers. Exhibited nuchal hypertension and other unusual posturing. Hand-flapping and, at times, darting and lunging movements, and body rocking.	Failed to imitate, avoided eye contact, and used other people's hands to accomplish his desires. Failed to develop anticipatory responses to being picked up.	Mute. Intermittent responses to simple, verbal commands such as "no."	
Stanley	3	Stared at his hands and inanimate objects. Scratched surfaces and felt textures. Unresponsive to loud noises. Mouthed and tasted objects.	Flapped hands and arms, whirled spontaneously and occasionally toe-walked. Rocked his body, banged his head, and flicked at objects.	Failed to imitate, avoided eye contact, lacked anticipatory responses to being picked up, used another person's hand as if it were an extension of his own, and stiffened when held.	Mute. Occasionally responsive to simple commands and the word "no."	

From E. R. Ritvo, A. Yuwiler, E. Geller, A. Kales, S. Rashkis, A. Schicor, S. Potkin, R. Axelrod, & C. Howard. Effects of L-dopa in autism. *Journal of Autism and Childhood Schizophrenia*, 1971, **1**, 190–205. With the permission of V. H. Winston & Sons, Publishers.

Table 4.4 LOTTER'S 24 BEHAVIOR ITEMS

Speech (speaking children only)
1. Speech not used for communication
2. Reversal of pronouns
3. Echolalia
4. Repetition of phrases

Social behavior
5. Visual avoidance
6. Solitary
7. Ignores children
8. Aloof and distant
9. Walks/looks through people

Movement peculiarity
10. Self-spinning
11. Jumping
12. Flapping
13. Toe walking
14. Other marked mannerisms

Auditory
15. Behaves as if deaf
16. Covers ears
17. Distress at noise

Repetitive/ritualistic
18. Elaborate food fads
19. Lines and patterns with objects
20. Spinning objects
21. Other elaborate ritualistic play
22. Carrying, banging, or twirling objects
23. Insistence on sameness (objects)
24. Insistence on sameness (events)

Adapted from V. Lotter. Epidemiology of autistic conditions in young children. 1. Prevalence. *Social Psychiatry*, 1966, **6**, 124–137.

later, he returned to his original position, rejecting the notion that the parent's behavior contributed to the disorder. Others, however, gave greater importance to parental lack of affection (Bettelheim, 1967) and stimulated a great deal of research on parent personality.

Bettelheim claimed the child reacts to his environment in an autistic manner because he is raised by indifferent parents. Because of this indifference, the child concludes his parents want him dead and fears for his life. In response, he gives up contact and communication with the outside world he believes is his enemy. Harlow (1969) reviewed the book in which Bettelheim presented his theory and stated that the theory, like the title of the book in which it was presented (*The Empty Fortress*), was empty, empty because there was no evidence that such rejection occurs or that rejection results in autism.

While Harlow's statements are unnecessarily harsh, they are nevertheless true. (The reader might be interested to know that Harlow is a comparative psychologist who has done extensive experimental research to prove that monkeys develop abnormally if brought up by automatons and so is certainly not theoretically predisposed to reject the significance of parental influence on the development of the child.) Bettelheim, a man deeply committed to disturbed children, has rarely seen fit to cite the work of others and is reluctant to work with the parents of the children he treats at his famous Orthogenic School in Chicago. Since removal from the home, even when parents are quite disturbed, can hinder the child's development (Ward, 1974), Bettelheim's position is unsound.

Rutter (1968) feels that Lotter's epidemiological survey provided convincing evidence that early infantile autism is not a variety of schizophrenia that occurs in very young children, but is an entirely different disorder. He cites seven factors that he feels supports this position. (1) The sex ratio is different—autism is much more common in males whereas schizophrenia is about equally common in the two sexes. (2) The parents of autistic children are often of above average intelligence and of superior socioeconomic status. (3) Schizophrenia is rare in the families of autistic children. (4) Whereas mental subnormality occurs in almost all autistic children there are often schizophrenics with average or above average IQs. (5) Autistic children display a pattern on IQ tests characterized by high scores on visual-spatial tasks and low scores on verbal tasks. (6) Whereas delusions and hallucinations are common symptoms in schizophrenia, they are rare in autistic children even after they reach adolescence and early life. (7) Marked remissions and relapses are observed in schizophrenia, but are rare in autism where a relatively steady course is more common.

Regarding Rutter's second point, both Kanner and Rimland reported that the majority of the parents of autistic children were bright professional people. Of the 100 fathers in Kanner's sample, 96 were high school graduates, 74 were college graduates, and the majority were in professional or business occupations. Goldfarb (1970a) feels that selective factors were operating in Kanner's sample. Two of these might have been his university setting and the fact that only wealthy people could afford to travel to his center for evaluation. Goldfarb states that centers other than Kanner's have treated children with features similar to those Kanner describes whose parents have been unintelligent, uneducated, and non-Anglo-Saxon. Lotter's (1966, 1967) studies indicate that parents of a group of children he called nuclear autistic were highly intelligent. The parents of those classified as less severely psychotic were also quite intelligent, but less intelligent than the parents of the nuclear group.

Rutter holds the view that the basic deficit in infantile autism is an impairment in the comprehension of sounds and is therefore closely akin to other developmental disorders of language (see Chapter 2). He cites convincing research in support of this thesis. Several Japanese researchers also hold this view (Ishikawa, 1970). To a child who is incapable of distinguishing between speaker and listener owing to some disturbance in perceptive-integrative mechanisms, his caretakers must appear as autistic to him as he does to them. Similarly, others believe that thought disorders result from an inability to process sensory data, especially heard speech, selectively or rapidly enough. Only confused information is relayed to the higher integrative centers, and this confusion is then manifested as a thinking disorder (Yates, 1966). Perceptual and neurobiological impairment is somehow involved in this data processing inability (Hingtgen & Bryson, 1972).

Des Lauriers and Carlson (1969) view infantile autism as a failure to develop normally rather than as an instance of abnormal development. They postulate that an internal barrier to normal levels of sensory and affective receptivity exists within the child. The autistic child is capable of attending to stimuli, but he is believed to be incapable of establishing associations between responses and reinforcements. The work of Lovaas (1967), who found that autistic children take an enormous number of trials to establish a conditioned response, supports this viewpoint.

Hutt and his colleagues (Hutt, Hutt, Lee, & Ounsted, 1965) believe that the stereotyped behaviors that autistic children display (e.g., twirling, hand flapping) are biological safety devices that protect the child from the deleterious effects of excessive sensory stimulation. Because of a failure of the reticular activating system, the autistic child is always in a state of high arousal. Consequently, stimuli that produce even higher levels of arousal (perhaps emotional contact with another person) are actively avoided.

Rimland (1964) also suspects that deficient functioning of the reticular activating system of the brain stem is responsible for infantile autism. Stimuli entering the brain are not sorted, segregated, or integrated with prior or subsequent input. Consequently, the child is unable to relate new stimuli to remembered experience. In short, he is unable to learn.

Goldfarb (1970a) states that theories regarding the role of the reticular activating system in autism have not been supported by empirical investigation. A more precise statement is that these theories are highly speculative, since little research has been undertaken in this area. Goldfarb did not mention, however, that the EEGs of autistic children do show a pattern that suggests a high state of physiological arousal (Hutt et al., 1965) and that often very large doses of sedative drugs are required before they have an effect on autistic children (Connell, 1966). Rutter (1968) suggests that high arousal may be a secondary rather than a primary defect and stresses the need for further study before this issue can be settled.

If a high arousal level does exist in autistic children, then autism may simply be schizophrenia at an early age, since our previous discussion stressed the seeming abnormality of the schizophrenic's autonomic nervous system. In this vein, Ornitz and Ritvo (1968) believe that early infantile autism is the same disorder as schizophrenia and that differences in symptoms seen at different ages, are due to the developmental level the child has reached at the time of the onset of the disorder. They state that the families of autistic children come from every socioeconomic class and that Rutter's failure to find schizophrenic parents among his population is not confirmed by other investigators. They claim that after the age of 5 or 6, symptom complexes of autism tend to merge with those of childhood schizophrenia. They presume a neurophysiological defect as the cause of the schizophrenias, more specifically, a breakdown of homeostatic regulation of sensory input resulting in a condition of perceptual inconstancy.

Hingtgen and Bryson (1972) emphasize that considerable disagreement still exists as to whether schizophrenia is a single disease entity or several pathological conditions with superficial similarities but different etiologies. They emphasize the need for more complete subject descriptions, independent of theoretical considerations, and caution against any premature false resolution of the problem of differential diagnosis of the childhood psychoses.

Learning theory and autism

Because of the increasing popularity of behaviorism and learning theory, brief mention will be made of the hypothesis generated from this viewpoint. Essentially, psychosis is viewed as the result of faulty conditioning (Ferster, 1961). This view is based on the favorable response of some autistic children to operant conditioning methods of treatment (to be discussed in a later section). However, no one has demonstrated that abnormal patterns of reinforcement existed in these children's backgrounds. Also, it does not follow that the nature of causation relates to the type of therapy that is effective. Rutter (1968, p. 391) stated that "One might just as well suggest that because depression frequently responds to electric shock treatment, therefore depression is due to a lack of electric shocks in childhood."

TRAINING AND TREATMENT

Special training programs

While many of the favorable responses to educationally oriented remediation programs have been situation-specific and short lived (Rutter, 1967), these efforts seem the most promising on the current scene. Biochemical and genetic explorations may open new vistas in the treatment of the autistic child, but educators can't wait. Faced with the task of teaching autistic children, many have developed specialized techniques for their instruction. Before we cite several examples of procedures in current use, some introductory remarks are in order.

In general, education of the autistic child is better conceived as training. The goal is to establish a basic repertoire of very simple behaviors. Once this repertoire is established, efforts are made to build increasingly complex chains of behavior and to establish their use in a variety of situations. The goal is to make the child easier to live with and to make him more competent in particular tasks. Behaviors that are important for the child to display are shaped; those that are undesirable are extinguished.

With self-destructive behavior (severe head banging, burning fingers, etc.), physical restraint is sometimes necessary. Lovaas (1967) has successfully used painful electric shock to extinguish self-destructive behavior that could have resulted in death (chewing through both tissue and bone). His view is that self-destructive behavior follows the laws of other learned behaviors; behavior is regulated by the consequences it has on the environment. The child who displays self-destructive behavior is one who had been initially rewarded for this behavior, either through increased attention to his needs or through the reactions of others. Consequently, he must learn that this behavior brings a new consequence. Lovaas summarized his position by stating the paradox that providing traditional treatment of support and affection to the self-destructive child is to aggress him, since it increases self-destruction; to deliver pain, which diminishes self-destruction, is to demonstrate affection.

Regarding training, Lovaas (1967) recommends that appropriate behaviors be shaped through a programmed environment. Discriminations should be taught in gradual steps, utilizing prompts. Adults can move the child physically through desired behaviors or tell the child correct verbal responses to stimuli. Gradually, prompts can be faded, until the child can produce the correct behavioral response to stimuli without an adult's guidance.

In this manner the autistic child can be taught to dress and feed himself and to take care of his own toileting. He may even be able to attain an acceptable level of decorum, so that he can accompany his family in public places. Although such changes may seem insignificant in terms of the overall clinical problem, they may facilitate the child's acceptance by his family (Churchill, 1969). Simply acquiring some control over his own behavior makes life easier for both the child and his family.

Although minimum self-control can be taught, the autistic child has a very limited response capability, even when his motivation is high. He also shows specific learning deficits that place an absolute ceiling on his ability to learn certain responses. For example, Churchill (1969, p. 441) describes the response of the autistic child to training on relatively simple tasks.

The child, after passing through the initial negativism and uncooperativeness, the tantrums and rituals, and after he has become hungry enough and appears to know that food is given contingent upon his responses, enters into a phase in which he is very highly motivated. His attention is riveted on the adult; the interfering behaviors drop away completely. Response latencies are extremely short and, indeed, if the adult is not quick enough the child tries to prompt him to present the next cue.

By now the child has been trained to give several different responses upon presentation of an adult model for that response—say, clapping hands and holding hands high over the head. If presented randomly with simply these two models to "imitate," the child may never achieve more than a chance number of successes. That is, with every indication of the highest possible motivation, the child may attentively watch the adult clap hands and then put his own hands over his head! He then looks for his reward and displays evidence of great frustration that it is not forthcoming. Similar examples could be presented in great number but the point is this: There is a situation of extremely high motivation and of astonishingly poor performance—astonishing, that is, in terms of our previous expectations. *(Copyright 1969, American Psychiatric Association.)*

Churchill reports that many autistic children can learn to write what they see and say what they hear, but they cannot write what they hear. "When this is observed, neither persistance nor ingenuity has produced association of information across the two sensory modalities" (1969, p. 443).

Keeping these remarks in mind, we will describe several procedures used to teach language skills to autistic children. Only 50 percent of children labeled autistic develop speech; the rest are mute. Of those who do develop speech, it is generally a peculiar, noncommunicative kind, produced in a high pitched, parrotlike monotone. The pronouns are absent until around the sixth year, followed by pronoun reversal (*you* for *I*). Literalness, part-whole confusion, delayed echolalia (repetition of phrases or sentences out of context), and metaphorical use of language are characteristic (Rimland, 1964).

A program designed to develop communication skills was initiated by the Day-Care Unit for Autistic Children at the University of Pennsylvania's School of Medicine. The program emphasized speech, language, and general communication. A worker was assigned to each child to vocalize his activities and ideas. When the child achieved a relationship with the worker, formal language training began. During training sessions, the worker remained until the child felt comfortable with the speech therapist. Implicit in this work was the development of basic trust between child and teacher.

Children were given tasks to perform in small increments. They first imitated nonhuman sounds, then the sounds of speech, and finally words. All attempts were immediately rewarded. The children echoed the words learned, but rarely used them to communicate. Echolalia was handled by making children repeat echoed phrases until they used the same phrases when it was appropriate for them to do so (Wolf & Ruttenberg, 1967).

Staff at the Neuropsychiatric Institute School, at the University of California at Los Angeles, attempted to teach speech to a 4½-year-old nonverbal, autistic boy named Peter. Candy, while somewhat effective as a reinforcer, did not hold his attention. A booth was constructed in which Peter occupied one half and the teacher the other. The teacher controlled a panel separating the two halves. When the panel was closed, Peter's side had no light; when raised, the light from the teacher's half flooded Peter's. In addition, a ball-drop device operated as follows. When the ball was released by the teacher, it went into a cup where Peter could pick it up and drop it into a box. When the ball was placed in the box, a bell would ring. The bell signaled the teacher to raise the panel. She then provided rewards such as candy, light, music, a ride on a revolving chair, cartoon movies, or games.

The training program required imitation of the therapist. Whenever Peter responded incorrectly or refused to try, he was isolated in his dark half of the booth. As he acquired certain words, he was required to use them in the living unit. For example, when time came for his training sessions, he had to say "go" before being taken. When he wanted water or food, he had to ask for them. Other children became interested in Peter and helped him to use his newly developed language. When speech developed to a level where he could make simple requests, Peter went home on visits. His parents were familiar with the training program and required him to use the words he knew. After weekend visits home, the therapist noted a great change in his attitude. When he first entered school, Peter showed no attachment to his parents, leaving them without hesitation. After several months in the program, he was reluctant to return from weekend visits. Peter eventually became an outpatient. He was enrolled in a private nursery-kindergarten where the speech therapist employed similar training procedures (Hewett, 1965).

Experimental programs to teach reading have also been initiated at the Neuropsychiatric Institute. Jimmy, a 13-year-old, could vocalize but could not speak. Like Peter, he was extremely distractible. Nevertheless, the therapists noticed that he spent hours working on jigsaw puzzles or copying letters, reproducing them accurately. Because Jimmy preferred self-directed activities rather than socially directed ones, conventional educational techniques were not employed. Instead, gumdrops were used to capture his attention and to reward his responses.

Jimmy was first taught that objects as well as pictures could represent words. The top rail of a word board contained a picture or object; the bottom rail contained the word, plus a glass box that contained a gumdrop. Jimmy was required to draw the object in order to get his gumdrop. The next step required his matching words and pictures. To assist him, a two-piece jigsaw puzzle was designed to help him associate words and pictures. Eventually, Jimmy worked because he wanted to, not just for candy. He communicated with the teacher using the words he learned and tried to describe events to his mother. Ultimately, he learned to write and to copy simple words. His teacher noted (Hewett, 1964, p. 618):

> In Jimmy's case, acquisition of rudimentary reading and writing skills seem to heighten his interest in the environment and make him more accessible to social control. On the basis of such a breakthrough experience with Jimmy, teaching reading and writing may offer a most promising means of furthering socialization and treatment of heretofore isolated autistic children.

The Neuropsychiatric Institute now places autistic and other atypical children in group learning situations. For forty-five minute sessions, five days a week, children attend an experimental kindergarten-primary program. The activities presented require skills that normal kindergarten children should have mastered. Tangible items, such as candy, are rewards for successful efforts. After three months the candy is replaced by tokens which can be traded for toys. Children are reported to make significant progress in this program (Rabb & Hewett, 1967).

Some investigators feel that language training should follow training in other areas. After several language sessions with autistic children, Pronovost and his colleagues (Pronovost, Wakstein, & Wakstein, 1966, p. 24) reported that "perceptual disturbances of the children became apparent and a nonverbal physical and gestural language developed." Sessions were, therefore, changed from language training to visual and auditory training. They (Pronovost et al., 1966, p. 24) found that

> as the structured stimuli were held within the limits of each child's frustration tolerance, his vocalization or speech became less explosive, less variable in pitch, intensity, and quality. . . . Thus, we tend to conclude that the perceptual problems of the children studied are the most significant factors contributing to the child's speech and language behavior.

Several factors must be taken into consideration when evaluating the results of special programs. First, when studies show that a child has improved his speech, the reader may be left with the false impression that the child converses more readily with others or is more spontaneous. What usually has improved is only imitative or rote speech; spontaneous speech may never develop (Hingtgen & Churchill, 1969; Weiss & Born, 1967).

Second, when a child does show substantial improvement, he may have been inappropriately labeled autistic. This possibility is quite likely considering the extensive use of this label without widespread agreement regarding the criteria for its use. For example, in an article entitled "A Social Learning Therapy Programme with an Autistic Child," the child described below was labeled autistic by Davison (1964, p. 151).

A little girl was chosen on the basis of four criteria: (1) she was not in individual therapy; (2) she had no known physiological damage; (3) she was not on medication; and (4) she accepted an M & M candy when it was offered to her. She was a pretty, frail-looking nine-year-old child. She was very talkative (although communicating little), and was characterized by withdrawal, various ritualistic behaviors, apparent hallucinatory activities, and general disobedience. Because the aim was to test the limits of a short-term programme, there was no inquiry made into the background of the child.

Comparing this description with Lotter's (1966) 24 behavior items reveals that she displays, at best, mild versions of only four of the symptoms and strictly fits none. The diagnosis is even more suspect after Davison remarks, "When it was time to leave, the child begged the therapist to stay a bit longer, telling him that she liked him" (p. 154).

Psychotherapy

Rimland (1964) reviewed the literature regarding psychotherapy with autistic children and concluded that conventional psychotherapy did not lead to significant improvement in autistic behavior. While this conclusion is correct (Eisenberg & Kanner, 1956), it is misleading because it implies that a significant number of therapists have attempted to do something "conventional" with the autistic child. This has not been the case; those major authors who describe psychotherapeutic techniques with autistic, or with all psychotic children for that matter, stress the need to modify therapy techniques in order to help these children. The modified techniques usually involve the use of considerable bodily closeness with the child, nonverbal participation with him, singing to him, and fondling him (Mahler, 1952; Rank & MacNaughton, 1950).

In addition, individual therapy of autistic children usually takes place within residential treatment centers where the total environment is organized to facilitate the development of the child's coping skills. In fact, without a programmed environment, individual psychotherapy may be useless. Goldfarb (1970a, p. 816) states, "Indeed it has seemed that only under the circumstances of a clearly articulated social environment does the psychotic child become aware of the conflictual aspects of his very frightened, unhappy existence."

As we will learn in Chapter 12, evaluating change is no easy task. Frequently, only global judgments about a child's progress are made rather than recording precise behavioral changes. An autistic child might improve in response to psychotherapy, but the improvement might be less than was expected by the therapist or parent. At present, no firm conclusions can be made about the value of individual psychotherapy in the treatment of autism (Goldfarb, 1970a).

Chemotherapy

Drugs are employed to alleviate anxiety that might interfere with learning or social responsiveness. They are adjunctive techniques to make the child more responsive to those ongoing social and educational activities that may help him (Fish, 1968). Some people fear that because medications diminish a child's anxiety, he may never learn to handle anxiety on his own. These fears have no solid foundation, however, for if medication works at all, it does so by facilitating the ability to focus attention and direct behavior. Medications, therefore, set the stage for improved future functioning.

INCIDENCE OF AUTISM AND SCHIZOPHRENIA

How frequent is psychosis in children? Considering autism as a separate group, Lotter (1966) cites the incidence as 2 per 10,000 for nuclear autism or as 4.5 per 10,000 if both groups are included. The sex ratio is cited as three or four boys to one girl (Anthony, 1958; Kanner, 1954; Keeler, 1957). Early infantile autism occurs primarily in first-born children. Rimland's (1971) analyses of check list data on 2,218 psychotic children indicated that 9.7 percent fit Kanner's original description of this syndrome. As we have seen, Kanner favors employing the term autism only for children displaying those behaviors he originally described. Rimland's (1964) results support Kanner's earlier statement that out of every 100 children referred to him as autistic, only about 10 actually fit his criteria. Most European researchers agree with Kanner and Rimland's position that autism is a unique psychosis. Most American researchers do not agree.

Taking child psychosis as a whole, the incidence of reported disorders is low. For every 1,000 children born, between 14 and 20 will be hospitalized for schizophrenia before age 21.

HOW DO THEY FARE?

What happens to the children who have been diagnosed as psychotic? Those researchers who have followed the development of psychotic children over a period of years indicate that most childhood and adolescent schizophrenics grow up to become adult schizophrenics (Annesley, 1961; Eisenberg & Kanner, 1956; Errera, 1957; Goldfarb, 1970b; Havelkova, 1968; Kanner, 1971; Menolascino & Eaton, 1967; Rutter, Greenfield, & Lockyer, 1968).

Although we would think that children afflicted early, such as those classified as autistic, would fare less well than those afflicted later, we would be incorrect. Autistic children with obvious organic involvement and those who lacked speech at age 5 fare considerably worse than other autistic children (Bender, 1969; Eisenberg & Kanner, 1956), but autistic children without those impairments function about as well as children whose psychoses appear later in life. For example, in a study of 61 autistic children followed over a 15-year period (Eisenberg, 1966), 30 were included who had not spoken prior to age 5. Of these 30, only 1 attained marginal social adjustment and even that marginal adjustment lasted only until age 20, at which time he was hospitalized for a psychotic episode. In contrast, of 31 with effective language, 16 attained some social adjustment accompanied by progress in school.

Similarly, Bender (1969) followed 30 children who met Kanner's criteria of infantile autism. The children were originally seen on the children's ward of Bellevue Psychiatric Hospital between 1935 and 1952 and at the time of follow-up ranged in age from 22 to 42. The life course of 17 patients who had organic involvement was one of progressive deterioration. By 1968 6 had died and the surviving 11 were chronically institutionalized, 8 in institutions for the retarded, 1 in a mental hospital, and 2 in hospitals for the criminally insane where they had been transferred from other institutions because they became dangerously violent during convulsions. Two of the deceased patients died in convulsive episodes, 3 died of cardiac difficulties, and 1 died of drowning. The 13 individuals without organic involvement did considerably better.

VIRGINIA

Virginia S., born September 13, 1931, had resided in a State Training School for retarded children since 1936. Dr. Esther L. Richards, who saw her there wrote in May 1941: "Virginia stands out from other children because she is absolutely different from any of the others. She is neat and tidy, does not play with other children, and does not seem to be deaf but does not talk. The child will amuse herself by the hour putting picture puzzles together, sticking to them until they are done. I have seen her with a box filled with parts of two puzzles gradually work out the pieces for each. All findings seem to be in the nature of a congenital abnormality."

Virginia was the daughter of a psychiatrist, who said of himself: "I have never liked children, probably a reaction on my part to the restraint from movement, the minor interruptions, and commotions." Of his wife he said: "She is not by any means the mother type. Her attitude (toward a child) is more like toward a doll or pet than anything else." Virginia's brother, 5 years her senior, when referred to us because of severe stuttering at 15 years of age, burst out in tears when asked how things were at home and he sobbed: "The only time my father has ever had anything to do with me was when he scolded me for doing something wrong." His mother did not contribute even that much. He felt that all his life he had lived in "a frosty atmosphere" with two inapproachable strangers.

In August 1938, the psychologist at the training school observed that

Virginia "pays no attention to what is said to her but quickly comprehends whatever is expected. Her performance reflects discrimination, care, and precision." With the non-language test items, she achieved an IQ of 94. "Without a doubt, her intelligence is superior to this. . . . She is quiet, solemn, composed. Not once have I seen her smile. She retires within herself, segregating herself from others. She seems to be in a world of her own, oblivious to all but the center of interest in the presiding situation. She is mostly self-sufficient and independent. There was no manifestation of friendliness or interest in persons. On the other hand, she finds pleasure in dealing with things, about which she shows imagination and initiative."

When seen on October 11, 1942, Virginia was a tall, slender, neatly dressed girl. She responded when called by getting up and coming nearer without ever looking up to the person who called her. She just stood listlessly, looking into space. Occasionally, in answer to questions, she muttered: "Mamma, baby." When a group was formed around the piano, one child playing and the others singing, she sat among the children, seemingly not ever noticing what went on, and gave the impression of being self-absorbed. She did not seem to notice when the children stopped singing. When the group dispersed, she did not change her position and appeared not to be aware of the change of scene. She had an intelligent physiognomy, though her eyes had a blank expression.

Virginia will be 40 years old next September. She has been transferred to the Henrytown State Hospital. "She is," the report from there, dated November 2, 1970, says, "in a program for adult retardates, with her primary rehabilitation center being the Home Economics Section. She can hear and is able to follow instructions and directions. She can identify colors and can tell time. She can care for her basic needs, but has to be told to do so. Virginia likes to work jigsaw puzzles and does so very well, preferring to do this alone. She can iron clothes. She does not talk, uses noises and gestures, but seems to understand when related to. She desires to keep to herself rather than associate with other residents."

From L. Kanner. Follow-up study of eleven autistic children originally reported in 1943. *Journal of Autism and childhood Schizophrenia*, 1971, **1**, 119–145. With the permission of V. H. Winston & Sons, Publishers.

While all had spent some time in special residential schools, institutions for the retarded, or state or private mental hospitals, by 1968 all were living at home in conditions ranging from psychotic dependency to financial independence.

The eventual status of autistic children who are free from organic involvement and who speak by age 5 is similar to the status achieved by other psychotic children; about one-third display what is considered marginal or fair adjustment.

Brown (1963) gave the current educational status of 129 children age 10 or older who were originally diagnosed "atypical disorder," a term often used synonymously with autism (Rank, 1955). Table 4.5 presents

Table 4.5 FOLLOW-UP OF "ATYPICAL CHILDREN"

Schooling	No.
Regular school	46
Special classes	14
Schools for mentally retarded	17
Schools for disturbed	10
Institutions	34
At home, no school	7

Adapted from J. L. Brown. Follow-up of children with atypical development. *American Journal of Orthopsychiatry*, 1963, **33**, 855–861. Copyright © 1963, the American Orthopsychiatric Association, Inc. Reproduced by permission.

this data. As we can see, about 35 percent of this group were attending normal classes. A similar figure was reported by Bender (1969) who followed 200 psychotic children seen at Bellevue Hospital between 1935 and 1952. By the age of 30, one-third of the group were doing fairly well, one-third were regressed institutionalized patients, and one-third fluctuated from poor to fair adjustment, most of them living in institutions. Bender (1968) also analyzed 12 reports that appeared in the literature between 1948 to 1968. These studies covered 759 cases followed from childhood to late adolescence or adulthood; 229 (31.5 percent) were said to have made an adequate social adjustment.

Some clarification of the word *adequate* is necessary, however, since former schizophrenics rarely are considered normal by other citizens. For example, even the relatively "successful" children in Eisenberg and Kanner's (1956) follow-up exhibited a lack of social perceptiveness best characterized by a lack of savoir-faire, that is, they made extremely untimely or inappropriate remarks without foreseeing their consequences. Similarily, even though 35 percent of Brown's (1963) group were attending regular classes, only 6 percent (7 children) of the total group were considered normal. The remainder of those attending school were classified as neurotic or schizoid.

In addition to speech and organicity, intelligence, original rating of the severity of disorder, and amount of schooling also relate to outcome (Havelkova, 1968; Rutter et al., 1968). The IQ is of value in differentiating those who will be rated "severe" at follow-up from those who will be rated "mild." The other two variables differentiate those rated as having made a good adjustment from those with fair adjustment. Reference to Table 4.6 further demonstrates the relationship of intellectual function to outcome. Note the tendency toward deterioration of intellect on follow-up, most marked in the least disturbed cases. Sixty-one percent of all subjects were functioning below 70 IQ at follow-up, whereas only 23 percent were below this score on the initial testing. None of these had much chance of independent functioning. Variables that seem to be

Table 4.6 RELATIONSHIP OF SEVERITY OF ILLNESS TO INTELLECTUAL FUNCTION—71 CHILDREN

Intellectual level	Severe—17		Moderate—29		Mild—25	
	Original	Follow-up	Original	Follow-up	Original	Follow-up
Dull normal, normal, or higher (from IQ 80 up)	0 (0%)	0 (0%)	16 (55%)	9 (31%)	21 (84%)	9 (36%)
Borderline (IQ 70–80)	6 (35%)	0 (0%)	9 (32%)	5 (17%)	3 (12%)	5 (20%)
Defective (IQ 50–70)	3 (18%)	1 (6%)	4 (14%)	9 (31%)	1 (4%)	10 (40%)
IQ under 50	8 (47%)	16 (94%)	0 (0%)	6 (21%)	0 (0%)	1 (4%)

From M. Havelkova. Follow-up study of 71 children diagnosed as psychotic in preschool age. *American Journal of Orthopsychiatry*, 1968, **38**, 846–857. Copyright © 1968, the American Orthopsychiatric Association, Inc. Reproduced by permission.

unrelated to outcome are sex, presence or absence of normal development prior to the onset of psychosis, and family situation (Rutter et al., 1968).

The finding that age of onset does not correlate with eventual outcome is surprising. Perhaps another developmental variable is more critical. Havelkova (1968) observed that a number of psychotic children show a change from autistic to pseudoneurotic behavior. The age of this change appears to be of considerable importance. Of those who changed before age 4½, 70 percent had a normal intellect on follow-up. Of those who changed between ages 5½ to 6½, none had a normal intellect. Thus children who changed earlier displayed better intellectual functioning. In Havelkova's study 22 of the 42 treated children changed prior to treatment efforts and two-thirds of those who improved did so without any formal treatment. Maturational processes, therefore, seem more important than therapeutic effort.

What about those whose psychosis appears at adolescence? Again we would assume that they would fare better than those impaired in childhood. Eaton and Menolascino (1967, p. 527) imply this when they state, "Children who have matured psychologically and physically in a relatively normal way but become psychotic as preadolescents probably have different prognoses than those who have histories of borderline or erratic psychological and physiological development prior to onset of psychosis." Unfortunately, research does not entirely support this assumption since the outcome for both groups is similar.

Errera (1957) reports a 16-year follow-up of adolescents. Excluded from the sample were those whose disorder started prior to adolescence. Onset in the sample cases was therefore sudden. Of 59 so classified, 29 percent received a rating of "good," 26 percent "mediocre," and 48 percent "poor"; 83 percent had one or more periods of hospitalization during the period covered. There was no relationship between improvement and treatment. As we can see, these figures are similar to those we reported for younger schizophrenics.

Age of onset, however, is significant when adolescents are compared with adults. For example, Annesley (1961) followed a group of 78 hospitalized schizophrenic adolescents and reported their adjustment as poorer than that for adult schizophrenics. Only 26 percent recovered; the recovery rate for adults was cited as 33 percent. Similar percentages were reported by Pollack, Levenstein, and Klein (1968).

The results of these follow-up studies suggest that schizophrenia, whether of sudden or gradual onset, is a severely disabling condition. When diagnosed, it is "not the onset which is being documented but rather the unmasking of the illness" (Pitt & Hage, 1965, p. 1095).

Bender's (1971) belief seems true; whether children start out as autistic or psychotic, either in childhood or adolescence, they run a life course of schizophrenia. During various periods of their life, they display a variety of clinical conditions depending upon both internal changes and experiential factors; ratings of their social adjustment and capacity to function independently will show episodic variation from good to fair to poor.

Relationship between treatment and outcome

Almost all the studies presented revealed no relationship between treatment and outcome. Havelkova's (1968) findings tentatively suggest that treatment helps to solidify maturational changes by improving the child's ability to attend school and by preventing deterioration of intellect.

Eisenberg and Kanner (1956) remark that psychotherapy is of little help. More important is a sympathetic and tolerant reception by schools. Those who improve are those exposed to sympathetic and patient teachers. Early investigators placed great stress on the treatment of social and behavioral disorders and considered educational efforts secondary; it was expected that intelligence would increase following psychotherapy, since these children were considered pseudodefective. Perhaps the current stress on educational efforts will bring about better results.

Institutions, as they were operated in the past, were of no help. Kanner (1971, p. 144) stated,

One cannot help but gain the impression that state hospital admission was tantamount to a life sentence, with evanescence of the astounding facts of rote memory, abandonment of the earlier pathological yet active struggle for the maintenance of sameness, and loss of interest in objects, added to the basically poor reaction to people—in other words, a total retreat to near nothingness.

The recent experience of several professionals who posed as mental patients indicates that conditions within state hospitals have changed very little in recent years. They experienced agitated boredom and fear of remaining institutionalized indefinitely (Goldman, Bohr, & Sternberg, 1970).

In America many psychiatrists consider drugs to be the "only treatment" for schizophrenia. The introduction of antipsychotic agents in the mid-1950s did produce a major revolution in psychiatric practice and was largely responsible for the rapid decline in hospital population over the last 10 years. Nevertheless, statistics on discharged schizophrenics reveal that American patients have a considerably higher readmission rate and display poorer overall community adjustment than those in Scandinavian countries where psychosocial aspects of treatment are emphasized (National Clearinghouse for Mental Health Information, 1970).

The Scandinavian experience reveals the need for careful study of the kinds of patients best suited for different types of treatment. For example, schizophrenic children who are free of neurological dysfunction and who come from highly deviant families make greater progress in residential than in day treatment (Goldfarb et al., 1966). With the more impaired, perhaps the increased emphasis on education and the encouraging results of language training programs (Hewett, 1967; Halpern, 1970) will permit more psychotic children to return to or remain in the community. Perhaps training to solidify maturational changes will result in different findings when children are followed in future studies. Let us hope so.

CONCLUDING REMARKS

While there is still much to be learned about the schizophrenias, there are some general conclusions that can be drawn. We can say that an individual's vulnerability to schizophrenia depends upon the interaction of six factors. These are: (1) genetic variables, (2) the modification by upbringing of the threshold for the appearance of the disorder, (3) the modification by age of the threshold, (4) the vulnerability of the child's nervous system to physical stress, (5) the vulnerability of the child to psychological stress, and (6) the ability of the child to monitor and avoid or to resolve stress.

Approximately two-thirds of schizophrenic children become severely incapacitated. Most live in institutions for considerable periods during their life. Others are enrolled early in special schools, later in sheltered workshops, and as adults live in halfway houses. Of those who live in the community, many are social outcasts considered peculiar by others. Treatment rarely brings about complete recovery. With adults chemotherapy is more effective than psychotherapy (May, 1968); with children the effect of drugs is unclear. Highly structured educational programs are the most promising form of treatment not only for disorders of early onset but also for cases of later onset, as they enable the individual to reintegrate and to gather the strength to return to society. When faced with stress, return to structure is necessary. In this fashion, the individual lives out his life, going from community to institution and from institution to community. If a child does recover, maturational changes are probably responsible. Treatment may help cement the positive effects of such maturational changes, but treatment by itself is relatively ineffective. Psychotherapy helps some children to function more effectively, but only while receiving treatment. As soon as it ceases and the child or family is again on their own, relapse usually occurs. Therapy serves to maintain the child, to give him support, but does not cure him.

Table 4.7 presents a summary of potentially helpful methods of treatment for schizophrenic youth at various age levels. Hopefully, future research will be directed toward finding the services most in keeping with the developmental needs of the child.

Table 4.7 POSSIBLE SOURCES OF VULNERABILITY, EARLY CHARACTERISTICS, AND POTENTIALLY HELPFUL METHODS OF INTERVENTION IN PRE-SCHIZOPHRENIA

Age and life stage	Possible sources of vulnerability	Relationships, experiences, symptoms	Potentially helpful methods of intervention
Before birth	genetic factors poor maternal health poor maternal nutrition attempts to abort		genetic counseling adequate prenatal care
0–2, infancy	birth damage postpartum depression early illness leaving permanent damage restriction and understimulation	overly dependent slow in developing speech poor coordination shy	adequate obstetrical care adequate pediatric care treatment for mother's depression early stimulation and training
3–6, early childhood	low IQ low social competence hyperreactive nervous system influence of disturbed family	shy, sensitive, irritable poor peer relationships speech problems awkward and rigid hyperactive	speech therapy physical training nursery school training in socialization
7–12, late childhood	low IQ low social competence poor school achievement disturbed family	shy poor peer relationships teachers report: indifferent, unlikable, stubborn, unhappy, lazy, scatterbrained	tutoring in speech, reading play therapy therapeutic camps and schools family therapy foster home or residential school placement

13–18, adolescence	sexual maturation in self and peers failures in adolescent developmental tasks	poor peer relationships withdrawal, tantrums, defiance feelings reported: vulnerability, anxiety, alienation, unreality some psychotic-like symptoms begin	reality oriented psychotherapy tutoring in school subjects vocational guidance into low-pressure jobs and areas foster home or residential school placement
19–25, early adulthood	failure in young adult social and vocational development	withdrawal despair apathy psychotic syndromes apparent but often not stabilized	drug treatment to minimize anxiety psychotherapy vocational guidance into low-stress areas and jobs institutional care vocational and social rehabilitation

From D. F. Ricks. Life history research in psychopathology: retrospect and prospect. In M. Roff & D. F. Ricks (Eds.). *Life history research in psychopathology*. Vol. 1. Minneapolis: University of Minnesota Press, 1970. Copyright © 1970, University of Minnesota.

References

Allen, M. G., Cohen, S., & Pollin, W. Schizophrenia in veteran twins: a diagnostic review. *American Journal of Psychiatry*, 1972, **128**, 939–945.

Annesley, P. T. Psychiatric illness in adolescence; presentation and progress. *Journal of Mental Science*, 1961, **107**, 268–278.

Anthony, J. An experimental approach to the psychopathology of childhood: autism. *British Journal of Medical Psychology*, 1958, **31**, 211–225.

Arieti, S. Schizophrenia, the manifest symptomatology, the psychodynamic and formal mechanisms. In S. Arieti (Ed.) *American handbook of psychiatry.* Vol. I. New York: Basic Books, 1959.

Arieti, S. Conceptual and cognitive psychiatry. *American Journal of Psychiatry*, 1965, **22**, 361–366.

Bateson, G., Jackson, D. D., Haley, J., & Weakland, J. H. Toward a theory of schizophrenia. *Behavioral Science*, 1956, **1**, 251–264.

Bender, L. Childhood schizophrenia: a clinical study of one-hundred schizophrenic children. *American Journal of Orthopsychiatry*, 1947, **17**, 40–56.

Bender, L. Twenty years of clinical research on schizophrenic children. In I. G. Caplan (Ed.), *Emotional problems of early childhood.* New York: Basic Books, 1955.

Bender, L. Schizophrenia in childhood. *American Journal of Orthopsychiatry*, 1956, **26**, 499–506.

Bender, L. Childhood schizophrenia: a review. *International Journal of Psychiatry*, 1968a, **5**, 211–220.

Bender, L. Discussion: prognosis of infantile psychosis and neurosis. *Excerpta Medica International Congress*, 1968b (Series No. 150), 124–126.

Bender, L. A longitudinal study of schizophrenic children with autism. *Hospital and Community Psychiatry*, 1969, **20**, 230–237.

Bender, L. Alpha and omega of childhood schizophrenia. *Journal of Autism and Childhood Schizophrenia*, 1971, **1**, 115–118.

Berkowitz, H. Effects of prior experimenter-subject relationships on reinforced reaction of schizophrenics and normals. *Journal of Abnormal and Social Psychology*, 1964, **69**, 522–530.

Bettelheim, B. *The empty fortress.* New York: Free Press, 1967.

Birch, H. G., & Hertzig, M. E. Etiology of schizophrenia: an overview of the relation of development to atypical behavior. Paper presented at the International Conference on Schizophrenia, Rochester, N.Y., March 1967.

Brenner, A. R. Effects of prior experimenter-subject relationships on responses to the Kent-Rosanoff word-association list in schizophrenics. *Journal of Abnormal Psychology*, 1967, **72**, 273–276.

Brown, G. W., Birley, J. L.. T., & Wing, J. K. Influence of family life on the course of schizophrenic disorders: a replication. *British Journal of Psychiatry*, 1972, **121**, 241–258.

Brown, J. L. Follow-up of children with atypical development. *American Journal of Orthopsychiatry*, 1963, **33**, 855–861.

Buss, A. H. *Psychopathology.* New York: Wiley, 1966.

Cameron, N. Reasoning regression and communication in schizophrenics. *Psychological Monographs*, 1938, **50** (1, whole No. 221).

Caputo, D. V. The parents of the schizophrenic. *Family Process*, 1963, **2**, 339–356.

Chethik, M., & Fast, I. A function of fantasy in the borderline child. *American Journal of Orthopsychiatry*, 1970, **40**, 756–765.

Churchill, D. W. Psychotic children and behavior modification. *American Journal of Psychiatry*, 1969, **125**, 1585–1590.

Claridge, G. The schizophrenias as nervous types. *British Journal of Psychiatry,* 1972, **121,** 1–17.

Connell, P. H. Medical treatment. In J. K. Wing (Ed.), *Childhood autism: clinical, educational and social aspects.* London: Pergamon, 1966.

Creak, E. M. Schizophrenic syndrome in childhood. Progress report of a working party. *Cerebral Palsy Bulletin,* 1961, **3,** 501–504.

Creak, E. M. Childhood psychosis: a review of 100 cases. *British Journal of Psychiatry,* 1963, **109,** 84–89.

Davison, G. C. A social learning programme with an autistic child. *Behavior Research and Therapy,* 1964, **2,** 149–159.

Des Lauriers, A., & Carlson, C. *Your child is asleep: early infantile autism.* Homewood, Ill.: Dorsey, 1969.

Des Lauriers, A., & Halpern, F. Psychological tests in childhood schizophrenia. *American Journal of Orthopsychiatry,* 1947, **17,** 57–67.

Despert, J. L., & Sherwin, A. C. Further examination of diagnostic criteria in schizophrenic illness and psychosis of infancy and early childhood. *American Journal of Psychiatry,* 1958, **114,** 784–790.

Douglas, K. B. The teacher's role in a children's psychiatric hospital. *Exceptional Children,* 1961, **27,** 246–251.

Eaton, L., & Menolascino, F. J. Psychotic reactions of childhood: experiences of a mental retardation pilot project. *Journal of Nervous and Mental Disease,* 1966, **143,** 55–67.

Eaton, L., & Menolascino, F. J. Psychotic reactions of childhood: a follow-up study. *American Journal of Orthopsychiatry,* 1967, **37,** 521–538.

Eisenberg, L., The autistic child in adolescence. *American Journal of Psychiatry,* 1956, **112,** 607–612.

Eisenberg, L. The classification of the psychotic disorders in childhood. In L. D. Eron (Ed.), *The classification of behavior disorders.* Chicago: Aldine, 1966.

Eisenberg, L., & Kanner, L. Early infantile autism, 1943–1955. *American Journal of Orthopsychiatry,* 1956, **26,** 556–566.

Ekstein, R. *Children of time and space, of action and impulse.* New York: Appleton, 1966.

Ekstein, R., & Wallerstein, J. Observations of the psychology of borderline and psychotic children. *Psychoanalytic Study of the Child,* 1954, **9,** 344–369.

Errera, P. A sixteen-year follow-up of schizophrenic patients seen in an out-patient clinic. *Archives of Neurology & Psychiatry,* 1957, **78,** 84–88.

Eysenck, H. J. *Dimensions of personality.* London: Routledge & Kegan Paul, 1947.

Farina, A. Patterns of role dominance and conflict in parents of schizophrenic patients. *Journal of Abnormal and Social Psychology,* 1960, **61,** 31–38.

Farnham-Diggory, S. Self, future, and time: a developmental study of the concepts of psychotic, brain damaged, and normal children. *Monographs of the Society for Research in Child Development,* 1966, **31**(1, Whole No. 103).

Feldman, R. C., & Mordock, J. B. A cognitive process approach to evaluating vocational potential in the retarded and emotionally disturbed. *Rehabilitation Counseling Bulletin,* 1969, **12,** 195–203.

Ferreira, A. J., & Winter, N. D. Family interaction and decision making. *Archives of General Psychiatry,* 1965, **13,** 214–223.

Ferster, C. Positive reinforcement and behavior deficits of autistic children. *Child Development,* 1961, **32,** 437–456.

Fish, B. Drug use in psychiatric disorders of children. In *Drug Therapy: Supplement to The American Journal of Psychiatry,* 1968, **124,** 31–36.

Fleming, P., & Ricks, D. F. Emotions of children before schizophrenia and before character disorder. In M. Roff & D. F. Ricks (Eds.), *Life history research in psychopathology*. Minneapolis: University of Minnesota Press, 1970.

Fraiberg, S. H. *The magic years*. New York: Scribners, 1959.

Freud, S. Negation. *Collected papers*, Vol. 5. New York: Basic Books, 1959.

Gelburd, A. S., & Anker, J. M. Humans as reinforcing stimuli in schizophrenic performance. *Journal of Abnormal Psychology*, 1970, 75, 195–198.

Geleerd, E. Borderline states in childhood and adolescence. *Psychoanalytic Study of the Child*, 1958, 13, 279–295.

Gittelman, M., & Birch, G. Childhood schizophrenia, intellect, neurologic status, perinatal risk, prognosis, and family pathology. *Archives of General Psychiatry*, 1967, 17, 16–25.

Goldfarb, W. *Childhood schizophrenia*. Cambridge, Mass.: Harvard University Press, 1961.

Goldfarb, W. Childhood psychosis. In P. H. Mussen (Ed.), *Carmichael's manual of child psychology*. Vol. 2. New York: Wiley, 1970a.

Goldfarb, W. A follow-up investigation of schizophrenic children treated in residence. *Psychosocial Process*, 1970b, 1, 9–63.

Goldfarb, W., Goldfarb, N., & Pollack, R. C. Treatment of childhood schizophrenia: a three year comparison of day and residential treatment of schizophrenic children. *Archives of General Psychiatry*, 1966, 14, 119–128.

Goldfarb, W., Levy, D. M., & Meyers, D. I. The verbal encounter between the schizophrenic child and his mother. In G. S. Goldman & D. Shapiro (Eds.), *Developments in psychoanalysis at Columbia University*. New York: Hafner, 1966.

Goldman, A. R., Bohr, R. H., & Sternberg, T. A. On posing as mental patients: reminiscences and recommendations. *Professional Psychology*, 1970, 1, 427–434.

Haley, J. *Strategies of psychotherapy*. New York: Grune & Stratton, 1963.

Halpern, W. I. The schooling of autistic children, preliminary findings. *American Journal of Orthopsychiatry*, 1970, 40, 665–671.

Haring, N. G., & Phillips, E. L. *Educating emotionally disturbed children*. New York: McGraw-Hill, 1962.

Harlow, H. A brief look at autistic children. Review of *The empty fortress* by B. Bettleheim. *Psychiatry and Social Science Review*, 1969, 3(1), 27–29.

Harrow, M., Himmelhoch, J., Tucker, G., Hirsh, J., & Quinlan, D. Overinclusive thinking in acute schizophrenics. *Journal of Abnormal Psychology*, 1972, 79, 161–168.

Havelkova, M. Follow-up study of 71 children diagnosed as psychotic in preschool age. *American Journal of Orthopsychiatry*, 1968, 38, 846–857.

Heston, L. L. Psychiatric disorders in foster home reared children of schizophrenic mothers. *British Journal of Psychiatry*, 1966, 112, 819–825.

Heston, L. L. Genetics of schizophrenic and schizoid disease. *Science*, 1970, 167, 249–256.

Hewett, F. M. Teaching reading to an autistic boy through operant conditioning. *The Reading Teacher*, 1964, 18, 613–618.

Hewett, F. M. Teaching speech to an autistic child through operant conditioning. *American Journal of Orthopsychiatry*, 1965, 35, 927–936.

Hewett, F. M., Mayhew, D., & Rabb, E. An experimental reading program for neurologically impaired, mentally retarded, and severely emotionally disturbed children. *American Journal of Orthopsychiatry*, 1967, 37, 35–48.

Hewett, F. M., Taylor, F. D., & Artuso, A. A. The Santa Monica Project. Evaluation of an engineered classroom design with emotionally disturbed children. *Exceptional Children*, 1969, 35, 523–529.

Higgins, J. Effects of child rearing by schizophrenic mothers. *Journal of Psychiatric Research*, 1966, 4, 153–167.

Hingtgen, J. N., & Bryson, C. Q. Recent developments in the study of early childhood psychosis: infantile autism, childhood schizophrenia, and related disorders. *Schizophrenia Bulletin*, 1972, **5**, 8–55.

Hingtgen, J. N., & Churchill, D. W. Identification of perceptual limitations in mute autistic children: identification by the use of behavior modification. *Archives of General Psychiatry*, 1969, **21**, 68–71.

Hutt, L., Hutt, S., Lee, D., & Ounsted, C. A behavioral and electroencephalographic study of autistic children. *Journal of Psychiatric Research*, 1965, **3**, 181–197.

Ishikawa, T. Structure of speech in autistic children. *Psychiatria et Neurologia Japonica*, 1970, **72**, 1159–1174.

Jourard, S. M. *The transparent self*. New York: Van Nostrand, Reinhold, 1964.

Kallman, F. J. Hereditary-genetic theory, analysis of 691 twin index families. *American Journal of Psychiatry*, 1946, **103**, 309–322.

Kanner, L. Autistic disturbances of affective contact. *The Nervous Child*, 1943, **2**, 217–250.

Kanner, L. To what extent is early infantile autism determined by constitutional inadequacies? *Proceedings of the Association for Research on Nervous and Mental Diseases*, 1954, **33**, 378–385.

Kanner, L. Follow-up study of eleven autistic children originally reported in 1943. *Journal of Autism and Childhood Schizophrenia*, 1971, **1**, 119–145.

Kantor, R. E., & Winder, C. L. Schizophrenia: correlates of life history. *Journal of Nervous and Mental Disease*, 1961, **132**, 221–225.

Keeler, W. R. In discussion. In *Psychiatric reports of the American Psychiatric Association*, 1957, **7**, 68–88.

Landau, R., Harth, P., Othnay, N., & Sharfhertz, C. The influence of psychotic parents on their child's development. *American Journal of Psychiatry*, 1972, **129**, 38–41.

Lidz, T., Fleck, S., & Cornelison, A. R. *Schizophrenia and the family*. New York: International Universities Press, 1966.

Lotter, V. Epidemiology of autistic conditions in young children: I. Prevalence. *Social Psychiatry*, 1966, **1**, 124–127.

Lotter, V. Epidemiology of autistic conditions in young children: II. Some characteristics of the parents and children. *Social Psychiatry*, 1967, **1**, 163–173.

Lovaas, I. I. A behavior therapy approach to the treatment of childhood schizophrenia. In J. P. Hill (Ed.), *Minnesota symposium on child psychology*. Vol. 1. Minneapolis: University of Minnesota Press, 1967.

Mahler, M. S. On child psychoses and schizophrenia. Autistic and symbiotic infantile psychoses. *Psychoanalytic Study of the Child*, 1952, **7**, 286–305.

May, P. R. A. *Treatment of schizophrenia*. New York: Science House, 1968.

McDermott, J. F., Jr., Harrison, S. I., Schrager, J., Lindy, J., & Killins, E. Social class and mental illness in children: the question of childhood psychosis. *American Journal of Orthopsychiatry*, 1967, **37**, 548–557.

Mednick, S. A. Birth defects and schizophrenia. *Psychology Today*, 1971, **4**, 48–50, 80–81.

Mednick, S. A., & Schulsinger, F. A pre-schizophrenic sample. *Acta Psychiatrica Scandinavica*, 1964, 40(Suppl. No. 180), 135–146.

Mednick, S. A., & Schulsinger, F. Factors related to breakdown in children at high risk for schizophrenia. In M. Roff & D. F. Ricks (Eds.), *Life history research in psychopathology*. Minneapolis: University of Minnesota Press, 1970.

Menolascino, F. L., & Eaton, L. Psychoses of childhood: a five-year follow-up study of experiences in a mental retardation clinic. *American Journal of Mental Deficiency*, 1967, **72**, 370–380.

Michael, S. M., Morris, D. P., & Soroker, E. Follow-up studies of shy, withdrawn children. I. Evaluation of later adjustment. *American Journal of Orthopsychiatry*, 1954, **24**, 743–754.

Mishler, E. G., & Waxler, N. E. *Interaction in families*. New York: Wiley, 1968.

Mordock, J. B., & Feldman, R. C. A cognitive process approach to evaluating vocational potential in the retarded and emotionally disturbed. *Rehabilitation Counseling Bulletin*, 1969, **12**, 136–143.

Mosher, L. R., Pollin, W., & Stabenau, J. R. Families with identical twins discordant for schizophrenia: some relationships between identification, thinking styles, psychopathology, and dominance-submissiveness. *British Journal of Psychiatry*, 1971, **118**, 29–42.

Myer, M., & Caruth, E. Inner and outer reality testing on the Rorschach. *Reiss Davis Bulletin*, 1967, **1**, 100–106.

National Clearinghouse for Mental Health Information. At issue: the psychosocial treatment of schizophrenia. *Schizophrenia Bulletin*, 1970, **3**, 4–5.

Ney, P. G., Palvesky, A. E., & Markely, J. Relative effectiveness of operant conditioning and play therapy in childhood schizophrenia. *Journal of Autism and Childhood Schizophrenia*, 1971, **1**, 337–347.

Offord, D. R., & Cross, L. A. Adult schizophrenia with scholastic failure or low IQ in childhood. *Archives of General Psychiatry*, 1971, **24**, 431–436.

O'Leary, K. D., & Becker, W. C. Behavior modification of an adjustment class: a token reinforcement program. *Exceptional Children*, 1967, **37**, 637–642.

Olson, D. H. Empirically unbinding the double bind: review of research and conceptual reformulations. *Family Process*, 1972, **11**, 69–94.

O'Neal, P., & Robins, L. N. The relation of childhood behavior problems to adult psychiatric status: a 30-year follow-up study of 150 subjects. *American Journal of Psychiatry*, 1958, **114**, 961–969.

Ornitz, E. M., & Ritvo, E. R. Perceptual inconstancy in early infantile autism. *Archives of General Psychiatry*, 1968, **18**, 79–98.

Payne, R. W., & Sloan, R. B. Can schizophrenia be defined? *Diseases of the Nervous System*, 1968, **29** (Gwan Suppl.), 113–117.

Pitt, R., & Hage, J. Patterns of peer interactions during adolescence as prognostic indicators in schizophrenia. *American Journal of Psychiatry*, 1965, **121**, 1089–1096.

Pollack, M., Levenstein, D. S. W., & Klein, D. F. A three-year posthospital follow-up of adolescent and adult schizophrenics. *American Journal of Orthopsychiatry*, 1968, **38**, 94–109.

Pollack, M., Woener, M. G., & Klein, D. F. A comparison of childhood characteristics of schizophrenics, personality disorders, and their siblings. In M. Roff & D. R. Ricks (Eds.), *Life history research in psychopathology*. Minneapolis: University of Minnesota Press, 1970.

Pollin, W., & Stabenau, J. Biological, psychological, and historical differences in a series of monozygotic twins discordant for schizophrenia. In S. S. Kety & D. Rosenthal (Eds.), *The transmission of schizophrenia*. London: Pergamon, 1968.

Pronovost, W., Wakstein, M. P., & Wakstein, D. J. A longitudinal study of speech behavior and language comprehension of fourteen children diagnosed atypical or autistic. *Exceptional Children*, 1966, **33**, 19–26.

Quinlan, D. M., Harrow, M., Tucker, G., & Carlson, K. Varieties of "disordered" thinking on the Rorschach: findings in schizophrenic and nonschizophrenic patients. *Journal of Abnormal Psychology*, 1972, **79**, 47–53.

Rabb, E., & Hewett, F. M. Developing appropriate classroom behaviors in a severely disturbed group of institutionalized kindergarten-primary children utilizing a behavior modification model. *American Journal of Orthopsychiatry*, 1967, **37**, 313–314.

Rank, B. Intensive study and treatment of preschool children who show marked personality deviations, or "atypical development," and their parents. In G. Caplan (Ed.), *Emotional problems of early childhood*. New York: Basic Books, 1955.

Rank, B., & MacNaughton, D. A clinical contribution to early ego development. *Psychoanalytic Study of the Child*, 1950, **5**, 53–65.

Reiser, D. Infantile psychosis, overview of studies at the James Jackson Putman Children's Center. *Mental Hygiene*, 1966, **50**, 588–589.

Ricks, D. F., & Berry, J. C. Family and symptom patterns that precede schizophrenia. In M. Roff & D. F. Ricks (Eds.), *Life history research in psychopathology*. Minneapolis: University of Minnesota Press, 1970.

Rimland, B. *Infantile autism*. New York: Appleton, 1964.

Rimland, B. The differentiation of childhood psychosis: an analysis of checklists for 2,218 psychotic children. *Journal of Autism and Childhood Schizophrenia*, 1971, **1**, 161–174.

Roff, M. Some life history factors in relation to various types of adult maladjustment. In M. Roff & D. F. Ricks (Eds.), *Life history research in psychopathology*. Minneapolis: University of Minnesota Press, 1970.

Rosenthal, D. A program for research on heredity in schizophrenia. *Behavioral Science*, 1971, **16**, 191–201.

Rutter, M. The influence of organic and emotional factors on the origins, nature, and outcome of childhood psychosis. *Developmental Medicine and Child Neurology*, 1965, **7**, 518–528.

Rutter, M. Psychotic disorders in early childhood. In A. J. Coppen & A. Walk (Eds.), *Recent developments in schizophrenia: a symposium*. London: Royal Medico-psychological Association, 1967.

Rutter, M. Concepts of autism: a review of research. *Journal of Child Psychology and Psychiatry*, 1968, **9**, 1–25.

Rutter, M., Greenfield, D., & Lockyer, L. A five to fifteen year follow-up study of infantile psychosis. In S. Chess & A. Thomas (Eds.), *Annual progress in child psychiatry and child development*. New York: Brunner-Mazel, 1968.

Sailor, W. S., Guess, D., Rutherford, G., & Baer, D. M. Control of tantrum behavior by operant techniques during experimental verbal training. *Journal of Applied Behavior Analysis*, 1968, **1**, 237–243.

Schuham, A. I. Power relations in emotionally disturbed and normal family triads. *Journal of Abnormal Psychology*, 1970, **75**, 30–37.

Schuham, A. I. Activity, talking time, and spontaneous agreement in disturbed and normal family interaction. *Journal of Abnormal Psychology*, 1972, **79**, 68–75.

Shields, J., & Gottesman, I. I. Cross-national diagnosis of schizophrenia in twins. *Archives of Psychiatry*, 1972, **27**, 725–730.

Shimkunas, A. M. Demand for intimate self-disclosure and pathological verbalizations in schizophrenia. *Journal of Abnormal Psychology*, 1972, **80**, 197–205.

Shimkunas, A. M., Gynther, M. D., & Smith, K. Schizophrenic responses to the proverbs test; abstract, concrete or autistic. *Journal of Abnormal Psychology*, 1967, **72**, 128–133.

Stabenau, J. R., & Pollin, W. Experimental differences for schizophrenics as compared with their non-schizophrenic siblings: twin and family studies. In M. Roff & D. R. Ricks (Eds.), *Life history research in psychopathology*. Minneapolis: University of Minnesota Press, 1970.

Stabenau, J. R., Pollin, W., & Mosher, L. A study of monozygotic twins discordant for schizophrenia: some biologic variables. *Archives of General Psychiatry*, 1969, **20**, 145–158.

Stevens, J. R., & Milstein, V. Severe psychiatric disorders of childhood: electroencephalogram and clinical correlates. *American Journal of Diseases of Children*, 1970, **120**, 182–192.

Sullivan, H. S. The language of schizophrenia. In J. S. Kasonin (Ed.), *Language and thought in schizophrenia*. Berkeley: University of California Press, 1944. (Reprinted: New York: Norton, 1964.)

Terris, M., Lapouse, R., & Monk, M. A. The relation of prematurity and previous fetal loss to childhood schizophrenia. *American Journal of Psychiatry*, 1964, **121**, 476–481.

Wahl, O., & Wishner, J. Schizophrenic thinking as measured by developmental tests. *Journal of Nervous and Mental Disease*, 1972, **155**, 232–244.

Walder, L. O., Breiter, D. E., Cohen, S. I., Daston, P. G., Forbes, I. A., & McIntire, R. W. Teaching parents to modify the behavior of their autistic children. Paper presented at the annual convention of the American Psychological Association, New York, September 1966.

Ward, A. J. Childhood psychopathology: a natural experiment in etiology. *Journal of Child Psychiatry*, 1974, **13**, 153–165.

Watt, N. F. Longitudinal changes in the social behavior of children hospitalized for schizophrenia as adults. *Journal of Nervous and Mental Disease*, 1972, **155**, 42–54.

Watt, N. F., Stolorow, R. D., Lubensky, A. W., & McClelland, D. C. School adjustment and behavior of children hospitalized for schizophrenia as adults. *American Journal of Orthopsychiatry*, 1970, **40**, 637–657.

Waxler, N. Parent and child effects on cognitive performance: an experimental approach to the etiological and responsive theories of schizophrenia. *Family Process*, 1974, **13**, 1–22.

Weakland, J. H. The "double-bind" hypothesis of schizophrenia and three-party interaction. In D. D. Jackson (Ed.), *The etiology of schizophrenia*. New York: Basic Books, 1960.

Weil, A. P. Some evidence of deviational development in infancy and childhood. *Psychoanalytic Study of the Child*, 1956, **11**, 292–299.

Weiss, H. H., & Born, B. Speech training or language acquisition? A distinction when speech training is taught by operant conditioning procedures. *American Journal of Orthopsychiatry*, 1967, **37**, 49–55.

Wender, P. H. The role of genetics in the etiology of the schizophrenias. *American Journal of Orthopsychiatry*, 1969, **39**, 447–458.

White, P. T., DeMyer, W., & DeMyer, M. EEG abnormalities in early childhood schizophrenia: a double-blind study of psychiatrically disturbed and normal children during promazine sedation. *American Journal of Psychiatry*, 1964, **120**, 950–958.

Wolf, E. G., & Ruttenberg, B. A. Communication therapy for the autistic child. *Journal of Speech and Hearing Disorders*, 1967, **32**, 331–335.

Yates, A. J. Data-processing levels and thought disorder in schizophrenia. *Australian Journal of Psychology*, 1966, **18**, 103–117.

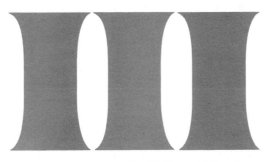

Identifiable handicapping conditions

In the first chapter in this part we discuss children with damage to their peripheral nervous system, damage that affects vision and hearing. As we will see, some of the same factors that damage the central nervous system also damage the peripheral system. We also discuss two speech disorders: cleft palate, a physiological condition, and stuttering, which has been attributed to emotional factors but also may be the result of peripheral or central nervous system impairment.

In Chapter 6 we discuss children with chronic diseases, conditions that will affect them throughout their life. These diseases require that the child carefully monitor his own behavior, a task that nonimpaired children master only after considerable practice. Consequently, parents are placed in a bind. If they pressure the child to demonstrate control beyond his capabilities or demand that he restrict his activities so as not to aggravate his condition, they may be overcontrolling, a child rearing attitude that stifles individuality and elicits negativism. Parents of ill children, like those of the deaf and blind, need considerable support from their community as they walk the thin line between being restrictive and overprotective and supportive and helpful.

The real criteria of success are in the enthusiasm a student shows, his movement toward self-reliance and the pride that is evident when he displays what he has produced.

—Joseph Ferdinand

5
Sensory and speech disorders

Surveys of school age children indicate that 2 or 3 in 1000 will be either blind or deaf (Rutter, Graham, & Yule, 1970). About 4 percent will have some hearing impairment (Robinson, Anderson, Moghadam, Cambon, & Murray, 1967). There are no adequate data regarding the incidence of visual difficulties other than blindness, although some estimates have been as high as 25 percent of all children (National Society for the Prevention of Blindness, 1961). We do know that the frequency of visual disorders in children experiencing educational difficulties is from two to four times higher than that found in children achieving at grade level (Eames, 1959; Paul & Proft, 1966). Although educational failure has been attributed to pathological eye conditions, the influence of these conditions has been overemphasized. Current data suggest that minor visual difficulties and academic failure are both part of a larger disorder affecting academic performance. In Chapter 8 we will discuss several syndromes that include visual disorders among their symptoms and that cause significant academic difficulty.

In the first two sections of this chapter we will confine our discussion largely to children with hearing and visual disorders known to produce difficulties that often require education apart from nonimpaired children. Following the discussion of children with sensory disorders, we will present two types of speech disorders. Perhaps 4 percent of school age children have some type of speech defect, with the largest number having defects in articulation (Johnson & Moeller, 1967). The two discussed in this chapter are cleft palate speech and stuttering.

Hearing loss

The teacher of a moderately retarded or psychotic child would not be surprised to find the results of a hearing, or audiometric, examination in the child's personal folder. As we mentioned in Chapters 2 and 3, many cerebral palsied, aphasic, and mentally retarded children have a hearing loss or are deaf. The autistic child discussed in Chapter 4 frequently responds inconsistently to sound and behaves as if he is deaf. Consequently, many of the children discussed in Part II are referred for an audiometric evaluation. A sample of an audiometric report appears below.

Informal communication testing on 6-23-72 revealed that Ann has minimal vocalization consisting of vowel sounds primarily. Her mother reported that Ann says "ma-ma."

Ann was constantly active during the evaluation. She rocked even when sitting or eating. She appears to have some receptive ability but was slow to perform the activity requested. She was unable to imitate sounds, words, or actions. She put everything she held into her mouth.

Audiological evaluation was accomplished on 6-6-72. Her mother reported that the child has had many upper respiratory infections, but no known ear infections. The child entered the testing booth by herself.

Ann could not be conditioned to conventional testing methods. She did respond to her name and to "no" at 50 db free field. An attempt was made to condition her to COR [conditioned orientating response] audiometry; however, after several responses, she lost interest and began banging her head against the wall. Responses were elicited to stimuli in the 50 to 60 db range. Ann exhibited bizarre behavior such as head banging and finger play. She engaged in some vocal play which consisted of vowellike utterances. She ceased vocal activity when the examiner imitated her at normal conversational levels. Testing was discontinued when the child began to cry.

Because of this child's lack of response to sound at low intensity levels, an ENT evaluation was recommended to rule out, if necessary, aural pathology.

The regular classroom teacher can also find herself faced with interpreting an audiometric report that uses terms she does not fully understand and mentions procedures with which she is unfamiliar. The technical terms used in Ann's evaluation—conditioned to conventional testing methods, 50 db, free field, conditioned orienting reflex, ENT— might be vaguely familiar, but the teacher must know their precise definitions in order to appreciate the effort that went into the evaluation and to comprehend the report's conclusions. Other reports might mention psychogalvanic skin resistance, bone conduction thresholds, play audiometry, or a host of other terms.

The following audiological report was taken from the record of a kindergarten child.

Communication status Michael was initially reluctant to remain alone with the examiner, but became interested in blocks and soon became very friendly, active, and talkative. Speech was unintelligible except for occasional words and phrases. Rate was often fast, as was his activity level. Voice quality and pitch were judged to be normal for his age and sex, as was syntax. Michael was able to match, but not name, colors. He was able to build a bridge and a train of blocks. He could not count to 10 correctly.

Michael achieved an Intelligence Quotient of 107 on the Peabody Picture Vocabulary Test; he used his nose to point to many of the pictures. During the Templin-Darley Screening and Diagnostic Tests of Articulation, he got up from his seat often to punch a balloon man. He achieved a score of 3 on the Templin-Darley test (norm for his age and sex is 34.7). Michael was very stimulable on many of his error sounds.

An oral peripheral examination revealed that Michael has a distoclusion (he is a thumbsucker). He was able to protrude, depress, and lateralize his tongue, but not elevate it. Diadochokinetic rates were judged to be within normal limits.

Audiological evaluation Michael was seen for an audiological evaluation on January 4, 1971. He was accompanied by his mother who reported that Michael has had a recent ear infection in his right ear. An otoscopic examination revealed clear eardrums. The results of pure-tone audiometry demonstrate the existence of normal hearing in the left ear and a mild conductive loss in the right ear. The speech reception thresholds are in good agreement with the three-frequency, pure-tone averages and show normal sensitivity for the reception of speech stimuli, bilaterally. Michael's speech discrimination ability is mildly reduced. Michael's articulation may be influencing the discrimination scores. Informal testing revealed good discrimination ability.

The report states that Michael has a conductive loss. What does this mean? Are there other kinds of losses? The apparent contradiction in the statements that his "speech discrimination ability is mildly reduced" and he has "good discrimination ability" is particularly confusing. The objective of this section, therefore, is not only to acquaint the reader with the deaf child and his educational needs but also to familiarize him with the various procedures and terms employed by the audiologist, the specialist in hearing evaluations.

AUDIOLOGICAL EVALUATION

Conventional audiological evaluation

Most sound waves are characterized by periodicity, that is, by repetitions of compressions and rarefactions (expansion by separation) that occur at the same rate over a period of time. One successive compression and rarefaction constitute one *cycle* of a sound wave. The frequency of a sound wave is the number of cycles that occur each second. The unit for expressing frequency is *cycles per second*, abbreviated cps. (An international abbreviation for cycles per second is Hz.) The frequency of a sound wave producing 1000 compressions and rarefactions in 1 second is 1000 cps. The higher the frequency, the higher the perceived pitch of the tone.

The human ear can perceive frequencies between 20 and 2000 cps. We call this the *audible range* of frequencies. The ear is not equally sensitive to all frequencies within this range; it is most sensitive to those between 1000 and 4000 cps. Sounds between 250 and 1000 cps and between 4000 and 8000 cps must be made somewhat more intense to be heard, and those below 250 and above 8000 must be made considerably more intense to be heard (Newby, 1964).

A child's hearing loss often is more impaired at one frequency level than at another. Consequently, testing evaluates the child's hearing for tones throughout a particular range of frequencies.

Pure-tone audiometry   A pure-tone audiometer is an instrument that electronically generates tones of essential "purity," such as those presented by a tuning fork, which are presented at various frequencies (cycles per second). The tones usually used for testing are 250, 500, 1000, 2000, 3000, 4000, 6000, and 8000, with 250 being a low, buzzing sound and 8000 a shrill whistlelike sound. The range of frequencies considered the speech range is 250 to 4000.

The pure-tone audiometer tests hearing by both air and bone conduction. In air conduction, sound waves travel through the air and enter the ear canal, strike the tympanic membrane (eardrum), and cause the ossicles of the inner ear to vibrate. The vibration sends impulses through the fluid in the inner ear to nerve endings that carry the sound to the brain. Tones produced by the audiometer can be delivered to the ear through earphones or introduced in a free field or sound field. In both field conditions, the child is placed in a soundproof room, and the tones are delivered through loudspeakers strategically placed in the room. In a free field, the effects of the room's boundaries, such as the floors, walls, and ceilings, are negligible over the frequency range of interest, whereas in a sound field the field is not free from the effects of bounding surfaces. The reasons for both earphone and field procedures will be discussed shortly.

An older child being evaluated by conventional pure-tone audiometry might be instructed as follows (Newby, 1964, p. 72).

We are now going to test your hearing. I am going to place an earphone over each ear, but we shall test only one ear at a time. The object of the test is to find the point where you can just barely detect the presence of the tone. We shall start each time with the tone off. Then I shall gradually introduce the tone until you can just hear it. As soon as you first hear the tone, signal me. Then

I'll make the tone louder so you can hear it well. I shall next make the tone softer until you signal me that you can no longer hear it. Then I'll make it louder and softer and turn it on and off while you tell me whether or not you can hear the tone each time, until I am satisfied that we have the point where you can just detect the presence of the tone. Then we'll shift to a different tone by pressing the button on the end of this cord, which will cause a light on the audiometer to turn on. Keep the button depressed as long as you hear the tone at all. When you no longer hear the tone, do not push the button. Do you hear any better with one ear than with the other? If so, we'll test the better ear first; if not, we'll begin with the right ear. Are you ready? Signal when you hear the tone by pushing the button, and hold it down until you cease to hear the tone. Here we go. . . .

The measure of intensity The intensity of the sound presented is measured on the *decibel* scale (abbreviated db). The decibel is not a measure of the actual intensity, that is, the *amplitude,* of the sound presented, but a measure of our sensory perception of the sound.

It has been known for some time that the perceived loudness of a pure tone increases proportionately to the logarithm of its physical intensity (Weber-Fechner law). When the sound amplitudes of a pure tone increase in steps of a geometrical progression, the first step of which may be any arbitrary amplitude, each additional step is obtained by multiplying the preceding step by a constant factor; for example, in the series 1, 2, 4, 8, 16, 32, 64, 128, 256, etc., each number differs from the previous one by the factor 2. However, when intensities graded in this way act upon our eardrum, we perceive the changes in intensity as if they occur in an arithmetic progression, such as 1, 2, 3, 4, etc. Thus the difference between steps appears to our hearing to be about the same, although the actual physical intensities always increase more rapidly from one step to the next. In contrast, if we increase the physical amplitude of a sound in arithmetic steps, we perceive the differences in loudness as increasingly smaller from one step to the next, so that eventually we would hardly notice any difference in loudness between steps.

The Weber-Fechner law demonstrates the relative insensitivity of our hearing to physical differences in intensity. This law clarifies how our hearing can encompass a wide range of physical intensities. The roar of an aircraft engine is physically about a million times stronger than the buzzing of a fly, but both are easily heard (Langenbeck, 1965). In order to allow for the difference between perceived and actual intensities, audiometer attenuators (the part of the audiometer that varies the intensity of the tone) are calibrated in logarithmic steps. When the intensity is increased in logarithmic steps, the testee perceives the intensities as increasing equally between each step.

This is especially important in testing individuals with hearing impairment because not only does the degree of impairment vary in each

Table 5.1 APPROXIMATE DECIBEL VALUES FOR CORRESPONDING INCREASES IN AMPLITUDE

Amplitude	Decibels (approximate)
1	0
2	6
3	10
5	14
10	20
20 (10 × 2) or (2 × 10)	26 (20 + 6) or (6 + 20)
30 (3 × 10) or (10 × 3)	30 (10 + 20) or (20 + 10)
40 (20 × 2)	32 (26 + 6)
50 (5 × 10)	34 (14 + 20)
100 (10 × 10) or (50 × 2)	40 (20 + 20) or (34 + 6)
200 (20 × 10) or (100 × 2)	46 (26 + 20) or (40 + 6)
300 (30 × 10) or (100 × 3)	50 (30 + 20) or (40 + 10)
400 (40 × 10) or (200 × 2)	52 (32 + 20) or (46 + 6)
500 (50 × 10)	54 (34 + 20)
1000 (100 × 10) or (500 × 2) *	60 (40 + 20) or (54 + 6)

* The astute observer will note that the db value for an amplitude of 900 (300 × 3) also would be 60 (50 + 10) in this table. This situation occurs because the values given are only approximate.

individual from one frequency level to another but also the tone intensities required to reach the threshold of hearing may vary widely among individuals.*

In order to interpret the significance of decibel values, it is helpful to know the db values for a few simple increases in intensity. These increases are presented in Table 5.1. We can see that doubling the amplitude always means 6 db more, that multiplying the amplitude by 3 means 10 db more, and that multiplying the amplitude by 10 means 20 db more. The decibel scale thus indicates *ratio of sound amplitudes* in steps that approximate our sensory perception of loudness. The base line intensity of 0 db is designated as 1.

The zero decibel hearing level at each frequency is the lowest intensity at which the average normal ear can detect the presence of the test tone

* Microphones do not measure sound intensity directly. Most are sensitive to sound pressure produced during compression and rarefaction in a longitudinal wave event. Since pressure is defined as force per area, sound pressure is given in dynes per square centimeter. Sound intensity is equal to the square of sound pressure (for example, doubling of intensity produces an increase of 3 db, while doubling the sound pressure produces an increment of 6 db). The mathematical definition of the decibel scale is as follows: $N(db) = 10 \log I'/I''$, $\therefore 20 \log p'/p''$. $N(db)$ refers to the number of decibels; intensities (I) are given in watts per square centimeter and sound pressures (p) in dynes per square centimeter. The constant, 20, in the case of sound pressure ratios, occurs because intensity is proportional to the square of sound pressure (an exponent behind a log sign becomes a multiplier in front of it, that is, $\log p^2 = 2 \log p$). The symbol p'' refers to the initial sound pressure amplitude and p' to sound pressure amplitude for which the value in db is sought. From this formula it can be seen that a 10-fold increase in the initial amplitude corresponds to an increase of 20 db, a 100-fold increase to an increase of 40 db, a 1000-fold increase to an increase of 60 db, etc., since the logarithm of 10 equals 1, 100 equals 2, 1000 equals 3. For the initial amplitude $p' = p''$ (no increase and no attenuation), the result is 0 db, as the logarithm of 1 = 0 (Langenbeck, 1965, p. 14).

50 percent of the time. If the intensity of a tone was decreased by another 5 db, the average child would no longer be able to hear the tone. The point at which he just hears the tone is considered the normal threshold for hearing that tone. This intensity varies with the frequency presented. As we have said, the human ear is more sensitive to frequencies between 1000 and 4000 cps than to lower and higher frequencies. The *zero hearing level* for each frequency, therefore, is the average zero level obtained by the population that serves as the norm group against which to evaluate an individual's hearing. *Hearing loss* is expressed as the number of decibels in excess of each zero point that the tone intensity must be increased in order for the impaired ear to just barely detect its presence (detection 50 percent of the time).

When we say that a tone is below a child's threshold, we mean that the tone is not intense enough for him to hear it. If we increase the intensity of the tone beyond the point at which he can just barely hear it, we say the intensity is above his threshold. If a child has less hearing loss for a tone of 250 cps than for a tone of 500 cps, we would say that his threshold for the 250 cps tone was lower, meaning that he can respond to a lower intensity of the 250 cps tone. If a child's threshold is lowered by some variable (e.g., a hearing aid), his hearing has improved. If his threshold is *raised*, his hearing has decreased.

A threshold of 40 db for hearing a particular tone means that a child requires an amplitude that is 100 times greater than the amplitude necessary for the average child to hear the tone, or, more briefly, 40 db corresponds to 100 times the normal threshold amplitude, 60 db to 1000 times the normal amplitude, etc. Consequently, if the attenuator must be set at 60 db before a child hears the tone, either on a headphone or in a free field, we would say that his hearing loss for that tone is 60 db. For another tone, a setting of 80 db may be required before we reach his threshold. If this were the case, we would say that the child has a lower threshold for the first than for the second tone. When an audiometer is calibrated in this fashion, it is calibrated for hearing loss, and the threshold for children with normal hearing is the decibel level for all tones. The child's threshold values are recorded on a graph known as an audiogram (see Figure 5.1). The frequency (pitch) of the tone varies along the abscissa and the intensity varies along the ordinate. Greater hearing losses are recorded in the lower regions of the graph. The graph also includes a −10 db value. This value does not reflect a hearing loss but indicates that the child has better than average hearing for a certain tone. Rabin and Costa (1969) present some data regarding the reliability of pure-tone audiograms.

Bone conduction thresholds Air conduction testing tells the examiner only the extent of a child's hearing loss; it does not tell whether the hearing loss results from dysfunction in either the outer or middle ear

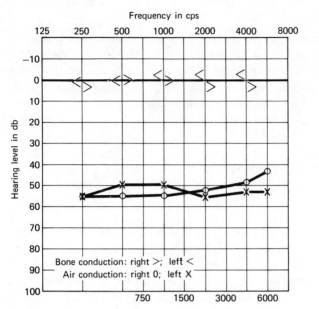

Figure 5.1 *Audiograph of a typical conduction loss.*

in the presence of a normal inner ear (difficulties in conduction of sound to the analyzing system) or from pathology in the inner ear or along the nerve pathway from the inner ear to the brain stem. Bone conduction testing helps establish the reason for a hearing loss revealed by air conduction testing.

In bone conduction, the outer and middle ear are bypassed. An oscillator (vibrator) is placed against the mastoid process of the temporal bone behind the pinna of the ear to be tested. The oscillator causes the bones of the skull to carry sounds directly to the inner ear where nerve endings pick up the impulse. Bone conduction tests are given only at the frequencies within the speech range.

If the bone conduction thresholds are normal, the disorder must exist in the outer or middle ear. Such a disorder is called a *conduction loss* (see Figure 5.1). If the bone conduction thresholds are high, the disorder is either in the inner ear or in the nerve pathway from the inner ear to the brain stem. Such a loss is called *sensorineural impairment*. A "pure" sensorineural impairment exists when the sound conducting mechanism is normal in every respect, but sound is not perceived properly after it is conducted to the fluid of the inner ear. In sensorineural loss bone conduction and air conduction thresholds are approximately the same.

Sensorineural impairments can be acquired through disease, injury, toxic effect of drugs, tumors, or changes in the ear due to the aging process. Diseases such as measles, mumps, scarlet fever, influenza, and many unnamed virus infections are chiefly responsible for sensorineural impairment. These diseases, however, more often cause conductive losses through *otitis media* (inflammation or infection of the middle ear) originating in an infection of the nasal passages that pass to the middle ear through the eustachian tubes. Sometimes, however, the disease process has a toxic effect on the sensitive nerve endings in the cochlea and sensorineural deafness occurs.

Air conduction in a free field There are several reasons for testing a child in a free field. First, many young children will accept all phases of a hearing examination except the wearing of earphones (Miller & Polisar, 1964). Second, other calibrated sounds can be employed when the child fails to respond to pure tones. Several studies have suggested that young children respond better to certain noisemakers and to narrow bands of white noise than to pure tones (Sanders & Josey, 1970; Thompson & Thompson, 1972). Third, in tight-fitting headphones, some of the sound's vibrations will be taken up by the head around the ear and transmitted to the cochlea by bone conduction. In some cases of severe conductive deafness, the thresholds of hearing would be found unduly low in earphone as compared to field testing. Fourth, the effectiveness of hearing aids are evaluated in field situations. Fifth, field testing also allows the examiner to evaluate a child's ability to localize a sound source. It should be emphasized that a field test is a bilateral test and yields information only about the functioning of the better ear. Dirks, Stream, and Wilson (1972) discuss the differential use of earphone and field procedures in speech audiometry.

Speech audiometry Imagine that you see someone speaking to a small audience at a considerable distance from you. As you approach the speaker, you hear his voice but cannot make out any words (threshold for hearing speech). If you go nearer, you can catch an occasional word and think that you understand the word's meaning (threshold for understanding speech). As you get closer, you understand more words until finally you can understand the meaning of single sentences (adequate understanding of meaningful speech). Finally, as you stand next to the speaker you catch every word correctly (effortless understanding of speech).

This experience can be duplicated in the laboratory, and it is possible to distinguish the threshold for (1) speech sounds, (2) understanding of isolated sporadic words, (3) understanding of sentences, and (4) full understanding of each word in a sentence. Such testing is called *speech audiometry*.

Speech audiometry measures a person's performance on speech reception tests and is, therefore, a direct measure of the difficulty a child experiences in communication. The reasons for performing both speech and pure-tone audiometry will become clear later.

The speech audiometer is a sophisticated way of measuring a person's response to voices. Employing microphones for live voice testing, turntables and tape recorders for recorded speech tests, and a white noise generator for masking purposes, the speech audiometer allows for the monitoring of speech materials presented to the patient. An attenuation system controls the output in one- or two-decibel steps over a range of hearing levels from −10 db to 100 db. With such equipment, the audiologist can obtain a speech reception threshold, determine tolerance for loud speech, and assess word discrimination ability.

The speech reception threshold (SRT) is a measure of how loud simple speech must be in order to understand it. The threshold differs from the pure-tone threshold, since the level at which a patient can repeat simple words or can understand simple running (connected) speech is determined, rather than the level at which he can barely detect the sounds of speech. The SRT is measured in db, the zero point being the level at which the average normal ear perceives speech.

The SRT for isolated words is usually determined by presenting a list of two-syllable words, (e.g., doorway, airplane) and is defined as the hearing level at which a patient can repeat 50 percent of the words correctly. An SRT for running speech can also be obtained. The child says "Yes" every few seconds as long as he can hear the connected discourse presented. The point at which the child can just barely understand the speaker is his SRT for running speech.

A second measure obtained in speech audiometry is the hearing level at which speech is most comfortable for the child (MCL). The MCL is measured by means of running speech. The child is instructed to signal when the speech is most comfortably loud for him as the examiner varies the intensity at suprathreshold levels. Both this threshold and the threshold of discomfort (TD) help determine the limits of amplification suitable for a child who is a candidate for a hearing aid. The TD is the level at which speech becomes uncomfortably loud. The child's *dynamic range*, the limits of useful hearing that the child has in each ear, is computed by subtracting the SRT from the TD.

In addition to measures of sensitivity to speech, the child's speech discrimination ability is often determined. This assessment is made because a hearing loss may not simply be a decrease in sensitivity to sound, but an impairment in understanding what is heard. The term *articulation* is employed to denote speech discrimination. An articulation test measures a child's ability to discriminate among similar sounds or among words that contain similar sounds. The term should not be confused with its use in speech, where articulation refers to a child's ability to pronounce discrete sounds. (Michael, the boy whose audiological report was presented earlier, had poor speech articulation.)

The articulation or discrimination ability is measured by administering phonetically balanced (PB) word lists well above the child's SRT. Each word list contains 50 monosyllabic words in which speech sounds occur in the same proportion as they do in English speech. The tests are scored in terms of the percentage of words heard correctly.

The chief reason for speech audiometry is that it gives exact information about the type of speech information that the child can and cannot hear, as well as the maximum intelligibility of speech that can be attained in a given child. The reader is referred to Schultz (1972) for a recent critique of speech audiometry. We will now examine how conventional audiometry contributes to the understanding of a child's behavior.

KATHY: HEARING LOSS DUE TO SENSORINEURAL DAMAGE

Kathy had been an excellent student until the seventh grade, at which time she began to make careless errors and to put less effort into her school work. Her mother reported that she also resisted going to her church group meetings, an activity she had always enjoyed. She said she didn't know what was going on at the meetings and therefore she wanted to stay home. Her father felt she was just irresponsible since her enthusiasm for chores around the house also had waned. Her teacher remarked that when girls reach this age they become preoccupied with their developing bodies and take more interest in boys, but don't always know how to act around them. Perhaps embarrassment could account for her emerging difficulties. Her mother wasn't convinced, but she agreed to a psychological evaluation, the results of which might clarify the reasons for Kathy's recent change in behavior.

During Kathy's testing, the psychologist noted that she asked him to repeat many questions. Cautious and insecure youngsters often ask for questions to be repeated, but in Kathy's case her requests usually occurred when the examiner spoke only certain words. While Kathy's test results indicated some interpersonal difficulties, the psychologist felt these difficulties were of recent origin. Because of her inconsistent responses to his questions, he suspected that she had a hearing loss and was missing much of her oral work at school and the instructions at her church meetings. He referred her to an audiologist.

Kathy's pure-tone test results revealed an audiogram of close to normal hearing up to frequencies of 500 cps and very poor hearing at higher frequencies. Typically, individuals with such records have no trouble hearing voices at normal intensities since their low-frequency hearing is unimpaired. Nevertheless, many consonants are characterized by high frequencies and weak intensities (such as *f, h, k, p, t, s*). Thus, Kathy's high-frequency loss might affect her ability to differentiate between words that sound similar but contain different high-frequency consonants. She might confuse the words *fake, cake,* and *sake* because she could not hear their initial or final consonant sounds; she might hear all the words as *a,* hearing only the vowel sounds. These were only speculations, however, since pure-tone measures allow only for an estimation of the effect of a hearing loss on speech reception. Close attention, therefore, would be paid to the results of speech audiometry.

Speech audiometry did reveal an inability to discriminate words containing high-frequency voiceless consonant sounds, particularly *s, sh, c, ch, t,* and *th.* Kathy heard the question "What time is it?" as "-a- -ime i- i-?" A hearing aid would be of little or no value to Kathy since an aid can only make sounds louder; it cannot make them clearer. Because Kathy heard low frequencies well and high frequencies poorly, she had what might be called a "confusion" deafness, that is, she could hear voices, but could not understand what they said. Her problem was magnified when she found herself in noisy surroundings.

Kathy's voice frequently was too loud because she did not hear her own voice normally, and in order to achieve what for her appeared as normal loudness, she talked louder than necessary. When her friends reminded her that she "Didn't need to shout, we're not deaf!" "she became embarrassed by her own unexplained behavior and was motivated to avoid crowds.

All Kathy's symptoms supported the diagnosis of reduced hearing sensitivity due to pathology in the inner ear or along the nerve pathway from the inner ear to the brain stem (sensorineural pathology). Since Kathy had had measles six months earlier, her deafness was attributed to this cause. While there are cases of progressive deafness that begin insidiously and progress slowly, they usually run in families. The hospital staff felt safe in attributing Kathy's loss of hearing to the measles attack.

JASON: POOR HEARING IN ONE EAR

For most of Jason's childhood he compensated for his poor hearing in one ear, compensations made without his or anyone else's awareness. Eventually, one teacher referred Jason for a psychological evaluation because of her concern about his poor academic functioning. At that time she noted that he turned one ear toward her when listening to her. Referral to an audiologist revealed very high thresholds in his right ear in addition to slightly increased thresholds in his left ear. Jason's speech audiogram appears below.

	Left	Right
Speech reception threshold	22 db	60 db
Most comfortable loudness	40 db	80 db
Tolerance level	100 db	98 db
Dynamic range	78 db	90 db
Discrimination	95 db	90 db

A hearing aid was placed on Jason's right ear, and he was tested with a speech audiometer in a sound-field situation. The benefit of the aid was measured by comparing these results with those obtained without the aid. The aid significantly improved Jason's hearing. A hearing aid must be tested at an audiology clinic to determine if it does, in fact, improve hearing at all and if the degree of improvement will have a significant effect on the patient. Aids are sometimes bought without an evaluation of their effectiveness and undue emphasis is placed on finding the "right aid" when no aid would ever be of benefit (Newby, 1964).

Play audiometry

Play audiometry is usually employed when evaluating the hearing of preschool children. A game is made of the testing situation when the child is considered too young to respond consistently in conventional audiometry where continued voluntary responding is required. While in a soundproof room, the child is conditioned to perform some playful act when he hears a tone. For example, he places rings on a toy peg or places toy cars in a box, drops blocks in a basket or bangs pegs into a board. Some children require periodic changes in the response required in order to maintain their interest and attention.

Lowell and his colleagues (Lowell, Rushford, Hoverston, & Stoner, 1956) have developed a conditioning procedure that is widely used. The child initially learns to make a response to the beat of a drum that he can see and also feel. Then the drumbeat is sounded with the drum out of sight. Finally, the tones from an audiometer are substituted for the drumbeat. The response required is changed frequently enough to maintain the child's attention.

An early technique that stimulated the development of other innovative play techniques is the "peep show" procedure developed by Dix and Hallpike (1947). A box with an open front is wired in series with an audiometer located behind a screen. Pure-tone stimuli are then presented through earphones in the conventional manner. When a tone is on, pressing a switch illuminates the interior of the box and permits observation of a picture. The child is conditioned to respond to the tone by pressing the switch. If the tone is not on and the child presses the switch, the stage does not light up. Variations on this procedure, while interesting, are not an essential part of the usual clinical accoutrement since the skilled clinician can usually do as well with less elaborate approaches (Miller & Polisar, 1964). Play audiometry was employed in the evaluation of the two youngsters described below.

LINDA: DEAF FROM GERMAN MEASLES

Linda, age 2½, was first seen by the public health nurse when she was brought to the county well-baby clinic for her measles immunization. After giving Linda's medical history, her mother verbalized her concern that Linda had not begun to talk; her brother was one year younger and was already talking.

The medical history indicated a full-term uneventful pregnancy and normal uncomplicated delivery. Linda's infancy had been trouble-free, with chicken pox her only illness. She ate well, and, because she seldom cried, she was considered a happy baby. She walked, climbed, and rode her tricycle at the normal ages. She fed herself at 15 months and was toilet trained at 2 years. Because of her delayed language development, the clinic staff suspected that she had reduced hearing sensitivity and recommended an audiological and psychological evaluation. Initially, they were puzzled about the possible cause since there was no deafness in the family history and there had been no complications during pregnancy or at birth. Then, as an afterthought, Linda's mother mentioned that she had had German measles during her second month of pregnancy with Linda. German measles (rubella) is known to produce deafness, as well as other abnormalities.

Linda readily accepted the wearing of earphones and, therefore, both air and bone conduction thresholds could be determined for both ears. Testing revealed both bone and air conduction thresholds of 70 db in each ear at all frequencies, a severe hearing loss. Extrapolating from Table 5.1, we can see that in order for Linda to hear sounds, she requires an amplitude approximately 3000 times that required by the normal ear (an increase in 10 db is equivalent to tripling the amplitude). Linda's psychological evaluation revealed normal intellectual functioning on nonverbal measures of intelligence.

Linda's hearing loss was attributed to damage to the inner and outer hair cells along the basilar membrane of the cochlea. This damage resulted from infection by German measles, infection passed from the mother to her fetus during the first trimester of pregnancy, a period when the developing nervous system is maximally affected by noxious agents and disease.

Children who contract rubella during their first trimester of growth *in utero* often show central as well as peripheral nervous system damage. Not surprising, then, is Vernon's (1967b) finding that more than half the children who are deaf as a result of the mother's rubella have multiple handicaps.

JAMMIE: CONDUCTIVE IMPAIRMENT

Jammie's motor development was similar to Linda's—everything proceeded normally. Nevertheless, his parents had felt uneasy about him since his early infancy. Many of the behaviors that concerned them would probably have gone unnoticed had he been their first child. During his first year, he would awaken only after being touched or shaken. He rarely was startled or frightened by loud noises, and he showed little interest in noisemakers or musical toys unless he held them. His mother's soothing voice provided no comfort until it was accompanied by her physical contact, and he usually ignored his own name unless looked at directly or motioned to when called.

By age 2, he still ignored the ring of the doorbell and telephone, and he seemed startled when he looked up from playing and saw someone in the room. He used gestures to express his needs and was not yet speaking. His parents brought him to a speech and hearing clinic for evaluation.

Audiometric evaluation revealed air conduction thresholds between 70 and 50 db, with better hearing at the higher frequencies, and bone conduction thresholds at normal levels. As we have indicated, pure conductive loss usually results from pathology or malfunctioning of the outer or middle ear with a normal inner ear. Because of the normal inner ear, bone conduction thresholds are at average levels. Usually, conductive impairment results from an inflammation of the middle ear, as in *otitis media*. An ENT (ear, nose, and throat) evaluation revealed that Jammie had no such condition. Further medical evaluation revealed that Jammie was born with only a rudimentary pinna (part of the ear that directs sound waves into the external canal), a malformed ear drum, and malformed ossicles in the middle ear. Corrective surgery would not restore Jammie's hearing.

Evaluating infants

Because the infant cannot give a voluntary response on command, neither conventional nor play audiometric procedures can be employed. Similarly, some retarded and severely disturbed children are unable to cooperate in an audiometric evaluation. Consequently, procedures that have been developed to evaluate infants are also used with older children. Let us examine how Ralph, a neonate, was evaluated for a hearing disorder. The procedure employed was suggested by Goldstein and Tait (1971).

Three infants, all in good health and born at approximately the same time, were brought to an examining room in their bassinets and placed alongside one another. Each child's identification bracelet was covered to prevent inadvertent recognition. Two nurses and an audiologist were present in the room. The audiologist took various noisemakers (clickers, bells, whistles) and held them a standard distance from each child. He presented to the three infants the quieter noises first, and then he proceeded to the louder ones. The nurses as well as the audiologist recorded their observations of each infant's response. Following this examination, each child's responsivity to light and touch was observed. A flashlight was shone in each child's eyes and air blown on its feet with an aspiration syringe. After all the testing was completed, each observer independently made two judgments. First, he judged which of the three children was least responsive to sound and, second, he judged whether the child displayed reduced responsivity to all types of stimuli or only to auditory stimuli.

In this examination all three observers felt that one child's auditory responses were noticeably different from those of the other two. The identification bracelets were uncovered and the child's identity revealed. The child was Ralph, previously considered a high-risk infant in terms of hearing impairment because of a family history of hearing loss. The degree of Ralph's hearing impairment was tentatively classified as profound, and he was scheduled for more definitive testing.

Several weeks later Ralph was seen alone. His responses to sound were observed both when he was awake and during stages of light and deep sleep. In general, the nature of a child's responses to sound depends upon his state of activity. If he is engrossed in play, he might turn his head in the direction of the sound. If he is asleep with a pacifier in his mouth, he might suck more vigorously on the pacifier. Ralph showed no consistent response to sound. He was therefore scheduled for electro-encephalic audiometry (EEA), sometimes referred to as evoked response audiometry.

Ralph was placed under induced sleep, electrodes were attached to his scalp with adhesive tape, and earphones were affixed to his head. Six series of stimuli were then presented. Each series consisted of 12 stimuli and 4 silent control intervals, so that for each series there were 16 segments of the record identified by a signal marker and numeral. In each series two frequencies were presented to each ear at three different intensity levels. The same frequencies and intensities were used in each series, but the order of stimulus presentation was randomized for each series. Goldstein, Kendall, and Arick (1963) describe this procedure in more detail, and Price (1969) presents a critique of EEA procedures.

Ralph's EEA record was then analyzed by an expert in electroencephalography. Research has established that electroencephalic responses to auditory stimulation consist of changes in the frequency and voltage of the brain's electrical activity that bear a definite time relation to the onset and completion of the stimulus. The task of the scorer is to judge whether an observable pattern change occurs in the segment of the child's record between the "on" and "off" points denoted by the signal marker. Scoring is done without knowledge of the stimulus that corresponds to the segment of the record studied. Scores for each stimulus condition are then compared with scores for each control condition. In Ralph's record significant differences between control and stimulus means occurred only at very high intensities. These findings corroborated those of the behavioral testing—the child had a hearing loss. The extent of his handicap could be determined more reliably when he was older and could be tested using behavioral audiometry.

Although we presented the testing of Ralph as if it followed a standard practice, infant screening for hearing disorder is actually a relatively recent procedure and has been the subject of considerable debate. Some investigators are not even certain that early screening programs are necessary, since they fail to identify children with mild or moderate hearing impairments as well as those whose hearing will deteriorate later. They suggest that screening should be done only when a hearing disorder is present in an immediate family member and deafness due to a genetic disorder is therefore expected (a high-risk infant).

It is beyond the scope of this chapter to discuss infant screening, but the interested reader is referred to several articles that review the literature in this area (Davis, 1965; DiCarlo, Kendall, & Goldstein, 1962; Goldstein & Tait, 1971). McCroskey and Cory (1969) have prepared an annotated bibliography of publications dealing with the topic.

Ralph's deafness was detected soon after birth, but only a small percentage of deaf children are identified that early. The largest number of congenitally deaf children are identified between the ages of 1 and 2. Konigsmark (1972) describes the various hearing disorders resulting from genetic causes. Other children become deaf following diseases that damage the middle or inner ear. Most diseases result in hearing loss rather than deafness, and the child's hearing impairment may go unnoticed for some time. Later, when a hearing impairment is suspected, the child is referred for audiometric evaluation.

Testing the difficult child

When the examiners presented the various sounds to Ralph, they were looking for some sign that he heard the sound. If Ralph moved his head in the direction of the sound (orienting reflex) or cried (startle response) and his response could be repeatedly demonstrated, they could conclude that the sound had elicited the response, that is, that he could hear the sound. Attempts to elicit the orienting reflex also are made with older children who fail to respond to play audiometry. Some clinicians have improved upon this simple technique by attempting to condition the orienting reflex. They use two loudspeakers, one to the child's right and the other to his left. If the child turns toward the loudspeaker that presents the tone, then a peep show is revealed to him. The audiological report on Ann, a severely retarded child, mentioned that conditioned orienting reflexes could not be elicited from her.

Galvanic skin response (GSR) audiometry also has been employed with both infants and children untestable by conventional methods. In this procedure the presentation of a tone is immediately followed by a slight shock. Following the shock, skin resistance decreases and this decrease can be measured electrically. After repeated shocks, a conditioned reflex is established and the tone alone will elicit the decrease in skin resistance.

Although the GSR technique has fallen into disuse in the last decade or so, it is still used occasionally. The GSR procedure could not be used with Ann since she would neither allow the administration of shock nor stay still during the conditioning procedure (activity results in changes in skin resistance). While EEA could have been used with Ann, its use was deferred until a later time. The audiologist preferred to try play audiometry again before resorting to the use of the EEA procedure.

When the audiologist wrote that Ann failed to respond to any conditioning technique, he meant that he had tried both classical and operant procedures without success. One of the problems in evaluating a neurologically impaired child such as Ann is that the audiologist has no way of knowing whether poor performance results from incapacity or from disinterest in sounds.

In most audiological procedures the child must "listen" for auditory stimuli. In the language-impaired child, it is difficult to instruct him to listen. Simply because the examiner points to his ears and nods his head to indicate the presence of sound does not mean that the child will pay attention to him (St. James-Roberts, 1972). Even the orienting reflex to sound may extinguish. Mark and Hardy (1958, p. 241) state:

> Continuously unreinforced stimuli, or auditory stimuli only inconsistently reinforced, serve to make for disorganized learning processes associated with auditory stimuli and have a general inhibitory effect on the auditory system. The child thus learns to "disregard" this sense modality completely, and a previously present OR [orienting reflex] is extinguished.

Obviously, then, some response measure other than the orienting reflex has to be used. When the retarded or psychotic child will work for some reward, operant audiometry can be employed. St. James-Roberts (1972, p. 52) describes his approach.

> The testee is seated in front of a screen on which three pictures are shown, one of which is "correct," in the sense that its appearance is accompanied by the presentation of a visual cue (for example, an illuminated bulb). If the testee pulls the lever in front of him when the cue appears, he is reinforced by a suitable reward. If he does not, the reward is omitted.
> The second, auditory stage of the test can be administered as soon as adequate response to the visual (or tactile) cues has been achieved. Pure tones or voices can be substituted for these cues, while the same rewards are retained.

St. James-Roberts's technique of employing a sensory modality other than the auditory in the first stage of an audiological evaluation has three advantages over other techniques. First, the child can be taught the necessary skill for proficient response in the test situation without recourse to cumbersome instruction. Second, his interest and involvement are established before auditory testing begins. Third, a base line measure of the individual testee's general ability to perform a matching task can be established. By comparing responses during the auditory stage of the test to this baseline, it can be determined whether poor performance at the auditory stage is due to auditory malfunction or to a general sensory, expressive, motor, or learning disability.

Results of evaluation in the cases presented

Linda and Jammie both showed the classic signs of hearing loss that can be observed prior to the age of 2. During their first year, they rarely awoke to sound and were not comforted by their mother's voice. Neither child showed much interest in noisemakers and neither responded to the mother's verbal commands if they were not looking at her. By the age of 2 neither child spoke. They never heard the doorbell or seemed interested in music.

Jason's turning his good ear toward the speaker and his inconsistent response to sound are characteristic responses of individuals whose hearing is poor in one ear. Kathy's reluctance to attend large gatherings and her loud speech are characteristic responses of those with sensorineural deafness. Such children often talk loud because they do not hear their own voice well, particularly when background noise is present.

Ralph, Linda, and Jammie were born deaf and were classified as *congenitally deaf*. Kathy was born with normal hearing but became hard-of-hearing through illness. If she had been rendered totally deaf through illness, she would have been classified as *adventitiously deaf*. The term deaf is typically reserved for those whose threshold in both ears is so low as to prevent the establishment of speech and language or those who had acquired speech but who could no longer speak or understand speech after damage to their ears. While those with a severe (60–75 db) or profound (above 75 db) loss are considered deaf, we will see later that the degree of language disability is not always a function of the threshold for hearing.

Kathy and Jason were classified as hard-of-hearing since their sense of hearing, although defective, was functional with or without a hearing aid. Jason's hearing loss in his good ear was considered a mild loss (29–40 db), but when combined with the moderate loss (40–60 db) in his bad ear, he had considerable difficulty in hearing what went on around him.

Ann, the retarded girl whose audiological report was presented at the beginning of the chapter, would be evaluated again. Perhaps when she was familiar with the audiologist, she would cooperate better with his efforts to evaluate her hearing.

After Linda's and Jammie's hearing disorders were discovered, they were referred to a preschool for the deaf, as Ralph would be when he was older. Kathy was given training in speech discrimination, and both she and Jason remained in the regular class setting.

REMEDIATION

Training techniques

Auditory training The preschool where Linda and Jammie were enrolled was patterned after the John Tracy Clinic in Los Angeles. The
program at the clinic remains one of the most highly regarded in the
world. Deaf children are given intensive, day-long oral instruction and
the best of modern amplification.

Auditory training is the featured approach of the preschool attended
by Linda and Jammie. Children who have a profound hearing loss (RT
above 80 db) do not hear the ordinary sounds of life well enough to
pay attention to them. Making them aware of the various sounds that
exist in the environment and of how the differences between sounds can
be used to identify them is the initial goal of training.

In the school the children use two types of auditory trainers. For seat
work, they use large headsets attached to individual student control boxes
and wired to a microphone used by the teacher (see Figure 5.2). When
they leave their seats, they used wireless trainers. The individual audiograms of each child are placed above the blackboard to remind the
teacher of the child's hearing level.

The first step in auditory training is to teach the children to make
gross discriminations between sounds. Linda and Jammie were trained by
the following technique. The children are shown that a bell and a horn
make different sounds. While they wear their earphones, the teacher rings
the bell and blows the horn alternately while they can see the noisemaker
that makes each sound. Then they turn away from the teacher and
guess which noisemaker is making the sound they hear through their earphones. When they can successfully discriminate between the two sounds,
a third sound is added, then a fourth, and so on. Once Linda and Jammie
had learned to pay attention to sounds, a portion of their learning proceeded without amplification.

The children are then taught to recognize the sounds of words. The
words are always presented with the objects they signify. Training proceeds from making discriminations between dissimilar speech sounds
(gross speech discrimination) to making discriminations between similar
speech sounds, such as /f/ and /th/ (fine speech discrimination).

When this training was well underway, Linda and Jammie were fitted
with hearing aids and given training in their operation. The school staff
believes that a hearing aid should be given to children only after they
have had prior experience with amplified sound. Without such experience, the children would have no notion of what they should hear and
might reject its use (Newby, 1964). The teacher prepares children for
aids by first giving them a carefully planned and controlled listening
experience with an auditory training unit. Training units provide high-

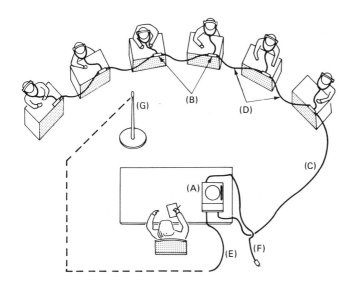

Figure 5.2 *Typical classroom layout for use of an auditory trainer. (A) Binaural amplifier or control unit located at teacher's desk; may be installed in any other convenient place. (B) Student control boxes equipped with dual volume controls for individual student sound level adjustment. (C) 12-foot interconnecting cable connects control unit to first student control box. (D) 4-foot interconnecting cables connect student control boxes. (E) 25-foot microphone cable connects control unit to ceiling-mounted microphones. (F) 8-foot AC cord, equipped with adapter where grounded 3-conductor wall socket is not available. (G) Ceiling-mounted microphones (floorstand is optional); for the ceiling-mounted microphones we recommend a height of approximately 7 feet above floor level. (From D. A. Sanders.* Aural rehabilitation. *Englewood Cliffs, N.J.: Prentice-Hall, 1970. Photo courtesy Ambico Electronics, Los Angeles, Calif.)*

fidelity amplification and have built-in protection against too great an intensity of sound. In contrast, the individual hearing aid amplifies over a limited frequency range and introduces distortion. Considerable adjustment is required to transfer from an auditory training unit to an aid. An even greater adjustment is required, however, to adapt to an aid without prior experience with amplification. Placing a child with a new hearing aid under the guidance of an audiologist usually results in better acceptance of the aid than when parents alone attempt to get their child to wear an aid (Newby, 1964).

Speech training Both Jammie's and Linda's hearing loss was reflected in their speech and voice patterns. When both started to speak, their speech was marked by the omission of many sounds and by substitutions of one sound for another. Both relied greatly on gestures for communication. Even children less impaired than they usually have speech disorders, because learning to speak is achieved by imitating the speech of others. The sounds a child produces are what he hears, not what is actually said, and thus any distortion in reception will be transmitted to the production of sound.

When Linda and Jammie did speak, their speech was dull and lifeless. Pitch was monotonous and higher than desirable. Linda's voice was too loud (characteristic of sensorineural losses), while Jammie's was too soft (usually characteristic of conductive losses where the child's own voice sounds very loud to him compared to the voices of others). Training to improve pitch and intensity involves making the child aware of both the kinesthetic sensations that accompany voice variations and the reactions of others in his environment to his speech.

Visual and tactual methods are employed to improve defective pronunciation of speech sounds (articulation). The speech therapist shows the child where the articulators (vocal organs—lips, tongue, jaw, etc.) should be placed to produce a particular sound. When movements of articulators are visible, the therapist has the child imitate him. When movements are not visible, the child is shown a cross-sectional drawing of the articulator placement and instructed to duplicate this placement with their own articulators. Children often have extreme difficulty learning the difference between voiced and unvoiced consonants that have the same articulator position, such as /t/ and /d/. To help them distinguish the sounds the therapist places a child's hands on his own larynx, to show that it vibrates when he says /d/ but does not when he says /t/. Plosives, sounds requiring the building up of breath pressure followed by a sudden explosion, as in /p/, /b/, /t/, /d/, /k/, and /g/, are equally hard to learn. The therapist places the child's hands in front of his mouth so they can feel the puff of air that occurs each time he says a word beginning with these letters. Nasal consonants, /m/, /n/, and /ng/, are demonstrated by the child's feeling the vibration in the therapist's nose (Newby, 1964). Other tactual techniques employed to help the child learn to articulate some of these sounds appear in Figure 5.3. Each time the child feels the sounds, he tries to imitate them.

Speech reading   Part of Linda's and Jammie's auditory training involved modeling lip and tongue movements after that of the teacher. Once children are proficient in this ability, they can be given practice in recognition of these movements. This training is called speech reading or lipreading. The major goal of this training is to enable the child to extract enough information from the visual characteristics of speech to predict what the speaker is saying. It is not necessary to identify each and every articulatory movement of the speaker; only enough words need to be recognized to identify the idea being communicated. The

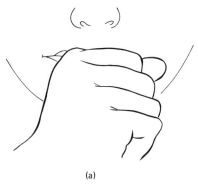

(a)

Make fist with right hand. Press against softly closed lips making b against last portion of index finger.

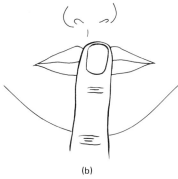

(b)

Place the right index finger over mouth; produce p through pursed lips, making a motion as if blowing the index finger away.

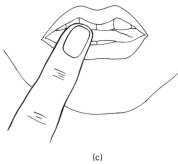

(c)

Open mouth exposing teeth together making the t sound. Tap teeth with the right index finger each time the t sound is produced.

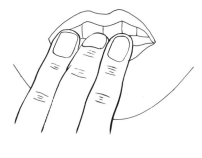

(d)

Open mouth exposing clenched teetch making the d sound. Tap teeth with three fingers of the right hand each time the d sound is made with the tongue.

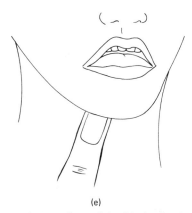

(e)

Push the index finger of the right hand under the chin. Make the hard c or k sound.

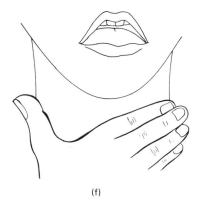

(f)

Place right hand in an outspread position (four fingers versus thumb) at the base of the throat. Make hard g sounds.

Figure 5.3 *Techniques of articulation training. (From R. O. Nelson & I. M. Evans. The combination of learning principles and speech therapy techniques in the treatment of non-communicating children.* Journal of Child Psychology and Psychiatry, *1968,* **9,** *111-124.)*

visual recognition of sounds can be made from various positions of the tongue, lips, and jaw; awareness of these positions is facilitated through mirror practice.

At the preschool level visual training emphasizes familiarizing the child with the role that vision plays in communication. At a later stage in training precise discrimination of speech sounds is stressed. Preschool activities include practice on visual matching of objects from memory and on predicting the probable nature of a message from nonverbal cues. The children are given pictorial materials and asked to derive meaning from them (see Figure 5.4) or to arrange them in sequence. Sanders (1971) presents visual communication procedures in detail.

The oral versus the manual approach to education

When Linda and Jammie reached age 5, they were enrolled in the public school system's special classes for the deaf. The system had three such classes, with about ten children in each class. Linda was placed with a teacher who continued to stress improving oral communication skills.

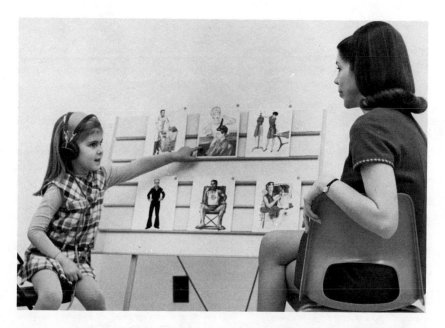

Figure 5.4 *The message to be speech read is easier if constrained by contextual material. Here, the pictures taken from the Peabody Language Kit help the child to predict the probable nature of the message. (Photo courtesy of Department of Speech Communication, State University of New York at Buffalo.)*

The oral approach devotes considerable time to the development of auditory and visual perception and to the production of speech sounds. Several pieces of equipment that present significant speech information visually may be used by the teacher. One piece of equipment is a vertical bank of lights wired so that more lights come on as the child's voice increases in intensity. Another device is a vertical bank of lights behind colored panes of glass. Particular color patterns of light correspond to particular speech sounds. The teacher demonstrates that a speech sound produces a pattern and asks the child to try to produce this pattern.

For older children, a more complex procedure, utilizing an array of 169 lights, is employed. Each speech sound has a particular configuration of lights associated with it. The configuration is intimately related to the articulatory configuration required to produce the sound. In essence, a configuration of lights for a sound approximates the configuration that would appear on a sound spectrograph (a photograph of a sound's wave lengths). The children are shown the manner in which the machine displays vowels, glides, and words. The teacher demonstrates the machine's use by saying a word into the machine and tracing its pattern with a marker pencil on the Plexiglas display screen that covers the array of lights. The children then try to match this pattern. The closer they can approximate the indicated pattern the more "acceptable" is their pronunciation of the particular word. (For a discussion of the visual portrayal of speech parameters, see Pickett & Constam, 1968; Potter & Peterson, 1948; or Thomas & Snell, 1970.) Children take turns using the machines, and the teacher keeps graphs of their progress. She uses a scoring system where points are earned for increasing approximations of the pattern, and she graphs the number of words "learned" each day. Back-up reinforcers are employed in addition to the reinforcement produced through feedback regarding success.

When children trained with these devices are compared with those receiving conventional training, equivocal findings result (Thomas & Snell, 1970). The view of teachers using the oral approach, supported by some research, is that students speak more intelligibly after using the device. How long these effects are sustained is still to be determined.

Jammie was placed with a teacher who believed that more stress should be placed on manual communication. In addition to oral communication skills, he was taught finger spelling and the language of signs. The difference in approach between Linda's and Jammie's teachers reflects an effort to resolve an educational conflict that has persisted for centuries—the conflict between the *oralists* and *manualists*. The oralists maintain that the deaf can be taught to talk and understand speech and can, therefore, learn to communicate with normal hearing people. The manualists maintain that the results of oral teaching do not justify the effort required of the child. The manual method of communication is relatively easy to teach. By this means, the deaf can communicate easily with one another and with teachers trained to use this approach. Teachers can, therefore, spend more time teaching subject matter rather than laboring to teach verbal communication skills. Vernon and Makowsky (1969) state that the oralists attempt to remake the deaf child into a fictitious version of the hearing child—a practice, they maintain, that emphasizes a denial of the handicap and makes deaf persons ashamed of manual communication and of certain aspects of themselves.

Historically, manual methods of communication were the first methods employed to educate the deaf. These methods, however, prevented the deaf child from integrating with society, leading to a separate society of deaf people and to the belief that the deaf could not learn to speak. A small group of professionals became committed to the idea that the deaf could learn to identify the visual aspects of speech and learn to speak. This group became larger, and in the early 1900s the tide began to turn in favor of the oral education of the deaf. Now, in the 1970s, manual methods are being reintroduced. This change has taken place primarily because research findings suggest that exclusive reliance upon oral methods may handicap the deaf child.

Research support for manual or combined manual-oral training   Vernon and Koh (1971) followed up every student who graduated from the Tracy Clinic Oral Preschool during the period between 1944 and 1968 and who went on to attend the California School for the Deaf. The orally educated children were matched with two groups of deaf children who had no preschool training: one group of deaf children of deaf parents and one of deaf children of hearing parents. This matching enabled comparisons of children given an oral preschool education (3 years) under optimal conditions both with children who had early manual communication but no oral preschool and with children who had neither oral preschool nor manual communication but who lived in an oral home environment. The average age of the subjects at the time of follow-up was 18. Comparison of Stanford achievement test scores revealed that higher scores were obtained by the children who had early training in manual communication. They were superior to the other two groups by nearly one full grade on all four subtests of the Stanford. The manual group scored at about the seventh grade level, while the Tracy group and those with hearing parents and no preschool experience scored at about the sixth grade level. Further comparisons indicated that the manual group also was superior in written language competence. An analysis of academic progress revealed that 90 percent of the children with early manual communication who were over 16 had passed college entrance exams or held high school or vocational school diplomas. Sixty-five percent of the Tracy oral preschool children achieved at this level.

There were no significant differences in speech intelligibility or speech reading among the three groups. These findings deserve special mention in light of the emphasis placed on the importance of an early oral environment (Elliott & Armbruster, 1967). The children of deaf parents had the most nonoral environment possible, while the Tracy children had an "enriched" oral environment. Yet, there were no differences in speech intelligibility between the two groups.

The achievement levels of the children in these three groups were considerably above the national norms for deaf individuals, of whom 30 percent are functionally illiterate, 60 percent never achieve beyond the fifth grade level, and only 10 percent achieve above a tenth grade level (Kronenberg & Blake, 1966; McClure, 1966). The Tracy graduates had an average IQ of 114. In order to match children in this group on intelligence test scores, equally bright children had to be selected from the other two groups. An IQ of 114 places a person in the upper 20 percent of the population. Data from other leading private oral facilities, such as the Clarke School and the Central Institute for the Deaf, indicate that those accepted are, on the average, also in the upper 20 percent. Those who graduate or are referred to regular public schools have an even higher IQ score (Vernon & Koh, 1971). Perhaps their success is more a function of their intelligence than "a tribute to the oralists' belief that with proper training the handicap imposed by deafness can be minimized" (Newby, 1964, p. 327).

Vernon and Koh's findings were not isolated ones. At least ten other American studies have demonstrated the superiority of groups given either manual or combined manual-oral training over groups given only oral training (Vernon, 1970a, 1970b). Vernon (1972) concluded that undue emphasis has been placed on oral methods of education in America and that a switch in emphasis is sorely needed.

In 1938 Russian investigators acknowledged the failure of purely oral methods and gave approval to teaching the written form of language at an early age and to the use of finger speech and sign language as legitimate methods of instruction (Moores, 1972). Research to support this position was disrupted by World War II and was not resumed until 1950. Morozova (1954) reported that through the use of finger spelling 3- and 4-year-old children could acquire in two years what it took three years to master using only oral methods. These findings have been replicated by other Russian investigators. In addition, their research demonstrated that finger spelling facilitated the separation of words into their phonetic composition and accelerated vocabulary growth (Moores, 1972).

Officers of the British Department of Education and Science who observed deaf children in Moscow schools, children who functioned without hearing aids or amplification, had this to say about the Russian methods.

It appeared to us, from what we were shown, that the Russians are more successful than we are in the development of language, vocabulary and speech in deaf children once they enter the education system. This seemed to us to be a strong point in favor of their method (use of fingerspelling from the very start as an instrument for the development of language, communication and speech), the investigation of which was the main object of our visit (Committee on the Education of Deaf Children, 1968, pp. 44–45).

The total communication approach   In spite of the Russian and American research, a great deal of which took place prior to 1968, Helen Lance, former president of the Alexander Graham Bell Association for the Deaf and principal of the Central Institute for the Deaf in St. Louis, reemphasized her faith in a predominantly oral approach when she delivered her presidential address to the Bell Association in 1968 (Lane, 1968). She concluded her speech with a quotation from Helen Keller: "A potent force within me, stronger than the persuasion of my friends, had impelled me to try my strength by the standards of those who see and hear." And in 1971, Northcott (1971, p. 29) remarked that

Today's educational focus . . . is on the development of . . . an independent child—one who depends on audition and oral communication as functioning social and cognitive skills for self-expression. . . . A major objective is the functional use of residual hearing as a primary modality for language acquisition and speech production *regardless of the severity of the hearing loss* [italics added].

Lane (1968) emphasized that the deaf should be evaluated using the same criteria as are used for the hearing. She has felt secure in placing a deaf child in a hearing school if his verbal IQ was within the normal range. She reached this conclusion after examining the intelligent quotients of 79 deaf children who received eighth grade diplomas from the Central Institute for the Deaf over a 15-year period. Their mean verbal IQ was 96.6 and their mean performance IQ was 119.8. Twelve of the group who graduated from hearing colleges had mean verbal and performance IQs of 103.6 and 126.8 respectively. She concluded that verbal abilities of deaf children can approximate normality as a result of education and good intelligence. This conclusion is an understatement. It would be more correct to say that verbal abilities can approximate normality if the deaf child is of superior intelligence, if he is among the brightest 10 percent of deaf children. What Lane does not state is how much general knowledge and special talent were sacrificed when predominantly verbal methods were used with less intelligent children. Northcott (1971) feels that every effort should be made to integrate deaf children into regular educational programs. Although past efforts at integration have been largely unsuccessful (Vernon, 1970a), there would be no quarrel with such efforts if both the normal hearing child and the deaf child were required to adapt to one another. This author has witnessed normal hearing children serving as interpreters for deaf children using finger spelling and the language of signs. In most classrooms there would be a youngster who would volunteer to learn sign language and who could serve such a function. In other instances hearing children of deaf parents, who already know manual methods of communication, could volunteer. The deaf child could attempt oral communication whenever possible, but on other occasions could communicate with methods that cause him less difficulty. There is currently a registry of interpreters for the deaf (Neesam, 1971); there is no reason why children couldn't be added to this list.

A number of investigators are now taking more seriously the total communication approach. This renewed interest brought about in 1971 a special conference devoted to the topic (O'Rourke, 1972).

FACTORS RELATED TO SCHOOL ACHIEVEMENT

We have discussed types of hearing loss and educational approaches used to help children compensate for their loss. Although a positive correlation exists between the extent of hearing loss and verbal deficit (Roach & Rosecrans, 1972), the relationship is not substantial enough to explain the diversity of language achievement obtained by the hearing impaired. In addition, individuals show a variety of methods to compensate for hearing impairment. Consequently, factors other than sensory loss must be evaluated before any definitive statements can be made about a child's ability to function in a classroom. Evaluation should focus on assessing skills basic to academic functioning, rather than on the extent of hearing loss (Jones & Byers, 1971). Attention has turned from the traditional classification of hearing loss in terms of pure-tone averages to an examination of how hearing impairment actually affects an individual. Current emphasis is on examining actual achievement in communication skills and the manner in which the deaf child acquires and retains language.

We know that age-appropriate academic achievement requires sufficient perceptual and conceptual skill, adequate memory, and average intellectual ability. Does being deaf or hard-of-hearing affect the development of these skills? To answer this question, we will examine the research that has compared deaf with hearing subjects on those skills or assets necessary for adequate academic achievement. These skills are: psycholinguistic efficiency, visual-perceptual ability, memory, intelligence, and emotional maturity.

Psycholinguistic efficiency

Because the study of the deaf's language acquisition is a recent endeavor, little information is available about this topic (Lowenbraun & Affleck, 1970). Early investigations were essentially nonlinguistic and examined either achievement test scores or performance on measures of written expression. These investigations were helpful, however, since they revealed the abilities and disabilities of deaf populations.

In 1917 Pintner and Patterson reported that median reading scores of the deaf at any age never reached the median of 8-year-old hearing children. Of the groups Pugh studied in 1946, none obtained scores higher than the sixth grade level or showed much improvement between the seventh and thirteenth years of schooling. A survey of 5307 deaf children between the ages of 10 and 16 revealed that only 8 percent of those tested read above the fourth grade level (Furth, 1966; Wrightstone, Aronow, & Moskowitz, 1963). The average reading score at age 11 was mid-second grade; five years later, at age 16, the mean was at mid-third grade—only one grade higher! The situation was no better in 1971, when Balow, Fultin, and Peploe reported reading scores at about the fourth to fifth grade level for a group between the ages of 13 and 21. Plotting scores by age revealed no significant increases in reading achievement with increasing age—the adult of 21 was no more proficient than the child of 12! Even these low reading test scores may be overestimations of the language capabilities of the deaf.

Reading tests usually require multiple choice responses, choices that include one of the five grammatical classes. Such a procedure requires recognition skill rather than recall for spontaneous use, and it limits selection to a grammatically correct subset. Thus, although a select group might score as high as the seventh grade level on reading tests, their written compositions, which require recall for use, may still be characterized as a "tangled web-type of expression in which words occur in profusion but do not align themselves in orderly array" (Fusfeld, 1955, p. 20). Even grammatically correct sentences produced by deaf children are often rigid, redundant, and stereotyped (Simmons, 1962). Moores (1970) matched deaf with hearing subjects on reading ability and had both groups read selected passages and fill in missing words that had been removed from the passages. Analysis of the words selected by members of each group revealed significantly more grammatical and semantic inadequacies in the deaf group.

In addition to inadequate morphological-syntactic integrations, the deaf have a lower level of vocabulary use. They write short sentences that are less complex, less flexible, and more stereotyped than those written by normal children. They also use fixed repetitive phrases that are grammatically incorrect (Fusfeld, 1955; Heider & Heider, 1940; Myklebust, 1960). Moores (1970, p. 651) concludes that "the majority of deaf children not only develop language skills at a lower rate, but also develop patterns and constructions which produce utterances not normally found in hearing children."

Although these studies confirm the presence of language deficiencies in the deaf child, they provide no information on how these deficiencies arise. What is needed is a description of the process of oral language development in deaf children. Several investigators have made a start in this direction (Lowenbraun & Affleck, 1970). Their initial findings suggest that the deaf child's receptive language ability is no better developed than his expressive language ability, and that educators who stress expressive skills before receptive control has been mastered may be responsible for the perpetuation of primitive error patterns. In other words, the teaching of language according to the rules of adult grammar, without awareness of the normal sequence of emerging language patterns, may preclude the grammaticality the teacher is trying to establish.

Study of psycholinguistic functioning of the deaf also involves isolating those morphological, syntactic, and semantic factors that present the most difficulties for deaf students. Moores (1970) has initiated research in this direction. He suggests that diagnostic test batteries be developed to help assess individual patterns of linguistic ability. Test results would provide the teacher with a basis for designing an individualized program of instruction or remediation. Testing need not be formal, however, since an individualized approach to diagnosis and instruction may reveal strengths and weaknesses as well as or better than formal tests (Osborne, Bellefleur, & Bevan, 1971).

Visual-perceptual ability and memory

Because of the emphasis on the deaf's verbal development, other facets of their development have been neglected. Studies have revealed that deaf children are inferior to hearing children on these visual-perceptual tasks that are prerequisites for reading, even though they equal hearing children on general perceptual ability (Clark & Leslie, 1971; Conrad & Rush, 1965; Doehring & Rosenstein, 1960; Van Zyl & Ives, 1971). For example, Marshall (1970) found that a group of preschool deaf children had a mean deficit of 15 months on subtests of the Frostig Developmental Test of Visual Perception and of 18 months on four subtests of the 1961 version of the Illinois Test of Psycholinguistic Abilities (visual decoding, manual expression, visual-motor sequencing, and visual-motor association). Similarly, Hartung (1970) found that a group of elementary age deaf children (7.5 to 9 years) could recognize unfamiliar Greek letters as well as hearing children, but were inferior to the hearing on tasks involving discrimination of nonsense syllables. These studies evaluated abilities that are learned skills, suggesting that the deaf lack appropriate learning experiences. This belief is supported by the finding that training not only increases visual-perceptual skill in the deaf, but also results in their showing improved reading achievement (Marshall, 1970).

Some years ago Gellermann (1931) hypothesized that humans use language to form symbolic representations of experience. Indirect support for this theory has come from the work of cognitive theorists who

have demonstrated the facilitating effect of verbal labels upon performance. For example, when children are trained to label visual stimuli,
their memory for the stimuli is facilitated (Spiker, 1956). The improved
memory is attributed to the children's use of the verbal labels to facilitate
rehearsal (thinking about the stimuli) during the interval between the
presentation and the recall of the stimuli. In other words, the verbal
label serves as a mediating response. In addition, the prior learning of
potential verbal mediating responses facilitates subsequent conceptual
learning (Lacey, 1961; Jensen, 1966; Kendler, 1963). Consequently, Kendler (1963) has postulated that a transition occurs in the course of human
development from unmediated, single-unit behavior to mediated behavior.

Because deaf children have poor verbal ability, verbal mediation is
not a natural mode of thought operation for them; their characteristic
mode is nonverbal (Furth & Youniss, 1964), primarily visual and tactual
(Blair, 1957). Because of verbal deficiencies they cannot employ verbal
mediators in problem-solving tasks, and, therefore, show a cumulative
deficit in learning as they get older. This theory has been used to explain
the poor memory of the deaf as compared to the hearing in memory
experiments (McCarthy & Marshall, 1969; Withrow, 1968).

The effect of this deficit, the lack of verbal mediation to facilitate
learning, is multiplied by the fact that inadequate verbal mediation not
only does not help the learner, but may hinder the learning process.
If names learned to label objects are similar and have not been learned
to a high criterion or are not adequately retained when required for
use in a second task, their use will result in interference with problem
solving or memory (Spiker, 1963). Perhaps this factor is responsible for
the poor showing of the deaf in some memory tasks; their use of poorly
learned verbal labels interferes with learning or memory, particularly
when the materials to be learned involve visual-motor activity (Chovan &
McGettigan, 1971). Since the primary teaching approach in the United
States has been an oral one, we may have prevented the deaf from con-
centrating on developing dimensional salience, that is, attending to certain characteristics (dimensions) in a task so that the "information" conveyed in these characteristics serves to mediate perceptions (Gibson, 1960).
Verbal labels may draw the deaf's attention away from the relevant characteristics of learning tasks.

When deaf children show memory deficiencies, it is often on tasks
involving sequential presentation of material (McCarthy & Marshall,
1969; Withrow, 1968). Withrow (1968) suggests that hearing children are
superior to the deaf in remembering sequentially presented stimuli because they have had more experience in coding and processing sequentially heard language material; their reception of language facilitates
the processing and coding of other materials presented in sequence. This
viewpoint is supported by the finding that when material is presented to

a manually communicating group of deaf children at a rate with which they are familiar, they do as well as or better than hearing children (Withrow, 1968).

Examining the research on verbal learning uncovers several facts that may relate to the learning of the deaf. Underwood (1969) has conceptualized the memory for a word as a collection of attributes about the word. These attributes are different types of uncoded information that serve to differentiate one memory from another in addition to serving as retrieval cues. Two attributes of a word are its *acoustic attribute,* or its sound pattern when pronounced, and its *verbal-associative attribute,* or the other words which may be elicited by it. At the time of learning these two attributes become part of the memory for the word. When the young child tries to remember newly learned words, the acoustic attribute predominates over the undeveloped verbal-associative. As the child grows older, the verbal-associative becomes dominant. Bach and Underwood (1970) found that in second grade children the acoustic attribute is still dominant, but by the time they reach sixth grade the verbal-associative is dominant. Also it has been found that the acoustic attribute is forgotten more rapidly.

Obviously, the deaf have a harder time employing the acoustic attribute and, therefore, more easily forget words. Because they acquire words slowly, they are not likely to have a large pool of words to employ when using the verbal-associative attribute. They may continue to use the less efficient acoustic attribute long after the hearing have progressed to the verbal-associative or they may use the acoustic almost exclusively. Hence, they would have an inefficient memory for words.

How can memory for words be facilitated? It has been suggested that verbal learning tasks are functionally indeterminant; that is, there is more than one way to process information or more than one strategy that can be utilized to remember items (Frederiksen, 1970). We know that pictures sometimes are learned better than words and that visual modes of learning predominate over verbal modes as a child grows older (Dilley & Paivio, 1968; Rohwer, 1970; Rohwer, Lynch, Levin, & Suzuki, 1967), suggesting that teachers should make greater use of visual materials when instructing the deaf.

Intelligence

Because of the sometimes facilitating effect of verbal mediators upon performance, verbal language has been considered the mediating symbol system for thought. Consequently, those with good verbal skills should show better conceptual reasoning than those with poor verbal skills. In other words, linguistic efficiency should correlate positively with intellectual efficiency. The deaf, therefore, present a "natural" control over the variable of verbal language, enabling researchers to examine more closely the role of language in thought. If a deaf group is matched with a non-deaf group on key variables such as age, IQ, sex, years in school, etc., so that the only variable on which the two groups differ is language skill, and both groups are required to do a multitude of problems involving conceptual reasoning, then such a study should be an ample test of the theory that thinking depends upon language skill. Several studies have been conducted in this manner, and the deaf have done as well as the hearing on the conceptual tasks employed. (Extensive reviews of correlations between linguistic and intellectual efficiency may be found in Furth, 1964, 1971; Vernon, 1967e, 1968b, 1972.)

The conclusion from this research is that language does not have a direct, general, or decisive influence on intellectual development. This conclusion implies that the current emphasis on linguistic skill, particularly in early education (see Chapter 9), may be an unsound practice (Furth, 1970). Piaget (Inhelder & Piaget, 1964, p. 293) has stated categorically that language is not essential for logical thinking; the research with the deaf provides strong support for this position. Yet, our schools currently emphasize learning through verbal modes; books are still the main medium through which knowledge is acquired in school, in spite of the vast improvement in audiovisual training materials or the easy access to "real" experiences, that is, visits, field trips, learning by doing. Consequently, our present educational approach demands superior linguistic skills in order to achieve academically. Thus, those students with adequate or even superior cognitive capacity, who are not verbal, may be earmarked for failure (Vernon, 1972).

Emotional maturity

One of the most frequently stated generalizations about the deaf is that they exhibit a high degree of emotional immaturity. They have been characterized as egocentric, irritable, impulsive, dependent, and indifferent to others (Altshuler, 1964; Levine, 1956; Myklebust, 1960). The consistency of these observations across a number of investigations lends credence to their reliability (Schlesinger & Meadow, 1972). We have discussed, and will discuss in other chapters, the relationship between a child's maladjustment and his parents' negative reaction to his handicap. Similar findings have been reported for deaf children (Neuhaus, 1969). The relationship, however, is not a simple linear one. A complex interplay of environmental factors, both school and family, are responsible for the emotional immaturity of deaf children.

Immaturity is more characteristic of children who attend residential schools, where development of independence and responsibility is often attenuated (Barker, Wright, Meyerson, & Gonick, 1953; Schlesinger &

Meadow, 1972). But even within residential settings, children with deaf parents act more mature than those with hearing parents (Meadow, 1968; Schlesinger & Meadow, 1972). In fact, those in institutions who have deaf parents act more mature than those who live at home with hearing parents, indicating that institutionalization is not necessarily detrimental. Vernon (1970a) suggests that deaf children with deaf parents are better adjusted because they can communicate more readily with their parents using manual means of communication. In support of this position is the finding that isolation and communication difficulties are more characteristic of the deaf than are other personality problems (Reivich & Rothrock, 1972).

Hearing mothers of deaf children often use child rearing techniques geared more toward keeping the child dependent than toward fostering independence. For example, they make infrequent use of verbal praise and rarely solicit the opinions and suggestions of their child. In comparison to parents of hearing children, they are more openly antagonistic toward and disagree more with their child (Goss, 1970). These child rearing practices may be partially responsible for the deaf child's immaturity.

In most studies of the deaf, they are compared to normal hearing children rather than to children with other disabilities. Most disabilities make it difficult for a child to master developmental tasks at a rate equivalent to that of the nonimpaired child. Erikson (1963, 1968) describes development as proceeding through a sequence of critical phases, each phase characterized by phase-specific problems that must be solved in order to move on to the next phase. Staats (1971) describes development as the acquisition of a repertoire of learned skills that proceeds in a hierarchical fashion. While the theories of Erikson and Staats differ considerably, both suggest that a child who is slow to acquire his basic behavioral repertoire is handicapped by educational procedures that fail to take his speed of acquisition into consideration.

In addition, the severity and type of emotional response that occurs in reaction to falling behind others is influenced by the point in development where the child falls behind. If future studies reveal that the deaf child is less mature emotionally than children with other disabilities, perhaps adequate communication is necessary to master the initial phases of development. Because the deaf child's behavior is not under the control of words, he cannot respond adequately to other's commands or internaliize their values. As a result of this inability to communicate, social, intellectual, and emotional learning is limited or distorted. Because of this deficit, other people respond to the deaf child in an atypical manner. Thus such a child encounters a continued social experience that cumulatively adds to his nonadjustive, abnormal behavior.

The finding that manually communicating children are better adjusted than orally communicating children suggests that this method of communication enables children to acquire appropriate behavioral repertoires at a level higher than can be attained when only oral methods are used.

THE DEAF WITH MULTIPLE HANDICAPS

Obvious disorders

Up to this point we have confined our discussion to deaf children who are relatively free of other disabilities. Unfortunately, many of the deaf suffer from multiple handicaps because some of the causes of deafness also cause other disabilities. About one-fourth of deafness results from hereditary factors, an etiology not usually associated with multiple handicaps; about one-third has an unknown etiology. The remaining cases are deafened as a result of maternal rubella, complications of Rh factor, meningitis, and premature birth (Vernon, 1967a, 1967b, 1967c, 1967d, 1968a). Vernon's studies indicate that, of those deafened by one of these four causes, 20 to 25 percent show aphasic behavior, 25 percent have visual defects, 4 to 18 percent are cerebral palsied, 8 to 17 percent are mentally retarded, and 2 to 9 percent have orthopedic defects. Over two-thirds of the children who are deaf as a result of complications of Rh factor or prematurity have at least one other disability in addition to deafness.

Other investigators also have reported substantial multiple handicaps among deaf children. Approximately half of a deaf group studied by Lawson and Myklebust (1970) had visual difficulties that warranted ophthalmological attention and that were expected to affect their learning adversely. Doctor (1959) reported that 40 percent of the multiply handicapped deaf in the United States are retarded. Estimates from studies of the mentally retarded suggest that anywhere from 13 to 49 percent are deaf, depending upon the criteria used to define hearing loss (Anderson & Stevens, 1969; Kodman, 1963).

Some of the behavior attributed to deafness can now be explained as resulting from an interaction between hearing loss and other central nervous system pathology associated with the condition causing the deafness. For example, language disabilities found in the deaf may result from both deafness and aphasia. Rainer and Altshuler (1966) report that symptoms among the deaf mentally ill are often similar to those seen in the minimally brain damaged (see Chapter 8).

The multiply handicapped deaf usually receive little or no formal education appropriate to their needs. Many remain dependent upon their families until the families can no longer provide for them. Then, they are sometimes admitted to state hospitals for the mentally ill or the retarded, or they get into trouble with the law and end up in correctional institutions (Vernon, 1967a).

Subtle disorders

Deaf children with comparable intelligence and no obvious related disorders can differ from each other in achievement in spite of similar motivation. For example, comparison of a deaf group achieving at expected levels with a deaf group more than three years retarded academically revealed that the underachievers had poorer muscular strength, slower motor speed, inferior motor planning, and less integration of neuromuscular control (Auxter, 1971).

Deaf children are not all equally adept at speech reading; some learn quickly and others experience considerable difficulty. In an effort to explain this difference in ability, researchers have examined variables such as chronological age, length of speech reading training, rate of speech, visual closure (the integration of parts to form a whole), visual memory span, short-term memory (visual sequential memory subtest of the ITPA), synthetic ability, movement closure (recall of patterns of gestures), conceptual and intellectual ability, stimulus material, educational achievement, and grade placement. Review of these studies indicates that lipreading ability can be related only to visual memory span (Costello, 1964; Simmons, 1959), visual closure (Kitson, 1915; Sanders & Coscarelli, 1970; Sharp, 1972), movement closure (Sharp, 1972), short-term memory (Sharp, 1972), and educational achievement (Simmons, 1959). The relationship to achievement is understandable as good lipreading ability should enhance academic ability when primarily oral methods of communication are utilized.

All the abilities relating to lipreading skill have in common what Thurstone (1940) has called visual closure, which is essentially a figure-ground function, the ability to differentiate a figure from the background in which it appears. This research makes it clear that lipreading is the ability to select relevant elements from among those that are irrelevant. To obtain meaning from lip movements, the movements must be remembered in correct sequence. It is no mystery, then, why children proficient in visual sequential memory are better at lipreading. Speech is also a rhythmic movement; those who are more proficient at perceiving and recalling movement patterns should be more proficient at lipreading.

These results suggest that tests should be developed to assess the abilities that relate to lipreading skill. If oral methods of instruction continue to be emphasized, the children selected for oral instruction should be those who are the most likely to profit from it.

HOW DO THEY FARE?

We already have learned that only a small portion of the deaf acquire the education that enables them to have a variety of vocational opportunities. The percentage of deaf students who attain college entrance is about one-tenth the percentage of those with normal hearing who attain entrance (Schein & Bushnag, 1962). Consequently, from 60 to 85 percent of employed deaf persons engage in unskilled or semiskilled work. About 85 percent of deaf adults are engaged in manual labor of various kinds, as contrasted to about 50 percent of the hearing population (Babbidge, 1964). Whereas 17 percent of the deaf are employed in white collar jobs, 47 percent of the hearing hold such positions (Crammatte, 1962; Rosenstein & Lerhman, 1963).

Many of the deaf find skilled work only after receiving a vocational-technical education from their local Vocational Rehabilitation Administration (VRA), a division of the Rehabilitation Service Administration. After the educational system has failed, the VRA helps them to attain some form of vocational competence, to learn to communicate with other deaf people, and to find appropriate social outlets; unfortunately, they are not always successful (Vernon, 1970a).

In addition to experiencing financial hardship, many of the deaf find themselves isolated from the mainstream of society, without close friendships and unable to exchange even rudimentary information with their families (Grinker, 1969; Rainer & Althuler, 1966). These discouraging findings indicate that we need to reevaluate our educational programs for the deaf. Even if we could justify the waste of talent that occurs when individuals with unrealized potential enter unskilled trades, we can no longer count on these trades to employ the deaf. Automation is eliminating many of the unskilled, semiskilled, and manual jobs in which the deaf have been employed (Tally & Vernon, 1965). Consequently, what is needed for the deaf is needed for other handicapped youth as well—better educational and vocational planning, counselors who can communicate with the client, a better relationship between schools and the Vocational Rehabilitation Administration, and more vocational-technical educational opportunities (Vernon, 1970a).

The visually impaired

The legal definition of blindness is a visual acuity equal to or less than 20/200 with corrective lenses. The child who has a central visual acuity of more than 20/200 but whose peripheral vision has contracted so that the visual field is no greater than an angular distance of 20 degrees is also considered legally blind (Hurlin, 1962). A visual acuity of 20/200 means that when the child is 20 feet from the Snellen chart he can see what the average child can see at a distance of 200 feet; 20/100 would mean that at 20 feet he can see what the average child sees at 100 feet, and so forth. If visual acuity is worse than 20/200, vision is measured at distances of less than 20 feet; the numerator then indicates the distance at which the child can see what the average child sees at 200 ft, for example, 5/200.

The definition of blindness from an educational viewpoint is a flexible one and only a minority of the children in classes for the blind have total loss of vision. Classes for the partially blind are a relatively recent development, and consequently, many partially sighted children (visual acuity between 20/200 and 20/70 have been enrolled in classes for the blind in order to enjoy better educational opportunities. Also, many multiply handicapped children have partial loss of sight and sometimes are admitted to schools for the blind when alternative educational facilities are inadequate (Fraser & Friedmann, 1967).

Within any legally blind group there is considerable variation among individuals. Some are totally blind (no light perception), others see light but cannot see visual images, while still others can read large-size print if it is brought close to their eyes or if they use magnifying glasses. Some wear glasses with extremely high magnifying power but still use a touch (braille) system to read because the reading of print is too time consuming an effort. Consequently, even when the 20/200 criterion of blindness is used to place a child in a special class or school for the blind, children who can actually see objects at a very close distance are grouped with those who cannot even distinguish darkness from light.

The 20/200 definition of blindness was more appropriate in the era when physicians considered it harmful for individuals with poor vision to use their eyes, particularly for close work such as reading. Since current evidence indicates that use does not damage the eye, this policy has changed. Children with visual handicaps are now encouraged to make maximal use of the vision they have remaining. Just as investigators in the field of hearing are defining hearing loss in terms of its effect on learning, those in vision research are attempting to determine the relationship between vision and educational attainment. For example, Barraga (1969) has outlined the stages in the development of visual discrimination and has proposed a sequence of educational activities for progressive training in learning through the visual system. This type of research may result in a new definition of blindness.

CAUSES OF BLINDNESS

Until 1957 the most frequent known cause of blindness was retrolental fibroplasia, a disorder resulting from the administration of high concentrations of oxygen over prolonged periods to prematurely born babies. Since 1954 the administration of oxygen in incubators has been carefully monitored, and the incidence of this disorder is now quite low.

As a result of accident prevention campaigns and improvement in medical care, the incidence of blindness due to accidents and infectious diseases also has decreased.

Some studies list the most frequent cause of blindness (approximately 50 per cent) as prenatal influences of unknown origin (Hatfield, 1963; Hurlin, 1962). Others list hereditary factors as the largest cause (about 38 percent) (Fraser & Friedmann, 1967). Close to 50 percent of blind children are born blind, and about 40 percent become blind during their first year of life (Hatfield, 1963). The reader interested in more detailed information about the causes of blindness is referred to Fraser and Friedmann (1967).

FACTORS RELATED TO SCHOOL ACHIEVEMENT

The use of visualization in thinking (visual imagery) is absent in those born blind and tends to disappear if sight is lost before 5 to 7 years of age (Blank, 1958; Schlaegel, 1953). Individuals who lose their vision later can usually retain a visual frame of reference, that is, they can feel an object and compare it mentally with their visual memory of other objects. Because the vast majority of the blind are either born blind or become blind during their first year of life, most of them cannot use visual imagery as they acquire knowledge about the world. As a result they must cultivate the senses that remain to them. The word *cultivate* is used because there is not the slightest shred of evidence to support the notion that the blind's other senses naturally acquire increased sensitivity to compensate for the visual loss (Fisher, 1964; Hayes, 1941). With considerable practice the blind can improve their ability to make auditory and tactual discriminations, and sighted individuals who have no need to do so might compare unfavorably with them. However, as a group the blind sometimes compare unfavorably with the seeing on measures of sensory discrimination (Fisher, 1964; Hayes, 1941).

While some of the blind do have subtle disorders that impair their learning, the majority without other obvious handicaps do remarkably well in the segregated classes in which they are enrolled. This was not true in the past, however, since studies completed in the 1940s found the blind to be from two to three grade levels behind their sighted peers (Hayes, 1941).

A recent sample of 100 fourth grade and 100 eighth grade blind students in local and residential schools for the blind was compared with seeing children at the same two grade levels. In the fourth grade the blind were approximately 1.2 years older than the seeing. In the eighth grade the age difference had dropped to no more than 3 months. The blind's reading comprehension scores on standardized achievement tests were approximately equal to those obtained by seeing children. Reading rate, however, was lower; it was half that of seeing children at the fourth grade level, but less than half by the eighth grade. This study concluded that blind children in local public schools were equal in reading rate and comprehension to those in residential schools and compared favorably with seeing youngsters on achievement tests. It was recommended, however, that older blind students need about twice the time as seeing children to read similar material (Lowenfeld, Abel, & Hatlen, 1969).

Because braille is a slow and cumbersome method of learning and because a limited range of materials is available in braille, many classes for the blind now rely more on aural study (listening) procedures. The better functioning of the blind in recent years has been attributed to the increased use of aural procedures. Brothers (1971) reviews the relevant factors included in aural study.

The reader interested in more detailed information about the education and achievement of the blind is referred to Franks and Baird (1971), Lowenfeld, Abel, and Hatlen (1969), and Scholl (1967). The training and preparation of teachers of the blind is briefly discussed in Weishahn (1972).

As we did with the deaf, we will examine the effect of blindness on the development of some of the prerequisites for adequate academic achievement: intelligence, cognitive differentiation, perceptual-motor skill, and emotional adjustment.

Intelligence

Does visual impairment have a detrimental effect on intelligence? Several investigators have spent the better part of their professional careers constructing intelligence or aptitude tests that they felt would help answer this question (Hayes, 1941, 1942, 1950; Newland, 1961). Some of the specially constructed tests are entirely aural, others depend upon touch, and some are given in braille for children competent in touch reading. In general, research findings, using special tests, adaptations of the Binet tests, and standard administration of the Weschler tests, reveal that the blind score only slightly below the seeing on IQ measures (Hayes, 1941, 1942, 1950).

This lower average IQ can be partially attributed to the disproportionate number of blind children in the severely retarded range. The overrepresentation of retardation among the blind is primarily because both loss of vision and intellectual impairment can result from the same cause, e.g., meningitis, rubella, hydrocephalus. Other retardation in the blind is attributed to environmental factors and restricted opportunity (Hayes, 1942). When conditions are more favorable, many of the blind display significant gains in measured intelligence (Elonen, Polzien, & Zwarensteyn, 1967; Komisar & MacDonnel, 1955).

On the WISC the blind score similarly to the seeing on measures of mental arithmetic, general factual information, and word defining skills. They perform more poorly on tests that measure the ability to relate words conceptually or to verbalize the appropriate response in selected social problem situations (Tillman, 1967). Further study of their WISC responses suggests that the blind often conceptualize events in a concrete and functional manner (Tillman, 1967; Zweibelson & Barg, 1967). A concrete response defines a relationship between two objects in terms of some common physical attribute, while a functional response defines relationships in terms of a common use. An abstract response, which the blind use far less than the seeing, relates objects on a representational level, for example, two objects might symbolize the concept of safety.

Rubin (1964) also found that the blind do less well than the seeing on tests of abstraction ability, particularly congenitally blind subjects or those who have been blind from an early age. The finding that age of onset relates to abstraction ability supports theories that stress the sensorimotor foundations of intelligence (Piaget, 1953). In our review of the intellectual functioning of the deaf, we mentioned that a great deal of emphasis, perhaps unwisely, has been placed on verbal factors in the reasoning process.

Keep in mind that the similarities in intelligence between the blind and the seeing far outweigh the differences, and that for all practical purposes the intellectual functioning of the blind is equivalent to that of the seeing. Moreover, blind children are as capable as the seeing on tests designed to measure divergent thinking ability (Tisdall, Blackhurst, & Marks, 1971). (Tests that measure divergent thinking are described in Chapter 10.)

We mentioned that the genetically deaf have a higher mean performance IQ than the general population. Similarly, those blind at birth due to retinoblastoma, a malignant tumor of the eye originating from immature retina cells, have IQs in the above average to superior range (IQ 110 to 142) (Williams, 1968). It is well recognized that the disorder is hereditary, although sporadic retinoblastomas account for the majority of cases. But even in the sporadic cases there is a good chance that the offspring will be affected. At present there is no adequate explanation to account for the intellectual superiority of these children. The most interesting speculation is that a genetic mechanism exists that is simultaneously responsible for both high intellectual development and retinal tumor.

Cognitive differentiation

The sighted child can learn a great deal without any effort on the part of the educator. The blind, however, require help in imposing an order on the discrete sensory experiences they encounter. Although the blind compare favorably with the sighted on tasks measuring verbal comprehension ability and are actually superior to the sighted on tasks requiring sustained auditory attention, they are inferior on tasks requiring competence in cognitive differentiation and articulation (Witkin, Birnbaum, Lomonaio, Lehr, & Herman, 1968).

A person's experience is articulated and cognitively differentiated if he can perceive parts of a field as discrete from background or if he can impose structure on an unstructured field and thereby experience the field as organized.

Adequate vision is necessary in order to develop a differentiated view of the environment. Because of vision, the parts of a field can be apprehended as a whole in one view. Visual access to objects during their manipulation enhances mental imagery (Wolff & Zevin, 1972) and, therefore, contributes significantly to differentiation of experience. A number of investigations have shown that the blind are inferior to the sighted on tasks requiring space perception and spatial orientation (Drever, 1955; Hartlage, 1969; Hunter, 1964; Worchel, 1951). Training can improve spatial orientation, but even with training, initially poor performers do not achieve the level of untrained good performers (Garry & Ascarelli, 1960). Because spatial ability is important for both adequate locomotion and body orientation, as well as for recognition and imaginal construction of forms and shapes, the blind are unable to obtain precise impressions of their experiences.

Visual inability is only one of several factors that contribute to undifferentiated perception. Sighted children who are unable to separate from their mother also show global, that is, undifferentiated, perception (Witkin et al., 1968). Consequently, the blind child most likely to show global perceptual functioning would be the child whose parents make little effort to help him achieve an articulated impression of his surroundings or to enhance and encourage his opportunity to function independently.

Perceptual-motor ability

Should a blind child have a subtle perceptual disorder superimposed on his already global conceptual style, then his perceptions of experience may be further distorted or his progress impeded on learning tasks. Research suggests that some blind children who fail to keep up with their blind peers are those who have subtle handicapping conditions.

Of the totally blind who are taught to read braille, approximately 15 percent evidence errors analogous to those found in sighted children often classified as dyslexic or as specific reading disability (see Chapter 8). Like the seeing child who reverses *b* for *d*, or *was* for *saw*, who displays mirror writing, and who shows right-to-left reversal of writing, this subgroup of blind show letter reversals, that is, ∴ for ∵ or ∷ for .∷ , confusion of letter placement in words, and poor orientation of fingers on paper. The errors appear in typing braille and in reading braille. In some instances these errors are so marked as to classify the child as a nonreader in spite of normal intelligence (Brodlie & Burke, 1971).

Study of legally blind children who could read special large-type books revealed that those who showed frequent reversal problems in reading type also had frequent letter reversals when they were taught braille.

Similarly, those who showed orientation problems with printed materials showed the same difficulty using braille (Brodlie & Burke, 1971).

Just as there are good and poor sight readers, there are good and poor braille readers. And just as there are studies designed to determine the characteristics of good and poor sight readers, there are studies of good and poor braille readers. These studies reveal that readers whose hands are equally effective read faster and are better readers than those with a dominant hand. This is probably because they read ahead on a lower line with the left hand before the right hand has finished the preceding line, whereas the poor reader keeps both his hands close together or reads with only one hand. Good readers move their fingers horizontally with a minimum of up-and-down motions, whereas poor readers interrupt their horizontal movements with frequent up-and-down movements, movements that may form loops. Good readers exert slight and uniform pressure, while poor readers employ strong and variable pressure (Lowenfeld et al., 1969). Although studies have revealed some of the differences between good and poor touch readers, few have related these characteristics to other variables. To what extent they are the result of other, more basic, deficiencies or of poor learning habits remains to be determined.

Berla (1972) required a group of blind children to discriminate between six raised-line metric figures. Those who performed poorly were those who scanned the figures in a seemingly random and unsystematic fashion rather than tracing the outline of the pattern and returning to the starting point. Poor learners also traced the outline in a clockwise motion with the right hand and in a counterclockwise motion with the left. These exploratory procedures could result in a different ordering of information received and a different spatial distribution of the distinctive features of each figure, and thus lead to erroneous integrations and comparisons of distinctive features. Unfortunately, Berla failed to relate these findings to reading ability.

Emotional adjustment

Because of the limitations imposed by their handicap, the blind show less variability and adaptability in behavior than do the sighted. They sometimes have been described as undifferentiated and rigid personalities (McAndrew, 1948; Witkin et al., 1968). Blind children placed in residential settings tend to have more difficulties adjusting to home and community than do those placed in integrated public school classes (Bauman, 1954), and the partially seeing and those with light perception show more maladjustment than the totally blind (Bauman, 1954; Hardy, 1968). Blind children are more dependent upon their mothers than are the sighted (Imamura, 1964) and could be expected, therefore, to show more maladjustment if parents prolong this dependent state. In studies of self-concept more blind than sighted subjects have either high-positive or high-negative self-attitudes, implying that the blind are less sure of themselves than are the sighted (Jervis, 1959). In all these studies, however, the differences were not pronounced. Cowen's research (Cowen et al., 1961) suggests that blind children who are accepted by their parents and viewed by them as well adjusted will develop adequate self-esteem and will be well adjusted. This statement could be said about most children, blind or otherwise.

THE NEED FOR PARENTAL ASSISTANCE

Many parents of the blind, like parents of other disabled children, over-indulge their child and thereby relieve him of the responsibility of learning for himself (Imamura, 1964). This overprotection may be why some blind and partially blind children use their low visual acuity less effectively than others. Nevertheless, a certain amount of parental assistance is necessary in order for the child to learn. We are aware from Piaget's research that active manipulation of materials in the environment enhances the child's use of his intellectual faculties (Flavell, 1963). Consequently, the blind child must be provided with varied experiences and playthings; he should be encouraged to use his remaining senses. His parents must label objects and describe the sensory attributes of objects that he has felt, and he must know where his playthings are so he can get to them easily. His parents must be his "eyes." Parents also must help their child to develop socially appropriate behaviors, because the child cannot model his behaviors after those he sees performed by others.

In addition to help in intellectual and conceptual development, the blind child needs help in learning to walk, since he cannot rely on visual cues, cues that are exceptionally important for the development of mobility. Anxiety must be kept at a minimum since it disrupts mobility (Cratty, Petterson, Harns, & Schöner, 1968; Harris, 1967).

The blind sometimes display mannerisms that others find annoying. These mannerisms have been called *blindisms*. Shaking and rolling the body, poking at the eyes and ears, or shaking the hands when excited are examples. Morse (1965) rejects the term blindism because it implies that these behaviors are peculiar to the blind rather than being normal behaviors displayed in an exaggerated form or with greater frequency. The most frequent mannerism, which often persists into adult life, is repeated rubbing of the eyes (Rae, 1962).

Parents often ask how they should respond to these mannerisms. It has been suggested that blind children should be encouraged to stop these mannerisms, so that they don't seem peculiar to those around them, particularly when they often are unaware that they are behaving in any unusual way (Bakwin & Bakwin, 1966).

Several investigators have suggested that these behaviors, especially eye rubbing, are efforts at self-stimulation in the absence of environmental stimulation. Thurrell and Rice (1970) hypothesize that when the neural portion of the optic apparatus is capable of any input whatsoever, eye rubbing could generate neural impulses via the retina, optic nerve, and visual pathways. As the amount of vision increases, the need for artificially induced optic stimulation would decrease. Since many of the totally blind cannot achieve visual pathway input by any means, they would not engage in eye rubbing. Data presented by these authors supports their theory. Significantly more eye rubbing was present in those blind who could perceive light or hand movement but could not discriminate the number of fingers held up by the examiner at a distance of 1 foot. The theory, however, does not indicate how or when eye rubbing should be extinguished. The authors' theoretical position is that a strong need to rub the eyes is usually present only during a limited period in development and that the habit is more easily modified at a later age when the need has diminished. In addition, plentiful substitution of other stimulation is known to diminish the need for self-stimulation. Consequently, keeping the blind occupied on other tasks should diminish their need to engage in these mannerisms.

It has been suggested that a blind child often fails to make himself clearly understood because he lacks visual feedback about the clearness of his communication, for instance, he can't see expressions of puzzlement or confusion. Without such feedback he cannot correct his communication unless the listener asks for clarification. This view may be overdone, however, since sighted children as old as 7 rarely reformulate their initial messages when faced with nonverbal expressions of listener noncomprehension (Peterson, Danner & Flavell, 1972). Normal 7-year olds also are unable to reformulate initial messages when verbal requests are limited to statements such as "I don't understand." What they need in order to reformulate their messages are prompts such as "Can you tell me more about it?" Research suggests that normal children up to age 10 may be unable to increase the amount of appropriate post-feedback modification when faced with implicit statements for help, such as, "I don't understand" (Glucksberg & Krauss, 1967). Investigators must be careful, therefore, to avoid mistaking normal behaviors for disability related behaviors. Otherwise, unsound advice may be given to the parents of blind children.

THE BLIND WITH MULTIPLE HANDICAPS

Multiply handicapped blind children have been said to outnumber "normal" blind children by almost 2 to 1 (Lowenfeld, 1968), primarily because a large number of children in institutions for the retarded and psychotic are blind. Other estimates are considerably lower. In 1968 Graham estimated that there were 15,000 multiply handicapped blind in the United States (Graham, 1968). Around that same period the total registration of legally blind students with the American Printing House for the Blind was 19,007 (Noland, 1967). Obviously, not all the blind were registered since the National Society for the Prevention of Blindness (1966) estimated in 1962 that there were about 39,000 blind individuals below 20 years of age in the United States. Using these figures, the estimate would be approximately 1 multiply handicapped blind child for every 2½ normal blind children. These other handicaps, however, are usually the obvious disorders, e.g., mental retardation, deafness, etc., rather than the subtle ones. With the recent upsurge of interest in subtle learning disabilities (see Chapter 8), perhaps future studies will determine the incidence of these disorders among blind children.

There have been several surveys of speech disorders among blind children. Some researchers suggest that anywhere from 30 to 50 percent of the blind have speech difficulties (LeZak & Starbuck, 1964; Miner, 1963; Stinchfield, 1933). The defects range from mild oral inaccuracies, such as letter substitutions and articulation errors, to lisping, stammering, and severe oral inaccuracies. Articulation errors are the most frequent disorders.

Other studies reveal that speech disorders are no more frequent in the blind than in the general population (Brieland, 1950; Rowe, 1958; Weinberg, 1964). Some observers may have been unduly sensitive to small defects in the blind and therefore viewed their speech with disfavor (Brieland, 1950). Another factor also could explain the inconsistent findings. Almost all the observations of speech disorders were made in residential settings where a large number of multiply handicapped blind children are enrolled (Lowenfeld, 1968; Wolf, 1967). The speech difficulties found, therefore, could have resulted from a related disorder rather than from blindness. If speech problems are found among the blind who are free from other disorders, speculations about the effects of vision on speech development would be on firmer grounds.

THE PARTIALLY SIGHTED

The partially seeing child is one whose visual acuity is between 20/70 and 20/200 after optimum correction or who has other visual disabilities and, in the opinion of a vision expert, can benefit from specialized instruction. He must be able to use sight as his main data gathering sense organ and to profit from the visually presented academic curriculum of a special class for the visually impaired (Hathaway, 1959). However, surveys of children in classes for the partially seeing indicate that less than one-third of those enrolled actually come within the defined visual acuity range. One-fifth were considered legally blind and two-fifths had visual acuity better than 20/70 (Kerby, 1952). The students with better vision were probably placed in the special classes for reasons other than visual acuity. Although this survey was done some years ago, when there was less emphasis on integration of the partially seeing into regular classes, a more recent survey indicates that the majority of the partially seeing are still in special classes (Birch, Tisdall, Peabody, & Sterrett, 1966). This survey did not indicate whether the composition of the classes was similar to those surveyed in 1952.

While the majority of the partially sighted are in special classes, some school systems maintain the child in the mainstream of education by employing the resource room (as discussed in Chapter 1) or the itinerant teacher. In the first approach the child receives most of his learning and instruction in the regular classroom and goes to the resource room for specialized instruction that cannot be offered in the regular class. In the itinerant teacher plan a specialist travels throughout the district to provide part-time individual instruction to students and to consult with teachers who have partially seeing students in their classrooms.

Advocates of each of the three plans, special class, resource room, and itinerant teacher, argue the merits of their approach. Nevertheless, research has failed to demonstrate the superiority of one plan over another (Stephens & Birch, 1969). Regardless of the educational approach, the majority of the partially sighted, unlike the blind, display significant educational retardation, which appears to be unrelated to the type of visual disability they display. By the time they reach the sixth grade, they are two and a half years retarded in academic achievement in spite of average intelligence.

Although many of the partially sighted are trained in special classes, the methods by which they are taught often are not particularly specialized. The methods typically include more practice in visual discrimination and word recognition, greater attention to reading habits, and more time allowed for completion of assignments. The typewriter is employed and braille is taught when necessary.

Similar to other children with disabilities, the partially sighted child's emotional adjustment depends largely upon his parents' reactions to his disability (Bateman & Wetherell, 1967). Lairy (1969) states, that when the child's visual impairment is not discovered until he is of preschool age, he probably will have been raised as a sighted child. If the impairment is discovered at birth or during the first year of life, then his development will be like that of the blind child.

Being raised as a sighted child when the child sees poorly further handicaps the child. We have already mentioned that the partially sighted fare less well than the blind. Why this is so remains undetermined. Perhaps the partially sighted child never learns to accept his handicap and thereby fails to develop compensatory behaviors.

Speech handicaps

Speech defects can be divided into four major types: (1) articulation defects—faulty sound production characterized by omissions, distortions, or substitution of speech sounds, (2) phonation defects—abnormal voice quality, loudness, pitch, variety, or duration, (3) disfluency—stuttering, stammering, cluttering, and (4) language dysfunction—delayed language development and aphasia. The most frequent speech disorders are articulation and disfluency defects.

A child may have more than one speech disorder. For example, the cerebral palsied child may show language delay, articulation errors, and poor voice quality as a result of organic damage. Faulty hearing can produce voice and articulation difficulties. In Chapter 8 we will see that delayed language development appears in the background of many children who experience severe reading difficulties. In this chapter, we will present two speech disorders, one clearly the result of organic factors and the other the cause of which remains an enigma. The first is cleft palate speech; the second is stuttering.

CLEFT PALATE SPEECH

A cleft palate is a congenital fissure in the palate (roof of the mouth), which forms a communicating pathway between the mouth and nasal cavities. Excessive nasality is the most common speech defect displayed by the child with a cleft palate.

At least one baby in every thousand is born with a cleft lip or palate or both (Johnson & Moeller, 1967). Successful habilitation of these children requires cooperative efforts among a variety of professionals. An oral surgeon, prosthodontist, orthodontist, plastic surgeon, psychologist, and speech therapist are usually involved. The cleft is either surgically repaired or an artificial plate (obturator) is constructed, teeth are straightened or repositioned, scars are removed and the nose is straightened, and the honking, snorting speech characterizing cleft palate speech is corrected.

Among the causes of cleft palate are those responsible for other disorders (e.g., fetal anoxia, malnutrition, etc.) and, therefore, other disorders often accompany cleft palate, with perhaps hearing loss the most frequent (Harrison & Philips, 1971; Pannbacker, 1969). Because cleft palate children are prone to middle ear infections *(otitis media)*, they experience fluctuations in hearing efficiency (Paradise, Bluestone, & Felder, 1969). In fact, Harrison and Philips (1971) suggest that the receptive and expressive language problems, as well as the deficient speech patterns noted in these youngsters (Philips & Harrison, 1969a, 1969b; Smith

& McWilliams, 1968), may be attributed to the adverse effects of fluctuating hearing levels. This supposition gains support from Owrid's (1970) findings that a relatively slight hearing loss has a marked effect on communication skills and verbal knowledge. Difficulties typical of those faced by children with a cleft palate are described in the case of Phil.

PHIL

When in elementary school, Phil did not participate in oral reading groups because no one could understand him. When he talked, he talked "through his nose." When he drank water, it sometimes came out of his nose, and the kids teased him. He was a tough little kid, however, and eventually the kids learned that teasing him was to their disadvantage. The teachers, too, eventually made allowances for his handicap. They let him run the motion picture projector and other audiovisual equipment since he had learned how to fix them when something went wrong. When he was older, he was given the job of showing films in all the classes. Consequently, he watched a lot of films and discovered he had learned a great deal as a result.

When Phil was not watching movies or visual presentations, he spent his time gazing out the window. Sometimes the maintenance men would be working near his window and he would daydream that he was out there with them. When Phil got mad at his teacher for reprimanding him for daydreaming, he would swear at her and then laugh because she couldn't understand him.

By the time he was 10, his family had saved enough money to have corrective surgery done to close the cleft palate and shut off the passageway to the nose. This operation enabled airflow and sound to pass through his mouth rather than his nose. Following corrective surgery, Phil was given speech therapy, and after several years he could be understood by most listeners in spite of his hypernasality and poor articulation. Therapy helped Phil improve his oral air pressure and oral airflow, eliminated abnormal foci of tension and abnormal nostril contractions, and improved his respiratory rhythms of speech and speech rate.

Because of Phil's articulation problems, his reading as well as writing suffered. He was a poor reader and made little effort to improve this skill. By the time Phil entered high school, his speech patterns were normal, but he still read and wrote at a second grade level. Some teachers gave him oral exams, exams that he passed. Others made him take written exams, exams he usually failed. At 16 Phil quit school and performed odd jobs until he found a full-time position as a limousine driver.

For a more detailed presentation of cleft palate, see Spriesterbach and Sherman (1968) or Westlake and Rutherford (1966).

STUTTERING

Stuttering occurs whenever the flow of speech is interrupted by repetition or prolongations of a sound or syllable. If these momentary lapses of fluency, or disfluencies, occur frequently in a child's speech, he is considered a stutterer. The terms stuttering and disfluency will be used interchangeably throughout this section because no definitional scheme has yet been proposed which unequivocally differentiates types of disfluent speech (Siegel, 1970).

Stuttering is considered by some as the "most complex disorganization of function in the field of medicine and psychiatry" (Bluemel, 1960, p. 30). Many theories of stuttering exist, the majority postulating that stuttering is a learned behavior. Several theories will be presented, with an attempt made to point out the shortcomings of each. No one position explains all the facts and in light of Eisenson's (1971, p. 200) statement that "any person with a bias can, by selective reading, find support for a position as to cause, concomitants, or treatments," only a cursory examination will be made of disparate findings.

Causes of stuttering

Behavioral theories One view posits that stuttering results from anticipatory tension that surrounds speaking; the child fears he will hesitate in speech and tries to avoid doing so. The avoidance is incomplete and stuttering results (Johnson, 1959). This hypothesis has been called the anticipatory struggle hypothesis (Bloodstein, 1972). It states that stuttering is a conditioned avoidance reaction.

There are various explanatory schemes to account for stuttering within this framework. These schemes differ in the roles they assign to conditioned emotionality and to positive and negative reinforcement processes in the regulation of disfluencies (Bandura, 1969). Wischner (1950) states that the anxiety elicited by specific words and situational cues results in a temporary blocking of a later portion of the word in an effort to postpone the anticipated social disapproval that would follow the saying of the word. The stuttering is reinforced because of its temporal proximity to the anxiety reduction that accompanies the successful completion of the anxiety arousing word. Similarly, Sheehan (1958) posits that stuttering is the resultant of competing urges to talk and not to talk. Whenever the conflicting approach and avoidance tendencies are equal, speech is interrupted. The momentary inhibition of speech reduces the fear generated by verbal communication, which both reinforces the disfluency and, by decreasing the avoidance gradient, releases the blocked word.

Several others conceive of stuttering as a form of behavioral disorganization rather than as an avoidance response. Disfluencies reflect the disruptive effects of emotional arousal that has been classically conditioned to certain situations or word cues through association with unpleasant experiences (Brutten & Shoemaker, 1967). This view is based on the finding that disfluencies increase in the presence of both noxious stimulation and stimuli previously paired with noxious stimulation (Hill, 1954; Savoye, 1959; Stassi, 1961). Even within this conceptualization, stutterers are assumed to adopt idiosyncratic speech designed to escape or avoid anxieties aroused by their disfluencies. These idiosyncrasies are instrumentally reinforced by subsequent word completion and the corresponding reduction of anxiety. Some support for this position comes from an intercorrelation study of the speech behaviors displayed by stutterers, suggesting that there are two types of stuttering behavior. Type I behaviors are prolongations, part-word repetitions, and eyelid oscillations. Type II behaviors are phrase repetitions, interjections, pauses, eyelid closures, jaw deviations, and left lip deviations (Prins & Lohr, 1972). Type I behaviors are believed to be the initial behaviors displayed by the stutterer and type II those learned in an effort to cope with type I behaviors. Whether type I behaviors are classically conditioned behaviors, as suggested by Brutten and Shoemaker (1967), or are inherited or developmental abnormalities is not yet clear.

In essence, each of the learning theories of stuttering postulates that the stutterer is a person who has learned to react in unfortunate ways to his own disfluent speech. (Disfluent speech regularly occurs in all speakers, particularly in the young child as he develops language skill.) Disfluencies, or thoughts of being disfluent, become cues that evoke the patterns of disruption characterizing stuttered speech (Siegel, 1970). Some believe that the stutterer blocks in an attempt to avoid stuttering, while others believe the block is a response to stuttering, and that eventually the stutterer reacts both to his own stuttering and to the context in which his stuttering occurs.

Findings that challenge behavioral theories   What are the cues that are believed to arouse anxiety and set the stage for stuttering to develop? Johnson (1959) states that all young children display disfluencies as they master speech, but that parents react differently to these disfluencies. Some accept them as natural phenomena. Others respond as if their child's speech is somehow defective and, as a consequence, frequently interrupt him to correct his speech and anxiously oversee his speech development. Because of the parents' negative speculations, anxiety reactions become conditioned to the act of verbal communication. This view implies that parents of stutterers are more critical, demanding, and perfectionist than parents of nonstutterers.

While some early studies corroborated the assumption of differences between parents of stutterers and nonstutterers, these differences could have occurred as a reaction to the child's continued disfluency, rather than as the cause of it. Several studies have suggested that stuttering is part of a larger communication disorder. The speech development of stutterers is usually delayed; they have a higher incidence of other developmental disorders; and they do poorly on tasks requiring phonetic ability and auditory-vocal sequencing (Andrews & Harris, 1964; Perozzi, 1970; Williams & Marks, 1972). Parents may react unfavorably to the communication disorder and, therefore, differ from parents of normal children.

Debate about whether parents are "reactors" or "causers" will probably continue. Nevertheless, two decades of research have failed to demonstrate convincingly that parents of speech-disordered children are maladjusted or have the distinctive personality pattern that is postulated to produce a stuttering child (Bloch & Goodstein, 1971; Goodstein, 1958a, 1958b).

In each of the behavioral viewpoints discussed, anxiety reduction is believed to maintain stuttering. From what we know about the stability (resistance to extinction) of conditioned avoidance reactions, we would expect stuttering to be an extremely persistent behavior, one that would persist until special consequences were interposed between the onset of blocking and completion of the word (Bandura, 1969). To the discredit of these theories, such resistance to extinction is not the case. To the contrary, stuttering has been referred to "predominantly as a disorder of childhood" (Bloodstein, 1969, p. 218), since a large number of children no longer stutter as adults and many recover without special intervention procedures (Cooper, 1972; Dickson, 1971; Shearer & Williams, 1965; Sheehan & Martyn, 1966, 1970; Wingate, 1964). Recovery usually occurs sometime between the ages of 12 and 21. Of those with a history of stuttering, 17 percent report recovery in the eighth grade (Cooper, 1972), 52 percent in the eleventh grade (Cooper, 1972), and 80 percent in college (Sheehan & Martyn, 1966, 1970). The later figure may be spuriously high, since stutterers as a group score lower than average on intelligence tests (Andrews & Harris, 1964) and, therefore, a college group may be an unrepresentative sample of stutterers. A familial incidence of stuttering was negatively related to recovery in Cooper's (1972) sample, but showed no such relationship in Sheehan and Martyn's (1970) study.

The finding that many outgrow their disorder suggests that a developmental variety of stuttering may exist and, because recovery sometimes relates to familial incidence (Cooper, 1972), there may be a hereditary component in some cases. It cannot be said, however, that those who "outgrow" their disorder are less severe cases since Cooper (1972) found no relationship between severity and recovery.

Physiological theories Stuttering also has been explained as a physiological deficiency, a faulty processing of information by the central nervous system. Within this viewpoint are several theoretical formulations. One suggests that stuttering is the result of minute physical imperfections in the feedback loop of the hearing mechanism (Dinnan, McGiness, & Perrin, 1970). A second holds that there is a discrepancy of feedback between air conduction and bone conduction of sound (Timmons & Boudreau, 1972). A third view is that faulty middle-ear muscle reflexes distort or momentarily cancel auditory feedback that is important for speech guidance (Webster & Lubker, 1968). In all three viewpoints, interference in auditory feedback is believed to produce involuntary pauses in the flow of speech.

Timmons and Boudreau (1972) review the research that supports the physiological position. In addition to research on physiological differences between stutterers and nonstutterers, they cite evidence to suggest a hereditary component in stuttering. A high frequency of stuttering exists among twins, with identical twins more concordant than fraternal twins, and, in some studies, boys outnumber girls as much as three to one.

Developmental theories Stuttering also has been conceptualized as a disturbance of the communicative functions of speech and, therefore, considered a developmental language disorder. This theory is based on the observation that declarative speech about concrete, visual objects or actions is the least difficult for the stutterer. For example, Cheveleva (1971) reports that: (1) sentences dealing with one action produce less disfluency than those dealing with several, (2) less disfluency occurs if reference is made to the near present than to the long ago, (3) less disfluency occurs if material is well known rather than recently learned, and (4) more disfluency occurs if utterances are about generalized or abstract statements. These findings are not necessarily in conflict with physiological theories. When words to be said are well understood or when they have been said before, that is, well-learned material, the individual may be less dependent upon proper auditory feedback for fluent speech.

Treatment

A number of treatment approaches have been used with stutterers and each has reported a modicum of success. We will examine those that have developed from the belief that stuttering is a learned behavior.

If stuttering is conceived of as a learned response, then it follows that punishing stuttering might decrease its occurrence. Several experimenters have reported positive results using "punishment" procedures. Siegal (1970) reviews these studies in detail. Both white noise and delayed auditory feedback of the person's own voice have been employed as punishments. Unfortunately, the positive results of punishment have not always generalized to outside the experimental laboratory, suggesting that the experimental situation becomes a place where the audience is not intimidating; the stuttering is not necessarily improved but the laboratory simply becomes an environment where the stutterer can speak more fluently (Bloodstein, 1949).

Several investigators are skeptical about the effects of punishment on stuttering. Webster and Dorman (1970) did a study in which they varied the onset of the punishing stimuli while four groups of subjects were reading. They presented white noise immediately after correct phonation (punishing fluency), had the noise on and turned it off after each correct phonation (rewarding fluency), presented the noise continuously, or did not present the noise at all. Compared to the group who read without any noise, all noise groups were significantly more fluent. Similar findings were reported using delayed auditory feedback (DAF), except that continuous DAF was more effective than response-contingent DAF (Webster, Schumacher, & Lubker, 1970). Cooper, Cady, and Robins (1970) said the words *wrong, right,* and *tree* after each disfluency or fluency said by the subject. They found that *tree* had as much effect as the other words. They postulate that fluency is increased in response-contingent experiments simply because the speaker pays more attention to his speech. Others have made similar statements (Siegel & Martin, 1968). After reviewing studies in which stuttering was punished, Siegel (1970) remarked that more was involved than just calling attention to stuttering speech, but that attention did play a substantial role in changing speech behavior.

Advocates of the anticipatory struggle hypothesis have suggested that both white noise and DAF, rather than calling attention to disfluencies, minimize the individual's auditory feedback of his stuttering so that he is less anxious about it. A second and more plausible explanation is that the stimulus causes the individual to reduce his rate of vocalization (Adams & Moore, 1972; Wingate, 1970). Self-reports of those recovering from stuttering reveal that many felt that learning to speak more slowly helped their recovery (Shearer & Williams, 1965; Sheehan & Martyn, 1966, Wingate, 1964).

Brady's (1969, 1971) finding that stuttering can be controlled through speech training with a metronome, and that miniaturized metronomes built into hearing aides enables speech control outside the therapist's office, supports the notion that a decreased rate of speech increases fluency. Brady theorized that continued use of the miniature metronome results in diminished anxiety through *in vivo* desensitization to those social situations that previously precipitated anxiety (in much the same manner as the treatment of phobics to be discussed in Chapter 7). Brady, therefore, undertakes desensitization in a hierarchical fashion in an effort to "wean" the individual from the metronome. The patient first uses the metronome in all situations and then does without it in increasingly demanding social situations—first with small gatherings of friends, then large gatherings, gatherings with business associates, meetings with strangers, and eventually in speeches. A social anxiety hierarchy peculiar to each stutterer is constructed for this purpose.

While anxiety reduction may partially account for increased fluency, the metronome probably serves to call the speaker's attention to his disfluencies and to slow down his rate of speech, a view more in keeping with other research findings. In this vein, Gray and England (1972) reported that stuttering can be reduced in the absence of a concomitant reduction in anxiety and vice versa. He found that desensitization to anxiety arousing situations can reduce stuttering, but the reduction is not dramatic.

A comparison of two types of speech therapy, one automated and emphasizing practice in language skills and the other oriented toward anxiety reduction and increased self-awareness, revealed that both were more effective than no treatment, but that the automated approach tended to be superior (Peins, McGough, & Lee, 1972). The results were attributed to the slower, controlled rate of speech established by the tape-recorded lessons. The teacher's taped voice served as a guide to establishing a slower rate of utterance. Wingate (1969) refers to this procedure as "pace setting."

Bloodstein (1972) has attempted to reconcile these findings with the anticipatory struggle hypothesis. He feels the metronome effect actually results from a simplification of motor planning that takes place when speech is reduced into smaller units. Whenever the stutterer can evaluate what he has to say as easier to pronounce, he will be less anxious and, therefore, more fluent. Since any novel speech pattern seems to reduce stuttering, distraction from anxiety is the metronome's chief effect. Both DAF and white noise are considered distracting stimuli. In addition, a slow rate of speech is necessary to resist the disturbance of DAF, and by slowing down, motor planning is simplified.

Because subjects show increased fluency whether or not they are instructed to pace their speech with the rhythmic effect of the metronome, perhaps distraction does play some part in the metronome effect (Greenberg, 1970). Nevertheless, other research casts doubt on Bloodstein's conclusions. First, stutterers may not anticipate when they will struggle with words when reading passages. When children were asked to predict the words they would stutter as they read each word of a 50-word passage, they varied considerably in their ability to do so (0 to 100 percent correct). Over half failed to predict the majority of their stuttering (Silverman, 1972). Second, stuttering can decrease without decreases in anxiety and vice versa, suggesting that anxiety does not play a crucial role in stuttering.

What can we conclude about treatment? The finding that there are two general classes or types of stuttering behavior brings a glimmer of light to the quagmire of theories and research findings about stuttering. Although the two types of stuttering behavior have not been analyzed separately in the research studies reviewed, it is suggested that anxiety reduction therapies most probably diminish type II behaviors, those behaviors learned in an effort to cope with stuttering. Almost any approach can be successful in diminishing these behaviors, since positive results have been reported using a variety of techniques, for example, using parents as play therapists (Andronico & Blake, 1971) or highly structured behavior therapy procedures. Whether other procedures, such as those that force the stutterer to slow down, modify type I or type II behaviors awaits further research. It is suggested that slowing down the rate of speech results in less disruption from deficient feedback and, therefore, affects type I behaviors.

At present, speech therapy should probably: (1) provide effective cues (antecedent events) designed to evoke correct responses, (2) make positive reinforcement contingent upon correct responses, since shaping fluency is considered a sounder procedure than punishing or extinguishing disfluency (Bar, 1971), and (3) teach the child to monitor his own responses (Mowrer, 1971). Remediation should proceed "visually," giving way gradually to increases in the use of abstract phrases. Material should cover what the child is certain about, what is meaningful to him, and what is of interest to him (Cheveleva, 1971).

Anxiety reduction techniques can be applied to help eliminate maladaptive behaviors developed in response to disfluency (type II instrumentally conditioned behaviors), but anxiety should be attacked on an individual basis since the unitary theories of the effect of anxiety on speech do not appear justifiable (Toomey & Sidman, 1970).

What we are suggesting, then, is that the anticipatory struggle hypothesis, as well as other theories that define stuttering as a learned behavior, explain only type II behaviors. Whether future research will support the view that type I behaviors also are learned or result from a physiologically based developmental or genetic disorder remains to be determined.

What should the teacher do? Considering the current state of knowledge about this disorder, the teacher would be safest if she adopted the following procedures with children who have been identified as stutterers. She can explain to the child that she is aware of his speech difficulties and of some of the conditions that can make his stuttering worse. If she has not observed these conditions herself, then she can make some generalizations from the research. First, he will be more fluent if he is reciting well-known material and if he is prepared for such recitation. Second, he will be more fluent if he recites slowly and carefully. Third, he will do better if he knows his stuttering will not be called to everyone's attention.

With this knowledge, the teacher can mark in advance the place where

the child will read when called upon in his reading group. He can practice reading this material at home so that it is well learned. The teacher
can also tell the child that if he stumbles she will simply ask another
child to continue where he left off, a procedure she practices in all
reading groups to keep children on their toes and following along in the
text as the material is read. She can assure him that she will never ask
him to recite unfamiliar material or call on him without advance notice
if she finds that these practices increase his stuttering. At first, abstract
sections in books should be assigned to other children, and the more concrete, explicit sections assigned to the stutterer. This approach can be
modified in keeping with the child's response and following the advice
of a speech therapist. As anxiety diminishes, the child's recitation can
be made more demanding.

OTHER SPEECH DISORDERS

While it is beyond the scope of this chapter to present other speech disorders, we should at least remark that, like stuttering, many speech disorders have been viewed in a simplistic fashion. Just as the stutterer has
been found to show language and linguistic deficiencies, so have children
with other speech disorders. For example, children with articulation disorders have traditionally been given treatment confined to remediation
of this deficit, such as, training in the production of individual speech
sounds. Many of these children, however, have other language deficiencies—underdeveloped syntax production (Marguardt & Saxman, 1972),
inability to synthesize phonetic components into whole words (Goldman & Dixon, 1971), deficient word-association skills, inability to discriminate possible from impossible phoneme sequences, and inability to
repeat sentences correctly (Whitacre, Luper, & Pollio, 1970). These findings suggest that these chlidren should be given remedial experiences in
many aspects of language usage, rather than just training limited to
improving articulation.

CONCLUDING REMARKS

Although specialized procedures have been developed to facilitate the
communication of the deaf and the blind, many educators have been
more willing to use these procedures with the blind than with the deaf.
The blind, and even the partially seeing child, are allowed to learn with
the help of a system specially designed to make learning easier for them—
the system of braille. In contrast, the deaf often are discouraged from
using systems designed for the same purpose—the language of signs and
finger spelling. Forcing the deaf to learn to communicate orally is anal-

ogous to forcing Puerto Ricans or Mexican Americans, who speak only Spanish, to learn in English. While Spanish-Americans are learning a second language, Anglo-Americans are going about the business of learning to read and write in a language already known to them. The deaf are exposed to the same experience. Even if they can learn to speak fairly intelligibly and to lipread, they are far behind hearing children of the same age by the time they master these basic skills. Why they aren't exposed to more visual learning experiences and allowed to communicate in a manner that should facilitate learning is a question without a satisfactory answer. The empirical evidence suggests that both these methods should be integral parts of their education. Similarly, the blind should be exposed to aural methods of instruction, particularly those who are not adept at braille.

Like the reluctance of the oralists to give up their position regarding the superiority of oral over manual methods of instructing the deaf, those who hold that certain speech handicaps are learned are reluctant to seriously consider the viewpoint that these handicaps may be developmental disorders. No one holds the view that cleft palate speech is a conditioned avoidance reaction, because they can see the cleft palate. Stuttered speech, however, has been attributed to all sorts of emotional factors. Perhaps stuttered speech also is the result of a structural disorder, but one that is unseen.

Scientists, while trained to apply objective methods to the study of phenomena, also are influenced by personal attitudes and opinions. Several of the well-known experts on stuttering are themselves stutterers and, therefore, may approach the topic with a different set than other professionals. Consequently, the student who plans to study a particular exceptionality must read more than one authoritative opinion. Hopefully, the interested reader will pursue these topics further.

References

Adams, M. R., & Moore, W. H. The effects of auditory masking on the anxiety level, frequency of dysfluency, and selected vocal characteristics of stutterers. *Journal of Speech and Hearing Research*, 1972, **15**, 572–578.

Altshuler, K. Z. Personality traits and depressive symptoms in the deaf. In J. Wortis (Ed.), *Research advances in biological psychiatry*. Vol. 6. New York: Plenum, 1964.

Anderson, R. M., & Stevens, G. D. Practices and problems in educating deaf retarded children in residential schools. *Exceptional Children*, 1969, **35**, 687–694.

Andrews, G., & Harris, H. *The syndrome of stuttering*. London: The Spastics Society, Heinemann, 1964.

Andronico, M. P., & Blake, I. The application of filial therapy to young children with stuttering problems. *Journal of Speech and Hearing Disorders*, 1971, **36**, 377–381.

Auxter, D. Learning disabilities among deaf populations. *Exceptional Children,* 1971, **37**, 573–577.

Babbidge, H. D. *Education of the deaf: a report to the secretary of Health, Education, and Welfare by his Advisory Committee on the Education of the Deaf.* Washington, D.C.: U.S. Department of Health, Education, and Welfare, 1964.

Bach, M. J., & Underwood, B. J. Developmental changes in memory attributes. *Journal of Educational Psychology,* 1970, **61**, 292–296.

Bakwin, H., & Bakwin, R. M. *Clinical management of behavior disorders in children.* (3rd ed.) Philadelphia: Saunders, 1966.

Balow, B., Fulton, H., & Peploe, E. Reading comprehension skills among hearing impaired adolescents. *Volta Review,* 1971, **73**, 113–119.

Bandura, A. *Principles of behavior modification.* New York: Holt, Rinehart & Winston, 1969.

Bar, A. The shaping of fluency not the modification of stuttering. *Journal of Communication Disorders,* 1971, **4**, 1–8.

Barker, R., Wright, B. A., Meyerson, L., & Gonick, M. R. *Adjustment to physical handicap and illness: a survey of the social psychology of physique and disability.* (Bulletin No. 55) (Rev. ed.) New York: Social Science Research Council, 1953.

Barraga, N. C. Learning efficiency in low vision. *Journal of the American Optometric Association,* 1969, **40**, 807–810.

Bateman, B., & Wetherell, J. L. Some educational characteristics of partially seeing children. *International Journal for Education of the Blind,* 1967, **17**, 33–40.

Bauman, M. K. *Adjustment to blindness.* Harrisburg, Pennsylvania: State Council for the Blind, 1954.

Berla, E. P. Effects of physical size and complexity on tactual discrimination of blind children. *Exceptional Children,* 1972, **39**, 120–124.

Birch, J. W., Tisdall, W. J., Peabody, R. L., & Sterrett, R. *School achievement and effect of type size on reading in visually handicapped children.* Pittsburgh, Pa.: University of Pittsburgh Press, 1966.

Blair, F. X. A study of visual memory in deaf and hearing children. *American Annals of the Deaf,* 1957, **102**, 254–263.

Blank, H. R. Dreams of the blind. *The Psychoanalytic Quarterly,* 1958, **27**, 158–174.

Bloch, E. L., & Goodstein, L. D. Functional speech disorders and personality: a decade of research. *Journal of Speech and Hearing Disorders,* 1971, **36**, 295–314.

Bloodstein, O. Conditions under which stuttering is reduced or absent: a review of the literature. *Journal of Speech and Hearing Disorders,* 1949, **14**, 295–302.

Bloodstein, O. *A handbook on stuttering.* Chicago: National Easter Seal Society for Crippled Children and Adults, 1969.

Bloodstein, O. The anticipatory struggle hypothesis: implications of research on the variability of stuttering. *Journal of Speech and Hearing Research,* 1972, **15**, 487–499.

Bluemel, C. C. Concepts of stammering: a century in review. *Journal of Speech and Hearing Disorders,* 1960, **25**, 24–32.

Brady, J. P. Studies on the metronome effect on stuttering. *Behavior Research and Therapy,* 1969, **2**, 197–204.

Brady, J. P. Metronome-conditioned speech retraining for stuttering. *Behavior Therapy,* 1971, **2**, 129–150.

Brieland, D. M. A comparative study of the speech of blind and sighted children. *Speech Monographs,* 1950, **17**(1), 99–103.

Brodlie, J. F., & Burke, J. Perceptual learning disabilities in blind children. *Perceptual and Motor Skills*, 1971, **32**, 313–314.

Brothers, R. J. Learning through listening: a review of the relevant factors. *New Outlook for the Blind*, 1971, **65**, 224–231.

Brutten, E. J., & Shoemaker, D. J. *The modification of stuttering.* Englewood Cliffs, N.J.: Prentice-Hall, 1967.

Cheveleva, N. A. Speech of stuttering children. *Defektologiya*, 1971, **3**, 17–21.

Chovan, W. L., & McGettigan, J. F. The effects of vocal mediating responses on visual motor tasks with deaf and hearing children. *Exceptional Children*, 1971, **37**, 435–440.

Clark, B. R., & Leslie, P. T. Visual-motor skills and reading ability of deaf children. *Perceptual and Motor Skills*, 1971, **33**, 263–268.

Committee on the Education of Deaf Children, Department of Education and Science. *The education of deaf children: the possible place of finger spelling and signing.* London: H. M. S. O., 1968.

Conrad, R., & Rush, M. L. On the nature of short-term memory encoding by the deaf. *Journal of Speech and Hearing Disorders*, 1965, **30**, 336–343.

Cooper, E. B. Recovery from stuttering in a junior and senior high school population. *Journal of Speech and Hearing Research*, 1972, **15**, 632–638.

Cooper, E. B., Cady, B. B., & Robins, C. J. The effects of the verbal stimulus words *wrong, right* and *tree* on the disfluency rates of stutterers and non-stutterers. *Journal of Speech and Hearing Research*, 1970, **13**, 239–244.

Costello, M. R. Individual differences in speech reading. In *Report of the International Congress on Education of the Deaf.* Washington, D.C.: U.S. Government Printing Office, 1964.

Cowen, E. L., et al. *Adjustment to visual disability in adolescence.* New York: American Foundation for the Blind, 1961.

Crammatte, A. B. The adult deaf in professions. *American Annals of the Deaf*, 1962, **107**, 474–478.

Cratty, B. J., Petterson, C., Harris, J., & Schoner, R. The development of perceptual-motor abilities in blind children and adolescents. *New Outlook for the Blind*, 1968, **62**, 111–117.

Davis, H. (Ed.) The young deaf child: identification and management. *Acta Oto-laryngologica*, 1965, Suppl. No. 206.

DiCarlo, L. M., Kendall, D. C., & Goldstein, R. Diagnostic procedure for auditory disorders in children. *Folia Phoniatry*, 1962, **14**, 206–264.

Dickson, S. Incipient stuttering and spontaneous remission of stuttered speech. *Journal of Communication Disorders*, 1971, **4**, 99–110.

Dilley, M. G., & Paivio, A. Pictures and words as stimulus and response items in paired-associate learning of young children. *Journal of Experimental Child Psychology*, 1968, **6**, 231–240.

Dinnan, J. A., McGiness, E., & Perrin, L. Auditory feedback: stutterers versus nonstutterers. *Journal of Learning Disabilities*, 1970, **3**, 209–213.

Dirks, D. D., Stream, R. W., & Wilson, R. H. Speech audiometry: earphone and sound field. *Journal of Speech and Hearing Disorders*, 1972, **37**, 102–176.

Dix, M. R., & Hallpike, C. S. The peep show. *British Medical Journal*, 1947, **8**, 719–723.

Doehring, D. G., & Rosenstein, J. Visual word recognition by deaf and hearing children. *Journal of Speech and Hearing Research*, 1960, **3**, 320–326.

Doctor, P. V. Deafness in the twentieth century. *American Annals of the Deaf*, 1959, **104**, 330–334.

Drever, J. Early learning and the perception of space. *American Journal of Psychology*, 1955, **68**, 605–614.

Eames, T. H. Visual handicaps to reading. *Journal of Education*, 1959, **141**, 1–34.

Eisenson, J. Speech defects: nature, causes, and psychological concomitants. In W. M. Cruickshank (Ed.), *Psychology of exceptional children and youth*. Englewood Cliffs, N.J.: Prentice-Hall, 1971.

Elliott, L. L., & Armbruster, V. B. Some possible effects of the delay of early treatment of deafness. *Journal of Speech and Hearing Research*, 1967, **10**, 209–224.

Elonen, A. S., Polzien, M., & Zwarensteyn, S. B. The "uncommitted" blind child: results of intensive training of children formerly committed to institutions for the retarded. *Exceptional Children*, 1967, **33**, 301–307.

Erikson, E. H. *Childhood and society*. (2nd ed.) New York: Norton, 1963.

Erikson, E. H. *Identity, youth and crisis*. New York: Norton, 1968.

Fisher, G. H. Spatial localization by the blind. *American Journal of Psychology*, 1964, **77**, 2–14.

Flavell, J. H. *The developmental psychology of Jean Piaget*. Princeton, N.J.: Van Nostrand, 1963.

Franks, F. L., & Baird, R. M. Geographical concepts and the visually handicapped. *Exceptional Children*, 1971, **38**, 321–324.

Fraser, G. R., & Friedmann, A. I. *The causes of blindness in children*. Baltimore: Johns Hopkins Press, 1967.

Frederiksen, C. H. Functional indeterminacy and cognitive processes in learning performance. Paper presented at the annual meeting of the Western Psychological Association, Los Angeles, April 1970.

Furth, H. G. Research with the deaf: implications for language and cognition. *Psychological Bulletin*, 1964, **62**, 145–164.

Furth, H. G. A comparison of reading test norms of deaf and hearing children. *American Annals of the Deaf*, 1966, **111**, 461–462.

Furth, H. G. *Piaget for teachers*. Englewood Cliffs, N.J.: Prentice-Hall, 1970.

Furth, H. G. Linguistic deficiency and thinking: research with deaf subjects 1964–1969. *Psychological Bulletin*, 1971, **76**, 58–72.

Furth, H. G., & Youniss, J. Color-object paired-associates in deaf and hearing children with and without response competition. *Journal of Consulting Psychology*, 1964, **28**, 224–227.

Fusfeld, I. The academic program of schools for the deaf. *Volta Review*, 1955, **57**, 63–70.

Garry, R. J., & Ascarelli, A. Teaching topographical orientation and spatial organization to congenitally blind children. *Journal of Education*, 1960, **143**, 1–48.

Gellermann, L. The double alternation. II. The behavior of children and human adults in a double alternation temporal maze. *Journal of Genetic Psychology*, 1931, **39**, 197–226.

Gibson, J. J. The concept of the stimulus in psychology. *American Psychologist*, 1960, **15**, 694–703.

Glucksberg, S., & Krauss, R. M. What do people say after they have learned how to talk: studies of the development of referential communication. *Merrill-Palmer Quarterly*, 1967, **13**, 309–316.

Goldman, R., & Dixon, S. D. The relationship of vocal-phonic and articulation abilities. *Journal of Learning Disabilities*, 1971, **4**, 251–256.

Goldstein, R., Kendall, D. C., & Arick, B. E. Electroencephalic audiometry in young children. *Journal of Speech and Hearing Disorders*, 1963, **28**, 331–354.

Goldstein, R., & Tait, C. Critique of neonatal hearing evaluation. *Journal of Speech and Hearing Disorders*, 1971, **36**, 3–18.

Goodstein, L. D. Functional speech disorders and personality: a survey of the research. *Journal of Speech and Hearing Research*, 1958a, **1**, 359–376.

Goodstein, L. D. Functional speech disorders and personality: methodological and theoretical considerations. *Journal of Speech and Hearing Research*, 1958b, **1**, 377–382.

Goss, R. N. Language used by mothers of deaf children and mothers of hearing children. *American Annals of the Deaf*, 1970, **115**, 93–96.

Graham, M. D. *Multiply-impaired blind children: a national problem.* New York: American Foundation for the Blind, 1968.

Gray, B. B., & England, G. Some effects of anxiety deconditioning upon stuttering frequency. *Journal of Speech and Hearing Research*, 1972, **15**, 114–122.

Greenberg, J. B. The effect of a metronome on the speech of young stutterers. *Behavior Therapy*, 1970, **1**, 240–244.

Grinker, R. R. (Ed.) *Psychiatric diagnosis, therapy, and research on the psychotic deaf.* (Final Report, Grant No. RD 2407S) Washington, D.C.: Social and Rehabilitation Service, U.S. Department of Health, Education, and Welfare, 1969.

Hardy, R. E. A study of manifest anxiety among blind residential school students. *New Outlook for the Blind*, 1968, **62**, 173–180.

Harris, J. C. Veering tendency as a function of anxiety in the blind. *Research Bulletin.* No. 14. New York: American Foundation for the Blind, 1967.

Harrison, R. J., & Philips, B. J. Observations on hearing levels of preschool cleft-palate children. *Journal of Speech and Hearing Disorders*, 1971, **36**, 252–256.

Hartlage, L. C. Verbal test of spatial conceptualization. *Journal of Experimental Psychology*, 1969, **80**, 180–182.

Hartung, J. E. Visual-perceptual skill, reading ability, and the young deaf child. *Exceptional Children*, 1970, **36**, 603–608.

Hatfield, E. M. Causes of blindness in school children. *Sight-Saving Review*, 1963, **33**. (Reprint)

Hathaway, W. *Education and health of the partially seeing child.* (Rev. ed. by F. M. Foote, D. Bryan, & Gibbons) New York: Columbia University Press, 1959.

Hayes, S. P. *Contributions to a psychology of blindness.* New York: American Foundation for the Blind, 1941.

Hayes, S. P. Alternative scales for the mental measurement of the visually handicapped. *Outlook for the Blind and the Teachers Forum*, 1942, **36**, 225–230.

Hayes, S. P. Measuring the intelligence of the blind. In P. A. Zahl (Ed.), *Blindness.* Princeton, N.J.: Princeton University Press, 1950.

Heider, F., & Heider, G. A. A comparison of sentence structure of deaf and hearing children. *Psychological Monographs*, 1940, **52**, 42–103.

Hill, H. E. An experimental study of disorganization of speech and manual responses in normal subjects. *Journal of Speech and Hearing Disorders*, 1954, **19**, 295–305.

Hunter, W. F. An analysis of space perception in congenitally blind and sighted individuals. *Journal of General Psychology*, 1964, **70**, 325–329.

Hurlin, R. G. Estimated prevalence of blindness in the U. S., 1960. *Sight-Saving Review*, 1962, **32**, 4–12.

Imamura, A. *Mother and blind child.* New York: American Foundation for the Blind, 1964.

Inhelder, B., & Piaget, J. *The early growth of logic in the child.* New York: Harper & Row, 1964.

Jensen, A. R. Verbal mediation and educational potential. *Psychology in the Schools,* 1966, **3,** 99–109.

Jervis, F. M. A comparison of self-concepts of blind and sighted children. In C. J. Bavis (Ed.), *Guidance programs for blind children.* Watertown, Mass.: Perkins Institution for the Blind, 1959.

Johnson, W. (Ed.) *The onset of stuttering.* Minneapolis: University of Minnesota Press, 1959.

Johnson, W., & Moeller, D. (Eds.) *Speech handicapped school children.* (3rd ed.) New York: Harper & Row, 1967.

Jones, M. C., & Byers, V. W. Classification of hearing impaired children in the classroom: a theoretical model. *Journal of Learning Disabilities,* 1971, **4,** 51–54.

Kendler, T. S. Development of mediating responses in children. *Monographs of the Society for Research in Child Development,* 1963, **28**(Whole No. 86), 33–48.

Keogh, B. K., Vernon, M., & Smith, C. E. Deafness and visuo-motor function. *Journal of Special Education,* 1970, **4,** 41–47.

Kerby, C. E. A report on visual handicaps of partially seeing children. *Exceptional Children,* 1952, **18,** 137–142.

Kitson, H. D. Psychological tests for lip reading ability. *Volta Review,* 1915, **17,** 471–476.

Kodman, F. Sensory processes and mental deficiency. In N. R. Ellis (Ed.), *Handbook on mental deficiency.* New York: McGraw-Hill, 1963.

Komisar, D., & MacDonnel, M. Gains in I.Q. for students attending a school for the blind. *Exceptional Children,* 1955, **21,** 127–129.

Konigsmark, B. W. Genetic hearing loss with no associated abnormalities: a review. *Journal of Speech and Hearing Disorders,* 1972, **37,** 89–99.

Kronenberg, H. H., & Blake, G. D. *Young deaf adults: an occupational survey.* Washington, D.C.: Vocational Rehabilitation Administration, 1966.

Lacey, H. M. Mediating verbal responses and stimulus similarity as factors in conceptual naming by school age children. *Journal of Experimental Psychology,* 1961, **62,** 113–121.

Lairy, G. C. Problems in the adjustment of the visually-impaired child. *New Outlook for the Blind,* 1969, **63,** 33–41.

Lane, H. S. What is our aspiration level for deaf students? *Volta Review,* 1968, **70,** 608–614.

Langenbeck, B. *Textbook of practical audiometry.* Baltimore: Williams & Wilkins, 1965.

Lawson, L. J., & Myklebust, H. R. Ophthalmological deficiencies in deaf children. *Exceptional Children,* 1970, **37,** 19–20.

Levine, E. S. *Youth in a soundless world: a search for personality.* New York: New York University Press, 1956.

Lezak, R. J., & Starbuck, H. B. Identification of children with speech disorders in a residential school for the blind. *International Journal for the Education of the Blind,* 1964, **14,** 8–12.

Lowell, E. L., Rushford, G., Hoverston, G., & Stoner, M. Evaluation of pure tone audiometry with preschool age children. *Journal of Speech and Hearing Disorders,* 1956, **21,** 292–302.

Lowenbraun, S., & Affleck, J. Q. The ability of deaf children to use syntactic cues in immediate recall of speech-read material. *Exceptional Children,* 1970, **36,** 735–741.

Lowenfeld, B. *Multihandicapped blind and deaf children in California.* Sacramento: State Department of Education, 1968.

Lowenfeld, B., Abel, G. L., & Hatlen, P. N. *Blind children learn to read.* Springfield, Ill.: C. C Thomas, 1969.

Lunde, A. S., & Bigman, S. G. *Occupational conditions among the deaf.* Washington, D.C.: Gallaudet College Press, 1959.

Marguardt, T. P., & Saxman, J. H. Language comprehension and auditory discrimination in articulation deficient kindergarten children. *Journal of Speech and Hearing Research,* 1972, **15**, 382–389.

Mark, H. J., & Hardy, E. G. Orienting reflex disturbances in central auditory or language handicapped children. *Journal of Speech and Hearing Disorders,* 1958, **23**, 237–242.

Marshall, H. R. Effect of training on visual perception skills and reading achievement in deaf children. *Experimental Publication System,* 1970, **8**(Ms. No. 281–283).

McAndrew, H. Rigidity in the deaf and the blind. *Journal of Social Issues,* 1948, **43**, 476–494.

McCarthy, R. J., & Marshall, H. R. Memory behavior of deaf and hearing children. *Journal of Genetic psychology,* 1969, **114**, 19–24.

McClure, W. J. Current problems and trends in education of the deaf. *Deaf American,* 1966, **18**, 8–14.

McCroskey, R. L., & Cory, M. W. An annotated bibiography of publications on testing the hearing of infants. *Volta Review,* 1969, **71**, 27–33.

Meadow, K. P. Early manual communication in relation to the deaf child's intellectual, social, and communicative functioning. *American Annals of the Deaf,* 1968, **113**, 29–41.

Miller, M. H., & Polisar, I. A. *Audiological evaluation of the pediatric patient.* Springfield, Ill.: C. C Thomas, 1964.

Miner, L. E. A study of the incidence of speech deviations among visually handicapped children. *New Outlook for the Blind,* 1963, **57**, 10–14.

Moores, D. F. An investigation of the psycholinguistic functioning of deaf adolescents. *Exceptional Children,* 1970, **36**, 645–652.

Moores, D. F. Neo-oralism and education of the deaf in the Soviet Union. *Exceptional Children,* 1972, **38**, 377–384.

Morozova, N. G. *Development of the theory of pre-school education of the deaf and dumb.* Moscow: Institute of defectology, Academy of Pedagogical Sciences, 1954.

Morse, J. L. Mannerisms, not blindisms: cautions and treatment. *International Journal for the Education of the Blind,* 1965, **15**, 12–16.

Mowrer, D. E. The management of consequent events in speech therapy. *Educational Technology,* 1971, **11**, 58–61.

Myklebust, H. R. *The psychology of deafness.* New York: Grune & Stratton, 1960.

National Society for the Prevention of Blindness. Vision screening in the schools: recommendations of the National Society for the Prevention of Blindness. *Sight-Saving Review,* 1961, **31**, 50–58.

Neesam, R. F. The registry of interpreters for the deaf. Paper presented at a special study institute, Psycholinguistics and Total Communication, Western Maryland College, June 28–July 23, 1971.

Neuhaus, M. Parental attitudes and the emotional adjustment of deaf children. *Exceptional Children,* 1969, **35**, 721–726.

Newby, H. A. *Audiology.* (2nd ed.) New York: Appleton, 1964.

Newland, T. E. The blind learning aptitude test. In *Report of proceedings of conference on research needs in braille.* New York: American Foundation for the Blind, 1961.

Noland, C. Y. A 1966 reappraisal of the relationship between visual acuity and mode of reading for blind children. *New Outlook for the Blind,* 1967, **61**, 255–261.

Northcott, W. N. The integration of young deaf children into ordinary educational programs. *Exceptional Children*, 1971, **38**, 29–32.

O'Rourke, T. J. *Psycholinguistics and total communication.* Washington, D.C.: American Annals of the Deaf, 1972.

Osborne, K. M., Bellefleur, P. A., & Bevan, R. C. An experimental diagnostic teaching clinic for multiply handicapped deaf children. *Exceptional Children,* 1971, **37**, 387–389.

Owrid, H. L. Hearing impairment and verbal attainments in primary school children. *Educational Research*, 1970, **12**, 209–214.

Pannbacker, M. Hearing loss and a cleft palate. *Cleft Palate Journal*, 1969, **6**, 50–56.

Paradise, J. L., Bluestone, C. D., & Felder, H. The universality of otitis media in 50 infants with cleft palate. *Pediatrics*, 1969, **44**, 35–42.

Paul, J., & Proff, H. Disturbances in the visual apparatus of children and adolescents with emotional difficulties. *Praxis der Kinderpsychologie and Kinderpsychiatrie*, 1966, **15**, 237–246.

Peins, M., McGough, W. E., & Lee, B. S. Evaluation of a tape-recorded method of stuttering therapy: improvement in a speaking task. *Journal of Speech and Hearing Research*, 1972, **15**, 364–371.

Perozzi, J. A. Phonetic skill (sound-mindedness) of stuttering children. *Journal of Communication Disorders*, 1970, **3**, 207–210.

Peterson, C. L., Danner, F. W., & Flavell, J. H. Developmental changes in children's response to three indications of communicative failures. *Child Development*, 1972, **43**, 1463–1468.

Piaget, J. *The origins of intelligence in the child.* (Translated by M. Cook) London: Routledge & Kegan Paul, 1953.

Pickett, J. M., & Constam, A. A visual speech trainer with simplified indication of vowel spectrum. *American Annals of the Deaf*, 1969, **113**, 253–258.

Philips, B. J., & Harrison, R. J. Language skills of preschool cleft palate children. *Cleft Palate Journal*, 1969a, **6**, 108–119.

Philips, B. J., & Harrison, R. J. Articulation patterns of preschool cleft palate children. *Cleft Palate Journal*, 1969b, **6**, 245–253.

Pinter, R., & Patterson, D. G. The ability of deaf and hearing children to follow written instructions. *American Annals of the Deaf*, 1917, **62**, 448–472.

Potter, R. G., & Peterson, G. E. The perception of vowels and their movements. *Journal of the Acoustical Society of America*, 1948, **20**, 528–535.

Price, L. L. Evoked response audiometry: some considerations. *Journal of Speech and Hearing Disorders*, 1969, **34**, 137–141.

Prins, D., & Lohr, F. Behavioral dimensions of stuttered speech. *Journal of Speech and Hearing Research*, 1972, **15**, 61–71.

Pugh, G. S. Summaries from appraisal of the silent reading abilities of acoustically handicapped children. *American Annals of the Deaf*, 1946, **91**, 331–349.

Rabin, I., & Costa, L. D. Test-retest reliability of serial pure-tone audiograms in children at a school for the deaf. *Journal of Speech and Hearing Research*, 1969, **12**, 402–412.

Rae, A. C. Report on investigations into eye-poking. *Teacher of the Blind*, 1962, **50**, 173.

Rainer, J. D., & Altshuler, K. Z., *Comprehensive mental health services for the deaf.* New York: Columbia University Press, 1966.

Reivich, R. S., & Rothrock, I. A. Behavior problems of deaf children and adolescents: a factor-analytic study. *Journal of Speech and Hearing Research*, 1972, **15**, 93–104.

Roach, R. E., & Rosecrans, C. J. Verbal deficit in children with hearing loss. *Exceptional Children*, 1972, **38**, 395–399.

Robinson, G. C., Anderson, D. O., Moghadam, H. K., Cambon, K. C., & Murray, B. A survey of hearing loss in Vancouver school children. *Canadian Medical Association Journal*, 1967, **97**, 1199–1207.

Rohwer, W. D., Jr. Images and pictures in children's learning. *Psychological Bulletin*, 1970, **73**, 393–403.

Rohwer, W. D., Jr., Lynch, S., Levin, J. R., & Suzuki, N. Pictorial and verbal factors in the efficient learning of paired-associates. *Journal of Educational Psychology*, 1967, **58**, 278–284.

Rosenstein, J., & Lerhman, A. *Vocational status and adjustment of deaf women.* New York: Lexington School for the Deaf, 1963.

Rowe, E. D. *Speech problems of blind children: a survey of the North California area.* New York: American Foundation for the Blind, 1958.

Rubin, E. J. *Abstract functioning in the blind.* New York: American Foundation for the Blind, 1964.

Rutter, M., Graham, P., & Yule, W. *A neuropsychiatric study in childhood.* London: Spastics International Medical Publications, Heinemann, 1970.

Sanders, D. A. *Aural rehabilitation.* Englewood Cliffs, N.J.: Prentice-Hall, 1971.

Sanders, J. W., & Coscarelli, J. E. The relationship of visual synthesis to lip-reading. *American Annals of the Deaf*, 1970, **15**, 23–26.

Sanders, J. W., & Josey, A. F. Narrow-band noise audiometry for hard-to-test patients. *Journal of Speech and Hearing Research*, 1970, **13**, 74–81.

Savoye, A. L. The effect of the Skinner-Estes operant conditioning punishment paradigm upon the production of non-fluencies in normal speakers. Unpublished masters thesis, University of Pittsburg, 1959.

Schein, J. D., & Bushnag, S. Higher education for the deaf in the United States—a retrospective investigation. *American Annals of the Deaf*, 1962, **107**, 416–420.

Schlaegel, T. F., Jr. The dominant method of imagery in blind as compared to sighted adolescents. *Journal of Genetic Psychology*, 1953, **83**, 265–277.

Schlesinger, H. S., & Meadow, K. P. Development of maturity in deaf children. *Exceptional Children*, 1972, **38**, 461–467.

Scholl, G. T. The education of blind children. In W. M. Cruickshank & G. O. Johnson (Eds.), *Education of exceptional children and youth.* (2nd ed.) Englewood Cliffs, N.J.: Prentice-Hall, 1967.

Schultz, M. C. A critique of speech recognition testing preliminary to hearing therapy. *Journal of Speech and Hearing Disorders*, 1972, **37**, 195–202.

Sharp, E. Y. The relationship of visual closure to speech reading. *Exceptional Children*, 1972, **38**, 729–734.

Shearer, W. E., & Williams, J. D. Self-recovery from stuttering. *Journal of Speech and Hearing Disorders,* 1965, **30**, 288–290.

Sheehan, J. G. Conflict theory of stuttering. In J. Eisenson (Ed.), *Stuttering: a symposium.* New York: Harper & Row, 1958.

Sheehan, J. G., & Martyn, M. M. Spontaneous recovery from stuttering. *Journal of Speech and Hearing Research,* 1966, **9**, 121–135.

Sheehan, J. G., & Martyn, M. M. Stuttering and its disappearance. *Journal of Speech and Hearing Research,* 1970, **13**, 279–289.

Siegel, G. M. Punishment, stuttering and disfluency. *Journal of Speech and Hearing Research,* 1970, **13**, 677–714.

Siegel, G. M., & Martin, R. R. The effects of verbal stimuli on disfluencies during spontaneous speech. *Journal of Speech and Hearing Research,* 1968, **11**, 358–364.

Silverman, F. H. Prediction of stuttering by school-age stutterers. *Journal of Speech and Hearing Research,* 1972, **15**, 189–193.

Simmons, A. A. Factors relating to lip reading. *Journal of Speech and Hearing Research,* 1959, **4**, 340–352.

Simmons, A. A. A comparison of the type-token ratio of spoken and written language of deaf and hearing children. *Volta Review,* 1962, **64,** 417–421.

Smith, R., & McWilliams, B. J. Psycholinguistic considerations in the management of children with cleft palate. *Journal of Speech and Hearing Disorders,* 1968, **33,** 26–33.

Spiker, C. C. Stimulus pretraining and subsequent performance in the delayed reaction experiment. *Journal of Experimental Psychology,* 1956, **52,** 107–111.

Spiker, C. C. Verbal factors in discrimination learning of children. *Monographs of the Society for Research in Child Development,* 1963, **28**(Whole No. 86), 53–69.

Spriestersbach, D. C., & Sherman, D. *Cleft palate and communication.* New York: Academic Press, 1968.

Staats, A. W. *Child learning, intelligence and personality.* New York: Harper & Row, 1971.

Stassi, E. J. Disfluency of normal speakers and reinforcement. *Journal of Speech and Hearing Research,* 1961, **4,** 358–361.

Stephens, T. M., & Birch, J. W. Merits of special class, resource, and itinerant plans for teaching partially seeing children. *Exceptional Children,* 1969, **35,** 481–485.

Stinchfield, S. M. *Speech disorders.* New York: Harcourt Brace Jovanovich, 1933.

St. James-Roberts, I. Why operant audiometry: a consideration of some shortcomings fundamental to the audiological testing of children. *Journal of Speech and Hearing Disorders,* 1972, **37,** 47–54.

Tally, N. L., & Vernon, M. The impact of automation on the deaf worker. *American Federalist,* 1965, **72,** 20–23.

Thomas, I. B., & Snell, R. C. Articulation training through visual speech patterns. *Volta Review,* 1970, **72,** 310–318.

Thompson, M., & Thompson, G. Response of infants and young children as a function of auditory stimuli and methods. *Journal of Speech and Hearing Research,* 1972, **15,** 699–707.

Thurrell, R. J., & Rice, D. G. Eye rubbing in blind children. Application of a sensory deprivation model. *Exceptional Children,* 1970, **36,** 325–330.

Thurston, L. L. *A factoral study of perception.* (Psychometric Monographs) Chicago: University of Chicago Press, 1940.

Tillman, M. H. The performance of blind and sighted children on the Wechsler Intelligence Scale for Children. *International Journal for the Education of the Blind,* 1967, **16,** 65–74, 106–112.

Timmons, B. A., & Boudreau, J. P. Auditory feedback as a major factor in stuttering. *Journal of Speech and Hearing Disorders,* 1972 **37,** 476–484.

Tisdall, W. J., Blackhurst, E. A., & Marks, C. H. Divergent thinking in blind children. *Journal of Educational Psychology,* 1971, **62,** 468–473.

Toomey, G. L., & Sidman, M. An experimental analogue of the anxiety stuttering relationship. *Journal of Speech and Hearing Research,* 1970, **13,** 122–129.

Underwood, B. J. Attributes of memory. *Psychological Review,* 1969, **76,** 559–573.

VanZyl, F. J., & Ives, L. A. Visual perception and eye-motor co-ordination in a group of young deaf children. *Developmental Medicine and Child Neurology,* 1971, **13,** 373–379.

Vernon, M. Meningitis and deafness: the problem, its physical, audiological, psychological and educational manifestations in deaf children. *The Laryngoscope,* 1967a, **77,** 1856–1874.

Vernon, M. Multiply handicapped deaf children: the causes, manifestations, and significance of the problem. Paper presented at the International Conference on the Oral Education of the Deaf, New York, June 1967b.

Vernon, M. Rh Factor and deafness: the problem, its psychological, physical, and educational manifestations. *Exceptional Children,* 1967c, **33,** 5–12.

Vernon, M. Prematurity and deafness: the magnitude and nature of the problem among deaf children. *Exceptional Children,* 1967d, **33,** 289–298.

Vernon, M. Relationship of language to the thinking process. *Archives of General Psychiatry,* 1967e, **16,** 325–333.

Vernon, M. Current etiological factors in deafness. *American Annals of the Deaf,* 1968a, **113,** 106–115.

Vernon, M. Fifty years of research on the intelligence of deaf and hard-of-hearing children: a review of literature and discussion of implications, *Journal of Rehabilitation of the Deaf,* 1968b, **1,** 1–12.

Vernon, M. Myths about the education of deaf children. Paper presented at the Communication Symposium at the Maryland School for the Deaf, Frederick, Md., March 1970a.

Vernon, M. Potential, achievement and rehabilitation in the deaf population. *Rehabilitation Literature,* 1970b, **31,** 258–267.

Vernon, M. Language development's relationship to cognition, affectivity and intelligence. *Canadian Psychologist,* 1972, **13,** 360–374.

Vernon, M., & Koh, S. D. Effects of oral preschool compared to early manual communication on education and communication in deaf children. *American Annals of the Deaf,* 1971, **116,** 569–574.

Vernon, M., Makowsky, B. Deafness and minority group dynamics. *The Deaf American,* 1969, **21,** 3–6.

Webster, R. L., & Dorman, M. F. Decreases in stuttering frequency as a function of continuous and contingent forms of masking. *Journal of Speech and Hearing Disorders,* 1970, **13,** 82–86.

Webster, R. L., & Lubker, B. B. Interrelationships among fluency producing variables in stuttered speech. *Journal of Speech and Hearing Research,* 1968, **11,** 754–766.

Webster, R. L., Schumacher, S. J., & Lubker, B. B. Changes in stuttering frequency as a function of various intervals of delayed auditory feedback. *Journal of Abnormal Psychology,* 1970, **75,** 45–49.

Weinberg, B. Stuttering among blind and partially sighted children. *Journal of Speech and Hearing Disorders,* 1964, **29,** 322–326.

Weishahn, M. W. Study of graduates in the education of the visually disabled. *Exceptional Children,* 1972, **38,** 605–612.

Westlake, H., & Rutherford, D. R. *Cleft palate.* Englewood Cliffs, N.J.: Prentice-Hall, 1966.

Whitacre, J. D., Luper, H. L., & Pollio, H. R. General languages deficits in children with articulation problems. *Language and Speech,* 1970, **13,** 231–239.

Williams, A. M., & Marks, C. J. A comparative analysis of the ITPA and PPVI performance of young stutterers. *Journal of Speech and Hearing Research,* 1972, **15,** 323–329.

Williams, M. Superior intelligence of children blinded from retinoblastoma. *Archives of Diseases of Childhood,* 1968, **43,** 204–210.

Wingate, M. E. Recovery from stuttering. *Journal of Speech and Hearing Disorders,* 1964, **29,** 312–321.

Wingate, M. E. Sound and pattern in "artificial" fluency. *Journal of Speech and Hearing Research,* 1969, **12,** 677–686.

Wingate, M. E. Effects on stuttering of changes in audition. *Journal of Speech and Hearing Research,* 1970, **13,** 861–873.

Wischner, G. J. Stuttering behavior and learning: a preliminary theoretical formulation. *Journal of Speech and Hearing Disorders,* 1950, **15,** 324–335.

Withrow, F. B. Immediate memory span of deaf and normally hearing children. *Exceptional Children*, 1968, **35**, 33–41.

Witkin, H. A., Birnbaum, J., Lomonaio, S., Lehr, S., & Herman, J. Cognitive patterns in congenitally totally blind children. *Child Development*, 1968, **39**, 767–786.

Wolf, J. M. *The blind child with concomitant disabilities.* New York: American Foundation for the Blind, 1967.

Wolff, P., & Zevin, J. R. The role of overt activity in children's imagery production. *Child Development*, 1972, **43**, 537–547.

Worchel, P. Space perception and orientation in the blind. *Psychological Monographs*, 1951, **65**, 332.

Wright, H. N. Viewpoint: hearing disorders and hearing science: ten years of progress. *Journal of Speech and Hearing Research*, 1970, **13**, 229–231.

Wrightstone, J. W., Aronow, M. S., & Moskowitz, S. Developing reading test norms for deaf children. *American Annals of the Deaf*, 1963, **108**, 311–316.

Zweibelson, I., & Barg, C. F. Concept development of blind children. *New Outlook for the Blind*, 1967, **61**, 218–222.

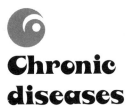

Chronic diseases

The child suffering from a chronic disease not only places a burden on his family but also displays behaviors that bring him to the attention of mental health practitioners. Whether these behaviors are part of the disease syndrome, a reaction to it, or the result of faulty parental management remains the subject of considerable research. In any case, we do know that emotional problems of children often have their onset following a serious medical disorder. Many mental health practitioners attribute this fact to the parents' wish to find an explanation for the child's emotional disorder that will absolve them of blame.

As we will learn in this chapter, diseases often precipitate an emotional disorder. Not only must the child deal with the physical aspects of his illness and the limitations it places on his life, but he must deal also with the way in which his parents are affected. Parents who might otherwise have used appropriate child rearing practices are sometimes rendered less effective by the child's illness. Even following his recovery, they may relate to him in an inappropriate manner. The child's illness may trigger latent conflicts between parents and generate disagreement about child rearing practices.

Children's reactions to different diseases have certain features in common, and these features, rather than the specific diseases themselves, are the main focus of this chapter. The chapter begins with a discussion of children's reactions to illness and hospitalization, their awareness of fatal illness, and the need for improvements in hospital practices on behalf of ill children. We then will familiarize the reader with some specific diseases. Finally, we discuss two disorders that present difficulties in diagnosis because the first symptoms can be mistaken for some other condition or attributed to emotional factors. We present these disorders not because the diseases themselves are so important, but to emphasize once again that interdisciplinary cooperation is necessary in the diagnosis and treatment of exceptional children.

CHILDREN AND ILLNESS

The child's reaction to disease

When children become seriously ill their life changes abruptly. They are exposed to limitations they often don't understand and to treatment that is sometimes more disturbing than the illness itself.

Illness usually includes bed rest and being cared for by others. Many children, particularly those who have just mastered independent mobility, resent bed confinement. Others, who have just mastered independence from parents after overcoming desires for passivity and dependency, are likely to react negatively to the dependency that accompanies illness. For example, toddlers who have recently learned to walk often stand up in their beds for the whole course of a severe illness (Freud, 1952). Motor restraint also increases restlessness and irritability regardless of age. Other children regress and have to relearn social skills after recovery.

The young do not understand why they are sick and are disturbed by the unfamiliar bodily changes that accompany illness. As will be seen in several cases to follow, they often feel responsible for having become ill; they feel they have brought the illness about because they were bad or did something they should not have done. Parents typically reinforce these attitudes by admonitions to "Wear a coat or you'll catch cold" or "Don't run in the street or you'll fall and hurt yourself." If an accident does occur, the parent often reacts first with anger and only later with concern—"I told you not to do that!" In addition, pain associated with treatment is often conceived of as a punishment for misbehavior (Freud, 1952).

Regression to an earlier level of functioning usually accompanies sickness. Regression is considered an adaptive device, serving to mobilize defenses against anxiety. The young child usually regresses more easily than the older. If the disease state is prolonged, regressions are more pronounced. Increased dependency often follows regression. Some children, particularly those whose relationships with parents are tenuous, attempt to prolong the immediate need satisfaction they experience when sick. When they are sick, their usually disinterested parents become solicitous, inadvertently reinforcing them for being ill. Children who develop hysterical disorders often are those who have gained from being ill (see Chapter 7).

Regression isn't confined to children. Hospital dietitians have observed that when anxiety is high in adults, the consumption of milk, bread, and cereal, particularly the cooked variety, goes up (Chappelle, 1972). These foods are considered security foods, foods associated with the love and affection experienced in infancy and childhood.

Parents also change when their child becomes ill. In their desire to follow the doctor's orders, they may force feed their child when he refuses to eat, restrain him when he wants to move about, and deceive him in order to induce cooperation with essential medical procedures (Wolff, 1969). These changes can cause the child to become rebellious or to blame his parents for his illness.

Parents may display irrational behavior toward their sick offspring. This irrationality usually results from anxiety related to their own past experiences, which are rekindled by the child's present illness. Blake, Wright, and Waechter present such a case.

When Mrs. A brought Ann into the hospital for cataract extraction, she was nervous and upset and therefore unable to support her child in the early part of her hospitalization. She fled from the ward as soon as Ann's history was taken, without heed to Ann's need for her. When the operation was postponed because Ann developed a respiratory infection, Mrs. A vented her anger on hospital personnel and on Ann. When she came to visit, she could not tolerate Ann's tears of rebellion. She said that she could not wait to get out of the hospital because, as she expressed it venomously. "It makes me jittery. I can't stay put. The quicker I can get out of here the better."

The nurse tried to find out what was troubling Mrs. A. She discovered that Mrs. A had cataracts extracted from both eyes when she was 4 years old. She remembered little about hospitalization, but from conversation it seemed evident that she had never made peace with her feelings about her eyes and the treatment she endured. She resented the fact that she had to wear thick glasses and felt she was unattractive in them. She felt guilty because she produced what she called a "defective" child. After her first child, Billy, was born, she sought medical advice and made sure that his eyes were perfect before she became pregnant again. "I'd never have had another child if I'd known it would have cataracts," she said. When her second child's eyes were found to be imperfect, she felt guilty and angry. Mrs. A's brother also had had congenital cataracts, but his children had normal vision. Mrs. A resented her brother's successful achievement.

After her operation, Ann cried and expressed anger toward her mother when she arrived late for visiting hours. Ann's response to discomfort and disappointment increased Mrs. A's guilt and also made her anxious and intolerant of frustration. She reacted with anger and inability to see anyone's problems but her own. It is highly probable that Mrs. A's memories of her own painful childhood hospital experiences were revived by her daughter's situation—hence, her anxiety, intolerance, and unintentional cruelty.

She knew that she was miserable, but she did not know why she acted as she did. In addition to feeling responsible for Ann's visual difficulties, Mrs. A was also ashamed of the fact that she was irritable, came late for visiting hours and had to leave Ann repeatedly to smoke cigarettes. *(From F. G. Blake, E. H. Wright, & E. H. Waechter.* Nursing Care of Children. *(8th ed.) Philadelphia: Lippincott, 1970, p. 23.)*

The child's reaction to hospitalization

David Levy was perhaps the first individual to emphasize the adverse effects of hospitalization on children. He observed that many young children displayed considerable fear and anxiety, as well as more nightmares, closely following operations. These symptoms were more pronounced in children between the ages of 1 and 3. He recommended that, whenever possible, surgery be postponed until after age 3 (Levy, 1945).

Somewhat later, Prugh and his associates investigated the effects of hospitalization upon behavior (Prugh, Staub, Sands, Kirschbaum, & Lenihan, 1953). While surgery was particularly disturbing to young children, all children under age 4 were manifestly disturbed regardless of the reason for their hospitalization. Those between 2 and 4 displayed panic attacks, outbursts of anger whenever parents left, depression, and eating and sleeping disturbances. Rocking and thumbsucking were common in those up and about. Although these behaviors occurred to a lesser degree in children given large amounts of individual attention, children under 4 displayed disturbances regardless of the quality of nursing care or of the sensitivity of the staff to the child's anxieties. Six-year olds, however, responded favorably to nursing practices in tune with their emotional needs.

Three weeks after discharge 50 percent of the children under 4 showed severe emotional reactions. Six months after discharge a number still displayed emotional disturbances. Prugh's findings were confirmed by Vaughan (1957), who also found that children under 4 displayed adverse reactions six months following discharge. It is important to note that the hospital stay of many of the children Vaughan studied was brief and was not associated with surgery. These findings emphasize the need to postpone all but the most urgent operations until after the age of 4.

Considering the animistic thinking of children under 4 (Piaget, 1928), many undoubtedly view their hospital experience as punishments for wrongdoings. At this stage children are concerned with body intactness and anxiety about this concern is easily stimulated. If Band-Aids are insisted upon for even a small cut, imagine the anxiety that must be generated by separation from the mother and an operation, the purpose of which they don't understand! Marlens's (1960) comparison of hospitalized with nonhospitalized ill children revealed that the hospitalized group felt more rejected, conceived of their hospitalization as punishment, and showed more somatic preoccupation, anxiety, and depression.

Marlens's research demonstrated that being ill is not as critical a factor as separation from the mother at a time when anxieties are increased by fantasies and fears of attack. The child is not sure he will return home and exaggerates the period of time between parental visits.

A one-year follow-up of children treated for burns revealed that hospitalization was a traumatic experience (Woodward & Jackson, 1961). Over 80 percent of the 198 children followed had emotional disturbances, compared to only 7 percent of their unburned siblings. The most common symptoms were phobias and anxiety, negativism and aggressiveness, eating and sleeping difficulties, and bed wetting. Over half of the mothers of burned children complained of their own nervous problems, and one in six had been treated for a "nervous breakdown." The unit in which the children were hospitalized provided the best possible medical treatment for the burn, but largely ignored the emotional needs of the child.

Some operations are more psychologically damaging than others. Children operated on for cryptorchism, or undescended testicle, a not uncommon condition, are quite susceptible to emotional disturbance. The disturbance starts with anxiety, restlessness, and regression and, if untreated, can develop into a character disorder with accompanying depression, passivity, poor self-concept, and confusion over body image and sexual identity. A dominant mother and a passive, withdrawn, or absent father are particularly predisposing to emotional difficulties in these children (see Chapter 7, the case of Leo). Unlike other operations, this operation is less traumatic when performed during the preschool years. An early operation cuts short the period of time during which the child shows concern over his atypical condition (Cytryn, Cytryn, & Rieger, 1967). This finding reflects society's concern with sexuality and the significance ascribed to the testicles.

Prugh's work also demonstrated that children who had prior traumatic experiences or whose relationships with parents were poor reacted to hospitalization with greater distress. The rejected child does not view his separation as temporary escape from an unhappy situation, but rather as further proof of his rejection. Unhappiness and insecurity impair the child's chances of an independent adjustment away from home. "He does not carry with him the firm inner image of a loving mother which can reassure him while he is parted from her" (Wolff, 1969, p. 59).

Children with known psychiatric disorders are hospitalized more frequently than normal children and stay for longer periods of time. The statistics of one outpatient psychiatric clinic revealed that 26 of 100 clinic attenders had spent three or more weeks of their life in a hospital because of physical problems. Only 7 of 100 of a nondisturbed group had been in the hospital for a similar period (Wolff, 1967).

It remains to be determined whether hospitalization results in or aggravates emotional difficulties or whether admission to a hospital and emotional difficulties both depend on a third factor (e.g., reduced tolerance to stress). In either case children admitted to hospitals are vulnerable children, forced to cope with both illness and the anxiety it arouses.

The child's awareness of fatal illness   The death of a child is particularly difficult to accept because it means unfulfilled promise and destroyed hopes. To defend ourselves against such pain, we may avoid children with fatal illness, leaving them to face alone their fears and anxieties.

Yet, several investigators report that fatally ill children do not usually experience or express anxiety about death until after age 10, and that prior to that time they are unaware of what is happening to them (Knudson & Natterson, 1960; Morrissey, 1965; Natterson & Knudson, 1960; Richmond & Waisman, 1955). More recently, however, Waechter (1971) demonstrated that children may express their awareness of and fears of death indirectly, particularly when adults are silent about their condition.

Waechter based her work on the hypothesis that, despite efforts to shield a child from awareness of his prognosis, the anxiety of adults is conveyed to him through their false cheerfulness or evasiveness. The child may feel that open expression of his fears may meet with disapproval. Consequently, research that relies on a child's overt expression of fear can get a distorted picture of the child's concerns.

Waechter administered to three groups of hospitalized children an anxiety scale adapted from Sarason's work (Sarason, Davidson, Lighthall, Waite, & Ruebush, 1960) and a modified version of the Thematic Apperception Test (see Figure 6.1). In addition, each child's parents were interviewed in order to gather data about variables that might influence the child's concerns about death.

Waechter's results revealed that children with fatal illness received scores on the anxiety scale that were twice as high as those received by children with chronic diseases who had favorable prognoses and by children hospitalized for brief illnesses. Of the 16 with a fatal illness, only 2 had been informed of their prognoses. Yet, children with poor prognoses told substantially more stories about threat to body integrity than did children in comparison groups. They discussed loneliness, separation, and death more frequently in their fantasy stories, although none had expressed these fears directly to hospital personnel. Characters in the stories often had the diagnosis and symptoms of the child telling it. (Several stories appear as sketches on the following pages of this chapter.) There was an inverse correlation between the amount of fear projected into the stories and the degree to which the child had been given the opportunity to discuss his prognosis and fears.

Some stories revealed that children saw the hospital environment as unsupportive; their sense of loneliness was revealed in their perception of time as stretching forever between parental visits. Other stories suggested that children felt responsible for having developed the illness and experienced guilt in addition to fear. Even more distressing was the belief that nobody cared, a belief resulting from misinterpretation of the parents' uneasy silence and feigned cheerfulness.

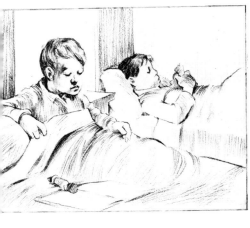

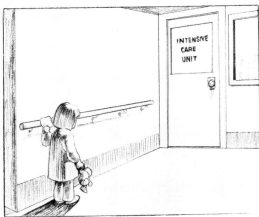

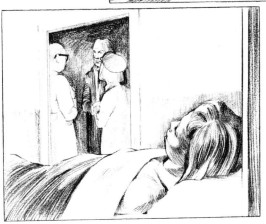

Figure 6.1 *In one of the projective tests to elicit the fantasies of dying children (age 6 to 10), Waechter asked them to tell stories about these pictures. They often gave the characters their own diagnoses and symptoms and 63 percent related their stories to death. (Courtesy of E. H. Waechter.)*

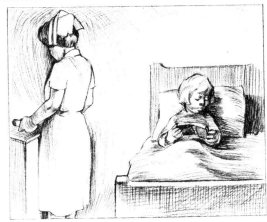

PROJECTED ANXIETIES

This is about a woman. She's somebody's mother. She's crying because her son was in the hospital, and he died. He had leukemia. He finally had a heart attack. It just happened . . . he died. Then they took him away to a cemetery to bury him, and his soul went up to heaven.

The woman is crying. But she forgets about it when she goes to bed. Because she relaxes and her brain relaxes. She's very sad. But she sees her little boy again when she goes up to heaven. She's looking forward to that. She won't find anybody else in heaven—just her little boy that she knows.

From E. G. Waechter. Children's awareness of fatal illness. *American Journal of Nursing,* 1971, **71**, 1168–1172.

PROJECTED ANXIETIES

One girl was reading a book in the hospital. The nurse was over by the bed. The girl's name was Becky. She had the bad coughing. She had trouble with her lungs. She had lung congestion. The nurse is looking at her chart. Becky is thinking they're going to do an operation. Becky is only 8 years old. She thinks they're going to hurt her and she doesn't want it. And they did give the operation. They gave her a sleeping shot. She didn't like shots. The same nurse always came in, because she knew what to do. Becky died. Then her mother came to see her and they told her she died. But the mother didn't like to hear that.

From E. G. Waechter. Children's awareness of fatal illness. *American Journal of Nursing,* 1971, **71**, 1168–1172.

Waechter's study indicates that denial and protectiveness does not prevent a child with a fatal illness from experiencing anxiety or even from obtaining knowledge of his diagnosis and prognosis. In fact, such attitudes increase feelings of isolation, alienation, and loneliness. What the child actually needs is support that allows for introspective examination of attitudes and fears related to death. Anxiety reduction not only eases the physical burden resulting from prolonged tension, but also may reduce perceived intensity of pain. Over twenty years ago, Hill and his colleagues (Hill, Flanary, Kornetsky, Conan, & Wikler, 1952) demonstrated that anxiety serves as a pain amplifier. This effect probably derives from the tendency of anxiety to narrow the focus of attention, thereby reducing the effect of peripheral, distracting stimuli and thus making the noxious sensation highly salient (Easterbrook, 1959).

Helping a child cope with anxiety As was mentioned earlier, the young child believes that every event occurs by intent—there are no impartial natural causes for events; logic is precausal. The child reasons from an internal model of the world rather than from observations of events (Piaget, 1928). Animistic explanations of illness, therefore, are usual in young children. Langford (1948) quoted several children who gave as the cause of their diabetes "because I ate too much sugar" and their rheumatic fever "because I ran too much."

PROJECTED ANXIETIES

The little boy had to stay in the hospital because the doctor wanted it. He got a shot in the back; a big needle. He was scared of shots, and didn't want it. And the doctor did it hard. His lungs are gone—he can't breathe. His lungs got worse and he didn't get well. He died and he was buried with a big shovel.

From E. G. Waechter. Children's awareness of fatal illness. *American Journal of Nursing,* 1971, **71**, 1168–1172.

The case of Mark, described by Wolff (1969, pp. 54-55), serves to emphasize how the young child's ideas can result in behavior that puzzles staff.

Mark, a little boy of six, was admitted to the hospital with an infectious osteomyelitis, affecting his thigh and the bones of his face. He bore weeks of hospitalization and immobilization in plaster stoically. Then he was moved to a convalescent home which he knew to be farther away from his home than the hospital. Here he refused his food and began to vomit. Extensive investigations failed to reveal a physical cause for his eating disturbances and the nurses and his parents became worried. "You must eat to get better," they said. But he refused. From being a favorite patient, easy to nurse, he became a problem. The more the nurses and his parents worried about him, the more pressure they put on the child. They were cross with him; they reasoned with him and they urged him to eat. When they asked him to explain why he would not eat, all he could say was "I don't like the peas."

At this stage outside help was summoned and I went to see Mark in his hospital bed. As an outsider, not directly responsible for his nursing care, and not therefore preoccupied with fears that unless I could persuade him to eat he would lose weight and go downhill, I was free to attend to what he had to say. When I asked him, "What is the matter with your face, why is it swollen?" he replied in matter-of-fact tones, "It's because I bite my nails." It was clear he accepted responsibility for his illness, thinking he had caused it by doing something naughty. The parents confirmed that he was a nail-biter and that they had often told him it was a "dirty habit." They also remembered the doctor saying that perhaps the infection had been caused by dirt getting into his mouth. They were shocked to think, however, that their son was blaming himself for being ill: *that* connection, between a naughty habit and his illness, was made by Mark himself. He has always been exceptionally "good" in the ward. His parents used to praise him and say that if he was good and did what the nurses told him, he would get better more quickly, a remark designed to reinforce the notions, magical and egocentric, that he already had about his own responsibility for his illness. When he was moved to the convalescent home against his will, he could not afford to protest openly, to make a fuss, to be "naughty." Instead he developed symptoms: food refusal and vomiting, over which he had no control.

It was now clear what had to be done. Rather than increase his sense of responsibility for his illness, by stressing that he must do his part to get better and demanding good behavior, we had to get across to him that nail-biting or indeed naughtiness of any kind did not cause illness; that illnesses happen "by accident" and it was the business of the doctors and nurses to get him well whatever he did. We had to convey to him that we understood that he refused the hospital food because he was angry with the doctors and nurses for sending him far away; that we did not mind his being cross because we knew that all children who are ill and in the hospital sometimes feel cross; and that this would not interfere with his getting better. *(From Sula Wolff, Children under stress, pp. 72–73. (Allen Lane The Penguin Press 1969) Copyright © Sula Wolff, 1969. Reprinted by permission of Penguin Books Ltd.)*

Because staff either are unaware of children's mistaken notions or cannot change them through verbal means, they sometimes employ operant conditioning techniques to alter regressive behavior (Berni & Fordyce, 1973).

Berni, Dressler, and Baxter (1971) describe the use of operant reinforcement procedures in the care of a child with a severe hereditary disease characterized by dilated capillaries, progressive cerebellar ataxia, and immunological defects which result in chronic infections, particularly of the respiratory tract. The patient, Billy, after passing through a period of crisis, grunted, whined, and pointed instead of talked. He refused to walk, reach for anything, eat or drink fluids well, and he continually turned on his call light. According to his medical report, Billy was capable of better functioning. His nurse encouraged Billy to do better, visited him frequently, and explained to him that he was improving and should do better. Nevertheless, his behavior remained unchanged.

PROJECTED ANXIETIES

She's in the hospital, and the doctor is talking to her mother and father. She's sick—she's got cancer. She's very, very sick. She's thinking she wishes she could go home. She had an operation at the hospital, but she didn't want it because she wanted to get out of the hospital. This little girl dies—she doesn't get better. Poor little girl. This girl at the hospital—she has cancer. Her hip is swollen and her bone's broken. This little girl in the picture died, and then they buried her. And then she went up to heaven. She didn't like it there—because God wasn't there.

From E. G. Waechter. Children's awareness of fatal illness. *American Journal of Nursing*, 1971, **71**, 1168–1172.

At a staff conference, the nurses concluded that, while acting on the physician's directive to make Billy happy and comfortable during what was to have been a terminal crisis, they had contributed to his excessive "sick" behavior. Without realizing it, they had produced Billy's current behavior by behaving in ways that reinforced it. The team decided, therefore, to use operant principles to reinforce "well" behavior. This meant ignoring Billy when his behavior was judged inappropriate. Several nurses expressed concern about forsaking traditional methods for one that seemed impersonal and perhaps inhumane. After consultation with the psychology staff, Billy's nurse wrote a nursing-care plan describing the course of action. Table 6.1 outlines this plan.

The first few days on this plan were traumatic for everyone. Billy interpreted the nurses' sudden removal of unconditional attention as rejection and became withdrawn and sullen. After two days of withdrawal, he finally asked the nurses why they were mad at him. At this point, the plan nearly fell apart.

A staff conference emphasized making more use of positive reinforcement rather than relying on extinction and time out from reinforcement to produce the needed changes in behavior. More emphasis would be placed on shaping desired behaviors by reinforcing approximations to the behavior. Billy began to respond favorably to the program and, in spite of congestive heart failure during the second week, was able to leave the hospital at the end of the third week of this treatment.

Six months later Billy was walking, breathing without oxygen for periods up to one hour, and was even yelling at his siblings. One year later Billy returned to the hospital in grave condition, but quickly rallied. Forewarned by their past experience, the nurses prevented dependent behavior from redeveloping and thereby facilitated a rapid discharge home.

Although Billy's nurses believed that their initial approach toward him had reinforced his dependency and maintained his regressive behavior, there is another explanation. Billy may not have verbalized his feelings about his illness because he was greatly frightened by his close bouts with death. Billy, like Mark, was 5 and at a level of conceptual development where animistic explanations of cause-effect relationships dominate thinking.

Improvements in hospital practice   During the 1940s some English hospitals admitted both mother and child when the child was under 3. This practice enabled the mother and nurse to learn from each other and freed the nurse to spend more time with older children (Spence, 1960). Beliefs that infections would increase because more adults were on the ward were proven false. Nevertheless, early arguments to humanize children's hospital treatment met with considerable resistance.

In 1952 James Robertson produced a film, entitled *A Two-Year-Old*

Table 6.1   PLAN FOR BILLY'S CARE

Week One

OVERALL GOAL: Teach the patient appropriate behavior in preparation for discharge by discontinuing attention on his excessively "sick" behavior and by reinforcing "well" behavior.

1. GOAL: reinforce ambulation and independence

Inappropriate behavior by patient: refusing to walk, wanting to be carried, and wanting to use wheelchair

Appropriate behavior by patient: walking

Extinction by removal of positive reinforcers: removing the wheelchair; reducing nurses' social contact, talking, and playing with Billy

Positive reinforcers: nurses smiling and joking with Billy within his physical capabilities

2. GOAL: teach verbal communication and extinguish pointing, grunting, and whining

Inappropriate behavior: grunting, pointing, whining, and not talking

Appropriate behavior: talking

Extinction by removal of positive reinforcers: nurses' refusing to comply with Billy's nonverbal requests after explaining the program to him; nurses' reducing their social contact, talking, and playing with him

Positive reinforcers: compliment his efforts to talk; smiling, talking, and playing with Billy when he talks

3. GOAL: reinforce "well" behavior by deemphasizing bad health and emphasizing positive factors

Extinction by: deemphasizing questions and remarks about his health status; not commenting in front of Billy about his condition; refraining from pointing out his blue nail beds whenever this occurs

Positive reinforcers: pointing out improvement in his activity; praising him for involvement in the occupational therapy program; praising him when he eats or drinks fluids well

Week Two

OVERALL GOAL: Make Billy's daily living experience as happy as possible by providing a feeling of security for him and by teaching him "well" behavior within his physical capabilities.

1. Omit ambulation goal of walking for the present

2. GOAL: verbal communication

Shaping: add, when Billy is not talking as he should; nurses' request verbal responses before complying with his request; go about necessary tasks in silence.

Positive reinforcers: add, take time to read to Billy

3. GOAL: reinforce "well" behavior

4. GOAL: maintain adequate fluid intake

Extinction by: nurses' neutral responses when Billy refuses the prescribed fluids

Positive reinforcers: place a plastic translucent cylinder at Billy's bedside, fill with colored water equal to the amount that Billy drinks, compliment Billy as the level of water rises

Table 6.1 *(Continued)*

Week Three

OVERALL GOAL: Make Billy feel worthwhile and needed with "a place in life," in addition to the goals of the first and second weeks.

1. GOAL: wheelchair ambulation

Positive reinforcers: arrange for portable oxygen tank; praise patient when he goes to the activity room

2. GOAL: establish verbal communication

3. GOAL: reinforce "well" behavior

Extinction by: neutral response to signs of health fluctuation.

4. GOAL: maintain prescribed fluid intake (500 cc.)

5. GOAL: maintain good nutrition

Extinction by: ignoring refusal to eat

Positive reinforcers: comment when he eats well; give him attention and choice at the time his menu is made out; be sure he is served small portions; schedule meals after pulmonary therapy; when he has a poor day, praise him for what he does eat

Adapted from R. Berni, J. Dressler, & J. C. Baxter. Reinforcing behavior. American Journal of Nursing, 1971, **71**, 2180–2183.

Goes to the Hospital, to demonstrate to pediatricians and nurses harmful practices that they overlooked or ignored. It demonstrated the typical reactions of a 2-year old admitted to the hospital, and it revealed the useless and harmful effects of what was then traditional hospital routine. The film showed that a child deprived of a continuing relationship with his mother reacts in a predictable manner. First, he protests by strongly expressing his distress. Second, he despairs, becoming less active in displaying his need for mother, but showing increasing hopelessness. He may become withdrawn and apathetic and cease to demand his mother's presence. The uninformed often believe that distress has lessened in this stage. In the third stage, denial, the child shows interest in his surroundings and appears sociable. Yet, when the mother comes, the child acts as if he doesn't know her and no longer cries when she leaves. He is even reluctant to leave the hospital. Robertson believes that extended hospitalization of young children produces serious emotional maladjustment (Robertson, 1970).

In 1954 the World Health Organization organized a study group to prepare a position paper on children's hospitalization. The study group concluded that the best place to care for an ill child is in his own home. If hospitalization is essential, a child should be prepared for the experience, and continuing close contact between mother and child should be encouraged (Capes, 1956). Under the age of 4 only the mother's actual presence in the hospital can alleviate a child's anxiety. Later reports encouraged hospitals to provide unlimited visiting to all children and to develop live-in facilities for mothers of preschool children. Hospitals in the United States have been slow in following these recommendations; however, in England hospitals are now required to develop live-in facilities for parents.

Other investigators varied the type of experience hospitals provided and studied the results of these variations. Prugh's staff studied two groups of children under two different ward conditions (Prugh et al., 1953). One group received special preparation for admission and an admission procedure designed to minimize anxiety. Parents visited daily and a special play period was provided. Special medical and nursing procedures were accompanied by extra attention and support. A single nurse was assigned to especially anxious children. In addition, weekly conferences were held to discuss the psychological problems of the children and of the staff in relation to the children.

The second group were cared for in the traditional manner. Visits from parents were weekly. Nurses with differing degrees of seniority were assigned specific tasks, which they performed for all the children. Under these conditions, no nurse was ever assigned the total care of a particular child and, therefore, the nursing staff never knew any of the children well.

Comparison of the behavior of the two groups, both during their hospital stay and after, showed that children in the experimental group manifested significantly less psychiatric disturbance. This finding, however, held only for those above age 4. Outward manifestations of distress, however, were greater in the experimental group while they were still in the hospital. Frequent visiting resulted in more tears following separations, and encouragement to express feelings led to more outbursts of anger and frustration directed at the staff.

Vaughan (1957) demonstrated that psychiatric interviews with the child have beneficial effects. The interviews he conducted were designed to help the child express his feelings about his hospitalization and the upcoming operation and to correct any misconceptions he held. The children interviewed displayed more disturbed behavior while in the hospital, but this situation was reversed following discharge. Six months after discharge only 3 of the 20 interviewed children showed disturbances compared to 11 of the 20 controls. Again, these findings were limited to those over age 4.

Psychiatric interviewing is beneficial even in hospitals where ward procedures are designed with children in mind (frequent visiting, one nurse for each child, preparation of the child for what is to happen, discussion groups with parents, and provision for school and play as part of each hospital day). The effect of interviews was demonstrated in the following manner. One group of children received only the normal ward routine, a second group took part in three weekly classes in which they were taught about their illness, and a third group was seen in three group sessions where they were encouraged to express their anxieties but were given no specific information unless they asked for it.

All three groups were reexamined at the end of three weeks following admission and at intervals up to two years following discharge. The children given group therapy were still as anxious after three weeks as they were at admission, while the other two groups were less anxious. After two years, however, the situation was reversed. Regarding information, the group given therapy knew as much as the lecture group at the end of the three weeks. Two years later, however, the lecture group had forgotten what they had learned, while the group given therapy was still well informed (Rie, Bovermean, Ozoa, & Grossman, 1964).

Counseling of parents also has a positive affect. Allowing mothers of burned children to air their feelings of distress and guilt helps them react more appropriately to their injured child. Without this opportunity, many mothers, overwhelmed with guilt, repress these feelings. As a result, they display irrational behavior toward their child. A child's accusations and aggressive behavior are hard for a mother to tolerate when she is burdened with guilt. When given an opportunity to ventilate these feelings, the mother's irrational behavior diminishes. A follow-up of 71 children whose mothers had met regularly with a psychiatric social worker revealed that only 20 percent displayed emotional disturbances one year after discharge as compared with 80 percent of 198 whose mothers had had no such opportunity (Woodward & Jackson, 1961).

The conclusion drawn from these studies is that encouraging children and parents to express their worries aids long-term adaptation to illness. Such expression is considerably more helpful than explanations or instructions. Without a psychotherapeutic program of some sort, many children regress temporarily, and a significant number sustain some

DEFENSES

Entrance of the medical staff into 4-year-old Suzie's room invariably caused her to withdraw into pensive contemplation while she fingered her lips. When her hand was free for this self-comforting activity, she was able to maintain control during frightening procedures. The defensive value of this gesture became apparent one day when the doctor removed her fingers from her lips as he examined her heart. With her defense gone, she was unable to control herself. She shrieked loudly and kicked until the doctor permitted her to resume her accustomed activity. Postoperatively, the nurse made sure that one arm was free so Suzie could comfort herself when she needed it.

From F. G. Blake, F. H. Wright, & E. H. Waechter. *Nursing care of children.* (8th ed.) Philadelphia: Lippincott, 1970. p. 409.

permanent maladaptive behavior. "For them the subjective meaning of the illness has become more disabling than the illness itself" (Wolff, 1969, p. 72).

What can be learned from these studies that can be applied elsewhere? First, there are many clinicians who place great emphasis on extinguishing maladaptive behavior. They do not view behavior as defensive or as symptomatic of underlying conflict. The finding that children can show less maladaptive behavior in the hospital than they do after discharge should be stressed in discussions with clinic staff. Second, the finding that age is a critical variable in program planning supports a developmental approach to children's treatment rather then a view that the same treatment approach can be applied at any age level (see Chapter 12). Third, training medical personnel to recognize psychological aspects of illness as well as to understand a child's conceptual development is immensely important. Wolff remarks,

> When a child's symptoms are not due to a physical illness, but are psychologically determined, doctors trained only to deal with organic illness may find that nothing they know of makes the situation any better. They have examined the patient and found nothing organically wrong but the complaint is still there. In this unsatisfactory situation drastic measures are sometimes resorted to. When bed-wetting or soiling in children does not respond to pills, regular toileting and encouragement, a period in hospital is still often recommended and many children are subjected to enemas and purgatives with only temporary improvement. Many children with abdominal pain due to anxiety have numerous physical investigations done because no explanation for the symptoms can be found on physical examination. In such a dilemma, the surgeon is often called in more readily than the psychiatrist and the child has an exploratory operation before his emotional state and his life history are examined. Such intensive physical investigations are likely to confirm the child's and the parent's view that there may be something physically wrong or, if not, that "nothing" is wrong. There is no reason for the child to do what he does. "Laziness" or "naughtiness" are adduced and this increases the child's guilt. *(From Sula Wolff,* Children under stress, *pp. 72–73. (Allen Lane The Penguin Press 1969) Copyright © Sula Wolff, 1969. Reprinted by permission of Penguin Books Ltd.)*

Since these initial studies, some hospitals have initiated additional procedures to ease a child's anxiety. Puppet shows depicting what the child will experience during his operation have been employed to allay anxiety (see Figure 6.2; Whitson, 1972). Hospital units have been developed where children are admitted in the morning, given minor surgery, and discharged in the evening. These units were developed primarily to reduce the emotional impact of hospitalization (Condon, 1972). Follow-up studies have demonstrated that preschoolers display less maladjustment when parents have stayed in the hospital with them (Brain & Maclay, 1968).

Nevertheless, current studies suggest that many hospitals still disregard both the child's and family's emotional reactions to hospitaliza-

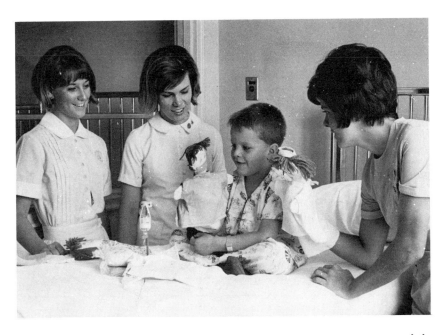

Figure 6.2 *A 5-year old tries his hand with the doctor puppet while one of the nurses brings the nurse puppet on stage. The IV pole is made from a toy construction kit. (Courtesy of B. J. Whitson.)*

tion. Many parents still feel they are kept in the dark regarding their child's illness. Table 6.2 categorizes the feelings of 25 mothers interviewed following their child's discharge (Freiberg, 1972). In addition, these mothers were not forewarned that their child might display maladaptive behavior upon return home (see Table 6.3).

Table 6.2 MOTHERS' REASONS FOR ANXIETY DURING CHILDREN'S HOSPITALIZATION

Reason given for anxiety	Number of mothers who mentioned
Fears about procedures and treatments	16
Lack of information about procedures and treatments	12
Lack of information about diagnosis	10
Fear about future health of child	8
Fears caused by sights of other hospitalized children	7
Fears about recovery of child from present illness	6
Fears about child having a fatal illness	5
Desire to have doctor visit more often	5
Feeling that child needed more medical treatment	4
Feeling that more diagnostic tests were needed	4

Adapted from K. H. Freiberg. How parents react when their child is hospitalized. *American Journal of Nursing*, 1972, **72**, 1270–1272.

Table 6.3 NEW NEGATIVE BEHAVIOR AFTER HOSPITALIZATION

Negative behavior	Number of children showing it
More demands for attention	15
Tics or mannerisms	8
New fears	7
Whining at separation from parent(s)	6
Jealousy of other family member(s)	6
Withdrawal and shyness	5
Insomnia	4
Angry behavior toward parent(s)	4
Joining parents in bed	3
Nightmares	3
Attachment to blanket or toy	3
Following parent everywhere	3
Temper tantrums	3
Hyperactivity	1

Adapted from K. H. Freiberg. How parents react when their child is hospitalized. *American Journal of Nursing*, 1972, **72**, 1270–1272.

Surveys of nurses and patients reveal that the two groups have quite different ideas about what information should be conveyed to the patient. The majority of patients are greatly concerned about reducing ambiguity about their condition; they want to know how serious their situations are, their chances of recovery and recurrence, the results of their operations and diagnostic work, and the complexity of their cases. In marked contrast, nurses are more concerned with conveying to patients what to expect regarding nursing care and hospital routines and practices (Dodge, 1972). The implication of these differences is that the alleviation of patient anxiety is not being dealt with in many hospitals. If a nurse is unaware of a patient's concern, her effectiveness in reducing his anxiety is limited.

SOME SPECIFIC CHRONIC DISEASES

There are many chronic disorders that affect children. Some disorders are visible and obvious and sometimes unpleasant, even repulsive, to the observer. Others become noticeable only on certain occasions; for example, when the epileptic has a seizure or when the asthmatic has an attack. Many are seldom apparent, for example, diabetes, heart disease, or hemophilia, and affected children must explain their inability to engage in certain activities.

Because of advances in medicine, many children live who once would have died from these disorders. Consequently, society is called upon to expend greater effort to help the growing numbers of handicapped children.

Observations based on epidemiologic surveys indicate that children with chronic illnesses fare less well than normals. The frequency of secondary disorders, educational retardation, behavior disorders, and behavioral maladjustment is higher in the diseased group (Pless & Roghmann, 1971).

The disorders with greatest frequency are respiratory disease, cancer (leukemia), tuberculosis, skin diseases, diabetes, heart disease (including rheumatic fever), sickle cell anemia in blacks, epilepsy, and asthma. We will discuss, only the last five, primarily because school and mental health personnel are more likely to be involved with children having these diseases.

Diabetes

Diabetes mellitus is a disorder in which the body is unable to metabolize carbohydrates, particularly sugar, because of insufficient production of insulin, a secretion of the pancreas. The disease is inherited as a recessive characteristic. Diabetes often is precipitated by some other illness, such as chicken pox. Early signs of the disorder are bed wetting, extreme hunger and unquenchable thirst, failure to gain weight in spite of eating, and extreme weakness. If untreated, these symptoms are followed by abdominal pain, nausea and vomiting, and finally by loss of consciousness (diabetic coma). The results of a glucose tolerance test and other laboratory studies substantiate the presence of the disease. The glucose tolerance test is performed by giving a certain amount of glucose to the patient, either orally or intravenously, and drawing blood samples at specified intervals. By this means, the patient's ability to metabolize glucose is determined.

Treatment includes the administration of insulin, a specially prepared extract of the pancreas which, when injected into the body, enables it to burn sugar. Urine is collected periodically to determine urine sugar level, which reflects blood sugar level, so as to guide modifications in insulin and carbohydrate dosage.

When a child is hospitalized following diabetic coma, part of his treatment includes attending group and individual instructional sessions where he learns to test his urine, use a syringe to measure and administer insulin, and review dietary procedures. The child's parents also attend these sessions. Before he leaves the hospital, the child has to demonstrate his knowledge of these procedures.

When the child returns home, his diet differs little from the rest of the family's, provided meals are well balanced and excesses are avoided, particularly excesses in carbohydrates. The child eats at regular intervals, has snacks at bedtime and between meals, and exercises after rather than before meals.

Usually the child has to rise an hour earlier than usual in the morning in order to void his urine and then, within an hour of emptying his blad-

IN THE HOSPITAL

(Poem by a 13-Year-Old Diabetic)
In the hospital there's just one thing that everyone minds
That is loads of shots in their behinds
One, two, three, away we go
Just three more shots. Oh no! Oh no!
No more shots for me, you see
My backside's as red as it can be
Oh well! Since his backside is so red
We'll have to let him just drop dead.

From J. E. Schowalter and R. D. Lord. The hospitalized adolescent. *Children*, 1971, **18**(4), 127–132.

der, urinate again to collect a sample for testing. This sample is tested both before eating and before taking insulin. Testing urine in the schools is sometimes a problem for the child since teachers do not always understand why the child has to visit the nurse twice. To avoid embarrassment, older children learn to take urine samples between school periods. Often the child can drop testing before lunch as a regular routine and test only when irregular events occur; such as special trips or minor illness.

The child must be aware of factors that change his need for insulin. First, adjustments have to be made when diet changes, such as when the child forgets his lunch and has to eat the school lunch (the child's packed lunches are high in protein, while school lunches are usually high in carbohydrates), when he goes on trips either with schoolmates or family, when he exercises excessively or irregularly (before eating), and when he is sick or upset about something.

Exercise results in a lowering of blood sugar level and can cause shock unless the insulin dose is reduced accordingly. The child can reduce his insulin dosage before planned exercise; he can be prepared for unplanned exercise by carrying a sugar cube to eat if he feels the beginning stages of shock resulting from too much insulin (see Table 6.4). It is not always easy to plan periods of exercise activity. Gym activities often change with the weather, and after school activities are frequently spontaneous happenings. School authorities will grant a request for gym after lunch, but the child doesn't always know how strenuous the activity planned will be. The child usually doesn't have to worry about what will happen if he does go into shock, since the school nurse knows what to do in such a situation. The child would be kept warm and injected with glucose if he were unconscious. While diabetics sometimes are excused from gym, this is not always necessary. Two of America's best tennis players, William Talbert and Ham Richardson, have been diabetic since childhood.

Table 6.4 SYMPTOMS OF INSULIN SHOCK AND DIABETIC COMA

	Insulin shock	Diabetic coma
Causes	Overdose of insulin	Infection
	Increase in exercise	Emotional agitation
	Reduction of diet	Nervous exhaustion
	Errors in insulin measurement	Excessive carbohydrates
Early signs	Pallor	Increased thirst
	Weakness	Increased urination
	Sweating	Increased hunger
	Sudden hunger	Loss of weight
	Mood change	Sugar in urine and blood
	Dizziness	Mood changes
	Tremor	Abdominal pain
	Dilated pupils	Vomiting
Severe reactions	Semiconsciousness	Dehydration
	Sugar-free urine	Acetone odor in breath
	Low blood sugar	Face flushed
	Coma	Lips cherry red
	Localized muscle jerkings	Little perspiration
	Convulsions	Coma
	Death	Death

When the child is sick, emotionally keyed up (adrenalin inhibits the activity of insulin), or menstruating, he or she has to take more insulin to prevent glycosuria (increased glucose in the urine) and eventual diabetic coma (see Table 6.4).

Some older children are bothered by being unable to sleep late on weekends. They must have their breakfast at a regular time each day, because a delay in meals may produce shock. If the child overextends himself during the week and plans to rest on the weekend, he has to decrease his insulin dose on Saturday morning.

Any cuts, bruises, wounds, or fractures the child receives heal just as easily as the normal child's and are no more likely to become infected. If cuts do become infected, however, a doctor's care is crucial because infections change the body's reaction to insulin.

Conflict in families with diabetic children   Family strife is often greater among families of diabetic children than among families of nondiabetics. Parents of diabetics have more marital discord and more disagreements about child rearing practices. The diabetic child, like the child with other disabilities, precipitates a family crisis (Crain, Sussman, & Weil, 1966). Because the disorder is hereditary many parents blame themselves unduly for their child's disorder. Perhaps this unresolved guilt causes them to be overprotective, a behavior that eventually leads to open conflict between parent and child. Joan, described below, serves as an exam-

A BASEBALL PLAYER

On two successive Sunday mornings one of our patients, a 10-year-old boy, was admitted in severe diabetic acidosis. On each occasion he responded well to treatment and was discharged in a few days. The following Saturday night his mother reported the presence of a third episode. . . . As repeated hospitalizations for treatment of acidosis were somewhat embarrassing for us *vis-à-vis* both parents and house staff, we elected to treat this episode at home. This was successfully accomplished but the pattern of decompensation was repeated on the next two Saturday nights. Inquiry as to the possible significance of the time pattern of these episodes revealed that the patient played Little League Baseball on Saturdays and began to show signs of arousal the day before. The parents volunteered the observation that they had never witnessed such intensely grim determination as was revealed by their son during the progress of the game on Saturday. When the family was informed that this reaction was the probable cause of their son's decompensation, they explained to him that the game was supposed to be fun and if he were unable to enter into it on this basis he would have to give it up. Happily for everyone, he accepted this point of view and continued playing without further incident.

From R. Kaye & L. Baker. Standards for control of the child with diabetes. *Medical Science*, February 1965, pp. 41–55.

ple of how poor parental management of diabetes can lead the child to using her disorder to control her parents.

Joan was a teenager who was overly disturbed by her condition. Her parents were overindulgent and overprotective toward her, and they displayed an overanxious attitude about her health. Joan complained about being unable to eat certain foods and about her parents spying on her to see that she kept to her diet. She dreaded giving herself injections and frequently persuaded the school nurse to give them to her.

Joan's parents wanted her to attend a camp for diabetic children hoping that she would learn to manage her disease better if around other diabetics. She didn't want to go. When her parents insisted, she stopped taking her insulin and went into a diabetic coma (acidosis). Thereafter, whenever her parents did something she didn't like she threatened to repeat this act. She also threatened to eat sweets or not to eat at all. Eventually, Joan was seen by a psychiatrist, and after a year in treatment she was enrolled in a boarding school. While in the school, she managed herself well, but when home on vacations her old problems recurred.

The type of dietary control required for diabetic children may be related to the degree of conflict in their families, although no study of this relationship has been made. Until recently, strict dietary management was employed in treatment. As we learned in Chapter 3 in our discussion of phenylketonuria, strict dietary regimentation places great strain on a family, and as the child approaches adolescence, he frequently rebels against what he conceives of as rigid parental control. Perhaps this strict dietary program partially accounts for earlier findings that diabetics fared poorly (Fischer, 1948).

Current practice advocates free diet management. Some sugar excretion in the urine is permitted and precise controls over diet and insulin are relaxed. Although an exact food intake is not prescribed, regularity and consistency in diet are urged, and frequent urine tests are encouraged. Advocates recognize that parents may become lax and casual in the regulation of the disease, but in the long run believe that most families can achieve a satisfactory regulation and avoid the emotional rebellion that the stricter regimen often produces (Blake et al., 1970).

Effect on future marriage and career A teenage youngster, particularly a girl, usually has disturbing thoughts and many questions about the disorder. What kind of a future will she have? Will she be able to complete her education? What sort of a professional career can she have? Questions regarding her sexual development and social life trouble her the most. Will it interfere with her physical development? Will it rule out motherhood? Should I tell my dates or not?

Eventually, the adolescent girl learns that most of her fears are unwarranted. Physical development proceeds normally, and with proper management of diabetes, dating and marriage are no more difficult than for the nondiabetic teenager. There is, however, a high rate of abortion, stillbirth, neonatal death, prematurity, and pregnancy complication in the pregnant diabetic (Babson & Benson, 1966).

Because the disease is hereditary, the offspring of a diabetic can be either afflicted or carriers of the disorder, depending on whether the spouse of the diabetic also is a diabetic or a carrier of the disease. If two diabetics marry, all their offspring would be diabetics. If one spouse is diabetic and the other a carrier, half their children would be diabetic and the other half carriers. If one spouse is diabetic and the other nondiabetic and not a carrier, all their offspring would be carriers. If an offspring married a carrier, the chances would be one in four that one of their children (grandchild of the original diabetic) would be diabetic.

Although practically all professions are open to diabetics, some fields remain closed. Some school districts will not hire diabetics as teachers, but this practice is rapidly changing. Policework, fire fighting, and other hazardous jobs are closed. The diabetic is not allowed to operate any public conveyances, such as taxis, buses, trains, or planes, because of the danger of insulin shock at a crucial moment. High school guidance counselors and teachers often are unaware of these facts and, in addition, have misconceptions about the effect of the disorder on the diabetic's ability to function professionally (Collier, 1969b). Comparisons of diabetic with nondiabetic adolescents indicate that the diabetic presents self-descriptions similar to his nondiabetic counterpart (Collier, 1969a).

About the only difference reported between diabetics and nondiabetics is that a greater number of diabetics than nondiabetics fall below the third percentile on a distribution of height (Farquhar, 1969).

Knowledge of his disorder Approximately 4,200,000 people in the United States have diabetes. Perhaps 1,600,000 are undiagnosed diabetics, and 5,600,000 are potential diabetics (American Diabetes Association, 1969). Approximately 250,000 new cases are diagnosed each year. These figures are rapidly increasing as blood screening tests are tripling the numbers diagnosed (Diabetes Detection Program, undated).

Many diabetics know very little about the disease and its care. A survey of patients at home found that many—even those with diabetes of long duration—made numerous errors in their disease management (Watkins, Roberts, Williams, Martin, & Cole, 1967). Studies done at camps for diabetic children showed that patients and their families often were ignorant of the most basic facts about diabetes.

Nickerson (1972) had 72 known diabetics fill out a questionnaire about their condition. The average duration of diabetes for all patients was 7.5 years. A patient who answered all the questions correctly would receive a score of 41 (43 if insulin-dependent). The average score was 17.4! More than half stated they had never learned much about their diabetes. Fifty patients could not name a single symptom associated with an insulin reaction or with low blood sugar, 59 could not name any signs of high blood sugar, 27 did not know that a person with low blood sugar should eat something sweet, 33 did not know that high blood sugar means they have not taken enough insulin, and 40 did not know what was needed if they became ill or pregnant. In fact, 47 had no idea why they took insulin but only knew it "was scary." Even more distressing was that 38 patients had no idea what diabetes actually was and feared they would die from it. Sixty-five were aware, however, that eating sweets was not good for them.

A study of diabetics from 3 clinics and 22 private practices revealed that 58 percent of 115 patients taking insulin made dosage errors, 35 percent of which were potentially serious (Watkins, Williams, Martin, Hogan, & Anderson, 1967).

These studies point out the need for more thorough educational programs for the diabetic and his family. Watkins and Moss (1969) describe the kinds of confusions that exist in disease management, and Nickerson (1972) presents an educational program that she believes meets the educational needs of diabetics.

Heart disorders

Acquiring mastery over one's body is a developmental task of childhood requiring large amounts of gross motor activity. In addition, physical movement is the young child's best defense against anxiety. Activity, therefore, is critical for normal development. Young children even equate life with movement and death with its absence (Piaget, 1926). Restriction of movement not only denies a child a defense against anxiety, but also impairs his ability to attain body mastery. If, in addition, the restriction must be imposed for reasons not directly obvious to the child, developmental difficulties are bound to occur. Heart disease imposes such restriction.

Up to age 7, children know little about the heart. (Table 6.5 shows children's answers to questions about their heart categorized into three stages of thought.) The young child with heart disease often does not feel sick and therefore sees no reason for his restriction. Consequently, management problems are likely to develop.

For the older child, restriction means loss of peer contacts. Anxieties about this loss often are more prominent than anxieties relating to ill health or death (Shirley, 1963). Other factors compound these difficulties. Some heart diseases are treated with steroids, resulting in increased appetite and obesity. This increased obesity affects not only body image and self-concept but also peer relations. Many children become depressed both as a response to teasing from others and to their own changed body image. Some heart diseases may result in severely stunted growth and abnormal skin color. These differences, in addition to restriction in activity, further isolate the child from others. This isolation contributes to low self-esteem, insecurity, and hostility.

Congenital heart disorders   Although the majority of congenital heart conditions are surgically corrected by the time the child is of school age, many teachers are anxious about having a child with a heart condition in their class, fearing they might mistakenly do something to aggravate

Table 6.5   **CHILDREN'S ANSWER TO THE QUESTION, "WHAT IS YOUR HEART?"**

Age	Characterization
4–7	It "drums," "hammers," "bumps," "ticks"; "Valentine shaped"; "Helps us breathe." Heart characterized by sound. Not certain whether animals and trees have hearts.
7–10	"It beats," "It makes you live," "Need it to stay alive," "Death results when it stops." No emotion shown when referring to life-death aspects of heart, still relate heart to breathing. Veins mentioned.
10–11	Can explain idea of veins, valves, circulation, and pumping action. Can begin to explain why death can result from heart problems, but the concept that death could result from a cardiac condition is not yet complete. Majority show no emotion when describing what happens when the heart stops.

Adapted from K. Reif. A heart makes you live. *American Journal of Nursing*, 1972, **12**, 1085.

the condition. In addition, mental health practitioners often are called upon to help the family cope with the distress caused by the disorder. For these reasons, we have included information about the types of disease and their treatment, as well as about their practical management.

After the first eight weeks of intrauterine growth, the heart is completely developed. Several abnormalities can occur during intrauterine development, either in the heart itself or in the blood vessels leading to or from it. These defects may be hereditary, that is, defects inherent in the genes or germ plasm, or they may result from vitamin deficiency or viral infections, such as rubella, during the first trimester of pregnancy. Bone abnormalities, particularly those of the spine, also can affect the development of blood vessels in the embryo (Robinson, Abrams, & Kaplan, 1965).

The diagnosis of heart defect is based on the mother's health during pregnancy and on signs displayed by the infant, such as heart murmurs, varying degrees of cyanosis, and, in later months or years, poor development and clubbing of fingers and toes. Weakness and irritability often characterize the infant. Special medical procedures, such as radiographic examination or electrocardiography, confirm the diagnosis.

As recently as thirty years ago the only available therapy for the child with a congenital heart disorder was regulation of activity according to the tolerance of his abnormal circulatory system. Today, with advances in corrective surgery, even the more complex disorders sometimes can be corrected. Nevertheless, many heart disorders cannot be corrected until the child reaches a certain age. For example, surgical repair of the aorta usually is delayed until the child has achieved maximal growth. This delay is necessary because the segment used as a graft will not grow as will the main structure of the aorta. Because of this delay, many children suffering from these disorders experience the psychological effects that accompany any chronic illness.

There are two types of heart defects: (1) cyanotic, with varying degrees of the cyanosis (bluish hue of tissues, instead of normal pink, caused by inadequate saturation of the tissues with oxygen) and (2) acyanotic, where cyanosis is not present.

In cyanotic disorders venous blood mixes in the arterial circulation because of abnormal connections between the pulmonary and systemic circulations. Consequently, blood delivered to the periphery of the body is never fully saturated with oxygen. Cyanosis may not be apparent at birth, but may develop during the first year of life. It becomes more marked as the child matures, due in part to an increase in the number of red blood cells per unit volume of blood, an increase that takes place in an effort to improve the oxygen carrying capacity of the blood. When there is a substantial increase in red blood cells, the mucous membrances of the body become distended with purple blood, body growth is retarded, the capacity for exercise is reduced, and various complications arise as a result of the thickened blood within the vessels (Blake et al., 1970).

The most common type of cyanotic congenital heart disorder that permits survival is tetrology of Fallot. The condition usually retards the child's growth. Exercise causes severe difficulty in breathing. Fainting spells and occasional convulsions may occur in children over 2 when the degree of anoxia is increased temporarily. Most children with the disorder are of normal intelligence in spite of chronic circulatory disturbance and diminished oxygen supply to the brain.

Treatment is surgical and may be corrective or merely palliative. The invention of the heart-lung machine has permitted more frequent use of corrective surgical techniques. If the condition is critical, the operation may be performed in infancy. More frequently, however, it is postponed until the child is 3 years of age or older.

A child with tetrology of Fallot, or a similar disorder, is likely to be irritable and overdependent upon others. Because of his condition, parents are likely to be concerned about him continually. If he becomes cyanotic while crying or during bouts of respiratory infection, he may sense his parent's fears and become increasingly anxious about his own safety.

Overprotection frequently is carried to extremes, not only because the parents know the hazards of respiratory infections, but also because such measures reduce their own anxiety about possible harm to the child. Everything possible is done for the child to lessen his distress and anxiety. Because he fatigues easily, the child often refuses to do things for himself and his parents do them for him. Because they wish him to remain calm, they avoid upsetting him or making him cry. The child quickly realizes that crying can get him his way. As a result, he develops less frustration tolerance and fewer opportunities for mastery than his condition actually dictates. Sleeping and eating problems, night terrors, and temper tantrums are common. As a result, lack of self-confidence and a low frustration tolerance are added to the existing sense of insecurity about his unhealthy body. It is only normal for children who have suffered frequent bouts of infection, fainting spells, weakness, and pain to compare themselves unfavorably with other children (Blake & Wright, 1963; Marlow, 1969).

I USED TO!

I used to be able to run around the house without stopping. Then I started getting bigger. Now I can walk only to the corner of the house before I have to rest.

A statement by a young boy with heart disease. Cited in F. B. Roberts, The child with heart disease. *American Journal of Nursing*, 1972, **72**, 1080–1084.

If the child's parents are inconsistent in handling him, his anxiety increases. To deal with this anxiety, he may attempt to control his environment by increasing his demands upon his parents. As these demands increase, so do his parent's anxieties. This anxiety reduces their ability to make correct decisions, and their inconsistency increases. Thus, a self-defeating cycle is perpetuated. This cycle is more easily prevented than corrected. Anticipatory guidance of parents as well as continual help is crucial for the family's well being.

In acyanotic disorders, abnormalities in the course or caliber of the blood vessels leaving the heart result in blood pressure changes, headache, fatigue, weakness of the legs, fainting spells, and, in severe cases, cerebrovascular accidents and interference with growth. Corrective surgery is the only treatment, and operations in early or middle childhood are preferred, except in some disorders where maximal growth is needed in order to perform graftings.

Rheumatic fever   Rheumatic fever is an inflammatory disease of unknown origin that causes damage to the connective tissue of organ systems, the most important of which is the heart. The disease usually is precipitated by infection from a streptococcus virus. The initial infection with the streptococcus is followed by a latent or nonsymptomatic period lasting several weeks, and then rheumatic fever occurs (Marlow, 1969).

This disease is one of the leading causes of chronic illness in children, particularly those between the ages of 5 and 15. The first attack occurs most frequently between the ages of 6 and 8. The incidence follows the curve of incidence of streptococcal infections. The disease occurs more frequently in temperate zones and in the spring months in the United States. It is more prevalent among lower socioeconomic groups where poor nutrition and crowded living conditions lead to respiratory infections and easy transmission of the causative organism. Because the disease has a high family incidence, a hereditary predisposition is suspected (Blake et al., 1970; Marlow, 1969).

The symptoms of the disease are extremely variable in type and severity. Some children are mildly affected, while others experience severe attacks. The chief problem in rheumatic fever is that it tends to recur. Each recurrence can result in additional damage to the heart. Correct diagnosis, therefore, is important in order to shield the child from additional harm. The early symptoms are muscle and joint pains, pallor, nosebleed, malaise, and attacks of abdominal pain. Major manifestations are arthritic joints, inflammation of the membranes that link the cavities of the heart, and the occurrance of nodules of varying size in the muscle tendons. Rheumatic nodules also form in the various heart structures. These growths eventually interfere with the function of the heart valves and thus, place a strain on the heart muscle as it attempts to maintain circulation. The strain causes the heart muscle to dilate and results in circulatory inadequacy. The affected child shows pallor, moderate anemia, poor appetite, loss of weight, and easy fatigue. When the heart inflammation is severe, the child runs a high fever and must remain in bed.

When outlying infections subside and when the heart's work is kept at a minimum through rest, the natural healing powers of the body check the cardiac inflammation. Penicillin is given to eradicate the streptococci, and other medications are given to relieve fever. These drugs, however, do not terminate the rheumatic process; they only suppress it.

After several months of bed rest, a child usually recovers from the first attack. However, because of the tendency for heart inflammation and other rheumatic manifestations to recur, repeated damage to the heart may cause death due to failing circulation or invalidism due to heart deformity and dysfunction.

Prolonged bed rest and restriction in activity can create many psychological problems. Once there is evidence that the infection has disappeared, normal activity can resume and these problems may diminish. If heart damage persists, doctors typically recommend continuing restriction of the child's activity. They do so, however, even when there is no actual proof that rest prevents or minimizes heart damage (Gasul, Arcilla, & Lev, 1966).

It is important to prevent the recurrence of attacks. Exposure to cases of upper respiratory infection is avoided. If the child does acquire a respiratory infection, a throat culture is taken immediately to determine if streptococci are present. As a prophylactic measure, penicillin is given indefinitely after the attack, either monthly by intramuscular injections or daily by mouth (Marlow, 1969).

Currently, a vaccine designed to prevent childhood streptococcal infections is being tested. Its effectiveness, however, will not be known for some time.

The school's role in rehabilitation of heart disease In some cities schools provide home instruction for the child confined to his bed or install a telephone connection between the child's classroom and his home so he can hear the instruction given to his classmates. The school's main function, however, is to help the child adjust to his illness after his return to school. Teachers, as well as the school nurse, should be aware of his health plan. Other children should be helped to understand why the child may have a routine that differs from theirs. This understanding can come after discussions about the heart and its function. Considering Reif's (1972) findings regarding children's lack of knowledge about the heart, such discussions might prevent the teasing and ridicule often directed at children who are "different."

Because the child cannot participate in strenuous activity, alternative activities must be planned for him. For example, the elementary school child can help the teacher keep score in games he cannot play or he can be assigned a role where exercise is kept to a minimum. The child should be encouraged to develop skills in music and the creative arts so that when he is older he can successfully participate in dramatics, in glee club, or in other high school activities that do not require strenuous activity for successful achievement. The most trying time for the child with heart disease is in late elementary school when physical prowess relates to peer group acceptance. If the child can maintain his self-esteem through this period, his chances for acceptance at a later age are greater. If a child does not like himself, other children usually will not like him either.

Personality characteristics of children with heart disease Comparison of cardiac patients with normals on measures of personality have produced contradictory results. At worst, cardiac patients show more behavioral disturbances, particularly withdrawal and passivity, than normals. These differences, however, may be due to illness per se or even to hospitalization rather than to heart disease, since comparisons were made with normal children rather than with children having other chronic disorders. In other studies, the children evaluated were in special classes for cardiacs. These classes are now considered unnecessary and undesirable, for it has been found that children who receive special instruction, either at home or in special classes, tend to score lower on measures of IQ and achievement than do those who attend regular classes (Wrightstone, Justman, & Moskowitz, 1953). The differences found between cardiacs and normals in studies of children in special classes may be a consequence of their isolation rather than a characteristic of heart disease.

Landtman (1968) studied 200 children with congenital heart disorders and 56 with "imaginary" heart disease. The emotional reactions of children with actual disorders were studied both before and after surgery, as were the reactions of their mothers. Those mistakenly thought to have heart disease were investigated both before and after "delabeling."

Both groups of children showed remarkably similar behavior before their operation or delabeling. The occurrence of behavioral disorders was related to the degree of maternal overindulgence. The majority showed improved behavior after surgical correction or delabeling. In cases of actual disorders, 30 of 100 showed higher IQs when tested following surgery. Children with imaginary heart disease all developed symptoms and complaints in keeping with the nature of the disease. In some cases delabeling failed to convince parents that there wasn't a disorder. The length of time the family had lived with the symptoms of the disease was related to the degree of emotional problems present and the acceptance of the new diagnosis.

Sickle cell anemia

Arleen's birth passed without incident, and she was judged to be in good health. She was the third child born into a relatively healthy family. Development proceeded normally until shortly after her first birthday. She seemed thinner and paler than other children and had more frequent colds. One cold hung on, and eventually she developed a deep chest cough, shaking chills, a sharp pain in her chest, and a high fever. She was admitted to the hospital with pneumonia and severe anemia. A blood study revealed a low red blood cell count and the presence of many sickle-shaped cells among the normal round cells. A screening test for sickle cell anemia was positive and hemoglobin studies showed sickle hemoglobin rather than normal hemoglobin.

Arleen was placed in an oxygen tent where she was given intravenous fluids to maintain normal body fluid level and electrolyte balance, penicillin to combat her pneumonia, and a blood transfusion. She improved rapidly. Tests of her parents' blood revealed that both were carriers of the sickle cell trait.

Her parents were shocked. Both their other children were normal— why Arleen? They had heard the physician explain the nature of the disease, that it was inherited as a recessive trait and was incurable, but somehow it didn't sink in. It all seemed over so quick. Arleen had just begun to be a personality in the family, no longer a dependent baby but a mobile into-everything kid. Now she would have to be dependent again.

After they took Arleen home, they explained the nature of the disease to their other children so they wouldn't fear for their own health and also so they wouldn't resent the extra attention and special care Arleen would need. They explained that the red blood cells in Arleen's body had changed in shape from fat doughnuts to elongated sickles, sickles that clumped together to cut off the blood circulation in Arleen's knees, ankles, shoulders, stomach, brain, and other areas. She would be in severe pain and could lose consciousness at any time (Pochedly, 1971).

Although Arleen's family took all the precautions recommended by the hospital physicians, Arleen was readmitted to the hospital with a high fever, nausea, and vomiting. She was pale and her eyes had a yellow tint. Treatment was similar to that administered on her first admission. She again improved, but her right hand lost its coordination and her right foot dragged when she walked. A pediatric-neurological examination revealed a right hemiparesis caused by a cerebral blood clot which had occurred during her last crisis. She was referred to the physical therapy department at the hospital. Four months later, Arleen was again hospitalized, treated with intravenous fluids, and discharged.

By the time Arleen was 7 years old, she had been hospitalized twelve times. Substantial damage occurred to her liver as a result of the repeated crises of sickle cell anemia. Each crisis was extremely painful. Obstructions of the vessels in her lungs brought episodes of severe chest pain, causing her body to twist and contort as she tried to breathe. As they witnessed these attacks, her parents experienced great anguish and, at times, perhaps wished she would die and thereby avoid such suffering.

Even though Arleen receives excellent treatment at the hospital, it is unlikely that she will live through adolescence. If she does, her crises may be less frequent and less severe since the disease seems to subside somewhat in adulthood.

The problems faced by Arleen's parents are not uncommon among black Americans. Perhaps one in every ten American blacks carries the trait. Most of the carriers have very little sickling in their blood and have no trouble with it during their lifetime. If two trait carriers marry, they can expect that one in four of their children will have the severe disease called sickle cell anemia. The other two will be carriers and the fourth will be free from the trait.

The sickle gene is believed to have been a spontaneous mutation that occurred thousands of years ago in equatorial Africa. The sickle cell trait produces an enhanced resistance to infection by the malaria parasite. This resistance increases survival in malarial areas, resulting in natural selection of persons with the trait. In regions of Africa where malaria is endemic, the trait is found in close to 40 percent of the population (Pearson, 1971). Blacks are not the only carriers of the trait. Italians, Greeks, and other peoples living around the Mediterranean also are affected, but not to the degree found in blacks. Today, its possible usefulness gone, sickle cell anemia is a torturer and killer of blacks.

Epilepsy

Jimmy smelled that familiar unpleasant smell, felt the tingling in his legs, and heard the teacher's voice fade, but before he could speak, he lost consciousness. The child in the seat next to him saw Jimmy's arm begin to quiver and then his whole body shake. The other children saw Jimmy fall from his seat and shake violently. He seemed to have difficulty breathing and saliva collected in his mouth and ran from his lips. He was having a seizure.

Mrs. Brown quickly moved to help Jimmy, shoved aside nearby furniture, loosened the clothing around his neck, turned him on his side so that he did not aspirate his saliva, and placed a stick between his teeth to keep him from biting his tongue. When Jimmy's jerking stopped, he looked very sleepy and was taken to the nurse's office to rest.

Mrs. Brown simply told her class that Jimmy had had a seizure; that he would need to take some medicine to prevent another attack, but if it happened again his friends could help him not to hurt himself during the seizure. Two students near Jimmy would be prepared to help the teacher place Jimmy on her coat, another asked to run for the nurse, and one of his close friends asked to sit and talk with him when he woke up. She added that Jimmy feels no pain and, in spite of the violent movements, slow breathing, and paleness, would not die, although he would need to rest when the seizure was over. She made it clear that, aside from the seizures, Jimmy is the same as the rest of the class and would continue to participate in all the regular activities.

Jimmy's teacher reacted without undue alarm. She explained his disorder simply and matter-of-factly, prepared her students for possible future attacks, and continued to treat Jimmy as she had before the attack. The nurse had cautioned her that although Jimmy was on medication to control grand mal seizures, he could have an occasional seizure in class, particularly if he became overly anxious.

Mrs. Brown was familiar with epilepsy. The year before she had become concerned about one child who sometimes stared into space and rolled his eyeballs. Unlike a normal child's daydreaming, these episodes were brief, perhaps no more than 30 seconds, and the child seemed confused following their termination. She discussed the child with the school psychologist who then referred the youngster to a pediatric neurologist. The neurologist identified the child's disorder as epilepsy (recurrent convulsive disorder). He had petit mal rather than the grand mal seizures that Jimmy experienced.

In addition to grand mal and petit mal epilepsy, some children have psychomotor seizures. During these seizures, the child performs motions that appear purposeful but which are irrelevant to the current task in which he is engaged; for instance, chewing, smacking lips, or fiddling with the buttons on clothing.

In about half the children who have recurrent seizures, there is no known reason for the disorder. Medication controls the seizures in about 85 percent of the cases (Marlow, 1969). The other half show signs of organic pathology traced to damage of brain tissue or structural malformations of the brain. A high percentage of retarded and cerebral palsied children and a small percentage of learning disabled children have recurrent seizures (see Table 8.2 in Chapter 8). Different types of organic epilepsy show a variety of EEG abnormalities. Epilepsy is not a specific disease entity, but rather a general term to embrace a variety of recurrent seizure patterns, both of known and unknown origin.

Teachers often are concerned when they learn they have an epileptic in their classes. This concern is primarily the result of ignorance about the disorder, how they should treat the child, and what to do in case of a seizure. Frequently, they fail to discipline the child for fear of eliciting a seizure. In addition, they attribute behaviors that are the result of other factors to his condition. For example, they may believe that temper tantrums or aggressiveness are part of his seizure pattern. Psychological consultation can help ease the teacher's anxiety, as well as assist her to find an appropriate course of action when the epileptic displays behavioral maladjustment.

Asthma

We have seen that children suffering from chronic illness are vulnerable children who have a greater likelihood of developing emotional problems. This maladjustment can, in turn, aggravate their illness. No one would postulate, however, that emotional maladjustment produced the chronic conditions we have considered so far. This is not the case with asthma. People have always been aware of the relationship between respiratory disturbances and emotional disturbances. The Hatha-Yoga system of breathing exercises, practiced for thousands of years in the east, was designed to control one's emotions. Thus, the study of asthma proceeds in two directions. First, the study of physical states to which the respiratory system is allergic and, second, the study of psychological states to which the respiratory system responds.

Asthma is defined as "breathing with difficulty." The difficulty results from a spasm of the bronchial muscle. The spasm is caused, in a mechanical sense, by an imbalance of the parasympathetic and sympathetic nervous systems; the action of the sympathetic fibers, which induces relaxation of the bronchial muscle, is overcome by the action of the vagus nerve, which causes constriction of the bronchial muscle. After the initial spasms, thick, tenacious mucus collects, causing further obstruction of the air passages. During the attack, not all the inspired air can be expired and some collects in the alveoli, thereby causing obstructive emphysema (enlargement, overdistention, and destructive changes in aveoli). Wheezing and rales (a hoarse sound in the lungs), due to the bronchial secretions, accompany the spasm. The attack may last for several hours or for several days. Eventually, the child coughs up the mucus, and the spasm diminishes.

The exact reason for the imbalance between the two nervous systems is unknown. The somatic, or physical, approach emphasizes abnormal antigen-antibody reactions. When an antigen or foreign substance enters the body, the body defends itself by creating an antibody to either destroy the antigen or render it harmless. The allergic individual produces histamine in large quantities in response to the antigen-antibody reaction, and this increased level of histamine causes the various manifestations of the acute allergic reaction. Logan (1962), after reviewing 121 research studies, describes in detail the changes in body chemistry that cause allergic reactions. As is the case with other disorders discussed in this text, more boys than girls (2 to 1) have asthma (Freeman & Johnson, 1964a).

Clinical evidence indicates that asthmatic attacks occur more often following a cold, vigorous activity, particular foods, respiratory infections, or contact with allergic substances. Nevertheless, it has not been determined whether illnesses such as colds, bronchitis, or pneumonia, trigger the asthmatic attack, aggravate allergic reactions already in progress, or sensitize the bronchial mucosa to other agents (Freeman & Todd, 1962).

In the psychosomatic approach (the term psychosomatic refers to an interaction between mind and body) the asthmatic attack is considered a body dysfunction caused primarily by emotional reactions, usually in combination with a physiological (somatic) condition. Most investigators who hold a psychosomatic viewpoint admit that the asthmatic has an allergic reaction to certain substances, but they believe that the frequency and perhaps intensity of asthmatic attacks are related to emotional stress. Metcalfe (1956) presents the case of a girl whose asthmatic attacks always occurred when she was reunited with her mother. Cases such as this substantiate the theory that asthmatic attacks occur in response to emotional stress (Garner & Wenar, 1959; Miller & Baruch, 1950; Prugh, 1962, Purcell & Metz, 1962).

A few investigators believe that asthma may be a learned behavior and unrelated to an allergic condition. One group believes asthma to be a classically conditioned response (Dekker & Groen, 1956; Dekker, Pelser, & Groen, 1957; Stubblefield, 1966). Turnbull (1962) postulated that asthma was a conditioned avoidance reaction, a learned way of avoiding stress.

Alexander's (1950) suppositions epitomize the psychoanalytic viewpoint of asthma. He suggests that a specific unconscious conflict arouses anxiety. The anxiety, a signal of danger to the patient's ego, sets in motion a series of specific unconscious psychological reactions involving psychological defenses and regressive phenomena. These emotional reactions have specific parasympathetic and/or sympathetic concomitants that affect specific visceral organs. The excessive autonomic organ innervation caused by the chronic tension of repressed conflicts leads to disturbances in function, which eventually lead to organic pathological changes in susceptible individuals.

Kaplan and Kaplan (1959, p. 1094) believe that psychosomatic diseases are a consequence of a breakdown of psychological defenses rather than of repressed conflicts.

We believe that as long as a patient can deal with unpleasant emotions and with the anxiety engendered by his conflicts by means of various psychological defenses and mechanisms, there will be no abnormal psychogenic functioning nor resultant psychosomatic illness. If, however, a patient's psychological defenses are inadequate to reduce his excited or anxious state, so that he is left in a chronic state of emotional tension, then a variety of psychosomatic diseases may be produced in constitutionally susceptible individuals as a result of the physiological concomitants of chronic tension.

Research into causation Studies indicate that the majority of asthmatic attacks occur prior to age 13. In approximately 80 percent of the children skin tests indicate that the asthma is due to allergy, sensitiveness to foreign substances in dust and occasionally to foods (see Table 6.6). In the majority of cases, eczema in infancy due to foods, especially to eggs and cow's milk, precedes the onset of asthma (Dees, 1957; Rackemann & Edwards, 1952a).

Follow-up studies indicate that over 60 percent of patients with childhood asthma are no longer asthmatic by their teens (Dees, 1957; Freeman & Johnson, 1964b; Pap, 1962; Rackemann & Edwards, 1952a, 1952b). Buffum's (1963) data suggests that the prognosis is less favorable for children who show allergic reactions to skin tests within the first two years of life than it is for those who display asthmatic symptoms during the same age period but whose skin tests are negative. In addition, children whose asthmatic attacks first occur after age 13 have a poor prognosis (Freeman & Johnson, 1964b; Rackemann & Edwards, 1952a, 1952b).

In approximately 20 percent of Rackemann and Edward's sample, skin tests were negative (see Table 6.6). Although the two investigators labeled these cases "bacterial asthma," perhaps the cause was psychosomatic in origin. If so, then we might expect that the follow-up data of this group would differ from that of the other groups. Examination of Table 6.6, however, reveals that a greater number of the bacterial group were cured by the time of the follow-up. Since conditioned avoidance responses are hard to extinguish and long-standing conflicts not easily resolved, the likelihood that these disorders were learned reactions or expressions of conflict is a remote one. More likely, these children had a less severe allergic disorder.

What about children whose asthma persists through adolescence? Perhaps they learn to use their asthmatic attacks to avoid stressful situations. Not likely. The children who retain their asthma more often have multiple allergies and, therefore, could be considered more serious cases (Freeman & Johnson, 1964b). While family history data suggests that asthma is hereditary, the family histories of adolescents who continue to display symptoms were similar to those whose symptoms had subsided (Freeman & Johnson, 1964b).

Since close to two-thirds of asthmatic children show other allergic manifestations, such as rhinitis (inflammation of nasal muscosa) and eczema (inflammation of the skin), and since the majority have diminished symptoms at adolescence, a time when emotional problems are magnified, it is unlikely that emotional factors greatly contribute to the incidence of the disorder. Perhaps a few isolated cases may fit the psychosomatic model. In those showing emotional maladjustment, the family's reaction to the child's disease probably is responsible for the maladjustment and may even intensify the disease process (Block, Jennings,

Table 6.6 ORIGINAL CLASSIFICATION AND PRESENT STATUS

Original cause of asthma	Total	"Cured"	Relieved; still sensitive	Other allergy	Mild symptoms	Trouble; no hospital	Trouble; hospital	Dead
Animal	114 (25.8%)	19	55	17	13	7	0	3 (1 of asthma)
Foods	36 (8.1%)	16	10	6	0	4	0	0
Pollens	21 (4.7%)	4	0	0	12	5	0	0
Hay fever	(86)	(2)	(11)	(25)	(42)	(3)	(0)	(3)
Mixed and unidentified	199 (43.3%)	50	22	60	26	24	9	8 (3 of asthma)
Negative tests ("bacterial"?)	79 (17.9%)	49	0	13	17	0	0	0
Totals	449 (100%)	138 (30.7%)	87 (19.3%)	96 (21.4%)	68 (15.1%)	40 (8.9%)	9 (2.0%)	11 (2.4%)
		(71.4%)				28.4%		

From F. M. Rackemann & M. C. Edwards. Asthma in children: a follow-up study of 688 patients after an interval of twenty years. *New England Journal of Medicine*, 1952, **246**, 815–823.

Harvey, & Simpson, 1964). The findings of many studies also could be reinterpreted to suggest that the severity of the disease intensifies family conflict rather than vice versa.

Recently, Resh (1970) suggested that adolescents and adults with asthma with an unknown origin (UO) are psychologically different from those whose asthma has an allergic basis. The UO group rated themselves as more severely ill and as being more limited because of their asthma. They also scored higher on the hypochrondriasis, hysteria, and depression scales of a personality inventory. The UOs had less family history of asthma and were rated as no more seriously impaired than the other asthmatics.

While there is evidence that some asthmatics use their disorder to manipulate others, the notion that the disease is the result of psychosomatic factors remains unsupported. Nor is there evidence that individuals without appropriate psychological defenses are more likely to show allergic symptoms since the incidence of asthma is the same among psychiatric patients, organically impaired individuals, and psychiatrically normal individuals (Spiegelberg, Betz, & Pietsch, 1970). Childhood hysterics, individuals whose chief defense is repression, seem to suffer from psychosomatic complaints in adulthood, but asthma is not one of their complaints (Brisset, 1970; Reyher & Basch, 1970; Robins, 1966).

We do know that a relationship exists between psychological factors and prognosis for recovery. In physiologically severe asthma neurotic anxiety is related to good prognosis, probably because it leads to verbalization about one's concerns, and emotional restriction is related to poor prognosis. In contrast, in physiologically mild asthma anxiety is related to poor prognosis, probably because it leads to overconcern and perhaps the use of illness as an excuse to avoid activities which raise anxiety (Schubert, 1969). We also know that psychotherapy, both behavioral and psychodynamic, sometimes results in improvement of the condition (Moorefield, 1971), but the manner in which it does so remains unclear.

Regardless of the outcome of future research, asthma remains one of the leading causes of absenteeism from school (Freeman & Johnson, 1964a). Both parents and teachers, therefore, need help to cope with children who have this disorder.

PROBLEMS IN DIFFERENTIAL DIAGNOSIS

We conclude our discussion of chronic diseases with the presentation of several disorders that can be mistaken for something else. We will present an actual case where the early symptoms of a fatal disease, muscular dystrophy, were attributed to minimal brain dysfunction, a disorder briefly mentioned in Chapter 1 and discussed more fully in Chapter 8. (The student might review this case after studying Chapter 8, for the discussion of minimal brain dysfunction may give him a greater appreciation of the reasons for the diagnostic mistakes.)

SCOTT: DEVELOPMENTAL LAG, BRAIN DAMAGE, OR MUSCULAR DYSTROPHY

Scott was referred to the social service department of his local community hospital. For some time this hospital had been providing diagnostic, treatment, and consultation services to families whose children displayed learning disabilities. Scott had been referred by his family physician after Scott's nursery school staff became concerned about his poor physical skills. His parents agreed with the observations of the school staff, although they always had felt that Scott was just lazy, and therefore had no strong urge to climb, swing, or ride a tricycle.

The social worker's interview of Scott's mother revealed the following information about Scott's birth. Pregnancy was uneventful, but Scott was born with his umbilical cord wrapped around his neck and he had difficulty initiating breathing. Nevertheless, oxygen was not administered nor was he placed in an incubator, indicating that the attending physician was not alarmed by the manner of his birth. He weighed 8 pounds.

Birth records obtained from the hospital where Scott was born revealed that, in addition to the delayed breathing, he experienced a mild left parietal hematoma (bleeding within the subdural space).

Scott's motor development was somewhat slow. He did not sit until 9 months and did not walk until 15 months. Speech developed early; he spoke his first words at 8 months. Toilet training was initiated at about 2 years, but was not yet completed since he was still a bed-wetter and soiled himself daily. His parents could not tell whether Scott didn't know when his bowels were going to move or whether he deliberately refused to use the toilet. His mother yelled, spanked, and ignored him, but could not get him to use the toilet spontaneously. Scott was able to dress himself, but because he was so slow to do so, his mother frequently dressed him herself.

A phone conversation with Scott's nursery school teacher supported his parents' feelings that his motor behavior was atypical and that he was socially immature. He related well to his teacher but not to his peers. He did not enter into group activities, such as singing, although his mother reported that he sang his school songs at home. On the playground, he simply watched others playing, stating that "Watching is what I like to do."

Although Scott had occasional sore throats and he once had a fever during a bout with bronchitis, he had had no severe illnesses, accidents, or operations and was described as a healthy child. He did have flat feet.

Scott was a quiet child who was neither overactive nor impulsive. Although he dominated his younger sibling, he was very shy in a group of peers. Except for his stubborn refusal to perform physical tasks, his parents felt he was easy to manage. Unless forced by an adult, Scott would not try to ride his tricycle nor would he use his wagon or sled unless pulled by an adult. He also was afraid to balance himself on his swings. He did enjoy fine motor tasks, such as puzzles or blocks, but preferred to play alone; if he was with peers, he tended to play alongside rather than with them.

Scott's younger sister greatly excelled him in physical agility and coordination, but they got along well. In fact, Scott's chief playmate was his sister as no children Scott's age lived in his immediate neighborhood. Both parents reported a relatively harmonious family that participated together in recreational activities. The father, however, because of his disinterest in nonphysical activities, spent little time alone with Scott. Both parents felt Scott's failure to excell physically resulted from their failures to press for and reward achievement in this area.

Scott's mother impressed the social worker as a warm and spontaneous person, but one who reinforced her children's dependency upon herself. The father was viewed as emotionally detached but motivated to help his son.

Following the interviews with the mother and the school staff, the social worker recommended a psychological evaluation. A week later Scott returned to the hospital and was seen by their staff psychologist. The psychologist described him as an extremely passive, seemingly fearful, and hypoactive child who sat in a hunched, stooped over manner. He usually looked to the examiner for possible cues to guide his action in each new testing situation. Failure was never followed by a renewed attempt, and initiative was conspicuously absent. Scott simply refused to try many test items, particularly motor and perceptual-motor items. His speech was difficult to understand, with poor articulation, elongation of word parts, and dropping of word parts. He would not hop, would run only while holding the examiner's hand, and was poor at bouncing and kicking a ball.

On the Stanford-Binet IQ test Scott achieved an average IQ, while on the Peabody Picture Vocabulary Test (a test where the child simply selects from four pictured objects the one the examiner names) his IQ was in the mildly retarded range. The examiner felt the poor Peabody suggested that Scott's receptive language skills were poor, perhaps explaining his imprecise expressive language.

Inconsistency was noted in visual-motor skill. On the Binet he failed visual-motor items at the 4-year level, yet passed one at the 6-year level. His drawing of a man was poorly conceptualized and perseveration destroyed the final configuration. A request to draw a dog resulted in a circle. Encouragement resulted in a larger, connected circle to represent the body, but legs and other features were absent.

The psychologist concluded that "While Scott had some neurological difficulties, it would be premature to suggest that the child's difficulty was anything more than a developmental lag." He suggested that attention be directed to the child's motor development within his present educational setting and that this attention be continued throughout kindergarten. If his motor difficulties persisted, then Scott should be reevaluated, perhaps also within the school setting where he could be observed. At that time an appropriate course of action could be suggested. The child's independence and initiative should be encouraged and, therefore, parental counseling was suggested.

A copy of the psychological report was sent to the family physician. One month later the physician received a letter from the psychologist stating that he had met with the social worker. After they had discussed the information that each had gathered on Scott, both felt that neurological and speech and hearing evaluations would be helpful. The speech and hearing evaluation could be performed at the hospital. Parental counseling, however, would not be necessary since the mother seemed amenable to suggestions to encourage Scott's independence.

For several reasons the family physician did not press the family to follow up on the recommendations for further evaluations. First, the psychologist's report suggested developmental immaturity or, at worst, minimal brain dysfunction, a condition the physician felt improved with age. If it were only developmental immaturity, why subject the family to the unnecessary expense of a neurological evaluation? It could always be done later, as suggested in the psychological report. The family was not concerned about Scott's language skills and felt a speech and hearing evaluation was unnecessary.

Second, the parents had been encouraged to concentrate on improving Scott's motor skills, the only real problem he displayed. Why not wait and see whether he improved? Often these same recommendations are made following a neurological diagnosis of minimal brain damage. Why pay for advice already given?

Scott's family followed the recommendations, but after two years he seemed to be getting worse. His family became increasingly concerned about him. They had Scott seen by a pediatrician associated with another hospital in the area. This doctor suspected that the previous diagnosis of developmental immaturity was in error and referred Scott to a pediatric neurologist.

The neurologist noted Scott's difficulty with large motor coordination, his stiffly held shoulder, and his clumsy attempts at running. He was now able to ride a tricycle, but if it got stuck or was difficult to move, he would not get off it. He had not tried to ride a two-wheeler. He was poor at climbing and still climbed stairs one at a time. He also walked on his toes with a slapping gait and had trouble getting up from the ground. He had just learned to button and zipper in the previous year.

The exam revealed atrophy and weakness in both shoulder girdle and pelvic girdle musculature, as well as in the speech musculature. In addition, there was marked enlargement of the calf muscles. The neurologist's impression was that Scott had Duchenne's dystrophy (muscular dystrophy). This impression was supported by elevated blood levels of the serum enzymes associated with this disease.

Forms of muscular dystrophy

Muscular dystrophies are inherited diseases characterized by progressive weakness due to degeneration of muscle fibers. Accompanying the degeneration of fibers is a change in muscle fiber size, an increase in connective tissue, and a deposition of fat. These changes affect skeletal muscle primarily, but cardiac muscle is sometimes involved. Classification of the disorder depends upon individual clinical and genetic patterns.

In the most common form, *Duchenne's* dystrophy, only males are affected. The disease is hereditary (sex-linked and recessive), but, as in Scott's case where there was no family history of the disease, sporadic cases frequently occur.

The musculature of the pelvic girdle is usually the first to be affected. Consequently, the first sign that something is wrong appears when the affected child begins to walk. A waddling gait, toe walking, difficulty rising from a prone position, and frequent falls are the early symptoms; these symptoms were observed in Scott but were initially attributed to something else. The shoulder girdle is affected later and the face is involved, although minimally even in advanced cases. Progression occurs throughout childhood, and by early adolescence the patient is usually confined to a wheelchair. Victims typically succumb in early adulthood to some intercurrent disease.

A second form of the disease, called *Landouzy-Dejerine* distrophy, affects both males and females. This form is also inherited (autosomal dominant). Its onset is later than Duchenne's, usually in adolescence. Weakness of the shoulder girdle is the first sign and is more prominent than leg weakness. The face muscles are also affected. Progression is variable and slower than in the Duchenne form. Some patients eventually become disabled, while others barely notice their symptoms throughout a normal life span.

Other than prolonging ambulation by muscle strengthening exercises, corrective surgical measures, and appropriate braces, there is no known treatment for either of these two common forms. Periods of bed rest are avoided because muscle strength deteriorates in the absence of activity.

There are other muscular dystrophies and a variety of other muscular disorders that affect children. The interested reader is referred to Farmer (1964) or Ford (1966) for a discussion of these syndromes.

Reasons for the error in Scott's diagnosis

Why did the staff of the first hospital fail to diagnose Scott's illness correctly? Perhaps it was because of set. Being interested in learning disorders that result from neurological impairment, they were primed to look for these conditions. Their theoretical orientation biased their observations; an investigator interested in proving a theory is likely to see signs that support his bias and overlook or misinterpret those that do not. As will be seen in Chapter 8, children with both neurological impairment and developmental immaturity frequently display coordination difficulties. Finding these difficulties in Scott and knowing of his early birth complications, the staff drew a conclusion in keeping with their own interests. Unfortunately, it was the wrong conclusion!

Perhaps the chief problem was that neither the social worker nor the psychologist viewed children's disorders from a developmental perspective. Several principles of child development were overlooked in Scott's assessment. First, the large muscles are the first muscular groups over which the growing child gains coordinated control. Second, there is a proximodistal trend in motor development, that is, parts of the body closest to the torso are brought under coordinated control before more distal portions. Third, there is a maximum-toward-minimum muscular involvement trend; the more immature the child, the greater will be his muscular involvement, expenditure of energy, and cross-purpose muscular involvement when he engages in motor activity. Immature children usually squirm excessively and display superfluous large muscle movements when performing on small muscle tests.

Scott's behavior was not characteristic of developmental lag. He was better at fine than at gross motor skills and was underactive during his testing rather than restless or squirmy. Some children fear falling because of disturbances in equilibrium. These disturbances can be due to a large variety of diseases, including middle-ear tumor, tumors of the cerebrum, hemorrhage, ocular imbalance, and cardiac failure. Scott seemed more awkward then afraid, but the presence of disease was a possibility and should have been considered. The code of ethics of the American Psychological Association includes this statement (1967, p. 65).

The psychologist recognizes the boundaries of his competence and the limitations of his techniques and does not offer services or use techniques that fail to meet professional standards in particular fields. The psychologist who engages in practice assists his client in obtaining professional help for all important aspects of his problem that fall outside the boundaries of his own competence.

This principle requires, for example, that provision be made for diagnosis and treatment of relevant problems and referral to or consultation with other specialists.

The psychologist did not violate the latter part of this principle since he did recommend referral to a neurologist and he had taken the referral from a physician. Nevertheless, his behavior was questionable on two counts. First, the psychologist who has not had wide exposure to children's diseases and yet works in a hospital setting where he is asked to look for signs of cerebral dysfunction should do so only as part of a team that includes a pediatrician or pediatric nurse associate, and then he should consider his test findings in the light of medical findings. Second, the practice of administering psychological tests to children and then referring them to a neurologist prior to a thorough pediatric evaluation is a costly procedure and should only be done after all other possibilities have been considered.

Regarding the first part of the code, the psychologist who independently evaluates children for possible concomitants of brain injury should have extensive experience with children and specialized training in neuropsychology. The social worker should have deferred action on the case until the child has been seen by a pediatrician. The proper procedure in Scott's case should have been similar to the procedure followed in diagnosing Art (case presented in Chapter 2). Physical diseases should have been considered first. The psychologist should then have been brought in to assist the physician in his diagnosis or to contribute data regarding the child's reaction to his disability. Like the physician who must not overlook the role of emotional factors in illness, the psychologist must not overlook the possibility of physical disease.

Behavioral changes as signs of disease

Although SSPE (subacute sclerosing panencephalitis) is a rare disease (1 in 100,000 children who have measles under the age of 4 will develop SSPE), it is mentioned here to emphasize that the first symptoms of some diseases are behavioral and, therefore, initially present diagnostic difficulties to non-medically trained personnel who may evaluate the child.

In the first stage of SSPE the child may become irritable, defiant, withdrawn, and shy. Lethargy, inappropriate affect, speech difficulties, and some drooling may occur. Often, neither the parent nor the teacher recognizes these behaviors as symptoms of a disease process. The child may run away from home when playing outside or wander around the house at night when his parents are sleeping. Occasionally, the child will scream and fight against ordinary activities of daily living, such as his bath.

In the second stage of the disease the child develops jerking movements involving the whole body. They may be mild, quick, jerking involuntary movements of the arms, or they may be so severe that the child is thrown from the bed or chair. When the child becomes excited, the jerking increases and disappears only with sleep. Occasionally a child will display other involuntary movements, hand tremors, or spasticity.

In the third stage the child becomes comatose and his response to pain is reduced. In the fourth stage there is a decrease in the jerking reactions and other involuntary actions, causing the parents to have false hopes, since the child usually dies in this stage from serious infections or, as in muscular dystrophy, from respiratory distress (Furr, 1972).

Children can get this disease at almost any age and live from three months to three years after onset (Jabbour et al., 1969). A study of eight children with the disease, ranging in age from 2 years, 5 months to 12 years, indicated that they all had measles antibodies in their blood serum and cerebrospinal fluid. They all had had measles from two to ten years before the onset of symptoms (Jabbour et al., 1969). The disease affects far more males than females (5 to 1 incidence). Canaday (1972) describes the support needed by a family in order to cope with this terminal disease.

Because the early signs of serious diseases can be behavioral disturbances, school staff should consult with the child's pediatrician or family physician before they take any action on a child's behalf.

CONCLUDING REMARKS

Common to all chronic childhood disorders is a disruption of family structure. Each disease discussed upsets the equilibrium of family life. Under pressure, parents often lose sound judgment and the family remains in a condition of unrest (Kottgen, 1969). Many times a physician's advice is ignored for no obvious reason. Sometimes parents simply blot it out by forgetting it or become confused and cannot follow it or change the advice into something they wanted to do in the first place or distort the advice so that it appears fallacious and can be justifiably ignored (Bird, 1964).

This paradoxical response to a physician's advice usually occurs when the physician concerns himself with the patient only. Unconsciously, parents often resent a doctor's preoccupation with their child and feel that he is overlooking their problems. When a parent's own fears are recognized and talked about, they usually follow advice well (Bird, 1964). Since it is unlikely that physicians will ever pay a great deal of attention to the needs of other family members or even to the total needs of the child (de Boer et al., 1970), a multidisciplinary approach is necessary in order to service the physically ill child.

Faced with illness and hospitalization, a child often regresses to an earlier mode of functioning; prolonged illness or hospitalization can result in arrestment at that level. Many patients with temporary illnesses continue to complain of being ill long after their physical symptoms have disappeared. The ill child often seeks undue attention from adults to compensate for the normal pleasures he has had to forego. Crying and complaining usually bring him his desired attention. When complaints don't work, he feigns illness or develops psychosomatic or hysterical disorders. If such behavior is reinforced in early childhood, psychosomatic complaints can persist as a way of maintaining interpersonal contact (Szilagyi, 1968) and can lead to high absenteeism from school (Frerichs, 1969). The occurrence of maladaptive behavior is a strong possibility in the child with a chronic disorder. Psychiatric and psychological assistance to both the child and his family can help prevent its development.

According to Kurt Lewin's field theory, illness occurs in a field consisting of social, cultural, biological, and psychological events. Since a disease arises in a social setting, reactions to it are culturally defined (Schwab, 1971). Community support systems often help determine the course of a disorder, and community attitudes affect parental attitudes. While these variables may play a stronger role in mental disorders, they should not be underestimated when attempting to understand reactions to physical disorders.

References

Alexander, F. *Psychosomatic medicine.* New York: Norton, 1950.

American Diabetes Association. *Detecting unknown diabetics: the labor leader's role.* New York: American Diabetes Association, 1969.

American Psychological Association. *Casebook on ethical standards of psychologists.* Washington, D.C.: American Psychological Association, 1967.

Babson, S. G., & Benson, R. C. *Primer on prematurity and high-risk pregnancy.* St. Louis, Mo.: Mosby, 1966.

Berni, R., Dressler, J., & Baxter, J. C. Reinforcing behavior. *American Journal of Nursing,* 1971, **71,** 2180–2183.

Berni, R., & Fordyce, W. E. *Be   .or modification in the nursing process.* St. Louis, Mo.: Mosby, 1973.

Bird, B. A mother's parad°   response to advice. *American Journal of Diseases of Children,* 1964, **107,** 383–385.

Blake, F. G., & Wright, F. H. *Essentials of pediatric nursing.* (7th ed.) Philadelphia: Lippincott, 1963.

Blake, F. G., Wright, F. H., & Waechter, E. H. *Nursing care of children.* (8th ed.) Philadelphia: Lippincott, 1970.

Block, J., Jennings, P. H., Harvey, E., & Simpson, E. Interaction between allergic potential and psychopathology in childhood asthma. *Psychosomatic Medicine,* 1964, **26,** 307–320.

Brain, D. J., & Maclay, I. Controlled study of mothers and children in hospital. *British Medical Journal,* 1968, **1,** 278–280.

Brisset, C. Hysteria and psychosomatic disorders: structural and historical relationships. *Evolution Psychiatrique,* 1970, **35,** 377–404.

Buffum, W. P. The prognosis of asthma in infancy. *Pediatrics,* 1963, **32**, 453–455.

Canady, M. E. SSPE—helping the family cope. *American Journal of Nursing,* 1972, **72**, 94–96.

Capes, M. The child in the hospital. *Mental Hygiene,* 1956, **40**, 107–159.

Chappelle, M. L. The language of food. *American Journal of Nursing,* 1972, **72**, 1294–1295.

Collier, B. N., Jr. The adolescent with diabetes and the public schools—a misunderstanding. *Personnel and Guidance Journal,* 1969a, **47**, 753–757.

Collier, B. N., Jr. Comparisons between adolescents with and without diabetes. *Personnel and Guidance Journal,* 1969b, **47**, 679–684.

Condon, S. R. Day-time hospital for children. *American Journal of Nursing,* 1972, **72**, 1431–1433.

Crain, A. J., Sussman, M. B., & Weil, W. B., Jr. Effects of a diabetic child on marital integration and related measures of family functioning. *Journal of Health and Human Behavior,* 1966, **7**, 122–127.

Cytryn, L., Cytryn, E., & Rieger, R. E. Psychological implications of cryptorchism. *Journal of the American Academy of Child Psychiatry,* 1967, **6**, 131–165.

de Boer, R. A., et al. An evaluation of long-term seminars in psychiatry for family physicians. *Psychiatry, Washington, D.C.,* 1970, **33**, 468–481.

Dees, S. C. Development and course of asthma in children. *American Journal of Disease of Children,* 1957, **93**, 228–233.

Dekker, E., & Groen, J. Reproducible psychogenic attacks of asthma. *Journal of Psychosomatic Research,* 1956, **1**, 58–67.

Dekker, E., Pelser, H. E., & Groen, J. Conditioning as a cause of asthma. *Journal of Psychosomatic Research,* 1957, **2**, 97–108.

Diabetes Detection Program. *Successful public screening—diabetes as a role.* New York: American Diabetes Association, undated.

Dodge, J. S. What patients should be told: patient's and nurse's beliefs. *American Journal of Nursing,* 1972, **72**, 1852–1854.

Duckett, C. L. Caring for children with sickle cell anemia. *Children,* 1971, **18**, 227–231.

Easterbrook, J. A. The effect of emotion on cue utilization and the organization of behavior. *Psychological Review,* 1959, **66**, 183–201.

Farquhar, J. W. Prognosis for babies born to diabetic mothers in Edinburgh. *Archives of Diseases in Childhood,* 1969, **44**, 36–47.

Farmer, T. W. (Ed.) *Pediatric neurology.* New York: Harper & Row, 1964.

Fischer, A. E. Factors responsible for emotional disturbance in diabetic children. *Nervous Child,* 1948, **7**, 78–83.

Ford, F. R. *Diseases of the nervous system in infancy, childhood and adolescence.* (5th ed.) Springfield, Ill.: C. C Thomas, 196

Freeman, G. L., & Johnson, S. Allergic disea adolescence. I. Description of survey; prevalence of allergy. *American Journal of Diseases of Children,* 1964a, **107**, 549–559.

Freeman, G. L., & Johnson, S. Allergic diseases in adolescence. II. Changes in allergic manifestations during adolescence. *American Journal of Diseases of Children,* 1964b, **107**, 560–566.

Freeman, G. L., & Todd, R. H. The role of allergy in viral respiratory tract infections. *American Journal of Diseases of Children,* 1962, **104**, 44–48.

Freiberg, K. H. How parents react when their child is hospitalized. *American Journal of Nursing,* 1972, **72**, 1270–1272.

Frerichs, A. H. Relationship of elementary school absence to psychosomatic complaints. *Journal of School Health,* 1969, **39**, 92–95.

Freud, A. The role of bodily illness in the mental life of children. *Psychoanalytic Study of the Child,* 1952, **7**, 69–81.

Furr, S. C. Subacute sclerosing panencephalitis—care of the child. *American Journal of Nursing*, 1972, **72**, 93–95.

Garner, A., & Wenar, C. *The mother-child interaction in psychosomatic disorders.* Urbana: University of Illinois Press, 1959.

Gasul, B. M., Arcilla, R. A., & Lev, M. *Heart disease in children.* Philadelphia: Lippincott, 1966.

Hill, H. E., Flanary, H. G., Kornetsky, C. H., Conan, H., & Wikler, A. Effects of anxiety and morphine on discrimination of intensities of painful stimuli. *Journal of Clinical Investigation*, 1952, **31**, 473–480.

Jabbour, J. T., et al. Subacute sclerosing panencephalitis: multidisciplinary study of eight cases. *Journal of the American Medical Association*, 1969, **207**, 2248–2254.

Kaplan, H. I., & Kaplan, H. S. Current theoretical concepts in psychosomatic medicine. *American Journal of Psychiatry*, 1959, **115**, 1090–1097.

Knudson, A. G., & Natterson, J. M. Participation of parents in the hospital care of their fatally ill children. *Pediatrics*, 1960, **26**, 482–490.

Kottgen, U. The sick child and his family. *Praxis der Psychotherapie*, 1969, **14**, 261–266.

Landtman, B. Emotional implications of heart disease: a study of 256 children with real and with imaginary heart disease. *Annales Paediatriae Fenniae*, 1968, **14**, 71–92.

Langford, W. S. Physical illness and convalescence: their meaning to the child. *Journal of Pediatrics*, 1948, **33**, 242–250.

Levy, D. M. Psychic trauma of operations in children. *American Journal of Diseases of Children*, 1945, **69**, 7–25.

Logan, G. B. Chemical mediators of acute allergic reaction. *American Journal of Diseases of Children*, 1962, **104**, 185–197.

Marlens, H. S. A study of the effect of hospitalization on children in a metropolitan municipal institution. *Dissertation Abstracts*, 1960, **20**, 3385–3386.

Marlow, D. R. *Textbook of pediatric nursing.* (3rd ed.) Philadelphia: Saunders, 1969.

Metcalfe, M. Demonstration of a psychosomatic relationship. *British Journal of Medical Psychology*, 1956, **29**, 63–66.

Miller, H., & Baruch, D. W. Emotional traumata preceding the onset of allergic symptoms in a group of children. *Annals of Allergy*, 1950, **8**, 100–107.

Moorefield, C. W. The use of hypnosis and behavior therapy in asthma. *American Journal of Clinical Hypnosis*, 1971, **13**, 162–168.

Morrissey, J. R. Death anxiety in children with fatal illness. In H. J. Parad (Ed.), *Crisis intervention.* New York: Family Service Association of America, 1965.

Natterson, J. M., & Knudson, A. G. Observations concerning fear of death in fatally ill children and their mothers. *Psychosomatic Medicine*, 1960, **22**, 456–465.

Nickerson, D. Teaching the hospitalized diabetic. *American Journal of Nursing*, 1972, **72**, 935–938.

Pap, L. F. Effect on bronchial asthma of female puberty and adolescence. A follow-up study of fifty-three cases. *Annals of Allergy*, 1962, **20**, 733–738.

Pearson, H. A. Progress in early diagnosis of sickle cell disease. *Children*, 1971, **18**, 222–226.

Piaget, J. *The language and thought of the child.* (Translated by M. Warden) London: Routledge & Kegan Paul, 1926.

Piaget, J. *The child's conception of the world.* (Translated by J. Thomlinson & A. Thomlinson) London: Routledge & Kegan Paul, 1928.

Pless, I. B., & Roghmann, K. J. Chronic illness and its consequences: observations based on 3 epidemiologic surveys. *Journal of Pediatrics,* 1971, **79,** 351–359.

Pochedly, C. Sickle cell anemia: recognition and management. *American Journal of Nursing,* 1971, **71,** 1948–1951.

Prugh, D. G. Toward an understanding of psychosomatic concepts in relation to illness in children. In A. J. Solnit & S. A. Provence (Eds.), *Modern perspectives in child development.* New York: International Universities Press, 1962.

Drugh, D. G., Staub, E. M., Sands, H. H., Kirschbaum, R. M., & Lenihan, E. A. A study of emotional reactions of children and families to hospitalization and illness. *American Journal of Orthopsychiatry,* 1953, **23,** 70–106.

Purcell, K., & Metz, R. Distinctions between subgroups of asthmatic children; some parent attitude variables related to age of onset of asthma. *Journal of Psychosomatic Research,* 1962, **6,** 251–258.

Rackemann, F. M., & Edwards, M. C. Asthma in children. A follow-up study of 688 patients after an interval of twenty years. *New England Journal of Medicine,* 1952a, **246,** 815–823.

Rackemann, F. M., & Edwards, M. C. Asthma in children. A follow-up study of 688 patients after an interval of twenty years (concluded). *New England Journal of Medicine,* 1952b, **246,** 858–863.

Reif, K. A heart makes you live. *American Journal of Nursing,* 1972, **72,** 1085.

Resh, M. G. Asthma of unknown origin as a psychological group. *Journal of Consulting and Clinical Psychology,* 1970, **35,** 429.

Reyher, J., & Basch, J. A. Degree of repression and frequency of psychosomatic symptoms. *Perceptual Motor Skills,* 1970, **30,** 559–562.

Richmond, J. B., & Waisman, H. A. Psychologic aspects of management of children with malignant diseases. *American Journal of Diseases of Children,* 1955, **89,** 42–47.

Rie, H. E., Boverman, H., Ozoa, N., & Grossman, B. J. Tutoring and ventilation. *Clinical Pediatrics,* 1964, **3,** 581–586.

Robertson, J. *Young children in hospitals.* (2nd ed.) London: Tavistock, 1970.

Robins, L. N. *Deviant children grow up.* Baltimore: Williams & Wilkins, 1966.

Robinson, S., Abrams, H., & Kaplan, H. *Congenital heart disease.* (2nd ed.) New York: McGraw-Hill, 1965.

Sarason, S. B., Davidson, K. S., Lighthall, F. F., Waite, R. R., & Ruebush, B. K. *Anxiety in elementary school children.* New York: Wiley, 1960.

Schubert, J. Rorschach protocols of asthmatic boys. *British Journal of Projective Psychology and Personality Study,* 1969, **14,** 16–22.

Schwab, J. J. Enlarging our view of psychosomatic medicine. *Psychosomatics,* 1971, **12,** 16–20.

Shirley, H. F. *Pediatric psychiatry.* Cambridge, Mass.: Harvard University Press, 1963.

Spence, J. *The purpose and practice of medicine.* London: Oxford University Press, 1960.

Spiegelberg, H., Betz, B., & Pietsch, B. Psychosomatic aspects of allergy diseases. *Nervenarzt,* 1970, **41,** 587–593.

Stubblefield, R. L. Psychiatric observations of asthma in children. *Southern Medical Journal,* 1966, **59,** 306–310.

Szilagyi, L. Complaining as a means of interpersonal contact. *Pszichological Tanulmanyok,* 1968, **11,** 493–506.

Turnbull, J. W. Asthma conceived as a learned response. *Journal of Psychosomatic Research,* 1962, **6,** 59–70.

Vaughan, G. F. Children in hospital. *Lancet,* 1957, **272,** 1117–1120.

Waechter, E. H. Children's awareness of fatal illness. *American Journal of Nursing,* 1971, **71,** 1168–1172.

Watkins, J. D., & Moss, F. T. Confusion in the management of diabetes. *American Journal of Nursing*, 1969, **69**, 521–524.

Watkins, J. D., Roberts, D. E., Williams, T. F., Martin, D. A., & Cole, V. Observations of medication errors made by diabetic patients in the home. *Diabetes*, 1967, **16**, 882–885.

Watkins, J. D., Williams, T. F., Martin, D. A., Hogan, M. D., & Anderson, E. A study of diabetic patients at home. *American Journal of Public Health*, 1967, **57**, 441–451.

Whitson, B. J. The puppet treatment in pediatrics. *American Journal of Nursing*, 1972, **72**, 1612–1614.

Wolff, S. Behavioral characteristics of primary school children referred to a psychiatric department. *British Journal of Psychiatry*, 1967, **113**, 885–893.

Wolff, S. *Children under stress.* London: Penguin, 1969.

Woodward, J., & Jackson, D. Emotional reactions in burned children and their mothers. *British Journal of Plastic Surgery*, 1961, **13**, 316–324.

Wrightstone, J. W., Justman, J., & Moskowitz, S. *Studies of children with physical handicaps. No. 1, the child with cardiac limitations.* New York: Board of Education, 1953.

IV

Subtle handicapping conditions

A child with a subtle handicapping condition is one in whom the casual observer can see no obvious reason for the behavior the child displays. There are no physical stigmata, no telltale signs of disability. Consequently, teachers and parents attempt to explain the child's learning or behavior problems by attributing them to factors they know operate in other cases: "He must be retarded!" "He must be emotionally disturbed!" "He must be brain-injured!"

After reading the chapters in this part, the reader will be more aware of the difficulties in categorizing children. Professionals, as well as laymen, sometimes give a child a label that is currently popular. For a long time the economically disadvantaged were thought to be dull. Before 1960 many children with learning difficulties were labeled emotionally disturbed in response to family disorganization. In the late 1960s many were labeled minimally brain-damaged and family disorganization was overlooked. The academic failure of many disadvantaged children with brain impairment was attributed to their family's disorganization, while many advantaged children were labeled brain-impaired when family disorganization was actually responsible for their failure.

Chapter 7 describes different socialization practices and their relationship to cognitive and learning style.

Parents who relate to their child in an autocratic manner often produce children with learning styles that differ considerably from parents who relate to their child in other ways.

Chapter 8 presents children with learning disabilities that result from central nervous system dysfunction. Keep in mind, however, that the functioning of these children is also influenced by parental child rearing practices. A brain-impaired child reared in an autocratic home is likely to display a pattern of strengths and weaknesses that differs from a similarly damaged child reared in another type of home.

Chapter 9 describes the effects of an impoverished environment on academic functioning. Again, many of the variables that produce mild central nervous system dysfunction (e.g., poor pre- and postnatal care, nutritional deficiencies, disease) are more prevalent among the poor. Similarly, some of the child rearing approaches discussed in Chapter 7 are used more often by less educated parents.

The autocratic leader is often the person who looks backward and downward so long that eventually he finds nothing there.

Leonard Green

7

Self-defeating behavior

In several of the preceding chapters we discussed the concepts of predisposing and precipitating factors in various disorders. In Chapter 4 we emphasized that schizophrenia seemed to result from an interaction between constitutional and environmental factors. The child with a particular constitutional weakness (a hypothesized deficiency in the autonomic nervous system) is likely to become schizophrenic if exposed to severe stress, the form of the disorder depending upon the developmental level of the child at the time of the precipitating event.

In Chapter 5 we learned that illness is reacted to, interpreted, and integrated differently as subsequent phases of development are reached. And in Chapters 5 and 6 we learned that the child from an unstable home (predisposing factor) was handicapped more by disease or sensory impairment (precipitating factor) than was the child from a stable home.

In this chapter we hope to show how particular child rearing practices, or a child's social-learning history, predispose a child to react in a particular manner when under stress or in conflict. We will discuss six disorders that are examples of extreme reactions to stress. Each reaction is believed to be an exaggerated expression of personality traits learned as a result of particular parental attitudes and behaviors. The disorders discussed are obsessive-compulsive neurosis, anorexia nervosa (inhibition of eating), severe depression, hysteria, phobia (extreme fear), and marked inhibition. The first four disorders are believed to occur in children raised in what has been called the autocratic household; the last two are postulated to occur in children raised in a protective-interdependent household. These two child rearing approaches—the autocratic and the protective interdependent—are by no means the only child rearing approaches; they are simply the two that we postulate lead to the disorders being discussed.

We will follow a similar format in presenting each disorder. First, we will describe the essential features of the child rearing approach. Second, we will describe the personality traits and the learning or cognitive style of children reared by that approach. Third, we will present a description of the disorder, the exaggerated form of the cognitive style. Fourth, we will mention other theories that attempt to explain the disorder. Fifth, we will discuss the various approaches to treating the disorder and their relation to the theories presented.

A major premise underlying our presentation is that deviant behavior is explained by reference to variables that are equally as important in the establishment of nondeviant patterns of response. The implication here is that deviant behaviors are simply exaggerated forms of nondeviant behaviors. This principle is basic to a social-learning approach to psychopathology (Bandura & Walters, 1963).

The reader is cautioned to remember that the relationships between parental child rearing practices and child behavior are far from complete. The hypotheses put forward in this chapter are supported by limited data. Nevertheless, they have led to fruitful investigations and have guided treatment approaches. Our chief reason for presenting these disorders in this fashion is to show how theory guides action, and how treatments derived from viewpoints that consider the child in the context of his family may be more beneficial than those that ignore family variables.

THE AUTOCRATIC FAMILY

A number of theorists have postulated that autocratic, authoritarian, or unilateral child rearing practices lead to particular personality traits and that extreme autocratic practices produce serious behavior disorders in children.

The strict authoritarian presents absolute criteria for behavior and rewards behavior directed toward absolute obedience to these criteria. Any deviation from the criteria is severely punished. Within the category of autocratic child rearing practices there are several variations. Some autocratic parents do not apply their absolute standards consistently. For example, some allow a degree of negativism, but discourage self-assertive resistance to their control. In addition to varying along the dimension of consistency-inconsistency in control, child rearing practices vary as to the degree of nurturance or warmth in the relationship. The high-controlling, low-nurturant parent is postulated to produce a different child than the high-controlling, high-nurturant parent.

Another way in which autocratic parents differ is the stability of demands, that it, the degree to which their demands upon the child remain the same. Some parents may change their demands so often that the child has difficulty knowing what is expected of him.

Each of these variables, consistency of attitude, nurturance, and stability of demands, is postulated to result in particular personality traits, different learning styles, and differential responsiveness to stress.

OBSESSIVE-COMPULSIVE BEHAVIORS

Consistent autocratic control

In the consistently autocratic household, active, open resistance to parental demands is selectively punished. However, research indicates that punishment does not extinguish a behavior; it merely suppresses it. Given the right conditions, oppositional behavior will reappear or it will be expressed in some altered or covert form. A child develops both his individuality and his self-control by opposing external control. Even if his opposition to control is punished, he will continue to experience pressures to express that opposition. However, if he knows such expression will be punished, he is made anxious by his impulse to disobey. The manner in which the child handles this anxiety and the degree to which anxiety is aroused undoubtedly depend upon a number of variables.

We stated above that autocratic parents vary along a dimension of warmth. The degree of warmth displayed toward the child by the autocratic parent could be one crucial variable in how the child deals with anxiety. High-controlling, nonnurturant parents display little warmth toward their child and might be described as hypercritical, intrusive, disapproving, and inconsiderate; they avoid communication with their child and suppress his efforts at self-assertion. The nurturant parent may use other techniques to control their child, such as reasoning, withdrawal of love, or deprivation of privileges, but the authoritarian nonnurturant parents rely almost exclusively on aversive control techniques of punishment and rejection.

The child exposed to aversive control techniques is likely to experience undue anxiety, not only because his self-esteem is continually threatened but also because his parents' attacks generate strong urges to retaliate, which, if expressed, would lead to further punishment. There are several ways in which the child can reduce this anxiety. One way is to try to avoid situations where others may encourage resistance to or independence from authoritarian control and to avoid situations where the control is so intense that internal pressures to resist also become intense.

Heilbrun (1968, 1972) refers to individuals who adopt this strategy as *closed-style* individuals. The closed style is a learned way of reducing or avoiding aversive cues. The child learns to avoid his mother's critical remarks by staying away from her or by withdrawing from her presence. As he grows older, he handles other potential criticizers in the same manner; he avoids them or reduces his exposure to them. This closed adaptive style involves both social detachment, which allows for avoidance of social evaluative cues, and a subtle ability to defend against censure cues when they occur.

Some children have difficulty adopting this strategy because the parent punishes even efforts at avoidance—"You come back here, young man, or you'll get a whipping!" This child can express his resistance to parental pressures only in covert ways. For example, he could think about disobeying or challenging his parent's authority, but never actually do either. Such thoughts, however, could raise his anxiety rather than reduce it. Clinical evidence suggests that when mildly assertive acts are forbidden and, therefore, are continually suppressed, these acts take more aggressive forms in fantasy. Children who are sent to their room for disobeying a parent usually fantasize retaliation that is stronger than simply redisplaying the disapproved act. Nonautocratic parents usually allow the child to vent his aggression in some manner or displace it; the autocratic parent does not. Consequently, the child begins to fear that his aggressive fantasies may be discovered or acted upon. Any stress or pressure to express independence, therefore, results in anxiety.

To handle this anxiety, the child who cannot avoid the critical parent may adopt strategies designed to reduce critical interaction between himself and the parent. For example, he might display an excess of behaviors least likely to get him into trouble (the result is rigidity in functioning) or display behaviors the opposite of what he feels, such as excessive kindness or excessive concern about pleasing the authoritarian adult. He may display extreme orderliness to avoid doubt about having mistakenly done something wrong or compulsive rituals designed to avoid the expression of a forbidden impulse. All these behaviors, however, demand that the child continue to suppress his anger, a demand that impairs normal personality development.

Heilbrun (1968, 1972) refers to individuals who adopt this strategy of trying to please the parent as *open-style* individuals. The child adopting the open style tries to reduce aversive cues by adopting social strategies designed to elicit the approval of the source of the evaluative cues. Heilbrun and his colleagues have demonstrated that open-style and closed-style individuals respond differently in learning situations.

In general, open-style individuals are especially vigilant to the manner in which others respond to them, have a low self-esteem, and judge social encounters in terms of whether they influence others to like them. Because of these characteristics, the cognitive functioning of open-style individuals is disrupted by evidence of rejection, rejection that they frequently overexaggerate or even fabricate. Open-style males also display considerable inflexibility of thinking, because they are fixed in their impressions of their social stimulus value. When this inflexibility is seen in its extreme form, paranoid ideation is likely (Heilbrun & Norbert, 1972).

Closed-style individuals, because they avoid social involvement and show decreased attentiveness to evaluative cues, are more likely to deny the importance of a negative evaluation than to see negative evaluations where they do not exist. Regardless of style, both groups show marked underachievement (Allaman, Joyce, & Crandall, 1972; Heilbrun & Waters, 1968).

Heilbrun has not yet investigated why one individual adopts an open style and the other a closed style. Perhaps one variable in the choice of style is the interraction between the parents in the child's upbringing. For example, in a maternally dominated family, does the father approve of his wife's critical behavior or does he try and shield his child from it?

Learning style

A child develops many of his own ideas by refusing to accept the ideas of others. A child never allowed to reject a parent's idea would be a relatively poor problem solver because he would know only his parents' way of solving the problem, the only "right" way. Consequently, those exposed to consistent authoritarian training may have high needs for achievement, but they tend to do well only in rote learning or on structured tasks and to do poorly on unstructured tasks demanding abstractness. They also would display a rigid approach to problem solving and adopt a "safe" approach to problem solution.

The intellectual functioning of authoritarian individuals is often characterized by concreteness, literal adherence to instruction, minimal creativity, a tendency to bifurcate events into black-white categories, and a tendency to view persons who are different as inferior (Harvey, Hunt, & Schroder, 1961). This pattern of functioning has been observed by many personality theorists, and individuals who function according to the pattern have been given many descriptive labels—melancholics (Pavlov, 1927), the authoritarian personality (Adorno, Frenkel-Brunswik, Levinson, & Sanford, 1950), dogmatics (Rokeach, 1960), externalizers (Rotter, 1966), rigid-inhibited (Rosenberg, 1968), and compliants (Ringwald, Mann, Rosenwein, & McKeachie, 1971).

Obsessive-compulsive neurosis

Suppose individuals with the personality patterns we have just discussed are exposed to considerable stress. What behaviors are they likely to display in exaggerated form? The closed-style individual could increase his resistance to control through increased withdrawal, but never actually show appropriate self-assertion. The open-style individual can reduce external control by doing more of what he feels is expected of him so that the additional controls are reduced. The open-style individual may also display increased covert resistance to control, thinking more about disobeying but never actually doing so. To do so would be to incur more punishment and more criticism, but the thoughts are there. To avoid expressing these thoughts as actions, the child may increase the behaviors that are incompatible with the thoughts. With continued pressures, he may show an exaggerated display of obsessive acts designed to prevent hostile thoughts from becoming hostile actions. Individuals displaying such behavior have been called obsessive-compulsive neurotics. The open-style individual would be more likely to develop this disorder than would the closed-style, since the latter would be expected to show increased withdrawal when subjected to increased control.

Obsessions are ideas that persistently obtrude into consciousness against the will and better judgment of the individual. The ideas interfere with normal trains of thought and are recognized by the afflicted person as abnormal and unhealthy; yet they cannot be ignored. Compulsions are the acts that result from these obsessions (Bakwin & Bakwin, 1966).

Mild obsessions and compulsions are common in children at particular ages and, therefore, cannot be considered abnormal. They probably are common because most children resist the control of parents even when the control is not overbearing. Because of their dependence upon their parents, some of this resistance is covert rather than overt. The compulsions help to avoid the active expression of too much resistance. Children feel compelled to touch certain objects, jump over cracks on sidewalks (the saying "Step on a crack, break your mother's back" implies that compulsions are employed to avoid hostile actions), eat only certain foods, smell objects, clean parts of the body, and so on.

In some children, however, compulsions consume a disproportionate amount of time and energy. The compulsions may so embarrass the child that he isolates himself from other children. Often the child develops compulsive acts to ward off other obsessive ideas that would lead to worse acts. When this happens, the child is said to have an obsessive-compulsive disorder.

LEO

Leo, a boy of 15, is an example of a child with a long-standing obsessive-compulsive disorder, a disorder aggravated by the stress of having to submit to many humiliating medical examinations.

As a young child, Leo's mother had been extremely perfectionistic; she was made nauseous by dirty diapers and made her disgust known by rigid efforts at early toilet training. She scolded Leo for behaviors that most children exhibit, and she demanded almost perfect behavior from him. She related to Leo as if he was a little adult who knew right from wrong and who misbehaved just to get her upset. She was also compulsive about his health, continually taking his temperature and having him examined by the doctor for minor ailments. She subjected him to enemas when he was constipated and force fed him when he was ill.

Psychiatric opinion was that Leo's mother was trying to avoid expressing her own aggressive impulses toward Leo. These impulses themselves were the mother's obsessive ideas, ideas that resulted in compulsive acts to ward them off. Preoccupation with his health served to bolster feelings that nothing had happened to him, that her hostile thoughts had not come true. By showing continual concern about his health, she could deny her aggressive obsessions.

Coupled with these maternal attitudes was Leo's early operation for undescended testicles. Not only was his mother obsessively concerned for his health, but actual trauma, perhaps conceptualized as symbolic castration, added injury to insult. As Leo grew older, he too became obsessively preoccupied with anticontamination acts. In addition, he would only eat certain foods and demanded that his mother perform a certain routine each night before bedtime. Eventually, most of his day was taken up with behaviors designed to ward off obsessive ideas or carry out compulsions.

Leo was enrolled in a residential treatment center after outpatient treatment failed to bring about change in his behavior. During the course of his stay in the center, staff helped channel his obsessions into intellectual pursuits.

Whenever Leo was interviewed as part of periodic evaluations of his progress, he was very responsive to questioning, elaborating freely, but in an automated fashion. Whenever he was asked about his family, he would give the exact birth dates of parents and siblings. His speaking vocabulary was extensive, but overembellished. He obviously enjoyed using grandiose words when simpler ones would do, not only to impress others but to convince himself of his own adequacy.

Obsessive-compulsive features were easily observed. He stacked materials around him neatly and symmetrically, answered questions in superfluous detail, and displayed considerable concern with intellectual striving. He was pleasant and well-mannered, but was robotlike when in control of his emotions.

Leo described his mother and her problems in a cold, abstract, and unemotional manner, as if she were a textbook case in abnormal psychology, but he rarely spoke of his father. His relationship with his mother seemed to be mutually sadomasochistic. She constantly invited from him compassion and understanding, but insisted upon humiliating him by having him submit to personal medical examinations. In the face of this behavior, Leo responded with a calm, detached, almost saintly air of tolerance for her difficulties, but was cruel in his criticism of her.

Leo was easily embarrassed and become distressed if he thought he had failed to convey a good impression. Consequently, he was cautious and condescending in social relationships.

Leo's intellectual functioning, as measured by the WISC, was at a high-average level in both the verbal and performance areas (IQ 118). However, his score was deceiving, because although he functioned at very superior levels in some areas, he functioned at just barely average levels in others. He recalled informational data only when it was academic in nature or commensurate with his past or present interests. When the items were those of an everyday variety or when judgments or estimations were required, he was less knowledgeable. His word defining skills were at superior levels, but were pedantic. His abstract-conceptual reasoning with words was also at an extremely high level. However, when confronted with a new, unfamiliar, problem solving situation that required differentiating as well as conceptual reasoning skill, his functioning was far below that expected from one with his intelligence. When asked to tell how everyday objects were alike, he could not find general terms to sum up all the essential common characteristics of the objects. His style of reasoning was rigidly fragmented; he could not handle more than two objects and would relate only two when three or more were presented for comparison. Diagnostic of an underlying thought disturbance was his response to a bottle of mercurochrome, thimble, and whistle. He said that the bottle of "mecurachrome has something to do with mercury, which is a metal, so they all have something to do with metal."

Similar inability to differentiate was seen in his relatively poor performance on a Wechsler subtest involving close scrutiny to details in pictures of common objects. Superior ability was noted when the details involved assessment of social situations.

Leo's uneven development resulted from intellectual strivings in certain areas to the neglect of others. Leo himself stated that, "you need an education to survive in the modern world . . . to get up there, to get anywhere." Upon close scrutiny, much of his intellectual achievement was seen as the frail superstructure of a shaky foundation. When asked how water and salt were alike, he credulously responded with "compounds"; yet, on another occasion, he definitely "knew" that water was an element. His confusion was most prominent on novel tasks. Leo's pattern of intellectual strengths and weaknesses and his approach to unstructured, problem-solving situations corresponded to descriptions of individuals subjected to authoritarian training.

The most recent administration of the California Achievement Tests found Leo's total achievement at the tenth grade level with little difference among the various areas measured. His academic grades in the special school were mostly B's, with most difficulty in social studies. The unit staff reported that he worked hard, was very cooperative, and had adequate peer relations.

The most striking feature of Leo's emotional functioning was his concept of himself as having been effeminized. Throughout his Rorschach tests, he made many references to humans or animals being dissected, spread open, cut, or ripped apart. His history of operations and medical problems in the genital areas, as well as his mother's continual preoccupation with his health, helped clarify the reasons for these feelings. He expressed unhappiness with his physical features in spite of his being rather masculine and rugged looking. Attempts to cast everything into intellectual realms and to superimpose generalizations on specific facts whether they fit or not resulted in reality distortion and restriction in spontaneity and flexibility.

As a result of his feeling effeminized, his heterosexual relations were disturbed. Masculine strivings were present, but were disrupted by feelings of inadequacy. Wishful thinking, therefore, served as a palliative, along with intellectual interests in sexology and obstetrics.

Not only was Leo's mother extremely autocratic, but she was rejecting as well. Leo seems to have reacted to her aversive behavior by adapting an open style of behavior. He showed the hyperalertness to criticism, the marked efforts to gain social approval, and the low self-esteem Heilbrun and his colleagues describe as characteristic of open-style individuals. In addition, his indirect oppositional tendencies represented the obsessive wishes (antisocial impulses) and his compulsions the self-corrective behaviors to counteract and set right his antisocial tendencies.

Other theories of obsessive-compulsive neurosis

We have conceptualized the development of obsessive-compulsive neurosis as the result of an interaction between a particular family climate and situational stress. Others postulate that the family climate is itself an inherited trait. They state that obsessive-compulsive personality traits are inherited. In one study monozygotic twins were concordant for obsessive-compulsive reactions in 8 of 10 cases, whereas dizygotic twins were concordant in only 1 of 4 cases (Inouye, 1965). These findings and others (Woodruff & Pitts, 1964) suggest a genetic origin for this personality trait. Other studies indicate that psychiatric illness occurs frequently among relatives of obsessional neurotics, but they do not support the notion that the obsessional personality is genetically determined (Rosenberg, 1967).

Investigators who believe the evidence supports a genetic origin of the disorder feel that it is inappropriate to label obsessive-compulsive behavior as neurotic. They prefer to use the term obsessional illness and to reserve the term neurosis for learned behavioral reactions to stress.

Nevertheless, without studies in which both monozygotic and dizygotic twins are compared with monozygotic twins reared apart, it is difficult to tell what is learned and what is the result of factors independent of environmental influences.

Many psychotic individuals also display obsessive-compulsive behavior. They differ from the obsessive-compulsive neurotic in that, unlike the neurotic, they are not aware of the inappropriateness of the obsessive thought or compulsive act (Despert, 1955). However, this distinction may be artificial, since psychotics in remission often behave like obsessive-compulsive neurotics, and neurotics sometimes have breaks with reality. Although Leo was disturbed by his obsessions, there were times when his behavior resembled the psychotic. Because of the seeming relationship between obsessive-compulsive behaviors and schizophrenia, several investigators have postulated that obsessional behaviors protect the individual from developing schizophrenia (Hare, Price, & Slater, 1972).

Because of the low incidence of the obsessive-compulsive syndrome (perhaps 0.05 percent of patients in psychiatric care) it is difficult to design research studies that will clarify the role of heredity in this disorder. Most likely, as in schizophrenia, there is a constitutional predisposition to particular personality traits, so that individuals born to obsessive-compulsive and autocratic parents are high risks to develop this disorder. Whether they do or not probably depends upon the extent to which the controlling parents cares for the child, the counterinfluence of the noninvolved parent, and the situational stresses to which the child is exposed. As we will learn in Chapter 12, children born to the same parents can have different temperaments. Perhaps the child most likely to develop a neurosis is the one whose temperament causes the controlling parent to increase controlling efforts or who is by temperament most like the controlling parent.

Treatment

How would you treat someone like Leo? The belief that obsessive-compulsive behaviors are designed to prevent the expression of hostile or even self-assertive acts gives the therapist some idea of where to begin. Guided by this belief, he would help the individual develop self-assertive behaviors. By considering the obsessive-compulsive behaviors to be conditioned avoidance reactions (learned ways to avoid anxiety), the therapist can introduce two procedures simultaneously. He can prevent the obsessive-compulsive child from engaging in behaviors that the child believes will forestall feared consequences. If the child is a compulsive hand washer, he would be restricted from this activity. If he is afraid to touch objects, he would be made to do so in order to learn that the feared consequences do not occur. These procedures are called *response-prevent techniques.* Response-prevent techniques have rarely been employed in clinical treatment, although Meyers (1966) reports some success with this approach. At the same time as response-prevent procedures are used, the therapist can help the individual develop appropriate self-assertive behaviors. When the latter behaviors are not followed by punishment, but are actually reinforced, assertive action arouses less anxiety and compulsive behaviors designed to avoid anxiety diminish. Walton and Mather (1963) report some success using assertive training procedures with obsessive-compulsive individuals.

If the individual still lives with his family and if they react negatively to his attempts at self-assertion, family therapy would be undertaken in an effort to change the autocratic atmosphere in the home. Hopefully, some compromise could be made between the child's needs for self-assertion and the parents' need for complete control.

How do they fare?

Because the frequency of this disorder is low, few follow-up studies of obsessive-compulsive children have been reported. Those published suggest that the disorder is a chronic one characterized by many relative remissions and exacerbations (Kringlen, 1965). Follow-up of adult obsessionals indicates that anywhere from 25 to 70 percent can be considered improved (Yates, 1970). Treatment, however, does not appear to have a significant influence since groups receiving no treatment are reported to show as high a recovery rate as those receiving a variety of treatments (Yates, 1970).

COVERT EXPRESSION OF NEGATIVISM

Inconsistent autocratic control

In our previous discussion, we described parents who were consistent in their controlling techniques. What about parents who are inconsistent and allow some negativism? Usually, the negativism allowed is not the type that leads to appropriate self-assertion. The child, although allowed to be somewhat negative, is never able to integrate autonomy with mutuality. Consequently, the child is threatened by pressures to submit to external control. He enjoys the little individuality he has developed and conceives of increased pressures to submit to parental demands as efforts to strip him of this individuality. The anxiety aroused by such pressures can be decreased by avoiding situations where acceptance of authoritarian control is required. If avoidance is blocked, the child might find that the only way to express his individuality is through covert or indirect negativism or contrariness.

Learning style

Children described as "the heroes"—resentful of authority, rebellious, and erratic, yet ambivalent toward teachers (Ringwald et al., 1971)—may have been reared by inconsistent autocratic parents. As pressures to conform increase, these children fail in school, display teacher-child antagonism, obesity, and speech problems as defenses against compliance (Levy, 1955).

If controlling pressures increase further, highly modified negativism occurs, developing to a point where such negativism provides immunity to control. Examples of extreme forms of indirect negativism are inhibition of effective performance (underachievement), inhibition of speaking (selective mutism), and inhibition of eating (anorexia nervosa) (Harvey et al., 1961).

Anorexia nervosa

The majority of anorexic children are shy, timid, and reserved and have difficulty making friends. Over half are described as conscientious and about a third as obsessional and anxious or hypochondriacal (Warren, 1968). This personality pattern might be expected from a child reared in an autocratic home. Several studies indicate that anorexics are overly dependent upon one member of the family and that a smaller number have hostile relationships with their mothers. The majority of mothers, while perhaps overprotective, are not considered domineering. Since the syndrome seems to appear in a variety of character types, some investigators have concluded that anorexia is not a discrete disorder, but rather a constellation of symptoms arising from severe but diverse psychopathology. If there is a common feature in the backgrounds of anorexics, it has yet to be clearly delineated. More detailed studies of interaction within families of anorexic children are needed to support our notion that a particular style of child rearing contributes to the development of this disorder.

The following case is an example of a child in whom extreme resistance to controlling pressures took the form of refusal to eat.

SANDRA

Although 18-year old Sandra had recovered from her viral infection, she still hung around the house and complained of not feeling well. Usually a light and finicky eater, her appetite had fallen off. She said she was too sick to eat. When the doctor assured her she was over the virus, she insisted that she now must have something else. Her older sister taunted her, claiming she wasn't really sick but afraid of being teased by boys and using her "illness" as an excuse to avoid them in school. True, Sandra had always been a shy and withdrawn girl who frequently was hypochondriacal, but in this instance she really looked sick. She continued to feel bad and refused to eat. Her parents insisted that she must be ill; perhaps she had some obscure illness. The physician insisted that he could find nothing physically wrong with her.

Eventually Sandra stopped eating altogether and became listless and inactive. Urging and reprimand had no effect, and after she lost 12 pounds her parents took her to see a psychiatrist. The psychiatrist insisted that she go to school; but after it was reported that she spent the day laying her head on the desk, he had her admitted to the local hospital.

Sandra was upset by hospitalization and insisted she should go home. Her appetite suddenly returned and she no longer felt sick. Although the psychiatrist felt she should stay for further observation, her bed was needed for other patients, and she was discharged. No sooner was she home then she again stopped eating. Her mother called the psychiatrist and expressed her utter helplessness in dealing with Sandra. She now was convinced that Sandra's problem was emotional and that both she and her husband were unable to handle her. The psychiatrist visited Sandra at home after she refused to come to the clinic. When he arrived, she locked and barricaded her door, refusing to let him in. After a week went by with Sandra staying in her room and refusing to eat, her parents agreed to hospitalization in a private psychiatric center.

Each time the family visited the center, Sandra insisted on being taken home. She said that she would "never eat if she had to stay in this crazy place," and that she was sorry for the trouble she'd caused and would start eating again when home. The family's first impulse was to accede to her request. They did not liked the idea of their daughter being in a psychiatric hospital, a fact they kept from friends and relatives. Sandra's father was worried about their image in the community should people find out, and her sister was worried she would lose her boyfriend.

Sandra's normal weight was around 104 pounds. At this time she weighed 84. She was told that she could go home when her weight reached 100 pounds and she was able to resume normal activities. In the meantime she would meet regularly with her therapist to discuss her feelings with him. If she continued to cry and fuss when her parents visited, visiting would be restricted.

Five months later, Sandra returned home. During this interval Sandra changed from a belligerent, omnipotent youngster to a very sad, depressed, and frightened one. She came to rely on her therapist, with whom she eventually shared her feelings of personal inadequacy, sadness, and fear. She had never made friends of her own and felt uneasy in social situations. In school she had been deathly afraid of speaking out in class and would be sick on days she had to give reports. She had not yet menstruated and became anxious when she thought about the eventual occurrence of this body change.

For a time during her treatment she regressed, staying curled up in bed and leaving it only to accompany her therapist to his office. She accepted help from no one else, and her day revolved around her therapist's visits. Hospital staff were encouraged to ignore her rebuffs and continue to make positive overtures toward her. Eventually, she became friendly with several nurses and could accept affection from them. During the last two months of her hospitalization, Sandra made visits home to take meals with her family.

After her return home, Sandra was seen twice a week in therapy for nearly two years. During this time she began to expand her activities outside the home and to establish several friendships.

Historical material, as well as interviews with the family and observation of their interaction with Sandra, suggested that Sandra was reared in an autocratic household, but that the parents differed in their handling of her. The father was somewhat seductive toward Sandra and forbade any back talk from her. He also limited her activities to those that the family did together. In contrast, mother tolerated some back talk from Sandra, but never took her seriously. Sometimes she let Sandra sneak out of the house without telling her husband, but then would stand by him if Sandra was caught. Both parents were intrusive, always wanting to know all about Sandra's school activities; yet they criticized her failures without rewarding her successes. As she got older, Sandra's father insisted that she stay away from boys and her mother disliked all of her friends. She would ask Sandra why she didn't bring more friends home, but when she did, she would find something wrong with each of them. Eventually, Sandra brought no one home. Her mother then would remark that she was a social "wallflower."

Other theories of anorexia nervosa

While early psychoanalysts viewed refusal to eat as a defense against fantasies of oral impregnation that occurred with the bodily changes of adolescence, later observations suggested that this explanation was an oversimplification. Rose (1943) emphasized the fear of growing up and of resistance to change. Historical material revealed that patients were resistant and aggressive at earlier, crucial points of change when new integrations were required. The specific syndrome was viewed as a response to the demands of puberty. More recently, the parents' subtle blocking of future development has been emphasized. In women, in whom this disorder is more frequent, the fear of growing up eventually reveals itself as rooted in anxieties about sexuality, particularly feminine functioning.

Treatment

Treatment is currently conceptualized as having two stages. The first stage includes management of the total situation and formation of individual supportive relationships with family and child. Emotional interactions rather than insight are stressed in this stage. Both child and family are protected from each other. The hospital is considered a corrective experience where emotional constancy is held through states of calm and states of excitement. Because of the hospital staff's readiness to protect and support the child, she is able to achieve security and to sort out confused feelings. The family also is protected from the child's manipulativeness and unspoken hostility (Rollins & Blackwell, 1968). Without hospitalization the child's manipulative control of the family through refusal to eat increases at the same time the family's aggressive tactics increase in direct proportion to their panic over that refusal.

The second stage involves providing outpatient psychotherapy designed to develop insight into reasons for the development of the disorder. Intensive psychotherapy while in the hospital is not helpful (Warren, 1968).

Sandra's treatment was based on the belief that since she had never been allowed to assert herself, a paralyzing sense of ineffectiveness pervaded all her thinking. This feeling was initially camouflaged by extreme negativism and stubborn defiance. Bruch (1970, p. 52) remarks that the oppositional phase of early childhood was absent in patients like Sandra: "The development of anorexia nervosa may be conceived of as shouting an unrelenting 'No,' which extends to every area of living, though most conspicuous in the food area." We would add that it is the first "No" which the family takes seriously.

When Sandra was acutely "ill," she showed disturbances in body image of delusional proportions. As Bruch (1971, p. 52) remarks, "The truly pathognomonic feature is a dramatic denial of illness, the absence of concern over the advanced emaciation, and the vigor and stubbornness with which the often gruesome appearance is defended as normal, and not too thin." Sandra also showed inaccurate perception and cognizance of stimuli arising in her body. Awareness of hunger seemed to be absent. When she said "I do not need to eat," it was probably an accurate expression of her nutritional disorganization (Bruch, 1971).

As treatment progressed and she began to feed herself, these delusions and distortions dropped out, suggesting that her delusional responses were the product, rather than the source, of her deviant behavior. By adopting a sick role, supported by delusional justifications, Sandra was initially successful in forcing attending and caretaking responses from others, demands that would otherwise have been ignored. At the same time her refusal to eat was the first self-assertive, albeit abnormal, act

Table 7.1 COURSE OF ANOREXIA NERVOSA

Case number	Pre-anorexia nervosa age of menarche Yrs	Mos	Age at start of anorexia nervosa Yrs	Mos	Pubertal development at start of anorexia nervosa	Age recovered from anorexia nervosa Yrs	Mos	Length of anorexia nervosa Yrs	Mos	Age at onset or re-onset of menses Yrs	Mos	Age at follow-up Yrs	Mos	Outcome
1	—		10	6		14		3	6	14	9	20		Healthy
2	—		11	2		*		3	2+			14	4	Not yet recovered anorexia nervosa
3	—		11	6	Pre-pubertal	*		5	9+			17	3	Not yet recovered anorexia nervosa
4	—		12					3	9 Died					Died from malnutrition
5	—		12	3				2	9 Died					Died from malnutrition
6	—		13			15	9	2	9	17		21		Healthy
7	—		13	6		16		2	4	18		28		Severe neurosis
8	—		14	3		15	10	1	7	16	7	26		Mild neurosis
9	—		12			12	10	0	10	14		20		Moderate neurosis
10	—		13		Pubertal	17‡		4		17		23		Continuing depression
11	—		14	3		*		5+		17		19	3	Not yet recovered anorexia nervosa
12	—		15			16	8	1	8	18		26		Schizophrenia

					Post-pubertal						
13	11†		11		14	6	3	6	—	18	Mild neurosis
14	9		11		15		4		16	20	Moderate neurosis
15	9	3	12	6	13	6	1		15	15	Severe neurosis
16	10	6	12	9	*		3	3+	—	16	Not yet recovered anorexia nervosa
17	11	6	13	6	15	6	2		N.K.	—	Not known
18	13		13	6	15	3	1	9	16	23	Mild neurosis
19	11		13	6	*		4	6+	—	18	Not yet recovered anorexia nervosa
20	14		15	9	18	9	3		N.K.	—	Not known

* Not recovered at follow-up.
† 1 period.
‡ Leucotomy.

From W. Waren. A study of anorexia nervosa in young girls. *Journal of Child Psychology and Psychiatry*, 1968, **9**, 27–40.

that was successful. While staff were instructed not to reinforce this sick role by feeding and attending to her on her terms, they were expected to encourage and reinforce assertive acts. Appropriate self-assertion was to take the place of the infantile refusal to eat. It was easier to apply the reinforcement contingencies necessary to bring this change about when Sandra was removed from her home.

How do they fare?   Anorexia nervosa is most common in adolescent girls. It is rare in boys. Although a number of cases have been reported in younger children, the majority range in age from 12 to 17 years.

Warren (1968) studied 20 adolescents who developed anorexia between the ages of 10 and 15. Table 7.1 presents the results of this follow-up. The girls remained in the hospital from 2 to 23 months (mean 6.7 months). After leaving the hospital, 16 had further inpatient treatment and 2 died from the disorder. Of the 16, 10 were readmitted for relapse of anorexia and 6 were readmitted for other psychiatric conditions.

Follow-up was carried out after anorexia had ceased in 11 out of 20 patients. The 11 recovered girls were between 15 and 28 years at the time of the follow-up. Two others who had recovered could not be located, 2 had died, and 5 were still suffering from anorexia. In 10 of those recovered, menstruation had been established between the ages of 14 and 18 years (mean 16 years, 3 months). All 11 showed psychiatric ill health. Sexual maladjustment was present in 4 girls, although most were still too young to determine sexual adjustment. Warren's data, which reveal the severity of the disorder, correspond to the findings of others, although the outlook was more favorable in one study (Lesser, Ashenden, Delsushey, & Eisenberg, 1960).

Bruch (1971) followed 64 patients over a 25-year period. Four died from the disorder and in others remission was often followed by relapse. Bruch remarked that caution is warranted when making claims for treatment effects, since arrest of the disorder may not mean recovery.

PSEUDOINDEPENDENCE

Accelerated autonomy and unstable demands

In order for a child to develop properly, he must be allowed to oppose external control through independent actions and yet still be able to seek external help and support when necessary. The small child who finds himself in a strange room stays by his mother until he feels safe enough to explore the room. The mother who reinforces the child's exploration but at the same time lets him return to her side if he gets into difficulty fosters development that integrates autonomy and dependence. In contrast, the child whose mother insists that he immediately explore the room and who rejects his overtures of dependence fosters development where autonomy is gained at the expense of dependency and where anxiety is aroused by internal pressures to express dependency needs.

Some autocratic parents not only attempt to accelerate the autonomous development of their child but also change their demands so often that the child has difficulty knowing what is expected of him. This instability of demands ignores the changing needs of the child and represents a form of indifference and neglect. The child is liked as long as he does what he's told, yet what he's told depends upon the parent's whim.

Learning style

Individuals consistently trained in such an accelerated fashion learn to avoid situations where they are likely to feel inadequate and to be in need of support from others. They strive to become independent of others, but do so at the expense of mutual interdependency; they cannot admit that they need help from others. They are pseudoindependents, individuals who handle their inadequacies by rationalizing them away or denying them altogether.

Should an individual with such a style be faced with revealing his deficiencies, he would be placed in considerable conflict. One way to handle this conflict would be to become "ill." When this happens we say the child has a hysterical or a conversion reaction.

Hysterical neurosis

When an individual cannot admit to himself or to others that he has dependency needs, the hysterical symptom serves both to avoid displays of inadequacy and to solicit attention and care. Poor Joe can't take the exam because he is ill and needs our loving care! Laybourne and Churchill (1970, p. 14) present a case which serves as an example of hysterical neurosis. In this case the child developed a conversion reaction, a somatic complaint with no known organic cause.

Betty, a twelve-year-old girl, was admitted to the University of Kansas Medical Center after four hospitalizations and an exploratory laparotomy for right-sided pain of three years duration. She had nursed her alcoholic father during the time he was dying from a cancer of the pancreas, which was manifested by increasing abdominal pain, and which was diagnosed only a few months before his death.

Following her admission to the pediatric ward, the child psychiatrist confronted Betty with the fact that her body was healthy. She admitted she knew this and said she was most likely to experience pain when she was tense or "nervous." Several days later she expressed bizarre ideas that her appendectomy scar bled with menses and that she was fifteen years old, not twelve. When this behavior was not reinforced and she was reassured that her body was healthy, it ceased.

It was noted that her mother would smile when Betty stated to her that her symptoms were physical, but was unhappy and cried when Betty would say they were emotional and that she wanted to be transferred to the psychiatric wards to work on her problem. The mother was asked about these responses and she said she thought the illness was organic, and reminded us that her husband had been diagnosed incorrectly as a psychiatric disorder. She was told her husband's problem was extremely rare and was reminded that Betty had had a three year illness with no signs of cancer, and furthermore, she had an exploratory laparotomy which had ruled out any organic disorder. The mother then agreed to transfer the child to the psychiatric wards.

On the psychiatric wards Betty had no pain but began to talk about her home which she regarded as intolerable. The symptoms she manifested on the psychiatric wards were those most impressive to the psychiatrists . . . hearing voices and suicidal ideation. She stated she wanted to be sick and/or crazy because the alternative was going home.

Laybourne and Churchill (1970, p. 1) state that "During twenty years of experience in such a setting [pediatric setting] we have seen children who have simulated blindness, deafness, aphonia, acute abdominal pain, paralysis, urinary infection, convulsions, amnesia, and psychosis."

Not much is known about the families of children with hysterical reactions. An increased incidence of hysteria has been found among female relatives and an increased incidence of alcoholism among male relatives (Arkonac & Guze, 1963), but a paucity of data exists regarding the child rearing practices of parents of hysterical children. Consequently, our theory regarding the role of child rearing factors in hysteria is not on very firm grounds. The theory, like other theories, points to directions that future research might take. It does seem clear that the hysterical symptom enables a child to resolve temporarily conflicts about expressing dependency needs, since his parents would be unlikely to reinforce direct expressions, while they might reinforce this indirect one. We do not know enough about the child rearing practices of these parents, however, to know whether they are inconsistently autocratic or vary along other dimensions. We do know, however, that children who develop severe headaches with no organic cause have parents who also have similar headaches (Ling, Oftedal, & Weinberg, 1970), suggesting that modeling plays a role in the development of hysterical disorders. We also know that the personalities of children who develop hysterical symptoms are in keeping with the learning style we attributed to an accelerated autonomy background. Prior to developing the hysterical symptoms, affected children display immaturity, superficiality, evasiveness, attention seeking, feigned poise, unmotivated mood swings, and emotional overreaction. They also are said to be great imitators, very suggestible, quick to form opinions, generally casual in the face of serious symptoms, and unconcerned about conflicts (Bakwin & Bakwin, 1966). Perhaps when overcompensatory forms of conflict resolution fail, avoidance reactions and eventually hysterical symptoms develop.

Other related theories

Learning theorists argue that conversion reactions are learned avoidance reactions to anxiety. They also emphasize the early learning experiences of the child regarding the role of being sick. Many children learn from their own experience or from observing others that fewer demands are made upon the sick. Solicitude and affection often accompany sickness, and threatening situations are frequently avoided. Conversion reactions are often precipitated by some minor physical trauma or by an organic illness that is self-limited (Laybourne & Churchill, 1970). Thus, the child can experience firsthand the advantages of a sick role. When the child is faced with a situation he considers insurmountable, he adopts the sick role to escape from this threatening reality conflict. A conversion reaction, therefore, is a conditioned avoidance reaction.

Kanner (1966, pp. 647–675), in his comprehensive textbook of child psychiatry, cites five cases illustrating that the sick role is rewarded by either solicitude or escape from unpleasant situations: (1) Margaret learned to avoid school difficulties by blind spells or hurting eyes; (2) Claudia, whose father had been very solicitous toward her the previous year when she had mastoiditis, developed earaches and could not sit, stand, or walk; (3) Miriam became unable to walk following the onset of a fear of failing in school; (4) Harry, whose father beat him when he didn't eat properly, developed hysterical dysphagia (eating difficulties associated with stricture of the esophagus, profound sore throat, etc.) and was thereafter treated well by his parents who were afraid he had a serious throat disease; and (5) Cecelia, who stated, "My mother is very good to me when I'm sick," was unable to get her tongue back inside her mouth.

Other authors have noted the presence of a minor illness just prior to the conversion symptoms. Forbis and Janes (1965) cite a case where upper respiratory infection preceded the symptom by a few days, and in all six of Gold's (1965) cases some minor trauma or orthopedic procedure preceded the hysterical contractures by several days.

The learning theorists provide an explanation of how hysterical symptoms can be learned avoidance reactions. However, they do not adequately explain why some children use these behaviors to resolve conflicts or reduce stress while others handle their conflicts in some other fashion.

Treatment Whether the therapist holds a classical psychodynamic or a behavioral view of neurosis, the treatment approach to hysteria concentrates on symptom removal through decreasing the gain from being ill (Kanner, 1966; Schulman, 1961; Yates, 1970). After symptoms disappear, their etiology can be dealt with. Classical psychotherapy appears to have little effect without symptom removal (Gold, 1965). Once the symptom is removed, the psychodynamic therapists would attempt to uncover the reason for its occurrence. Hysterical or conversion reactions have a strong tendency to remain stable over a considerable period of time (Woodruff, Clayton, & Guze, 1971) and to spontaneously appear and disappear (Yates, 1970). Unless the child learns more appropriate ways to deal with his anxieties, relapse can occur.

Treatment in keeping with social-learning theory would stress helping the child develop coping strategies within the framework of supportive relationships. Once the symptoms had been removed and the child returned to his prior pseudoindependent state, efforts would be directed toward getting him to accept help from others. Working with others and accepting their support would be reinforced. The child's deficiencies would not be ridiculed, but neither would his denials or rationalizations be accepted; they would be ignored while relationships with others were strengthened. At the present time the effects of such a therapeutic approach have not been evaluated.

How do they fare?

In Robins's (1966) sample the childhood behavior of women who displayed hysterical symptoms resembled the early behavior of women diagnosed as having character disorders, or sociopathic personalities (see Chapter 9). They tested low on IQ measures, had a high rate of grade failures in school (72 percent), and very few (7 percent) completed high school. The girls with hysterical syndromes had a high rate of juvenile sexual offenses. A third of the girls had been raped before age 18 (a higher rate than that of the sociopathic group) and three-fourths had had a voluntary premarital sexual experience.

The girls diagnosed as hysterics showed their first symptoms earlier than the sociopathic group; 41 percent had symptoms reported before age 8, whereas only 17 percent of the sociopathic girls had such an early onset. As teenagers, many were incorrigible, associated with undesirable companions, ran away from home, and violated parental authority. As adults, they were verbally aggressive and unable to hold jobs. Nevertheless, they had fewer arrests than the sociopathic group; only 35 percent had been arrested after age 18, whereas 86 percent of the sociopathic group had been arrested after this age. Three-quarters of the hysterics were married and living with their husbands at the time of the follow-up. About half had been divorced at some time, and two-thirds reported behavior problems in their husbands. By the time they had reached middle age, almost all had ceased their antisocial activity.

About half perceived themselves as sick and had displayed a multitude of symptoms since the age of 30. They complained of nervousness, dizzy spells, sexual indifference, menstrual problems, and a lump in the throat. They also had frequent nausea, inertia, palpitation, headache, and bowel difficulty. None of the hysterics had recovered at follow-up, and very few had shown improvement. They had a high rate of medical care and one-third had taken tranquilizers (Robins, 1966).

Because Robins's sample was drawn from patients treated at a child guidance center, it is likely that acting out, aggressive children were over-represented in the study. Follow-ups of children treated privately or in general hospitals have not been reported.

HELPLESSNESS

Because depression correlates highly with low self-esteem, depression in children usually occurs in conjunction with the disorders already mentioned. It is discussed here because research suggests that depression is a learned feeling of helplessness that develops in children whose parents are autocratic at the same time they are rejecting.

All children are subjected to environmental setbacks of one form or another. Why is it that some children become depressed while others emerge from these setbacks relatively unscathed? Before examining the environmental contingencies that can produce a state of depression, we will examine how depression is conceived and then how it is manifested in children.

Characteristics of helplessness

Helplessness as a factor in depression has been obvious to observers for some time. Bibring (1953) and Lichtenberg (1957) see the basic mechanism of depression as the awareness of helplessness and hopelessness regarding the attainment of goals. The individual gives up the effort to obtain his goals because he has learned to expect failure.

Schmale (1958) adds that helplessness is felt after an individual senses a lack of external support for his activities. He feels he is neither responsible for his dilemma nor capable of changing it. With continued feelings of helplessness, the individual eventually withdraws from contact with the unsatisfying environment.

Intercorrelational studies of personality inventories also reveal a factor of hopelessness as a central theme in depression (Friedman, Cowitz, Cohen, & Granick, 1963; Grinker, Miller, Sabshin, Nunn, & Nunnally, 1961; Hunt, Singer, & Cobb, 1967; Overall, 1962). Associated with this factor are feelings of unworthiness, failure, indecisiveness, doubt, perplexity, and loneliness.

Perhaps the chief characteristic of helplessness is the inability to act. Beck (1967) refers to a "paralysis of will." This inability to act is rooted in the expectation that actions will be unsuccessful: "No matter what I do, it's no use." Beck (1967) found this complaint in 78 percent of depressed adults. This attitude pervades the individual's thinking to such an extent that he perceives even his adequate performances as failures. Depressives are known to underestimate their actual performance on cognitive, perceptual, vigilance, and psychomotor tests (Friedman, 1964; Loeb, Beck, & Diggory, 1971). This pessimism and devaluation of ability underlie their apparent lack of motivation to succeed.

A second feature of helplessness is the belief that one has no control over the situations that lead to depression. A generalized expectation that outcomes are contingent upon what one does (internal control) versus an expectation that outside forces are responsible (external control) defines a locus of control variable that has promoted considerable research in recent years. The concept was introduced by Rotter in 1954 and elaborated in 1966. Rotter (1966) differentiates skill orientation from chance orientation. Those who believe that rewards are contingent on their own actions are more likely to engage in goal-directed behavior than are those who believe their fate is determined by chance or is beyond their own control. In addition, a belief in the efficacy of one's actions gives rise to a feeling of competence. This belief in one's capabilities is a large component of self-esteem; disbelief is a fundamental component of feelings of helplessness. It would seem, therefore, that external locus of control, helplessness, and depression go hand in hand (Abramowitz, 1969).

In adult depressives the observer often finds it difficult to appreciate how a person whom they perceive as competent can feel so helpless in the face of trauma. It is important to realize that the feeling of helplessness is subjective and often contrary to objective facts. In addition, the specific trauma that precipitates the feeling is not itself responsible for the inability to respond to future traumas, but rather it is the experience of having no control over the trauma's occurrence. The depressive seems to say, "Since what happens to me is beyond my control, and the rewards and punishments I receive are determined by others, I am helpless to effect any changes in my environment because the abilities I possess are inadequate. There is, therefore, no sense in my trying to change my situation; others will have to solve my problems for me."

Analogue in animal experiments Although experiments with animals may not tell us why a man acts as he does, they do help us to look for factors that might control his behavior. Ferster (1966) presents a functional analysis of depression by describing the kinds of variables that decrease an animal's responsiveness to his environment. One variable is the amount of work required to obtain a reinforcement. If large amounts of energy are required to obtain food reinforcement, long pauses occur following the attainment of the food. These pauses can be so long that the animal will starve to death. In other words, the rewards are not worth the effort, so the animal stops trying.

A second factor that reduces responsive behavior is aversive stimuli. A buzzer previously paired with shock will eventually disrupt an animal's ongoing behavior as effectively as the shock. In human terms the anxiety connected with certain assertive acts is enough to stop the individual from doing the acts.

A third variable in reducing behavior is a sudden change in the environment. A bird conditioned to receive food when it pecks a green key will not peck if the color changes to red. Similarly, a person may lose his repertoire of behaviors if someone on whom he was dependent dies or if he is forced to separate from that person.

Punishment is a fourth variable in behavior reduction. The manner in which punishment is delivered is critical. If animals are exposed to shock from which they cannot escape and are subsequently exposed to shock from which they can escape, they frequently make no effort to escape. The more trials of inescapable shock to which the animal is exposed, the poorer is the subsequent escape or avoidance behavior. In other words, the original learning that they were helpless to change their situation interfered with new learning where active coping was necessary for success (Overmier, 1968; Overmier & Seligman, 1967; Smith, Cohen, & Turner, 1968).

Vicarious learning Learning can result not only from direct experience, but also from observing what happens to others. Learned helplessness, therefore, can be the result of vicarious processes through which the individual adopts the attitudes, feelings, and behaviors of others who are prime models in his environment. These vicarious processes have been referred to as imitation, copying, modeling, role playing, observational learning, social facilitation, contagion, and identification.

Depression reaction

Depression manifests itself differently in children than in adults (Toolan, 1962). Depression in infancy is manifested in eating and sleeping disturbances, colic, crying, and head banging. These behaviors occur when the mother herself is depressed or the child is rejected. In the older child expressions of inadequacy, self-derogatory remarks, poor peer relations, listlessness, complaints of fatigue, loss of interest in activities, and loss of satisfaction if the child does participate in activities are characteristic behaviors of the child who gives in to his feelings of helplessness (Poznanski & Zrull, 1970). If the child fights these feelings (masked depression), then behavior problems, poor school performance, or psychosomatic complaints are seen (Glaser, 1967; Hollon, 1970).

A high percentage of children complaining of stomachache have no organic cause for the ache. Usually such children also display labile mood swings, changes in sleep patterns, and misery, and they are frequently relieved by antidepressive medications (Frommer & Cotton, 1970). An examination of 25 children who complained of headaches, but who had no apparent reason to do so, revealed that 10 showed six or more symptoms of depression; 9 of the 10 also had a history of depression in the family as well as a history of headache and showed improvement after being treated with antidepressive medication (Ling et al., 1970).

Rejecting autocratic control

From the preceding review we can postulate that parents who use autocratic controls and who reject their child, either overtly or because of their own depression, are likely to produce a child who feels that much of what goes on around him is beyond his control. If the child is separated from those adults who direct his behavior or is exposed to other trauma, he is likely to show symptoms of depression.

Studies of the parents of depressed children reveal a high incidence of depression, problems in handling aggression, and violent outbursts of control (Poznanski & Zrull, 1970). Parents of depressives are also seen as controlling, critical, and overprotective toward their child and disappointed in his functioning (Cofer, 1970; MacDonald, 1971).

Depression is more frequent in females than males. Perhaps this is because women in our society are expected to fill a helpless, dependent role. Consequently, the usual child rearing practices for females tend to predispose them to depression (Wittenborn, 1965).

While we would theorize that depression underlies all the disorders previously described, we also know that depression can be manifested in other forms. If the child has rejecting and inconsistent autocratic parents who display many problems of their own, his depression is likely to be expressed in a disorganized, inconsistent manner.

Jack, a 9-year old referred to a residential treatment center, sometimes displayed behaviors designed to ward off depressive feelings and at other times gave into these feelings. Consequently, he displayed masking as well as direct symptoms.

JACK

Child care worker's report When Jack first entered the residence, he was a rather quiet, pathetic, withdrawn boy. Much of his verbalization consisted of sheer fantasy; he talked to door knobs or to imaginary people. He would spend much time whispering to our dog, letting him know in advance what I had planned for the group. His abnormal closeness to the dog is still predominant today. His rationalization for this behavior is simply, "Dogs are happier than people." He is no longer completely withdrawn. He will not participate in most games because he fears competition. He has mentioned that he fails at everything, that he is not as "good as others," and that he is a "born loser." Jack anticipates the worst from every event and every encounter with another person. His low self-concept and belief that he is "doomed to failure" prevent healthy interaction in the group setting. I have tried to show Jack that he is not inadequate, but when I think he has made gains, he will revert to his expression of helplessness and magnify his shortcomings.

When he is not feeling depressed, Jack is bright and witty, even by adult standards. At present he is esteemed by the boys and holds a high place in the group (as seen in a recent sociometric test). Nevertheless, he takes no credit for these achievements. On the negative side, Jack's jokes and talk stimulate the other children. He becomes silly and starts a contagion cycle in the group. He mimics and teases other children when they are upset, but reacts strongly if he is teased. If the boys tell Jack to stop his silliness, he sometimes becomes even louder.

When Jack is corrected, he either flutters his eyelashes and says, "OK, anything you say" or becomes sullen and storms off muttering to himself. Jack has insight into reasons for other's behavior, but he cannot apply such insight to himself. He philosophizes a great deal and says people are hypocrites. In short, Jack is a boy who thinks little of himself (refers to himself as a dog, a specimen, a failure) and who is fearful and mistrusting of others, especially adults. He is a hurt boy hiding behind his humor. His relationship with his mother and her overwhelming influence on him are still crucial problems. He is notably more agitated before and after each contact with her.

When Jack goes home on vacations, his parents are always critical of his Negroid features. His mother cuts his hair close each time he arrives home and before he visits his grandparents who are even more intolerant of blacks. No wonder Jack frequently requests to have his hair straightened and shows confusion about his racial identity. Both parents still threaten each other with divorce but neither has ever acted on these threats.

Social history Jack was born out of wedlock to a white, Irish Catholic mother and black father. His mother refused to marry his father because he was a "selfish, Godless man who wanted her to work for him." He had seen the boy only once when he was 2 months old.

During his early infancy Jack spent the weekdays at a school for women where he was used to demonstrate proper mothering techniques. Despite the stress of this period, his mother spoke of it with great pride and joy.

Mother and child then moved in with her parents. Jack's presence disturbed the family and his mother was severely mistreated by her family during this stay. Her ambivalence about Jack intensified during this time. When Jack was 2½, his mother began to take care of her sick father. Jack was boarded out during the week with an Italian family who took care of his physical needs but expected him to "toe the line." Jack spent the weekends with his mother and reacted strongly to separation each time he left her to return to the Italian family. Jack was toilet trained early by the Italian family but was enuretic on weekends at home. During this period Jack had his first asthmatic attack. Since then he has had frequent hospitalizations for asthma (see Chapter 6). His mother resented taking him to the hospital because of the inconvenience it caused her. During his hospital stays Jack tended to drift into dreamland, and hospital records described the boy as apathetic.

At age 4, Jack was put in a day nursery, and he and his mother moved to their own apartment. Jack responded poorly to the nursery school placement. When Jack was 7, his mother quit her job and admitted herself to a day care hospital. She was there for six months. Jack felt deserted by this act and both his disruptive behavior and his enuresis intensified. One year later, his mother had him admitted as a day patient to the psychiatric division of a children's hospital. After three months in this program, primarily because his mother no longer could bring him every day, he switched from a day patient to a five-day-a-week patient, going home on weekends. Jack adjusted to hospital routines, but his mother's behavior worsened; she began to resist the treatment offered her at the children's hospital. After one therapy session, she became drunk and attempted to take Jack from the ward.

Jack's progress at the children's hospital prompted his referral to the residential treatment center. Destructive behavior ceased and his behavior became more appropriate. Peer and adult relationships improved as did school performance. Hospital staff felt, therefore, that the child would profit from treatment in a more open setting. After Jack's admission to residential treatment, his mother became engaged to a man who made limited contact with Jack one condition for marriage. She felt torn between this man and her son. With a sense of high drama, his mother said "This is my last chance." Jack's placement acted as a partial release, enabling her to at least think about the satisfaction of her own needs.

Treatment

Treatment of the depressed child would be guided by the theory that depression is helplessness learned within the context of an overcontrolling and rejecting family environment. The child would be positively reinforced for the emission of assertive behaviors (Lewinsohn & Shaffer, 1971), while the family would be helped to alter their style of relating to the child and to model more self-assertive behaviors themselves. Any depression in other family members would have to be lifted and alternative coping styles developed in that member. Lazarus (1968) presents various techniques that help to disrupt the emotional inhibitions characterizing depressed adults.

One obstacle to the treatment of depressives is our emphasis on procedures designed to lift the depression (e.g., medication) and our relative disinterest in helping the client develop a life style that will enable him to learn that he can influence his environment to his benefit. Simply discharging a patient from the hospital after medication or psychotherapy has made him feel better is not very helpful. Until we appreciate the stresses a patient will have to face when he returns home and prepare him to cope adequately with these stresses, we are likely to see him return again for treatment.

How do they fare?

At present there are no studies that have followed a group of depressed children over a period of time. One reason for this gap in our knowledge is that many depressed children probably never come to the attention of mental health professionals. A child who is withdrawn but who voices no complaints and stays out of trouble does not usually get referred to a child guidance clinic because he causes no one any real concern. A child with stomachaches or headaches is usually taken to a family physician or pediatrician and is reassured that it is just "nerves."

A second reason for this gap in knowledge is that depression in childhood is often masked by behaviors not recognized as depression. As clinicians become more aware that depression underlies other behaviors, perhaps a group of depressed children could be followed into adulthood.

One approach to this problem would be to identify children who are a high risk to develop depression. This could be done in two ways. First, children of women hospitalized for depression could be followed to see how many develop symptoms of depression and under what conditions these symptoms appear.

A second approach would be to examine the early childhoods of adults who have become depressed. There is some evidence that when depressed adults were seen as children they displayed anxiety, depression, and somatic complaints (Pritchard & Graham, 1966). Nevertheless, adults with disorders other than depression were more often seen in childhood than were those with depression. As we have already implied, these findings could mean that they were overlooked as children rather than that they were not depressed. In addition, the stresses these patients faced in childhood may not have been substantial enough to have precipitated severe depression at that time. As they became older and were required to face more responsibilities, their background of learned helplessness may have culminated in a depressive reaction. Hopefully, future research will shed some light on these speculations.

SUMMARY OF DISORDERS PRECIPITATED BY THE AUTOCRATIC FAMILY

The preceding review has suggested that parents who insist that children always follow the standards they set and severely punish any minor deviation from these standards predispose a child to develop certain behavior disorders when the child is faced with stress beyond his ability to handle. These behaviors are seen as exaggerations of behaviors that characterize the child prior to his adverse reaction to stress. Within the atmosphere of a rigidly controlling family environment, the child develops limited coping strategies and displays a rigid-inhibited approach to problem solving. When faced with stress, stress that serves to restrict the choice of alternative coping strategies even in normal individuals, the autocratically reared child becomes fixed in nonproductive, stereotyped patterns of behavior. We have labeled these behaviors as obsessive-compulsive behaviors, covert expressions of negativism, pseudoindependence, and helplessness. Extreme forms are called obsessive-compulsive neurosis, anorexia nervosa, hysterical neurosis, and depressive reaction. The adoption of these particular behaviors is considered a function of the degree of both the consistency of control, the stability of standards, and the warmth displayed toward the child.

If the control is rigidly consistent, we postulated that obsessive-compulsive behaviors would characterize the personality. If the control is inconsistent, covert expressions of negativism, such as intellectual inhibition or contrariness will predominate in the personality, with refusal to eat as an extreme expression of indirect negativism. If the standards the child is to obey fluxuate according to whim and the child is pushed to achieve beyond his ability, pseudoindependent functioning will typify his behavior, with hysteria a reaction to a failure of this type of functioning to reduce stress.

If the child is outwardly rejected by the autocratic parent, either because the parent is depressed and therefore self-preoccupied or because the child is disliked, then the child is likely to become depressed. Being disliked or ignored and forced to comply to rigid standards, he never learns that he can effect change in his environment. The extent to which depression underlies obsessive-compulsive neurosis, anorexia nervosa, and hysteria is theorized to relate to the degree of rejection present. We would add that some rejection underlies the behavior of most autocratic parents since they lack respect for the child as a developing individual: to be liked, the child has to be just like his parents.

THE PROTECTIVE-INTERDEPENDENT FAMILY

In contrast to the autocratic parent who provides absolute criteria for behavior and who rewards and punishes his child in terms of these criteria, the protective-interdependent parent is one who helps the child to achieve independently but who anticipates that he will fail and supports him in his activities before failure occurs (Harvey et al., 1961). In a general sense, both autocratic and protective-interdependent training could be called overprotective training. In consistent autocratic training, however, overprotection takes the form of parental control to meet externally established criteria; failure to meet these criteria is a transgression. In protective-interdependent training overprotection takes the form of parental support of the child's instrumental behavior to achieve internally determined goals, but the parents' help prevents the development of autonomy.

The child whose activities are always carefully monitored by his parents and who is rarely allowed to fail achieves conditional dependence at the expense of autonomous independence (Hogan, 1973; Harvey et al., 1961). The course of his development is also affected by the fact that considerable time may pass before the child realizes that he is not self-sufficient, that his achievements were not due to his own efforts but rather to the efforts of his parents.

Protective-interdependent training sensitizes the child to other people's reactions to his behavior and increases his tendency to rely on the support of others in unstructured situations. The child's prime motive is to maintain positive relationships with others so as to avoid the withdrawal of their support. Such a child becomes anxious when threatened with loss of support or when pressured to function autonomously. When the child reaches negativisitic stages of development (when he asserts his individuality), his oppositional tendencies enlist the support, attention, and interest of his parents. Because oppositional tendencies are in conflict with learned tendencies to look to others for support and assistance, they are never serious efforts nor are they taken seriously by the parent. The child, therefore, never learns how to master a challenging task alone because others always help him. Consequently, he is threatened by pressures toward autonomy and separation. Under such threat, the individual avoids situations where autonomous or independent actions are required. On other occasions, he overstrives to keep his self-image positive in the eyes of others. Neither of these strategies is ever totally successful. Consequently, the child exhibits a high level of anxiety whenever he is forced to be independent.

Learning style

When a child raised in a protective-interdependent environment goes to school, his parents can no longer effectively intercede on his behalf. Consequently, he is likely to become anxious and seek out the support of the teacher. He may be said to have an anxious-dependent learning style, displaying high achievement anxiety, reliance on others, and need for closeness to the teacher (Mordock, 1968–1969). If he is a particularly bright child and if pressures for achievement are low, he may show relatively little anxious dependency. If pressures for achievement are high and if the material to be learned is difficult, his anxiety may reach panic proportions. Because of the continually high anxiety level of the anxious-dependent child, he is prone to develop conditioned fear reactions, or phobias.

PHOBIAS

In 1920 Watson and Rayner (1920) demonstrated that a child can learn to fear neutral objects that are present when fear is aroused by something else. Little Albert had no fear of white rats, but the rat was present when a loud unexpected noise frightened him This noise occurred nine times in the presence of the white rat. When the rat was presented alone, Albert cried, fell over, and crawled away with all his might. A week later this same fear reaction had generalized from the white rat to a friendly white rabbit and to white furry objects. He even showed fear to a Santa Claus mask.

Several years later Jones (1924) demonstrated that deconditioning of a feared object can take place by pairing the object with a pleasant situation. She deconditioned a 3-year-old boy's fear of furry objects by pairing a white rabbit with a pleasant affect. The rabbit was placed in a wire cage across the room from where the child, Peter, was eating. Each day the rabbit was brought a little closer, until Peter could eat with one hand while stroking the rabbit with the other.

Prior to the work of Watson and Jones, phobias had been explained quite differently. In 1909 Freud published the first case of a child's psychoanalysis. The child presented had a phobia of horses and would not go out into the street for fear of being bitten by a horse. Freud noticed that prior to the development of this fear the child, Hans, had been generally irritable and fretful in the presence of his parents. Once the fear developed, however, these signs of anxiety disappeared. Freud concluded that by substituting the conscious fear of a horse for the unconscious fear of his father, Hans was relieved of his anxiety in the home (Freud, 1950).

Why did Hans fear his father? Freud postulated that this phobia represented displaced anxiety associated with the Oedipus complex. According to this theory Hans desired to possess his mother all to himself and was jealous and hostile toward his father. He therefore feared his father and dreaded the possibility of retaliation from or even castration by him. Since he also loved his father, this fear was unacceptable; displacing the fear of his father onto the innocuous horse resolved this dilemma (Wangh, 1967). Castration fears and Oedipal anxiety were heightened in Hans because of his mother's seductive behavior. The horse was selected as the feared object because the father used to play "horsie" with Hans. The phobia also served to keep him home with his beloved mother. Psychoanalytic theorists, drawing on this early work, have considered phobias as displaced fears, and they have designed their treatment to uncover the source of the "real" fear. For example, a man who fears that he may lose his job develops an elevator phobia, making it impossible to get to his office and hence protecting him from the embarrassment of being fired. Phobias also can develop as a defense against a dangerous impulse, for example, a husband develops a fear of lakes, ponds, and other bodies of water because he has ideas of drowning his wife (Coleman, 1964).

In a critique of Freud's case of little Hans, Wolpe and Rachman (1960) concluded that Hans probably learned to fear horses in the same manner as Albert learned to fear white furry objects—a conditioned fear reaction. On three occasions Hans had been frightened in situations where horses were involved. Hans's recovery from the phobia could have resulted from gradual deconditioning over time. Many children's phobias decline and disappear over time when parts of the feared stimulus (generalized phobic stimuli) evoke anxiety responses weak enough to be inhibited by other emotional responses aroused in their presence. The interpretations of the source of his fear, which were presented to Hans in the course of his analysis, were probably irrelevant in his recovery; rather, the repeated presentation of phobic stimuli in a variety of emotional contexts may have inhibited the anxiety and thereby diminished its habit strength. The gradualness of Hans's recovery is consonant with this explanation.

Although phobias are learned responses, they are more prevalent among children in families who use protective-interdependent training techniques and who thereby produce anxious-dependent children (Al Salih, 1968; Andrews, 1966; Bates, 1970; Fazio, 1972). Phobic children are described as dependent children who are eager to please their overprotective parents. Perhaps the phobia that presents the greatest challenge to teachers is a fear of school. We said earlier that if achievement pressures are high and the material to be learned is difficult, the anxious-dependent child may become so anxious that a state of panic results. This panic attack has been called school phobia. School phobia is believed to be an extreme reaction to fears of failure and potential loss of support.

School phobia

The term school phobia refers to a state of acute anxiety about going to school. The word phobia implies that the anxiety is localized, its focal point being an irrational fear of attending school. Nevertheless, the reason for the acute panic is not readily apparent if just the school itself is examined as a source for the anxiety (Levison, 1962; Olsen & Coleman, 1967). From our theoretical conceptions regarding protective-interdependent training, we would postulate that school phobia is actually an extreme form of achievement anxiety, anxiety precipitated by increased pressures to achieve autonomously (Malmquist, 1965). Within this framework school phobia could appear at any time, but it would be most likely to appear when anxiety about autonomous functioning is maximal. During the first few years in school most children would perform satisfactorily since relatively little independent functioning is demanded and teachers are quite helpful. Material to be learned is concrete and requires convergent rather than divergent thinking ability.

After third grade the situation changes. The student is expected to read directions and perform assignments independently. Independent projects in social studies are undertaken and dictionary skills should have been mastered. In addition, the child moves from the stage of concrete operations to the stage of symbolic reasoning at about the same time.

Children raised in a protective-interdependent environment are not necessarily aware that their achievements are "arranged" for them. When they finally realize that they are not as competent as they originally conceived, their anxiety quickly mounts. Should some external (precipitating) event make it harder for them to retain the facade of competence and should their failures become apparent to others, school phobia may develop. Let us examine the evidence that bears on this theory.

Examining their own as well as other reported cases, Leventhal and Sills (1964) cite the following descriptive findings: (1) ages cover the school years, but the greatest frequency is among 10- to 12-year olds; (2) there is an equal number of boys and girls; (3) intelligence is usually average and school grades at least satisfactory; (4) there are high academic standards and concern about achievement; (5) personality traits noted are willfulness, domination of mother but closeness to her, manipulative tendencies, and nonaggressiveness bordering on timidity outside the home; (6) mothers overindulge the children; (7) parental rejection is noticeably absent; (8) the most frequent precipitants are change in schools and illness; (9) most children maintain their social activities outside the home, except for those at school; and (10) a wide range of pathology is represented, varying from adequate functioning to the verge of a psychotic break.

Leventhal and Sills postulate from this data that school phobics are children who overvalue themselves and their achievements. When their unrealistic self-image is threatened in the school situation, they suffer anxiety and retreat to another situation where they can maintain this narcissistic self-image. In terms of a social-learning theory approach the overevaluation of self may be the result of early parental indulgence; the omnipotence of the child, fostered and not challenged in early home experiences, persists into later years and results in the child's continual struggle to maintain a lofty self-image. Unprepared for the frustrations and demands of the outside world, the indulged child may see himself as suffering constant failure and defensively falls back on attempts to recapture the infantile narcissistic position. Because the self-image is not securely held, it is extremely sensitive to threat; thus, the child with high achievement needs is markedly sensitive to imagined school failure. Switching schools or return after a prolonged absence may signal challenges that the child senses he cannot master; remaining home allows him to avoid the anxiety generated by the thought of such failure (Leventhal & Sills, 1964). Such an explanation of school phobia is consistent with predictions generated from our notions of the effects of protective-interdependent training.

Because school phobia is usually precipitated by some environmental event (Smith, 1970), the predisposing conditions are often overlooked. The case of Dora serves as an example of school phobia that didn't seem to fit the expected pattern because of the unusual manner in which the phobia was precipitated. Further evaluation, however, revealed a family pattern of protective-interdependent training.

DORA

The school guidance counselor called the local child guidance clinic about a 10-year old girl who sat in her office and refused to go to her classroom. The principal had tried to take her to class, but she turned white with fear and almost passed out. Clinic staff said to bring her and her mother to the clinic and they would see what assistance they could provide.

The mother revealed that Dora's phobia had followed her father's admission to the state hospital. He had brandished a gun and had threatened to kill all the police in town (his father was chief of police). Dora's adolescent brother was described as a highly nervous person who had been hospitalized several times. The mother verbalized that perhaps Dora was afraid that her father might kill her mother and felt that she should be home to protect her. However, Dora denied that this was her fear, insisting that she feared school but didn't know why. Clinic staff initially felt the reason for this denial was because of her love for her father; perhaps it was too painful to admit fearing him.

Historical material revealed that Dora had been somewhat fearful upon entering kindergarten and often had unexplained absences. Clinic staff then began to see that her mother actually wanted Dora home because of an interdependent relationship with her. The parents had fought violently in the past and Dora had often called her older brothers to come and intervene. Dora was also her mother's "baby." Her two other children had left home and her husband was emotionally divorced from her. Dora, therefore, was her only source of close emotional support. Dora's mother had always emphasized that Dora should do well in school and stressed that Dora had always been a good student. Nevertheless, her style of relating to Dora suggested protective-interdependent training strategies. The father's own loss of control and threatened attacks on those who represented his own father (Dora liked her grandfather a great deal) made it clear to Dora that people could lose control over their actions. Perhaps she felt that she too might lose control in school, that she might react to her mounting anxieties about continued success in school in the same way as her father had reacted to his anxieties. Admittedly, the precipitating factor which led to this phobia was not the typical one; nevertheless, the family pattern was considered one of mutual interdependence.

Dora's treatment took two directions. The mother was helped to extend herself into the community, encouraged to find a job, and given a great deal of support through case work. Dora was required to attend school for increasing amounts of time, but remained in the principal's outer office until she could attend class.

The first classes that Dora attended were taught by females. In the clinic Dora refused to relate to one male therapist and was transferred to a second, much older therapist, who, according to the mother, resembled the grandfather to whom Dora was quite attached. Eventually, the mother took a job and all appointments ceased. Dora by then had returned to all her classes.

When Dora's fear subsided, her mother was no longer interested in continuing treatment. Since the fear was gone, she was under no pressures and could see no need for any further assistance. Her response is typical of many parents—once the crisis has passed they reject the notion that another crisis might occur in the future.

Other theories of school phobia Not all theorists ascribe to the view that school phobia represents a retreat from threats to a lofty self-image. Some consider school phobia a problem of separation anxiety related to an ambivalent attitude toward one or both parents (Olsen & Coleman, 1967). The mother is usually the dominant figure in the relationship with the child. Unsuccessful in resolving her own dependency and separation anxieties, the mother unconsciously prescribes and reinforces the child's dependency on her. Attempts to understand a school phobia will fail if efforts are confined to investigation of the school situation itself.

Leventhal and Sills feel that findings do not support the dependency-separation-fear theory. If this theory were correct, then the greatest frequency of school phobia should be at kindergarten age rather than at 10 to 12. In addition, children would be expected to have difficulty separating from the mother in many areas of life. This was not always the case, and in older children, about 12 on, was rarely the case. Most published cases report that children maintain their outside social activities. The willfulness and controlling personality traits and their academic success and achievement motives are also not consonant with a formulation of a complete lack of independence.

The learning theory approach postulates that if intense fear occurs in the presence of a neutral stimulus (the school), the stimulus acquires the ability to evoke fear subsequently. If the fear at the original conditioning situation is of high intensity or if conditioning is repeated, the conditioned fear will show the persistence that is characteristic of neurotic fear. There will also be generalization of fear reactions to stimuli resembling the conditioned stimulus (Wolpe & Rachman, 1960).

A third theory, based on operant principles (instrumental conditioning), postulates that the phobia arises because of undue attention given the child following a fear response. Should the child desire more attention, he would display the fear.

The actual reason for school phobia is probably a combination of all the various factors mentioned. Threatened by demands for autonomous functioning, the child displays continual anxiety in school. Various properties of the school get conditioned to the fear and acquire the ability to evoke fear independently. When at home, the child anticipates having a fear reaction in school and attempts to avoid the feared situation. If the child is kept home, this avoidance reaction is reinforced and therefore becomes a conditioned avoidance reaction, i.e., whenever the child's fear of school is aroused, his initial response will be to avoid school. Conditioned avoidance reactions are extremely difficult to extinguish since extinction can take place only in the presence of the feared stimulus.

Soloman and Wynne (1954) demonstrated the marked resistance to extinction of conditioned avoidance reactions. Dogs were shocked in half of a cage separated from the other half by a wall. Eventually the dogs learned to escape the shock by jumping the wall into the safe half of the cage. An auditory signal then preceded the shock by a brief interval, and the dog learned to jump the wall immediately after the signal and thereby avoid the shock. The shock was then turned off, but the signal continued. Some dogs continued to jump the wall over 1000 times in the absence of shock. The only way to eliminate this fear was to force the animal to remain in the feared half in order for him to learn that he would no longer be shocked.

School phobia seems to follow a similar pattern. If the child is allowed to remain out of school, successful treatment is less likely. Before much was known about school phobia, children were allowed to remain at home. The symptom frequently persisted for months and even years after treatment. The child's prolonged absence from school disrupted his education, hampered his social adjustment, and distorted his family relationships. It was not until 1959 that the relation between remission of the symptom and the promptness of treatment initiation was elucidated.

Research has also revealed that school phobia in children beyond the fourth grade was considerably more serious and occurred among those with more serious family pathology (Waldfogel et al., 1959). In many of these cases signs of trouble had appeared earlier, but had been ignored. All investigators indicate that school phobia in adolescence is a very serious disorder. The symptom's onset is preceded by a long history of unmet needs that have seriously interfered with development. The phobia is usually an expression of panic in the face of adolescent pressures and usually accompanies a return to infantile behavior (Coolidge, Willer, Tessman, & Waldfogel, 1960; Robinson, Dalgleish, & Egan, 1967).

Treatment Regardless of whether one holds a psychodynamic or behavioral viewpoint, treatment emphasizes getting the child back in school as soon as possible. The difference between the two theoretical positions lies in the manner in which the child is approached. Psychodynamic practitioners provide insight oriented therapy designed to free the parent and child from their unhealthy dependency upon each other. During therapy the child remains in the school building as long as possible, even if only in the library or an office.

An investigation of 26 cases of school phobia revealed that when treatment was initiated shortly after the symptom appeared, in most cases school attendance resumed after a few weeks. When treatment was postponed for a semester or more after the phobia's onset, the sympton continued long after treatment had begun (Waldfogel, Tessman, & Hahn, 1959).

The Judge Baker Guidance Center arranged to identify cases of incipient school phobia in order to provide preventive help within the school. Over a two-year period a total of 36 children with symptoms of school phobia were identified in the school. Of these, 16 received therapy in the school, 4 received therapy in the clinic, 5 made a spontaneous recovery, and 11 received no therapy. Every effort was made to keep the children in school during treatment. Follow-up one year after treatment revealed that 14 of the 16 treated in school were symptom free, as were all 4 treated in the clinic. Four of the 5 who had made a spontaneous recovery were still symptom free. Of the 11 who had received no treatment, only 3 were symptom free at follow-up (Waldfogel et al., 1959). Similar findings were reported by Robinson, Dalgleish, and Egan (1967).

Medication has also been used in combination with insight oriented family guidance. The drug (Tofranil) is postulated to lower the anxiety and block the panic attack. Comparison of a group of 16 children given medication with 19 given a placebo revealed the superiority of the drug-treated group. Although no differences were apparent after three weeks of treatment, after six weeks 13 of the 16 on medication were attending school (81 percent), while only 9 of the 19 on placebos were attending (47 percent). All of the drug-treated group reported feeling much less anxious, while only 4 of the placebo group felt this way.

Rather than using medication to lower anxiety, behavior therapists attempt to do so by instituting procedures that require the child to face anxieties he can master. A widely used method among behavioral therapists is systematic desensitization (Wolpe, 1969), or gradual habituation, to the anxiety arousing stimulus. In most cases desensitization takes place in the actual school situation (*in vivo*). The child is accompanied to school by the therapist and he stays for a short period, perhaps 15 minutes. The next day the period of stay is longer. With each successive day the time in school is increased, until the child remains for the full day. The reason for such a procedure is that the child is required to cope with only a small amount of anxiety on each occasion (he knows he only has to stay 15 minutes). Initially 15 minutes is feared. Then 15 minutes is no longer feared, but it is an additional 15-minute period that is feared. Then a half hour is no longer feared, but the last 15 minutes of a 45-minute period is feared, and so on. In this fashion the amount of anxiety generated remains the same. Requiring the child to face a whole day usually generates anxiety too high to cope with successfully. The child is reassured and rewarded for each successful performance so that staying in school is reinforced (instrumental or operant conditioning).

Lazarus, Davison, and Polefka (1965) describe the use of systematic *in vivo* desenisitization with a boy of 9 who had been absent from school for about three weeks. This case, too long to present here, is perhaps the best published example of the use of various behavioral techniques in the removal of a rather serious school phobia.

Desensitization can also take place to an imagined stimulus through the use of anxiety inhibiting emotive images. Emotive images are those images assumed to arouse feelings of self-assertion, pride, affection, and mirth, emotions assumed to have autonomic effects which are incompatible with anxiety.

Lazarus and Abramovitz (1962, p. 459) describe the steps employed in this procedure.

a. As in the usual method of systematic desensitization, the range, intensity, and circumstances of the patient's fears are ascertained, and a graduated hierarchy is drawn up, from the most feared to the least feared situation.
b. By sympathetic conversation and enquiry, the clinician establishes the nature of the child's hero-images—usually derived from radio, cinema, fiction, or his own imagination—and the wish-fulfillments and identifications which accompany them.
c. The child is then asked to close his eyes and told to imagine a sequence of events which is close enough to his everyday life to be credible, but within which is woven a story concerning his favorite hero or *alter ego*.

d. If this is done with reasonable skill and empathy it is possible to arouse to the necessary pitch the child's affective reactions. (In some cases this may be recognized by small changes in facial expression, breathing, muscle tension, etc.)

e. When the clinician judges that these emotions have been maximally aroused, he introduces, as a natural part of the narrative, the lowest item in the hierarchy. Immediately afterwards he says, "If you feel afraid (or unhappy or uncomfortable) just raise your finger." If anxiety is indicated, the phobic stimulus is "withdrawn" from the narrative and the child's anxiety-inhibiting emotions are again aroused. The procedure is then repeated as in ordinary systematic desensitization until the highest item in the hierarchy is tolerated without distress.

They then illustrate its use with the following case (1962, p. 461).

An eight-year-old girl was referred for treatment because of persistent nocturnal enuresis and a fear of going to school. Her fear of the school situation was apparently engendered by a series of emotional upsets in class. In order to avoid going to school, the child resorted to a variety of devices including temper tantrums, alleged pains and illness and on one occasion she was caught playing truant and intemperately upbraided by her father. Professional assistance was finally sought when it was found that her younger sister was evincing the same behavior.

When the routine psychological investigations had been completed, emotive imagery was introduced with the aid of an Enid Blyton character, Noddy, who provided a hierarchy of assertive challenges centered around the school situation. The essence of this procedure was to create imagined situations where Noddy played the role of a truant and responded fearfully to the school setting. The patient would then protect him, either by active reassurance or by "setting a good example."

Only four sessions were required to eliminate her school-going phobia. Her enuresis, which had received no specific therapeutic attention, was far less frequent and disappeared entirely within two months. The child has continued to improve despite some additional upsets at the hands of an unsympathetic teacher.

Although behaviorists claim their treatment procedures are superior to other approaches, there have been no meticulous follow-up studies of cases treated by behavioral approaches. Reports of school and social adjustment have been omitted from the studies made (Hersen, 1971).

How do they fare? In spite of the recent optimism of behavioral therapists (Patterson, 1965; Smith & Sharpe, 1970), follow-up studies of phobic children reveal many manifest symptoms traceable back to the original phobia. Former phobics displayed chronic apprehension about attending school or exaggerated and unwarranted concern about studies or exams. These concerns were expressed as Monday morning anergia, vague aches and pains, or absences due to feigned illnesses. Absences for minor illnesses were more frequent and of longer duration than usually expected. Many showed a cautious approach to new situations. In one study of 47 children, only 13 (10 girls and 3 boys) were progressing satisfactorily toward normal adulthood, 20 (13 girls and 7 boys) showed a definite limitation in emotional and intellectual growth, characterized by a stifling of achievement in all the important areas of adolescence or uneven growth where there was adequate development in one area at the expense of others, and 14 (5 girls and 9 boys) had given up realistic attempts to move into psychological adulthood and were considered seriously disturbed. Of these 14, 10 had character disorders with 9 borderline psychotic and 1 overtly psychotic. Of the total group of 47 children, 48 percent were judged unusually dependent.

In the total sample more than half were leading colorless, restricted, unimaginative lives, with delayed or absent heterosexual development, excessive dependency, blunted affect, and lack of mood swings. They were primarily home centered in their activities and extremely cautious in their pursuits. Even the relatively successful cases exhibited this trait, evidently guarding against anxiety aroused in new situations (Coolidge, Brodie, & Feeney, 1964). Similarly, Weiss and Burke (1970) report that the majority of their subjects were relatively constricted, affectively cool, and unable to relate to others deeply and intimately.

In adulthood school phobics approach situations requiring autonomy with extreme caution or avoid them altogether by restricting their activities. Radin (1972) reports that severe anxiety about work—job phobia—has its antecedents in school phobia.

The degree of restriction in activity is probably related to the amount of anxiety generated by threats to self-esteem or to the extent to which parental child rearing practices were exclusively protective-interdependent. Additional pressure for autonomy in adulthood may come from parents. Although encouraging dependency in childhood, parents may not be able to tolerate a dependent adult. Consequently, they may pressure the young adult to leave home and be more autonomous, unaware that their earlier attitudes have ill-equipped their child for such functioning.

Other phobias

Anxious-dependent children show a variety of phobias, with maturational factors playing an important role in the selection of the feared object. In a study of 129 adult phobic patients almost all animal or insect phobias had started prior to age 5. Other phobias (heights, closed spaces, crowds, etc.) were noticeably absent prior to age 10 (Marks, 1966). These findings suggest a period in childhood when certain fears are more readily acquired.

Treatment We saw in our discussion of school phobia that one way to treat this disorder is to arouse emotions incompatible with anxiety. If these positive emotions (e.g., mirth, affection) can be paired with school, then school becomes less aversive. This same principle is used to treat other phobias.

Both Jones (1924) and Wolpe (1958) postulated that deep relaxation can inhibit mild anxiety and diminish its habit strength. Wolpe calls this process reciprocal inhibition. Frequently, however, the individual cannot remain relaxed in the presence of the fear object because the anxiety aroused is to strong. Wolpe (1969), therefore, developed a procedure where the individual could imagine the feared object in such a manner that only mild anxiety would be aroused. For example, a child who feared dogs would be trained to relax and asked to imagine scenes previously ranked according to their anxiety arousing properties. The first scene imagined might be looking out a car window at a little dog standing 100 yards from the car. When the child could imagine this scene without feeling anxious, the therapist would ask him to imagine the next scene on the list, which might be the dog standing 90 yards from the car. In each scene the child would imagine the dog a little closer until it stood right outside the car. This scene might be repeated except that the car window would be opened and the dog a little bigger. Next the child might imagine himself on a bike and then standing. Eventually he would pat the dog in his imagination. When the child could imagine the most distressing situation on the list without anxiety, the therapist would introduce a real dog in a similar manner.

Sometimes emotive imagery is used to arouse emotions incompatible with anxiety. Molly, a young girl who was a good swimmer, was treated with emotive imagery in combination with systematic desensitization. Molly would make believe she was swimming and had to save drowning dogs of increasing sizes. She knew that dogs swam poorly and imagining such a scene raised little anxiety. She saved the dog first by pushing a large surfboard under it, then by using a smaller board, and finally by placing a ring over the dog's head. Molly eventually learned to touch dogs in real life.

For children who cannot or will not use their imagination, some rather ingenious manipulations of the environment have been performed to accomplish *in vivo* desensitization. McNamara (1968–69) describes an unusual approach to eliminate a child's fear of the bathroom. Although the child would visit the bathroom if accompanied by her teacher, she would not go alone. Individual therapy sessions in the classroom, while the other children were on the playground, utilized sequential presentation of fear-associated cues in the presence of preferred toys and candy. A model bathroom situation was set up in the room in alignment with the bathroom but 15 feet from it. A 6-foot square was set off by four small rectangular dividers. Preferred toys were placed in the area along with candy. The child played with the therapist inside this space until no apprehension was noted. A cardboard toilet was then placed in the model area and play continued for several sessions.

Three large outdoor blocks were set in a line running from the model area to the bathroom. The child gradually learned to sit on the block in the bathroom. She was then rewarded for sitting on the toilet and then for wetting. At this time the teacher and aides were instructed to take her to the bathroom but not to hold her hand. They gradually withdrew physically and started closing the door. The therapist's involvement ceased after 11 sessions when the girl was spontaneously going to the bathroom alone during regular class. A follow-up three months after treatment indicated no return of phobic symptoms.

Miller and his colleagues (Miller, Curtis, Hampe, & Noble, 1972) compared the effect of systematic desensitization, insight oriented psychotherapy, and no treatment (a control group on the clinic's waiting list). Sixty-seven children between the ages of 6 and 15 were studied. The evaluation revealed that both treatments were equally effective for young phobic children (23 of the 24 children between the ages of 6 and 10 improved, compared to 8 of 14 in the waiting list control group), but that neither treatment had much effect on the older children (ages 11 to 15).

Because the younger children improved regardless of the treatment method employed or the experience of the therapist, Miller concluded that the crucial variables affecting change are unknown. It was obvious, however, that the strategies available to influence young children had no effect on the older. Factors such as the child's increased capacity for information processing combined with a shift from concrete thinking to formal logical operations could be a factor in the choice of therapy. Recall the principle presented at the beginning of this chapter that traumatic events in childhood are reacted to according to the developmental level of the child at the time of the events. Evidently, a child's response to treatment is also affected by developmental age. Another explanation is that the child's increased social anxieties combined with the adult's intolerance for infantile coping mechanisms when they are used by older children contribute to treatment failure.

Miller's statement regarding our lack of knowledge about what actually helps the phobic child to overcome his fears reflects the state of knowledge regarding the psychotherapy of phobic conditions. Behavioral therapists directly attack the fear, either through graded exposure (Wolpe, 1969) or through forced prolonged exposure to the feared situation. It is postulated that exposure results in extinction of the fear since no real pain occurs to the patient. While autonomic reactivity (heart rate and skin resistance) does decrease after desensitization (Mathews, 1971), the decrease does not occur faster to weak than to strong stimuli (Van Egeren, Feather, & Hein, 1971), suggesting that graded and massive exposure to the feared object are equally effective (Mealiea & Nawas, 1971; Wilson & Davison 1971). However, support plus encouragement is often more effective than behavioral approaches (Fazio, 1972). In fact, Wilkins (1971), in a review of the behavioral therapies, concludes that neither muscle relaxation, graded hierarchy of fear-relevant scenes, or concomitance of instructed imagination to muscle relaxation are necessary conditions for treatment success. What seems more critical are the social and cognitive variables in the patient-doctor relationship, that is, the patient's expectations of cure, the feedback given him regarding his success, the training in control of attention, and the vicarious learning of the contingencies of behavior. The fact that these variables are common to both behavioral and insight oriented or cognitive therapies perhaps explains why Miller and his colleagues (Miller et al., 1972) found both behavioral and cognitive treatments equally effective in treating young phobics. This finding, as well as others, suggests that the differences between cognitive and behavioral perspectives have been exaggerated by the proponents of both approaches (Nawas, 1970).

If protective-interdependent training leads to anxiety states that render the child susceptible to conditioned fear responses, treating each fear as it occurs is only a partial treatment. A more appropriate approach would be to change the manner in which the family relates to the child so that he is more autonomous, less anxious, and therefore less susceptible to fear responses (Davidson, 1960; Malmquist, 1965; Mendell & Cleveland, 1967).

How do they fare?   Do phobic children grow up to be phobic adults? We do not yet know the answer to this question. Our best clue at present as to whether or not a phobic disorder will be permanent seems to be the number of symptoms accompanying the phobia and the incapacitation it causes. In general, individuals who had relatively isolated phobias as children seem to be free of phobias as adults. Follow-up studies of anxious, fearful children show that most improve with time; only those with numerous symptoms show signs of emotional disturbance as adults (Robins, 1970).

EXTREME INHIBITION

Another behavior pattern that is associated with protective-interdependent child rearing practices is extreme inhibition. If a family's protective-interdependent style of child rearing is extreme and the child is given the covert message that he can be secure only within the home, marked inhibition in functioning can occur outside the home while within the home the child appears normal.

The term inhibition is used here to refer to children who handle anxiety by restricting their range of behavior. People often handle overstimulation or anxiety by narrowing their spatial range. An adult entering a party where he knows few people rarely stands in the center of activity; he usually stands near the wall and searches for a familiar face. Similarly, the young child often copes with a unfamiliar room by going to one corner and taking out play materials. Eventually, however, he ventures out and explores the room. After he becomes familiar with the room, he makes use of the total space or those areas interesting him most. If a child continues to go to the same corner and remains there, he would be considered inhibited. Continued withholding, ignoring, shutting out, turning away from, or not giving in to others are examples of inhibition.

A specific pattern of child rearing practices that is predisposing to inhibition has been called infantilization (Sharlin & Polansky, 1972). The concept of infantilization was first described by David Levy (1943). He listed it as one of four forms of maternal overprotection, the others being excessive contact, prevention of independent behavior, and lack or excess of maternal control. Infantilization is a process where mothers encourage their child to become, or to remain, less competent and self-sufficient than the child might otherwise be. Mothers who infantilize transmit three distinct messages: "You are part of mother"; "You are fragile"; "You are special."

The infantilizing mother cannot change herself by a simple act of will. Her own needs are too strong. In most cases the mother's clinging to her child is a direct expression of her horror of loneliness, an unresolved problem in her early development. The case of Denise presents a pattern of behavior characteristic of restriction due to extreme insecurity resulting from exposure to infantilizing child rearing practices.

DENISE

Psychological evaluation of Denise was requested by her first grade teacher because of her failure to respond to the classroom routine during the first week of school. She was described as "extremely quiet and timid." Academic productivity was very low. The teacher noted Denise's inability to work on her own; she copied from peers and exhibited no independent work. She even copied during crayon coloring exercises. She had no friendships among her class peers, although she was frequently dependent upon a deskmate for companionship.

When picked up for psychological evaluation, Denise greeted the examiner with a big smile. She readily followed him to the testing office, but, once seated, became frightened and tearful. She was reassured and coaxed into cooperation by drawing tasks. Her fear appeared to subside and the WISC was begun. However, she began to sob during the administration of the second subtest of WISC. Cessation of testing and efforts at establishing rapport and cooperation loosened a flood of tears, deep sobs, and near hysterical pleas for return to the classroom. Denise was returned to the classroom after a long period of comforting from the office secretary.

Testing was again attempted a week later, with Denise's school principal delivering her to the examiner and promising to remain with her. Denise again burst into tears and sobbed her way back to the classroom.

One week following this incident Denise's mother accompanied her to school and attempted to deliver her to the examiner. Mother, child, and psychologist met in the hall and Denise again burst into tears and sobs. The mother was unable to persuade her daughter to cooperate, and as the volume and ferocity of Denise's resistance increased, the mother appeared increasingly incapable of controlling or altering her daughter's behavior; she became deeply embarrassed. The examiner left them and noted that Denise's sobs than began to become screams of anger directed at the mother.

The following week the mother wrote that Denise had agreed to testing, but only in her presence. Denise reported that she felt singled out in the class for examination and feared something was wrong with her. The night before the next testing date she again refused to agree to psychological evaluation. Consequently, Denise's mother was interviewed regarding her opinion of Denise.

Denise had a long history of temper tantrums. Like the behavior exhibited in school, such emotional outbursts served both an expressive and manipulative function. Her screams expressed her fear, her anxiety, and her anger as well as effectively blocking any adult's efforts to control or direct her behavior. Her mother alluded to a year in Denise's life when one screaming episode followed another. Denise may have learned to scream her way through conflicts from her mother, who admitted periods of intense anger, expressed vocally. Reluctantly, with a depressed sigh, Denise's mother recognized the manipulative effects of Denise's temper tantrums. She had responded differently at times to such behavior, sometimes ignoring it for long periods of time, but Denise could scream longer, in many instances, than she or other family members could tolerate.

The mother emphasized Denise's insecurity and shyness. She feared all males, even relatives, except for immediate family members. She refused to play outside, remaining near her mother as much as possible. Only in the last year had she ventured beyond her mother's side.

The father was described as the dominant person within the family system, although he rarely communicated with the mother. He was quite protective of Denise's feelings and his relationship with her was close and secure—she was "Daddy's girl."

Denise's mother believed that Denise's development suffered a traumatic blow when she left abruptly to give birth to her fifth child when Denise was 3 years old. Although she had been prepared for a new sibling, delivery was early, and upon her mother's return from the hospital, Denise refused to leave her side.

The mother reported that Denise liked school, indeed, looked forward to it. Each evening she chose clothing for the next day, and each morning was eager to go to school. She often requested that her older sister play "school" with her, with the sister acting as teacher and Denise as pupil. Denise frequently reported her liking for her classroom teacher and her efforts at making new friends.

After six months in school, Denise's teacher reported that she was beginning to display some expressive behaviors. She raised her hand to offer answers, spoke up in some group situations, and was more receptive to peer relationships. The teacher rewarded this coping behavior and, in some instances, provided opportunities for more self-expression. Nevertheless, although allowances were made for Denise's excessive shyness, she was incapable of regular first grade work. The classroom aide gave Denise individual tutoring in letters and numbers, but retention was minimal. Within minutes of learning some material, she was unable to perform accurately.

Two years later Denise was still shy and withdrawn but with daily tutoring was able to cope with some first grade material. She had repeated first grade, since even daily tutoring had not enabled her to keep pace with other children. Concentration was totally disrupted if a stranger watched her during a tutoring session. Learning was still characterized by lapses in attention, rapid forgetting of material, and resistance to new material. Nevertheless, she was more spontaneous in relations with both her teacher and peers and was liked by others.

Treatment   Treatment for extreme inhibition involves rearranging the environment so that the child can become assertive. Although some changes can be made without involving the family, total personality reorganization can take place only if the parents cooperate in the treatment venture. Often they must be made more autonomous and assertive themselves before they can encourage these traits in the child.

How do they fare?

While follow-up studies of severely inhibited children have not been reported, a cycle of infantilization has been found in many disorganized families (Sharlin & Polansky, 1972). If children such as Denise do eventually marry and have children, their child rearing approach is likely to be similar to their mother's (Jenkins, 1968). They will mother as they were mothered. Their own immaturity will pervade their mothering and their children in turn are likely to emerge as childish people.

NEUROTIC REACTIONS AND PARENTAL DOMINANCE

In discussing the role of child rearing attitudes in the development of learning styles and of psychopathology, we did not consider whether one parent was more responsible than the other for establishing the family's child rearing approach. We did imply that the mother was a crucial figure because of her greater initial involvement in child rearing. We would assume that when both parents approach the child similarly, he would be more likely to display a "purer" form of the learning style associated with the particular child rearing approach than the child whose parents differ in their approach. For example, when both parents are autocratic or when one parent allows the autocratic attitude of the other parent to predominate, the child is more likely to be a concrete learner with a more rigid-inhibited learning style than is the child whose parents display two different attitudes, with neither parent dominating the other.

When the parents' attitudes differ and the child identifies with the parent of the same sex, he tends to display the learning style resulting from that parent's influence. Furthermore, a child will tend to imitate the dominant parent (Hetherington & Frankie, 1967). Should the dominant parent in a family with serious conflicts be the opposite-sex parent, the cross-sex identification may place further stress on the child (Kagan, 1964) and thereby precipitate a neurotic reaction. Some support for this supposition comes from the research of Gassner and Murray (1969). These investigators found that neurotic boys tend to come from maternally dominated homes marked by parental conflict and neurotic girls from paternally dominated homes marked by parental conflict. Evidently, overtly hostile parental conflict is not solely responsible for neurotic difficulties in children; it is rather conflict interacting with cross-sex parental dominance that seems to be responsible. Gassner and Murray (1969, p. 41) state:

Let us assume that the child is drawn into the husband-wife conflict. Now, if the child is the same sex as the dominant parent, he very likely follows the lead of that parent in resolving the conflict with no consequent sex-role problem, although with some alienation from the non-dominant parent. Depending on the characteristics of the dominant parent, such a child may show nonconforming behavior but is not likely to show up in a neurotic child guidance clinic population. On the other hand, if the child is of the opposite sex of the dominant parent, he cannot follow the lead of that parent without entering into a sex-role conflict. Thus, a boy with a pro-achievement dominant mother may try to do well in school but fail because he does not want to be a sissy. At the same time he does not become a truant because this involves identification with the anti-achievement non-dominant father who is disparaged by the mother.

Let us see how these findings fit our cases. Leo, the obsessive-compulsive youngster, never mentioned his father; it was his mother with whom he seemed to identify and whose aversive influence over his life was not softened by a positive relationship with his father. Sandra, who refused to eat, came from a paternally dominated home where neither parent had ever taken her seriously. Betty, who had pains in her right side with no organic cause, was treated behaviorally with little information given about her parents. Dora, who turned white with fear at the thought of going to school, had a mother who babied her and a rigid, overbearing father whose children and wife feared him. Denise, the extremely anxious and inhibited child, came from a mutually interdependent family dominated by the father.

While our cases follow the trend noticed by Gassner and Murray, the children they studied were not classified into the categories used in this chapter. Perhaps only a subgroup of neurotic behaviors results from identification with a dominant parent of the opposite sex who relates poorly to the other parent. Future research is needed to clarify this issue.

CONCLUDING REMARKS

Although the term neurosis could have served as the title of this chapter, it was rejected because of its historical roots. The *American College Dictionary* (1960, p. 978) defines psychoneurosis as "an emotional disorder in which feelings of anxiety, obsessional thoughts, compulsive acts, and physical complaints, without objective evidence of disease, in various patterns, dominate the personality." *Webster's New Collegiate Dictionary* (1973, p. 772) defines neurosis (used interchangeably with the term psychoneurosis) as "a functional nervous disorder without demonstrable physical lesion." Neither of these definitions consider the disorders as learned. However, current evidence suggests that the disorders are learned reactions to stress, adaptive mechanisms that are self-defeating because they restrict further emotional growth at the same time they ward off anxiety. Most likely, these behaviors are the only behaviors the child's immediate environment would tolerate without undue censure.

The child who becomes obsessive-compulsive, anorexic, hysteric, or depressed is a child who cannot express his rebellion against restrictive child rearing practices; his only alternative is to modify direct expression. Through such modification, he develops particular strategies to cope with stress and particular ways of assimilating information about his environment (which we have labeled his cognitive or learning style).

When faced with severe stress, the individual will cope in the only way he knows how; he will display an exaggerated form of his particular style. Because these behaviors appear to outsiders as abnormal, we label the child who displays them as neurotic.

Not all children raised in autocratic families develop neurotic reactions. The child's temperament, the parents' temperament, the behaviors modeled by the parents, the behaviors punished by the parents, the degree of parental conflict in the home, and the sex of the controlling parent all interact to produce a neurotic child. The same can be said of the children raised by protective-interdependent parents. The degree to which they are impaired is also undoubtedly due to a host of interrelated factors. What we have done in this chapter is present the skeleton of a theory, and we're not even sure the "bones" are in the right place! Only research can help us to rearrange the bones that are out of place and to add organs and flesh.

One thing we do know is that follow-up studies of children displaying maladaptive coping strategies reveal the remarkable persistence of extreme forms of these behaviors. Once learned, behaviors are more difficult to alter than we perhaps realize. As any golf professional will tell you, it's easier to teach a beginner the proper form than to correct the improper swing of a self-taught golfer. The result of not improving one's golf game, however, does not wreak havoc upon the individual and his society.

References

Abramowitz, S. I. Locus of control and self-reported depression among college students. *Psychological Reports,* 1969, **25,** 149–150.

Adorno, T. W., Frenkel-Brunswik, E., Levinson, D. J., & Sanford, R. N. *The authoritarian personality.* New York: Harper & Row, 1950.

Allaman, J. D., Joyce, C. S., & Crandall, V. C. The antecedents of social desirability response tendencies of children and young adults. *Child Development,* 1972, **43,** 1135–1160.

Al Salih, H. A. A general practitioner's approach to phobia and childhood phobia. *Journal of the Iowa Medical Association,* 1968, **58,** 39–43.

Andrews, J. Psychotherapy of phobias. *Psychological Bulletin,* 1966, **66,** 455–480.

Arkonac, O., & Guze, S. B. A family study of hysteria. *New England Journal of Medicine,* 1963, **268,** 239–242.

Bakwin, H., & Bakwin, R. M. *Clinical management of behavior disorders in children.* (3rd ed.) Philadelphia: Saunders, 1966.

Bandura, A., Ross, D., & Ross, S. A. A comparative test of status envy, social power, and secondary reinforcement theories of identification learning. *Journal of Abnormal and Social Psychology,* 1963, **67,** 527–534.

Bandura, A. & Walters, R. H. *Social learning and personality development.* New York: Holt, Rinehart & Winston, 1963.

Bates, H. D. Relevance of animal-avoidance analogue studies to the treatment of clinical phobias: a rejoinder to Cooper, Furst, and Bridger. *Journal of Abnormal Psychology,* 1970, **75,** 12–14.

Beck, A. T. *Depression, clinical, experimental and theoretical aspects.* New York: Harper & Row, 1967.

Berg, I., Nichols, K., & Pritchard, C. School phobia—its classification and relation to dependency. *Journal of Child Psychology and Psychiatry,* 1969, **10,** 123–141.

Bibring, E. The mechanism of depression. In P. Greenacre (Ed.), *Affective disorders.* New York: International Universities Press, 1953.

Bruch, H. Psychotherapy in primary anorexia nervosa. *Journal of Nervous and Mental Disease,* 1970, **150,** 51–67.

Bruch, H. Death in anorexia nervosa. *Psychosomatic Medicine,* 1971, **33,** 135–144.

Cofer, D. H. Depressive symptomatology as a function of perception of parental attitudes, feelings and reactions. Unpublished master's thesis, Rutgers, The State University, 1970.

Coleman, J. C. *Abnormal psychology and modern life.* (3rd ed.) Chicago: Scott, Foresman, 1964.

Coolidge, J. C., Brodie, R. D., & Feeney, B. A ten-year follow-up study of sixty-six school-phobic children. *American Journal of Orthopsychiatry,* 1964, **34,** 675–684.

Coolidge, J. C., Hahn, P. B., & Peck, A. L. School phobia, neurotic crisis or way of life. *American Journal of Orthopsychiatry,* 1957, **27,** 296–306.

Coolidge, J. C., Willer, M. L., Tessman, E., & Waldfogel, S. School phobia in adolescence: a manifestation of severe character disorder. *American Journal of Orthopsychiatry,* 1960, **30,** 599–607.

Davidson, S. School phobia as a manifestation of family disturbance: its structure and treatment. *Journal of Child Psychology and Psychiatry,* 1960, **1,** 270–287.

Despert, J. L. Differential diagnosis between obsessive-compulsive neurosis and schizophrenia in children. In P. H. Hoch & J. Zubin (Eds.), *Psychopathology of childhood.* New York: Grune & Stratton, 1955.

Fazio, A. F. Implosive therapy with semiclinical phobias. *Journal of Abnormal Psychology,* 1972, **80,** 183–188.

Ferster, C. B. Animal behavior and mental illness. *Psychological Record,* 1966, **16,** 345–356.

Forbis, O. L., & Janes, R. H. Hysteria in childhood. *Southern Medical Journal,* 1965, **58,** 1221–1225.

Freud, S. *Collected papers.* Vol. 3. London: Hogarth, 1950.

Friedman, A. S. Minimal effects of severe depression on cognitive functioning. *Journal of Abnormal and Social Psychology,* 1964, **69,** 237–243.

Friedman, A. S., Cowitz, B., Cohen, N. W., & Granick, S. Syndromes and thesis of psychotic depression: results of factor analysis. *Archives of General Psychiatry,* 1963, **9,** 504–509.

Frommer, E., & Cotton, D. Undiagnosed abdominal pain. *British Medical Journal,* 1970, 4, 113–114.

Gassner, S., & Murray, E. J. Dominance and conflict in the interactions between parents of normal and neurotic children. *Journal of Abnormal Psychology,* 1969, **74,** 33–41.

Gittelman-Klein, R., & Klein, D. F. Controlled imipramine treatment of school phobia. *Archives of General Psychiatry,* 1971, **25,** 204–207.

Glaser, D. Masked depression in children and adolescents. *American Journal of Psychotherapy,* 1967, **21,** 565–574.

Gold, S. Diagnosis and management of hysterical contracture in children. *British Medical Journal,* 1965, **1,** 21–23.

Grinker, R., Miller, J., Sabshin, M., Nunn, N., & Nunnally, J. *The phenomena of depressions.* New York: Harper & Row, 1961.

Hare, E. H., Price, J. S., & Slater, E. T. O. Futility in obsessional neurosis. *British Journal of Psychiatry,* 1972, **121,** 197–205.

Harvey, O. J., Hunt, D. E., & Schroder, H. M. *Conceptual systems and personality organization.* New York: Wiley, 1961.

Heilbrun, A. B., Jr. Cognitive sensitivity to aversive maternal stimulation in late-adolescent males. *Journal of Consulting and Clinical Psychology,* 1968, **32,** 326–332.

Heilbrun, A. B., Jr. Style of adaptation to perceived aversive maternal control and internal scanning behavior. *Journal of Consulting and Clinical Psychology,* 1972, **39,** 15–21.

Heilbrun, A. B., Jr., & Norbert, N. Style of adaptation to aversive maternal control and paranoid behavior. *Journal of Genetic Psychology,* 1972, **120,** 145–153.

Heilbrun, A. B., Jr., & Waters, D. B. Underachievement as related to perceived maternal child rearing and academic conditions of reinforcement. *Child Development,* 1968, **39,** 913–921.

Hersen, M. The behavioral treatment of school phobia. *Journal of Nervous and Mental Disease,* 1971, **153,** 99–107.

Hersov, L. A. Refusal to go to school. *Journal of Child Psychology and Psychiatry,* 1960, **1,** 137–145.

Hetherington, E. M. A development study of the effects of sex of the dominant parent or sex-role preference, identification, and imitation in children. *Journal of Personality and Social Psychology,* 1965, **2,** 188–194.

Hetherington, E. M., & Frankie, K. Effects of parental dominance, warmth, and conflict on imitation in children. *Journal of Personality and Social Psychology,* 1967, **6,** 119–125.

Hogan, R. Moral conduct and moral character: a psychological perspective. *Psychological Bulletin,* 1973, **79,** 217–232.

Hollon, T. H. Poor school performance as symptom of masked depression in children and adolescents. *American Journal of Psychotherapy,* 1970, **25,** 258–263.

Hunt, S. M., Jr., Singer, K., & Cobb, S. Components of depression. *Archives of General Psychiatry,* 1967, **16,** 441–447.

Inouye, E. Similar and dissimilar manifestations of obsessive-compulsive neurosis in monozygotic twins. *American Journal of Psychiatry,* 1965, **121,** 1171–1175.

Jenkins, R. The varieties of children's behavioral problems and family dynamics. *American Journal of Psychiatry,* 1968, **124,** 1440–1445.

Jones, M. C. Elimination of children's fears. *Journal of Experimental Psychology,* 1924, **7,** 382–390.

Kagan, J. Acquisition and significance of sex typing and sex role identity. In M. L. Hoffman & L. W. Hoffman (Eds.), *Review of child development research.* Vol. 1. New York: Russell Sage, 1964.

Kanner, L. *Child psychiatry.* (3rd ed.) Springfield, Ill.: C. C Thomas, 1966.

Kennedy, W. A. School phobia: rapid treatment in 50 cases. *Journal of Abnormal Psychology,* 1965, **70,** 285–289.

Kringlen, E. Obsessional neurotics: a long term follow-up. *British Journal of Psychiatry,* 1965, **111,** 709–722.

Laybourne, P. C., Jr., & Churchill, S. W. The treatment of hysteria in childhood and its relationship to a behavior modification model. Paper presented at the annual convention at the American Association of Psychiatric Services for Children, Philadelphia, November 1970.

Lazarus, A. A. Learning theory and the treatment of depression. *Behavior Research and Therapy,* 1968, **6,** 83–89.

Lazarus, A. A., & Abramowitz, A. The use of "emotive imagery" in the treatment of children's phobias. *Journal of Mental Science,* 1962, **108,** 191–195.

Lazarus, A. A., Davison, G. C., & Polefka, D. A. Classical and operant factors in the treatment of a school phobia. *Journal of Abnormal Psychology,* 1965, **70,** 225–229.

Lesser, L. I., Ashenden, B. J., Delsuskey, M., & Eisenberg, L. Anorexia nervosa in children. *American Journal of Orthopsychiatry,* 1960, **30,** 572–580.

Leventhal, T., & Sills, M. Self-image in school phobia. *American Journal of Orthopsychiatry,* 1964, **34,** 685–695.

Levison, B. Understanding the child with school phobia. *Exceptional Children,* 1962, **28,** 393–397.

Levy, D. M. *Maternal overprotection.* New York: Columbia University Press, 1943.

Levy, D. M. Oppositional syndromes and oppositional behavior. In P. H. Hoch & J. Zubin (Eds.), *Psychopathology of childhood.* New York: Grune & Stratton, 1955.

Lewinsohn, P. M., & Shaffer, M. Use of home observations as an integral part of the treatment of depression. *Journal of Consulting and Clinical Psychology,* 1971, **37,** 87–94.

Lichtenberg, P. A definition and analysis of depression. *Archives of Neurology and Psychiatry,* 1957, **77,** 516–527.

Ling, W., Oftedal, G., & Weinberg, W. Depressive illness in childhood presenting as severe headache. *American Journal of Diseases of the Child,* 1970, **120,** 122–124.

Loeb, A., Beck, A. T., & Diggory, J. Differential effects of success and failure on depressed patients. *Journal of Nervous and Mental Disease,* 1971, **152,** 106–114.

MacDonald, A. P., Jr. Internal-external locus of control: parental antecedents. *Journal of Consulting and Clinical Psychology,* 1971, **37,** 141–147.

Malmquist, C. School phobia: a problem in family neurosis. *Journal of the American Academy of Child Psychiatry,* 1965, 4, 293–319.

Marks, I. M. Ages on onset in varieties of phobias. *American Journal of Psychiatry,* 1966, **123,** 218–221.

Mathews, A. M. Psychophysiological approaches to the investigation of desensitization and related procedures. *Psychological Bulletin,* 1971, **76,** 73–91.

McNamara, J. R. Behavior therapy in the classroom: a case report. *Journal of School Psychology,* 1968–1969, **7,** 48–51.

Mealiea, W. L., & Nawas, M. The comparative effectiveness of systematic desensitization and implosive therapy in the treatment of snake phobia. *Journal of Behavior Therapy and Experimental Psychiatry,* 1971, **2,** 85–94.

Mendell, D., & Cleveland, S. E. A three-generation view of school phobia. *Voices,* 1967, **3,** 16–19.

Meyers, V. Modification of expectations in cases with obsessional rituals. *Behavior Research and Therapy,* 1966, 4, 273–280.

Miller, L. C., Curtis, L. B., Hampe, E., & Noble, H. Comparison of reciprocal inhibition, psychotherapy, and waiting list control for phobic children. *Journal of Abnormal Psychology,* 1972, **79,** 269–279.

Mordock, J. B. The use of behavioral rating scales in the in-service training of teachers. *Journal of School Psychology,* 1968–1969, **7,** 10–12.

Nawas, N. M. Wherefore cognitive therapy? A critical scrutiny of three papers by Beck, Bergin, and Ullman. *Behavior Therapy,* 1970, **1,** 359–370.

Olsen, I. A., & Coleman, H. S. Treatment of school phobias as a case of separation anxiety. *Psychology in the Schools,* 1967, **4,** 151–154.

Overall, J. E. Dimensions of manifest depression. *Psychiatric Research,* 1962, **1,** 239–245.

Overmier, J. B. Interference with avoidance behavior: failure to avoid traumatic shock. *Journal of Experimental Psychology,* 1968, **78,** 340–343.

Overmier, J. B., & Seligman, M. E. P. Effect of inescapable shock upon subsequent escape and avoidance responding. *Journal of Comparative and Physiological Psychology,* 1967, **63,** 28–33.

Patterson, G. R. A learning theory approach to the treatment of the school phobic child. In L. Ullman & L. Krasner (Eds.), *Case studies in behavior modification.* New York: Holt, Rinehart & Winston, 1965.

Pavlov, I. P. *Conditioned reflexes.* London: Oxford University Press, 1927.

Poznanski, E., & Zrull, J. Childhood depression: clinical characteristics of overtly depressed children. *Archives of General Psychiatry,* 1970, **23,** 8–15.

Pritchard, M., & Graham, P. An investigation of a group of patients who have attended both the child and adult departments of the same psychiatric hospitals. *British Journal of Psychiatry,* 1966, **112,** 603–612.

Radin, S. S. Job phobia: school phobia revisited. *Contemporary Psychiatry,* 1972, **13,** 251–257.

Ringwald, B. E., Mann, R. D., Rosenwein, R., & McKeachie, W. J. Conflict and style in the college classroom: an intimate study. *Psychology Today,* 1971, **4,** 45–47, 76–79.

Robinson, O. L., Dalgleish, K. B., & Egan, M. H. The treatment of school phobic children and their families. *Perspectives in Psychiatric Care,* 1967, **5,** 219–227.

Robins, L. N. *Deviant children grown up.* Baltimore: Williams & Wilkins, 1966.

Robins, L. N. Follow-up studies investigating childhood disorders. In E. H. Hare & J. K. Wing (Eds.), *Psychiatric epidemiology.* London: Oxford University Press, 1970.

Rodriguez, A., Rodriguez, M., & Eisenberg, L. The outcome of school phobia: a follow-up study based on 41 cases. *American Journal of Psychiatry,* 1959, **116,** 540–544.

Rokeach, M. *The open and closed mind.* New York: Basic Books, 1960.

Rollins, N., & Blackwell, A. The treatment of anorexia nervosa in children and adolescents: stage I. *Journal of Child Psychology and Psychiatry,* 1968, **9,** 81–91.

Rose, J. Eating inhibitions in children in relation to anorexia nervosa. *Psychosomatic Medicine,* 1943, **5,** 117–124.

Rosenberg, C. M. Familial aspects of obsessional illness. *British Journal of Psychiatry,* 1967, **113,** 405–413.

Rosenberg, M. B. *Diagnostic teaching.* Seattle: Special Child Publications, 1968.

Rotter, J. B. Generalized expectations for internal versus external control of reinforcement. *Psychological Monographs,* 1966, **80** (1, Whole No. 609).

Schmale, A. H., Jr., Relationship of separation and depression to disease. I. A report on a hospitalized medical population. *Psychosomatic Medicine,* 1958, **20,** 259–277.

Schulman, J. L. The management of acute conversion reactions in children. *Current Psychiatric Therapies,* 1961, **1,** 34–38.

Sharlin, S. A., & Polansky, N. A. The process of infantilization. *American Journal of Orthopsychiatry,* 1972, **42,** 92–102.

Smith, J. A., Cohen, P. S., & Turner, L. M. Short-term interference effects of inescapable shocks upon acquisition of subsequent escape-avoidance responding. *Proceedings of the 76th Annual Convention of the American Psychological Association,* 1968, **3,** 145–146.

Smith, R. E., & Sharpe, T. M. Treatment of school phobia with implosive therapy. *Journal of Consulting and Clinical Psychology,* 1970, **35,** 239–243.

Smith, S. L. School refusal with anxiety: review of 63 cases. *Canadian Psychiatric Association Journal*, 1970, **15**, 257–264.

Soloman, R. L., & Wynne, L. C. Traumatic avoidance learning: the principles of anxiety conservation and partial irreversibility. *Psychological Review*, 1954, **61**, 353–385.

Stampel, T. Implosive therapy: an emphasis on covert stimulation. In D. J. Lewis (Ed.), *Learning approaches to therapeutic behavior change*. Chicago: Aldine, 1970.

Sullivan, H. S. *Conceptions of modern psychiatry*. New York: Norton, 1953.

Toolan, J. M. Depression in children and adolescents. *American Journal of Orthopsychiatry*, 1962, **32**, 404–415.

Van Egeren, L. F., Feather, B. W., & Hein, P. L. Desensitization of phobias: some psychophysiological propositions. *Psychophysiology*, 1971, **8**, 213–228.

Waldfogel, S., Tessman, E., & Hahn, P. B. A program for early intervention on school phobia. *American Journal of Orthopsychiatry*, 1959, **29**, 324–333.

Walton, D., & Mather, M. D. The application of learning principles to the treatment of obsessive-compulsive states in acute and chronic phases of illness. *Behavior Research and Therapy*, 1963, **1**, 163–174.

Wangh, M. The aim of the psychoanalyst's treatment in phobia therapy. *American Journal of Psychiatry*, 1967, **123**, 1075–1080.

Warren, W. Relationship between child and adult psychiatry. *Journal of Mental Science*, 1960, **106**, 815–826.

Warren, W. A study of anorexia nervosa in young girls. *Journal of Child Psychology and Psychiatry*, 1968, **9**, 27–40.

Watson, J. B., & Rayner, R. Conditioned emotional reactions. *Journal of Experimental Psychology*, 1920, **3**, 1–14.

Weiss, M., & Burke, A. A 5- to 10-year follow-up of hospitalized school phobic children and adolescents. *American Journal of Orthopsychiatry*, 1970, **40**, 672–676.

Wilkins, W. Desensitization: social and cognitive factors underlying the effectiveness of Wolpe's procedure. *Psychological Bulletin*, 1971, **76**, 311–317.

Wilson, G. T., & Davison, G. C. Processes of fear reduction in systematic desensitization: animal studies. *Psychological Bulletin*, 1971, **76**, 1–14.

Wittenborn, J. R. Depression. In B. Wolman (Ed.), *Handbook of clinical psychology*. New York: McGraw-Hill, 1965.

Wolpe, J. *Psychotherapy by reciprocal inhibition*. Stanford: Stanford University Press, 1958.

Wolpe, J. *The practice of behavior therapy*. New York: Pergamon, 1969.

Wolpe, J., & Rachman, S. Psychoanalytic "evidence": a critique based on Freud's care of little Hans. *Journal of Nervous and Mental Disease*, 1960, **130**, 135–148.

Woodruff, R. A., Jr., Clayton, P. J., & Guze, S. B. Hysteria: studies of diagnosis, outcome, and prevalence. *Journal of the American Medical Association*, 1971, **215**, 425–428.

Woodruff, R., & Pitts, F. N., Jr. Monozygotic twins with obsessional illness. *American Journal of Psychiatry*, 1964, **120**, 1075–1080.

Yates, A. J. *Behavior therapy*. New York: Wiley, 1970.

*I am a watermelon. I am lying on the sidewalk. There is
a crack on my side, and the pink is running out.
I cry Help! Help! but nobody hears.*

—Bert K. Smith

Learning difficulties:
central process dysfunction

In Chapter 2 we learned that damage to the brain can have both primary
and secondary effects. We learned that a lesion that destroys portions
of the brain responsible for the control of motor or language behavior
does not cause just a loss of that specific function but results in
disturbances of all functional systems linked to the specific area.
Consequently, when children are classified according to the primary
effect of a brain lesion, many children who display a variety of secondary
disorders are grouped together. For example, children classified as
cerebral palsied show many secondary disturbances, the number and
the type depending upon the extent and the location of the lesion
causing the motor abnormalities. In addition, the damage can be diffuse
rather than focal; it can include portions of the frontal or parietal
lobes, as well as the motor strip, so that functions subserved by these
areas also would be impaired (for example, verbal fluency or short-term
memory subserved by the frontal lobe or spatial construction and
spatial orientation subserved by the parietal). The damage might affect
intelligence and leave motor behavior intact, or both intelligence and
motor behavior might be impaired.

In Chapter 3 we learned that dysfunction may occur not because of
damage to the brain but rather because of malformation of the brain
due to abnormal growth patterns. Sometimes these malformations
produce identifiable signs (e.g., Down's syndrome, hydrocephalous),
while in other cases there are no easily observed neurological
abnormalities (e.g., mental retardation of unknown origin). However,
autopsies of those with intellectual quotients under 50 usually reveal
brain abnormalities.

Although brain dysfunction can, and frequently does, cause a global reduction in intelligence, as shown by the positively skewed IQ distribution (many low scores) of children with brain disorders, IQ is a poor indicator of brain disorder in children with scores above 50. Studies of monozygotic twins, where one twin was brain-damaged, indicate that the effect of damage on IQ can be very slight (Bradway, 1937; Jenkins, 1935). We have learned that cerebral palsied children who have normal IQs sometimes display perceptual-motor deficiencies and attentional disorders. We have also observed that aphasic, as well as palsied children, often exhibit perseverative activity, that is, they seem unable to stop abruptly an activity they have initiated. For example, if asked to copy 10 dots on a paper, they might make dots until they reach the edge of the paper and end up with 20 instead of the 10 assigned. Some aphasic children are also hyperactive and very distractible.

Suppose a child displays these behaviors but has no noticeable motor, language, or intellectual deficit? In the past, he might have been labeled emotionally disturbed. With increasing knowledge of brain-behavior relationships, we now know that brain damage can affect cognitive and attentional skills and leave other behaviors relatively intact.

In this chapter we will discuss children whose brains do not seem to function normally, but whose intelligence is average or better. The children are sometimes classified as minimally brain-damaged, particularly when a thorough neurological exam reveals minor neurological abnormalities (e.g., reflex abnormalities or sensation loss). The use of this term has been criticized, however, because neurological studies sometimes reveal that children so classified may actually have considerable brain damage. What is minimal is the behavioral consequences of the damage. For this reason the terms minimal brain dysfunction (MBD) or minimal cerebral dysfunction (MCD) are currently used to classify children with subtle signs of neurological abnormality.

DIAGNOSIS OF MINIMAL BRAIN DYSFUNCTION

Children are often given the diagnosis of MBD even when the routine neurological exam is negative if they display the cognitive and perceptual deficits discussed in Chapter 2 and 3 that are known to accompany brain damage. Table 8.1 presents clues from both neurological and psychological evaluations that suggest neurological dysfunction in certain regions of the brain. Behaviors suggestive of neurological dysfunction often occur only in the psychological exam. For example, errors in spatial construction and poor memory for visually presented material are suggestive of

Table 8.1 CEREBRAL DYSFUNCTION: CLUES TO ANATOMIC LOCALIZATION OF DEFICIT

Area of the brain	Neurological examination	Psychological examination
Frontal lobe	Loss of initiative Diminution in range of interest Stereotyped behavior Perseveration Speech loses regulatory role Dissociation between speech and motor activity Impaired synthesizing ability Poor comprehension of written text Disturbances in selective organization of mental activity Auditory suppression	Figure-ground difficulties Interference with the perception of illusions Interference with organization of movements directed toward specific goals Deterioration of planned activity Perseveration of answers to test questions Impaired synthetic ability Impulsive and fragmented responses on problem solving tasks
Parietal lobe	Tactile extinction Tactile agnosia (inability to discriminate objects by touch) Stereognosis (inability to recognize the form of objects by touch) Loss of kinesthetic sensitivity Motor apraxias (failure to perform certain familiar movements) Impairment in fine motor skill	Spatial construction (right lobe) Inability to utilize kinesthetic methods of instruction Poor writing skill

Parietal-occipital	Visual imperception (inability to distinguish clearly visual forms)
	Sharply reduced visual attention
	Visual extinction
	Hemianopsia (visual field defect)
	Disturbance of visual fixation or gaze
		Primarily left lobe dysfunctions
		  impaired recognition of symbols
		  writing letters backwards
		  impaired organization of oral communications
		  spatial imperception and directional confusions
		  confusion in performing practical activities
		  nonrecognition of visual shapes
		  poor synthesis of individual stimuli into groups
		  inability to understand complex logicogrammatical constructions (e.g., "Draw a circle to the right of the cross")
		  impaired mathematical ability
		  inability to remember the elements in an execution of an act

Temporal	Speech imperception
	Isolated Babinski (an infantile reflex)
	Poor emotional control
	Disturbed interpersonal relations
	Slowed motor speed
		Primarily left lobe
		  low scores on speech perception and phonetic skills tests,
		  inability to pronounce words smoothly, especially nouns
		  difficulty in naming objects
		  poor in mental arithmetic
		  poor memory for recent events
		  impaired ability in writing to dictation and spontaneous writing
		Primarily right lobe
		  inability to arrange pictorial materials in sequence
		  visual suppression (reproduction of only part of a visual field)
		  musical inability

parietal lobe dysfunction. If tactile agnosia and stereognosis are also present, brain injury is strongly suggested. If they are not present, the evidence is less conclusive.

The terms MBD and MCD, therefore, are used to categorize children whose cerebral dysfunction does not produce gross motor or sensory deficit or generalized impairment of intellect, but who exhibit impairment in perception, conceptualization, language, memory, or control of attention, impulse, or motor function (Clements, 1966).

The difference between MBD and other brain disorders is that in most instances the diagnosis is merely presumptive, because physiologic, biochemical, or structural alterations of the brain have not been demonstrated. This is also true, however, for a large number of severely retarded children. Neurologists are now beginning to accept this presumptive evidence in diagnosis, that is, certain categories of deviant behavior, learning disorders, and visual-motor-perceptual irregularities are considered valid indices of brain dysfunction. These indices are perhaps more meaningful than previous signs, such as reflex or sensory abnormality, and reflect disorganized brain functioning at a higher level. It is no longer acceptable to consider learning and behavior as distinct from other neurological functions (Clements, 1966). Table 8.2 depicts brain disorder as a continuum from minor to major dysfunction.

Although children subsumed under the category of MBD are a heterogeneous group, numerous authors have noted similarities in the clinical picture. Ten characteristics most often cited by clinicians, in order of frequency, are: (1) hyperactivity, (2) perceptual-motor impairments, (3) emotional lability, (4) general coordination deficits, (5) disorders of attention (short attention span, distractibility, perseveration), (6) impulsivity, (7) disorders of memory, (8) specific learning disabilities, (9) disorders of

Table 8.2 CNS DYSFUNCTION SYNDROMES

Minimal dysfunction	Major dysfunction
1. Impairment of fine movement or coordination	1. Cerebral palsies
2. Nonperipheral impairments of vision, hearing, haptics, and language	2. Severe aphasias (autism?)
	3. Mental retardation
3. Specific and circumscribed perceptual, intellectual, and memory deficits	4. Childhood psychosis and autism
	5. Epilepsies
4. Deviations in attention, activity level, impulse control, and affect	
5. Electroencephalographic abnormalities without actual seizures, or possibly subclinical seizures, which may be associated with fluctuations in behavior or intellectual function	

speech and hearing, and (10) equivocal neurological signs and electro-encephalographic irregularities (Clements, 1966).

While these behaviors have been observed by practicing clinicians, actual research supporting clinical impressions is less often cited. Mordock's (1971, p. 404) survey suggested that "several of these behaviors were no more frequent in brain-impaired youngsters than in emotionally disturbed children, and, when present in the brain impaired were characteristic of those with secondary emotional disturbance. Physical inadequacy, social inadequacy, and coordination deficits, however, were present in the majority of brain-impaired youth." Rutter and his colleagues (Rutter, Graham, & Lule, 1970) reported that there is a very high rate of reading retardation in children with all kinds of neurological difficulties and that this retardation is perhaps their major handicap.

We said earlier that children with MBD were often mistakenly diagnosed as emotionally disturbed as a result of intrafamily psychopathology rather than as a result of brain impairment. Clinicians began to have second thoughts when children with attentional, perceptual, and reading disorders appeared in families that functioned normally. Historical material sometimes revealed that the child's birth had been complicated by obstetrical difficulties or that language development had been delayed. These findings led to some rethinking about attributing the abnormal behaviors to family variables. Perhaps an environment that is adequate to meet the needs of a normal child may be inadequate to meet the excessive requirements of a child who has a short attention span or who is distractible, emotionally labile, or hyperactive. Such a child may be the catalyst that triggers conflicts among other family members or he may actually create conflicts because of differences of opinion about his management. Because nothing seems to work, the family may eventually regard the child as an outcast. Professionals who evaluate the child after a family's energies have been exhausted may regard the child as disturbed because of his parents' reactions toward him—and they would be partially correct. The child may have many emotional problems, but these problems would not have developed had his brain functioned normally in the first place.

Studies in one residential center for emotionally disturbed children revealed that about a fifth to a quarter of the children in residence showed relatively little improvement in achievement during the course of their stay (Talmadge, Hayden, & Schiff, 1969). Initial speculation was that lack of improvement was related to particular kinds of emotional disturbance. A test of this hypothesis failed to establish such a relationship. Although the admitting policy of the center was to reject children with obvious organic involvement, a thorough evaluation with refined neurological and psychological techniques disclosed that over a third of the children displayed minor signs of neurological dysfunction (Mora,

Talmadge, Bryant, Amanat, Brown, & Schiff, 1968). A significantly larger proportion of the organic group than of the nonorganic group failed to make substantial academic improvement.

Why weren't these children originally diagnosed as having an organic inefficiency? Probably because signs often associated with emotional disturbance also are associated with organicity (e.g., hyperactivity, distractibility, poor coordination, awkwardness in mobility, rigidity of behavior). Routine evaluative techniques frequently fail to differentiate between the two disorders, and even with more refined procedures differential diagnosis is often difficult (Kenny & Clemmens, 1971).

Examination of the test battery employed in the residential center gives a picture of the tools used to evaluate organic integrity. This battery was administered by a multidisciplinary team and therefore represented an interdisciplinary effort. In other words, the various professionals evaluated the children together rather than separately as described in Chapter 1.

The test battery included an evaluation of the following functions: (1) orientation to time, place, and person, memory, level of consciousness, motor activity, attention, and intellect; (2) cortical sensory interpretation and cortical motor integration; (3) language; (4) cranial nerve functioning; (5) cerebellar functions; (6) the motor system; (7) reflexes; (8) the sensory system; and (9) perceptual-motor functioning. Some specialized procedures were also utilized to evaluate orientation, eye dominance, eye movement, skilled acts, and double sensory stimulation. These tasks are described in detail in Goldfarb (1961). The evaluations of the sensory system and perceptual-motor functions are not generally utilized in standard neurological examinations. These procedures were developed by Birch and Lefford (1964) and their use provides information about the intersensory organization among the visual, kinesthetic and haptic systems. These sensory studies included tests of double sensory stimulation, localization, stereognosis, graphesthenia, and intersensory functioning. Perceptual-motor studies included perceptual analysis, perceptual synthesis, and motor coordination.

The staff of the residential center sought to determine whether neurological findings would correlate with scores on Birch and Lefford's tasks, intellectual functioning (WISC), perceptual-motor coordination (Bender-Gestalt), gross motor movements (Lincoln-Oseretsky Motor Development Scale), overt behavior (Devereux Child Behavior Rating Scale), and with an overall judgment of cerebral dysfunction made from psychological protocols. On the basis of the standard neurological evaluation, children were classified into one of two groups, brain impaired or non-brain impaired. The number of children in each who performed poorly on the supplementary evaluative procedures was then tabulated to see if any items discriminated between the two groups.

Items that did discriminate between the groups were measures of intersensory functioning, perceptual synthesis, and perceptual-motor functioning. Intersensory visual-kinesthetic functioning was tested by first moving the subject's hand, while he held a pencil, through eight geometrical designs carved on a Seguin form board and then asking him to identify visually blocks that would fit into these forms. Intersensory haptic-kinesthetic functioning was tested by a similar method, except that the child was asked to identify tactually the blocks corresponding to the geometrical designs. Perceptual synthesis was studied by asking the child to select one of four sets of lines corresponding to a given whole figure. The perceptual-motor studies were performed by asking the child to copy several letter designs, proceeding from very simple to more difficult designs. Table 8.3 describes in more detail the tasks that discriminated between organic and nonorganic groups.

HARRY

Five months in residence. Age 9-3. Full scale IQ 78, verbal IQ 81, performance IQ 79.

Areas of neurological weakness. (1) Harry displays mixed dominance, as well as confusion between left and right. (2) Bender-Gestalt reveals reversals (sometimes reversals are mirror images). (3) Drawing and writing are poor. (4) Perceptual analysis and synthesis are extremely inadequate, that is, his ability to draw conclusions about specific aspects of a stimulus are limited. (5) Intersensory studies suggest a great deal of inadequacy. Specifically, he cannot feel an object, for example, a triangle, with eyes blindfolded and then describe what he is feeling; he is unable to translate material presented by touch into a concept.

Educational recommendations. Harry is able to translate material presented visually to other senses. He is better able to form concepts about material presented visually than material presented in other sense modalities. Since Harry's strength is in the visual sphere, vision is the modality through which Harry should be approached in the classroom. Exercises in form consistency, fine motor coordination, spacial relations, and visual-motor sequencing are suggested. Tracing, drawing with a wet finger on the blackboard, and following a sandpaper pattern might be beneficial exercises to teach writing.

DORIS

Recent admission. Age 7-3. Full scale IQ 77, verbal IQ 75, performance IQ 83.

Areas of neurological weakness. (1) Field of vision is restricted (child was referred for eye examination). (2) Bender-Gestalts are distorted and rotations frequently noted. (3) Comprehension is very poor. (4) Perceptual synthesis is very poor; what she perceives she cannot translate and relate to

Table 8.3 NEUROLOGICAL ITEMS THAT DIFFERENTIATED IMPAIRED FROM NONIMPAIRED CHILDREN

Eye movement (Goldfarb)	1. Schematic—move eyes in various directions without moving the head 2. Command—fixate on a target in space 3. Pursuit—follow a moving target right, left, up, and down 4. Convergence-divergence—follow a moving object at eye level from beyond far point to beyond near point and from near to far point 5. Ability to dissociate movements of eye and hand and body
Skilled acts (Gold)	1. Coordination of perioral muscles, demonstrated by whistling 2. Coordination of fine muscles of the fingers in doing simple and complicated tasks, demonstrated by thumb touching each of the four fingers in succession 3. Coordination of large muscles, demonstrated by walking on tip toes, walking on heels, walking backward and forward, walking on line, hopping and skipping on each foot, throwing and catching
Intersensory visual-kinesthetic (Birch)	Blocks from a Seguin form board were placed on a table directly in front of S. Ss arm was placed behind a screen and was passively moved through a path which fitted the geometric form. This was accomplished by placing a stylus in Ss hand. E gripped the stylus above the point and moved it through the path of the tract which fitted the geometric form
Intersensory-haptic kinesthetic (Birch)	The Ss hand was placed behind an opaque screen and he explored the form of the blocks with his hands outside his field of vision. His ability to match up the blocks that had first been presented to him was the measure of this task
Perceptual-motor synthesis (Birch)	S had to select from a number of isolated pieces four sets of lines that would reproduce a given figure. A series of letter designs were offered similar to written es, les and the same letters in a different direction. Scoring was based upon difficulty in shifting angles and on making errors similar to those found on the Bender

other perceptions. (5) Spatial perception is poor. (6) Motor coordination is poor.

Educational recommendations. One strong point is adequate performance on perceptual analysis tasks where geometric figures are presented and she has to perceive the component elements. Her favorable performance indicates some ability at visualization and abstraction. Exercises in visual decoding (to help comprehension and perceptual synthesis) and visual-motor sequencing, as well as eye-motor coordination are suggested.

ISOBEL

Four months in residence. Age 8-7. Full scale IQ 88, verbal IQ 95, performance IQ 82.

Areas of neurological weakness. (1) Poor angulation on the Bender-Gestalt. (2) Fine motor coordination is quite poor; because of this Isobel has difficulty writing. (3) Weakness is evident in the haptic-kinesthetic sphere; she is unable to translate material presented by touch into concepts (such as a triangle felt while she was blindfolded into the idea of a triangle).

Educational recommendations. Isobel's inadequate performance in the motor sphere stands in sharp contrast to perceptual functioning, and motor problems should be regarded as her most serious area of weakness. Her intact perceptual functions should be used as vehicles to present school material. She needs work in eye-motor coordination. Exercises in spatial relations and figure drawing are suggested.

DOUGLAS

One year in residence. Age 10-9. Full scale IQ 91, verbal IQ 89, performance IQ 94.

Areas of neurological weakness. (1) Douglas manifests confusion between right and left. In addition, he is left-eye dominant, but uses his right hand and foot. (2) Coordination is very poor. (3) Perceptual synthesis is very poor (ability to look at discrete parts of a geometric design and visualize them as a completed whole).

Educational recommendations. One strong point is a better-than-average performance in perceptual analysis (ability to look at a completed geometric design and visualize it in discrete parts). The discrepancy in performance between perceptual analysis and perceptual synthesis indicates that in learning concepts, particularly in the perceptual sphere. Douglas will learn more efficiently if he starts with the whole and then proceeds to the discrete component parts, rather than vice versa. He clearly needs work in coordination, especially fine coordination. The Frostig training procedures to improve eye-motor coordination are recommended.

Bender-Gestalt scores and behavioral ratings did not distinguish between organic and nonorganic groups, nor did WISC subtest scores. The organic group did score lower on the Lincoln-Oseretsky Motor Development Scale and on the WISC performance IQ. Global judgment of organic or nonorganic made by independent psychologists agreed with the refined neurological evaluation in 16 of the 22 organic cases. In only 7 of the 57 cases was there disagreement (Mora et al., 1968).

The intersensory inabilities displayed by these children were similar to those displayed by moderately retarded children, IQ 40 to 60 (Hill, McCullum, & Sceau, 1967; Knights, Hyman, & Atkinson, 1967; Knights, Hyman, & Wozny, 1966). Perhaps intersensory functioning is more often affected by brain injury than is general intellectual functioning.

Determining which items discriminate between groups, however, is important only when undertaking differential diagnosis. When attempting to tailor an educational program to a child's specific needs, analysis of his unique patterns of strengths and weaknesses is what is important (the sketches—digests of the profiles of four children studied at the residential center—illustrate such analysis of the individual).

TYPES OF MINIMAL BRAIN DYSFUNCTION

The sketches of Douglas, Harry, Doris, and Isobel suggest that the category of MBD is a heterogenous one. In other words, there is no unitary MBD syndrome. For this reason, we have chosen to title this chapter "Central Process Dysfunction" to emphasize that the brains of some children function differently from the brain of the average child but the causes of this different functioning may vary widely. There is evidence that some forms of the MBD syndrome are inherited metabolic dysfunctions (Wender, 1971, 1972) and that some children who represent temperamental extremes are erroneously classified as MBD (Thomas, Chess, & Birch, 1968).

Before attempting to divide the syndrome of MBD into different subtypes, it is worthwhile to emphasize our earlier presentation of the word syndrome (Chapter 2). Minimal brain dysfunction and its cognates (the hyperactive behavior syndrome, minimal brain damage, postencephalitic behavior disorders, the learning disabled child, the neurologically handicapped, and so on) have been applied to a broad and poorly delineated spectrum of behavior. In addition, there is no agreement about the limits of the syndrome. A typical MBD child is inattentive, uncoordinated, and hyperactive and displays perceptual and cognitive difficulties. Should the child who is inattentive, clumsy, and hyperactive but has no perceptual-cognitive difficulty be classified as MBD? How about the child who has perceptual-cognitive deficits but is not hyperactive, clumsy, or inattentive? At present, there are no satisfactory answers to these questions.

Recently, increased precision in diagnostic techniques has made possible the finding that specific biological abnormalities exist in behaviorally defective children (Wender, 1972). In addition, Luria (1966) states that defects in different areas of the central nervous system may result in superficially similar syndromes. For example, the inability to read noted in MBD children may be due to (1) poor auditory analysis of word sounds, (2) dysfunction of the "kinesthetic analyzer," (3) abnormality of the "visual-spatial analyzer," or (4) disturbances of the general cerebral neurodynamics. Each of these deficiencies results in poor reading achievement, but each would need a different approach in order to help a child overcome his reading deficiency.

Conners (1973) expresses the view that factor analytic (intercorrelation) studies are necessary in order to undertake syndrome analysis, or the clustering of groups of neurologically handicapped persons according to profile similarities. Factor analytic procedures involve administering a number of tests, both neurological and psychoeducational, to a sample of children diagnosed as MBD, and then identifying children who score differently on the various tests, that is, those who score high and low on the different tests. In this fashion, Conners (1973), Crinella (1973), and Crinella and Dreger (1972) have identified six to eight clusters or types on the basis of intragroup profile similarities. Crinella's studies included children with verified neuropathology who served as "marker" subjects. Cluster determinations were related to both location and severity of brain lesion, and MBD children were included on each cluster. The marker subjects were those known to have structural pathology of the CNS, pathology identified either by neurosurgical observations of the brain itself or through diagnostic techniques that provide visual evidence of the locale and nature of a lesion (e.g., angiography, which is the examination of the vascular system by X-ray). The MBD children were those who satisfied two or more of the criteria set forth by the Clements (1966) task force report.

Crinella administered to each child a number of psychological and neuropsychological tests and also had the child's parents and teachers rate him on a child behavior rating scale. The scores of all the children on all 90 test variables were intercorrelated and factor analyzed.

The first group of children isolated from Crinella's larger group displayed right-left disorientation (inability to perform tasks requiring differentiation of right from left for successful completion), mirror-reversal writing, dyscalalia (inability to perform simple arithmetical calculations), and poor coordination. Children with known brain injury included in this group had damage to parts of the left hemisphere, particularly the frontal-temporal area. Many of the children in this group had marked reading difficulties preceded by delayed speech development.

A second group of children displayed spatial disorientation (marked inability to perform tasks requiring appreciation of external spatial relations), perseveration, poor attention, poor coordinatión, clumsiness, and general academic and intellectual retardation. The brain-damaged (BD) children in this cluster had relatively early injuries to the frontal or temporal regions. Their behavior was characterized by general academic retardation, inattention, and hyperactivity.

A third group displayed marked defects in fine manual coordination and in general cognitive ability. Within this group were two 7-year olds with athetoid movements of the upper limbs and a child who suffered traumatic injury to the posterior cerebral areas. Mordock and DeHaven (1968) isolated a similar factor in MBD children called deficits in distal alternate motion rate. Children in this group could not adequately control the smaller muscle groups of the hands and feet, resulting in poor writing, clumsiness, and slowness on tasks requiring fine motor skill.

A fourth group showed greater than average irascibility, that is, they displayed aggressive and antisocial outbursts, as well as hyperactivity and restlessness in school. They also had fine motor incoordination and often became excessively fatigued. Only one BD child was in this group. He was given to aggressive, violent outbursts, possibly secondary to damage in the brain stem (his damage was in the septal-anterior hypothalamic area).

A fifth group was characterized by a general weakness of excitation and lethargy. They were also more irritable than other MBD children and had poor kinesthetic awareness (awareness of their body's position in space). All showed severe academic retardation. The two BD individuals included in this group had both sustained injury to their nondominant temporal lobe.

A sixth group displayed visual-sequential disorganization (could not adequately remember the sequence of visually presented material), spatial defects, and lowered intellectual functioning. Their fine motor coordination and bodily awareness was better than the average score of the total sample.

A seventh group demonstrated a number of specific deficits in the presence of near normal intellectual development. They displayed visual-spatial problems, lethargy, and irritability. They tended to be confused and concrete thinkers and to have a poor body image (appreciation of body boundaries). The BD child in this group had, at age 4, sustained a depressed skull fracture with penetration into the cortex in the area of the brain associated with speech functions (left angular gyrus). As a consequence, the child had a severe expressive speech disturbance marked by awkward grammar usage and the inability to imitate tongue and lip positions in order to form correct speech sounds. In addition, he was unable to recognize letters (alexic), could not perform simple calculations, and could not appreciate tactile or kinesthetic stimuli emanating from his right side.

While factorial studies of MBD children are of recent origin, several of the groups isolated by Crinella have been described in the clinical literature. Crinella's fourth group, the irascible group, is perhaps the syndrome most frequently associated with MBD and has been the subject of considerable discussion and research in recent years.

The irascible

About 40 percent of children referred to mental health clinics display the behaviors characteristic of Crinella's irascible group—overactivity, impulsivity, low frustration tolerance, short attention span, distractibility, and overaggressiveness (Patterson, 1955; Rogers, Lilenfeld, & Pasamanick, 1955). Although it is not known how many children display this syndrome in reaction to family disorganization, rejection, or anxiety, clinicians are beginning to recognize that a significant proportion of hyperactive children are so because of brain dysfunction rather than because of environmental factors. Their opinion is supported by reports that some children with this syndrome have sleep problems characterized by difficulty in falling asleep, frequent awakenings, short duration of sleep, and difficulties associated with known brain dysfunction (recall Art's sleep problems presented in Chapter 2). The presence of one brain-damaged child with a subcortical lesion in the group in Crinella's sample suggests that the hyperactive-aggressive MBD child may have subcortical abnormalities, perhaps biochemically induced, that affect the activating systems of the brain, as has been suggested by Wender (1971, 1972).

Wender feels that the absence of neurological abnormalities in many MBD children, rather than reflecting the imprecision of current neurological techniques, suggests that the MBD syndrome may be produced without brain injury. He suggests that the syndrome may arise from a congenital defect in the metabolism of biochemicals responsible for maintaining normal levels of arousal. There are two sources of evidence that suggest that one form of the MBD syndrome can arise from congenital factors. The first stems from clinical observation that congenital abnormalities (strabismus, cranial size, and features seen in mongolism) frequently appear in MBD groups (Daryn, 1960; Milman, 1956; Waldrop & Halverson, 1971).

The second source of evidence that MBD may arise on a genetic basis comes from studies that indicate a familial clustering of the syndrome. A large proportion of hyperactive children demonstrate a constellation of factors associated with disturbance or disruption of the family situation (Clarkson & Hayden 1971, 1972; Morrison & Stewart, 1971; Owen, Adams, Forrest, Stolz, & Fisher, 1971). Although the hyperactivity might be a response to a frustrating home life, it might also reflect a family syndrome of hyperactivity, hyperactivity that keeps the family situation unsettled.

Support for the genetic hypothesis comes from Shafer's research (cited in Wender, 1971). Shafer studied the behavioral characteristics of the siblings and half-siblings of MBD children raised in foster homes. He found a greater incidence of the syndrome among the sibs than the half-sibs. In addition, the syndrome occurred with greater frequency in both groups than in the general population. Because the sibs and half-sibs had been raised in a different environment than the index MBD children, the findings are clearly compatible with a genetic mechanism of transmission.

Wender feels that metabolic factors are primarily responsible for the behavioral abnormalities seen in this group of MBD children. He feels that this MBD syndrome is characterized by two primary functional deficits: (1) an abnormality in arousal (hyperactivation) that produces increased activity and an inability to concentrate, focus attention, or inhibit irrelevant responses and (2) a diminished capacity for positive and negative affect.

As we mentioned in Chapter 4, arousal is partially a function of lower brain stem systems, particularly the reticular activating system (RAS). Wender postulates that the RAS functions inadequately and, therefore, the child is continually overaroused. The RAS is affected, however, by the higher cortical centers. These centers have a dampening or inhibitory affect on the RAS. If for some reason these centers fail to inhibit the RAS, it may function abnormally because of this cortical inadequacy.

Electroencephalographic, psychophysiological, and reaction-time studies of MBD children have isolated a group of MBD children whose cortical centers appear to be underaroused. These children exhibit a slowing of brain wave activity in the occipital region (Stevens, Sachdev, & Milstein, 1968; Wikler, Dixon, & Parker, 1970). If brain wave activity is a measure of arousal, then this group of MBD children are under- or hypoaroused. Similarly, a subgroup of MBD children show galvanic skin responses (GSR) that are assumed to indicate low arousal, that is, greater skin resistance, fewer and smaller nonspecific GSRs, and smaller specific GSRs than normal children (Satterfield & Dawson, 1971).

This hypoactivity of the higher cortical centers of the nervous system may be one reason why some MBD children are unable to make rapid discriminations in reaction-time experiments. Studies have revealed that they take longer to develop and maintain a state of readiness to respond (Czudner & Rourke, 1971) and to process information (Dykman, Walls, Suzuhi, Ackerman, & Peters, 1970).

Since the higher cortical centers have an inhibiting effect on the RAS, the hyperarousal of the RAS could be due to the hypoarousal of these centers. Perhaps this is why stimulant drugs, drugs that should increase hyperactivity, actually decrease it in some MBD children. Perhaps these drugs stimulate the inhibiting action of the cortical centers involved with the RAS. However, the manner in which they do so not only is too involved to present here but also is imperfectly understood.

Wender (1971) postulated that these two primary defects, the defects in arousal and in the capacity to experience positive and negative affect, can account for a host of other behaviors that form this particular MBD syndrome. For example, diminished sensitivity to positive reinforcement can cause increased pleasure seeking. Because of the child's already increased attentiveness to the environment but diminished reaction to positive experiences, he requires more intense stimulation to experience positive affect; he is less satiable. He also becomes bored and stimulus-hungry more quickly. The MBD child's demands for attention can also result from his diminished ability to experience positive reinforcement. Disobedience and perhaps delinquency are a reflection of his insensitivity to social reinforcement.

When clinicians speak of the hyperactivity of the MBD child, it sometimes sounds as if they consider activity level a relatively stable dimension of behavior, which, when measured over a period of time, is characteristic of the individual. There has been relatively little research performed in an effort to support this hypothesis.

What makes hyperactivity so conspicuous is not the elevated level of activity itself but rather the inappropriateness of its situational quality. Parent and teacher complaints about the hyperactive child's behavior are always made in reference to a particular situation (Werry, 1968). Eisenberg (1964, p. 63) commented that the usual complaints about the hyperactive child—that he is always on the move, into things, and difficult to restrain—are applicable to most normal children, at times, for instance, when they are playing on the school grounds during recess.

Several studies have investigated the nature of situational influences upon the hyperactive behavior of MBD by attaching accelerometers (a modified self-winding wristwatch used to measure motor activity) to both normal and MBD children and recording their activity under different conditions. If hyperactivity is defined as excessive total motor activity, then these studies indicate that there is no difference in activity level between MBD and normal children (Pope, 1970; Schulman, Kasper, & Thorn, 1965). These same studies have revealed, however, that MBD children display more restlessness than normal children under certain conditions. For example, Pope (1970) observed the children's behavior in a playroom while they performed several activities. She recorded the number of locomotions made across quadrants of the observation room, how much time was spent in locomoting, standing, or sitting, and how often and for how long they were in contact with a variety of toys. In undirected activity in the playroom the MBD group did not show significantly greater total motor activity than the normals, as determined by the accelerometer readings. They did, however, make a significantly greater number of contacts with the toys and made these contacts for significantly shorter periods of time. They also spent more time without any toys and more time locomoting than the normals. When children from the two groups performed a simple task on the Seguin form board, there was again no significant difference between them in total motor activity. However, the MBD children spent a larger proportion of their time standing. Finally, during the performance of a more difficult task on the Seguin form board, the MBD spent a greater proportion of the time locomoting and made more contacts with objects (toys left from the first part of the experiment).

There are probably a number of different reasons for a child's hyperactivity. He may have a neurological impairment or he may simply be a child whose temperament is not suited for sedentary activities. He may be a child who makes decisions too rapidly, decisions as a reflection of cognitive style rather than neural dysfunction (Keogh, 1971). In addition, there is hyperactivity associated with emotional disturbance and anxiety, and hyperactivity that results from the direction of excess energy into socially inappropriate behaviors (Marwit & Stenner, 1972).

When associated with brain impairment, hyperactivity is greater in those who display a secondary emotional reaction (Mordock, 1971). Children have only a few ways to avoid frustrating situations. If a child with a learning deficiency is continually given tasks beyond his ability, one way to avoid them is simply to leave the situation. Hyperactivity, therefore, can be a learned defensive or avoidance reaction to anxiety arousing situations. Without adequately assessing the reasons for the hyperactivity, as well as the situations under which it occurs, remedial efforts may be misguided and may place the child under undue stress. We suspect that stress has a more debilitating effect on brain-impaired than on other children (Mordock, 1969).

Exceptionally poor readers

One group isolated by Crinella showed right-left disorientation, mirror reversals, dyscalculia, and poor coordination. This group seems similar to children described by Gerstmann (Benton, 1959). Children with Gerstmann's syndrome demonstrate bilateral finger agnosia, right-left disorientation, writing inability (agraphia), and inability to discriminate numbers (acalculia). A child with finger agnosia cannot differentiate, correctly name, or indicate specific fingers on command nor can he imitate given finger postures. Gerstmann showed that finger agnosia tends to occur in association with right-left disorientation, agraphia, and acalculia. Kinsbourne and Warrington (1966) also identified a group of backward readers they called a Gerstmann group.

Many children who display this syndrome are unable to remember letters and words and are, therefore, very poor readers. Children who display a seeming inability to learn to read have been labeled dyslexic (Critchley, 1970) or word blind (Bannatyne, 1966a). Others employ the terms specific reading disability (Silver & Hagin, 1967) or primary reading disability (Rabinovitch, 1959). Orton (1937) used the label strepho-symbolia, which means twisted symbol, because these children seem to twist the order of letters and words. Some investigators believe that the disorder is primarily a language disorder that involves the secondary symbol system, the visual language system. Written language is a symbol of a symbol, or, as Johnson and Myklebust (1967) have indicated, a symbol twice removed from experience. If there are difficulties in the primary auditory symbol system, the classification would be aphasia.

Nevertheless, Crinella's study, as well as several others to be cited later, reveal that the majority of children diagnosed dyslexic display other developmental disorders, such as delayed language development, suggesting that dyslexia may be a less extreme form of aphasia. Let us see how children with this disorder might function in the normal classroom.

DICK AND JACK

Mrs. Jones's first year as a third grade teacher had been relatively successful. She related well to the children and had fewer discipline problems than other teachers. Her second year, however, was another matter. She had two children in her class she just couldn't reach; neither could read. She had tried a little of everything, giving them special help both in class and through the aide whom she supervised. Nevertheless, neither youngster had made any substantial progress.

Mrs. Jones had talked with both sets of parents and initially felt she had benefited from each parent conference. Now, she was no longer sure. Jack's parents impressed her as completely disinterested in his welfare. They weren't interested in her viewpoint, simply stating that she should punish Jack for being lazy. As a result of this conference, Mrs. Jones attributed Jack's language difficulties to inadequate stimulation at home, a poor self-concept, and passive resistance toward authority figures such as herself. She had decided to avoid power struggles with Jack, to give him more attention and affection, and to decrease her demands upon him. Nevertheless, after three months of this approach Jack could read no better than before.

Her conference with Dick's parents resulted in no new understanding. They were as concerned as she. Although the father was a little distant and withdrawn and the mother a little overbearing, she didn't feel these behaviors could explain Dick's failures. Other parents displayed these characteristics to an even greater degree and yet their children could read. Because Dick's parents were both interested in his welfare and in helping him in any way possible, Mrs. Jones suggested they give him extra help at home. Since Dick was a bright but immature youngster, perhaps home tutoring would help him to catch up. She outlined Dick's deficiencies as follows: ignores punctuation, substitutes and omits words, transposes letters, repeats words and phrases, and has difficulty understanding what he reads. Dick's father agreed to give him extra help in these areas. Perhaps tutoring would help improve the strained relationship he had with his son because of absences due to business obligations.

Several months passed, however, without substantial gain in Dick's academic functioning. Perhaps his parents had not followed through on the decision to provide extra help; she decided to call them and see how things were doing at home. After the phone conversation Mrs. Jones wished she hadn't called. Yes, Dick had been tutored, tutored religiously for one hour each night and sometimes more. His father had decided that if a little extra help would be of value, then a lot of help would be even better. However, the hour had usually ended early, with Dick in tears and his father in anger. Each evening Dick's father resolved not to lose his patience, but each evening Dick would not recognize a word known on one page when confronted with it on another. Such behavior simply wasn't logical! His father began to feel that Dick simply liked to make him angry, perhaps as an expression of Dick's resentment of his father's absences from home. This suspicion was supported by Dick's eventual rejection of his father's help and an increase in his misbehavior. The father became more engrossed in his work, as if to say to his wife, "I give up. He likes you better. You help him!"

The mother wished they had never started the tutoring since their family was more united before its initiation. She now believed what she had secretly feared all along—that Dick was really retarded and that his teachers were wrong in assuming him bright. Mrs. Jones reassured Dick's mother that he wasn't retarded, but said she would ask the school psychologist to evaluate him anyway; perhaps his findings would shed some light on the problem.

Dick's evaluation   Administration of the Wechsler Intelligence Scale for Children revealed Dick's verbal IQ to be 118 and his performance IQ to be 106. Examination of the scaled scores indicated relative weakness in immediate recall, coding, and comprehension. His scores on the Wide Range Achievement Test (WRAT) were at the following grade levels: 1.3 in word reading, 1.3 in spelling, and 2.4 in arithmetic.

Dick's arithmetic ability was deficient in spite of the 2.4 grade level on the WRAT arithmetic subtest. He was able to add numbers only by counting dots. For example, to solve the problem $6 + 2$, he would use his fingers; to calculate $6 + 8$, he would write eight dots, then six, and then count them. To subtract 3 from 9 in his head, he would use his fingers and count backwards; if the problem were $17 - 11$, he couldn't do it consistently. He could correctly count blocks serially in small groups, but he was usually unable to sum the same set of written numbers. He frequently demonstrated strephosymbolic errors; for example, when he added 9 + 7, he would write 61. He was aware of this tendency and would often correct his errors by reversing the order of numbers; for example, if told that 9 + 6 was not 16, he would write 61.

Phonic skills were limited to some knowledge of simple consonant sounds. Sight vocabulary was better for distinctive words such as *red* or *dog* than for words such as *this, their, them, these,* or *that.*

To support the initial impression of specific reading disability and to reveal the extent of the disorder, the psychologist evaluated Dick with further tests. He followed an approach modified from Betts (1954), Boder (1971), and Silver and Hagin (1967).

Since Dick demonstrated almost no reading ability, the usual tests of reading comprehension were of no value. Tests selected, therefore, were those that would give some idea of how Dick had learned what he did know and those that measured the ability to learn and remember material presented through different sense modalities. These tests included measures of vocabulary determined in several ways:

1. Does the child know the *auditory symbol for a visual symbol*? The child simply reads the words on a vocabulary list.
2. Does he know the *meaning of auditory symbols*? The child gives the meaning of the words he has read successfully on the prior list and is then asked to give or demonstrate (manual expression) the meaning of additional words presented auditorily. (WISC or Binet vocabulary tests can be used.) If the child shows significant deficiency, he is given further tests.
3. Can he find the *pictured object that is denoted by a written word*? The child selects from among four pictured objects the one that is denoted by a given written word.
4. Can he select the *pictured object or event that is denoted by an auditory symbol*? The child selects from among four pictured objects or events the one for which a given word is the symbol, that is, the examiner says, "Which one is raking?" (The task is similar to the Peabody Picture Vocabulary Test.)
5. Can he identify the *written symbol for a pictured object*? The child selects from among four written words the one which denotes a pictured object (visual-to-visual learning).
6. Can he identify the *auditory symbol for a pictured object*? The child is asked to give the name of a pictured object (recall); the child selects from among four orally presented words the one which is the name of a pictured object (recognition).

Most children do more poorly on task 5 and on the first part of task 6 than on tasks 3 and 4 because recognizing the objects that words represent is easier than recalling the word that stands for an object or event. The degree of difference between scores for recognition and scores for recall is diagnostically important in assessing associative learning disorders.

After the six measures of vocabulary have been administered, the child is asked to spell the words he could recognize (his sight vocabulary) and then to spell words well above this level (unknown words).

If the child shows a poor memory for words, but can give the meaning of words orally or manually, he is given the word opposites test from the Botel Reading Inventory and the associative learning tests from the Gates Reading Diagnostic Tests (Betts, 1954).

The word opposites test from the Botel consists of words given to the child for which he must respond with the opposite. Like the automatic subtests of the ITPA, the ability to give a word's opposite is believed to be an associative skill that becomes automatic in most youngsters. A very poor score on this test suggests that the child cannot make automatic associations to words and is therefore not likely to make rapid progress in remedial reading. It is suggested that the word opposite test taps the associative attribute of words that we discussed in our presentation of the deaf, an important attitude in advanced language learning. Some items from the Botel appear below.

	a	b	c
white	yellow	black	back
work	funny	happy	play
day	play	red	night
take	away	give	find

The Gates associative learning tests are actually measures of learning ability. The tasks presented require the child to learn to associate pictures of objects and sounds with geometric forms and symbols (wordlike patterns). In the visual tasks the child is shown cards on which either a symbol or a geometric form is presented on one side and the pictured object on the other. When the child is shown the symbol or the form, he is required to identify the object that goes with it (visual-to-visual paired-associates learning). Similarly, a number of nonsense sounds are paired with symbols and forms, and the child then has to tell which symbol or form goes with the sound (auditory-to-visual paired-associates learning).

The examiner presents the pairs in each list until the child has learned all the pairs. The number of trials taken to learn the list is recorded. There are eight paired associates in each of the four conditions (eight geometric forms paired with eight pictured objects, eight symbols paired with eight pictured objects, eight nonsense sounds paired with eight geometric forms, and eight nonsense sounds paired with eight symbols).

While it is possible for the child to adopt an auditory strategy to learn what the examiner thinks are visual tasks, (e.g., the child can covertly name the geometric forms or wordlike symbols and associate these sounds with their corresponding pictured object in the former task or the sounds in the latter task), the astute examiner would assess for this possibility by simply asking the child what strategy he employed to learn the paired-associate tasks.

A memory span battery is also given. The battery includes memory for digits, spans of letters, syllables, lists of words that are conceptually related (e.g., *dog, cat, pig*), lists of words with no conceptual relationships (e.g., *dog, hammer, that*), sentences, pictures, and directions. Sequencing, tactile discrimination, laterality, and body image are then assessed.

Analysis of Dick's test results revealed the following. On the vocabulary tests testing proceeded in a backward manner until Dick did well. Not until he was given the auditory symbol for an object (task 4), could he select the object it represented. When given the pictured object, he could not select the written word representing it (task 5), but he could usually give the name for a pictured object (task 6). In addition, he could define words in his sight vocabulary, but could not always define well words in his speaking vocabulary, primarily because he had difficulty recalling adequate synonyms or words to describe the object. Nevertheless, Dick had a far greater understanding of words than he displayed in reading tasks. He was quite expressive and had a good speaking vocabulary.

He could spell correctly only 10 percent of the words in his sight vocabulary. He had no idea how to attack unknown words and his attempts were dysphonetic. Normal readers can usually spell correctly over 70 percent of the words in their sight vocabulary and can write good, readable phonetic equivalents for over 80 percent of the words not in their sight vocabulary (Boder, 1971).

Dick received an extremely low score on the word opposites test from the Botel and the Gates associative learning tests. Auditory-visual associations were markedly superior to visual-visual associations, but geometric forms were associated better than were symbols (wordlike patterns). On the memory span tests Dick had significantly better memory for related words than for unrelated words, for visual objects than for unrelated words, and for visual objects than for visual letters. His memory for sentences and for oral directions was poor and perseveration was noted. Dick's Bender Visual Motor Gestalt Test performance and his drawing of a human figure revealed some difficulties in spatial arrangement.

Temporal sequencing of sounds also was defective. Although Dick could understand words presented auditorily, he could not place sounds in temporal sequences (recall from Chapter 2 that aphasics display this difficulty). More basic was his inability to perceive similarities and differences in auditory configurations, in blending a sequence of sounds into a word pattern, and in isolating and matching initial and final sounds of words. No deficits were present in tactile or kinesthetic perception or in coordination.

While Dick was being evaluated by the psychologist, the school nurse met with his parents to gather information about Dick's early development and about his family. This structured interview revealed that Dick developed speech relatively late, and that, when developed, it was not clearly articulated at the expected time. Baby talk, sound substitutions and omissions, and cluttered speech (words uttered so rapidly that they run into each other) were characteristic. These delays were not dramatic and, while they caused some concern at the time, they were forgotten when he grew older and his speech became normal. Both his father and his father's brother had had difficulty reading as youths and avoided reading as adults; both his uncle and grandfather were left-handed. Other than these factors, Dick's development was considered normal and included the usual childhood diseases.

When each staff member presented his findings at a child study conference held at the school, the combined information substantiated the earlier impression of an associative learning disorder. While auditory deficits were paramount, visual-integrative functions also were impaired. Perhaps Dick could be considered alexic, a term coined by Betts to denote complete inability to read, because he could read neither by sight nor by ear.

Dick's remediation   Dick was tutored forty-five minutes each day by a remedial reading specialist associated with a private psychoeducational center in the community. Since Dick had some sight vocabulary and could recognize letter forms, initial remedial goals were to improve his perceptual discrimination of details within words, to develop stable association of short vowel sounds for each vowel, and to make word recognition an automatic process rather than a figuring out process (Bryant, 1965).

Phonic associations were stabilized incidently by starting off with words with short /a/ sounds. Small words were used to reduce the number of units to process at one time. Only when Dick could correctly and quickly recognize every short /a/ word given was another vowel introduced. Calling attention to the details within words was an important aspect of his remedial teaching. Writing and tracing of words was featured since his tactile-kinesthetic abilities were intact. Words were presented with one or more letters left out in order to force reproduction of missing parts and to produce a stable memory image. Tachistoscopic practice to develop rapid recognition was included. Each time a word was written, a letter filled in, or a word briefly exposed Dick pronounced it aloud to practice symbol perception and sound association. Words were chosen so that the particular sound association was the only process requiring effort for Dick. Until each basic symbol-sound association was established, no new words were presented. The goal was to develop automatic responses to common combinations of letters. During each remedial session, the learning experience was programmed so that nearly all of Dick's responses were correct (Bryant, 1965).

Jack's evaluation   Mrs. Jones became concerned that perhaps Jack also had an associative learning disorder. Her initial impression that his poor reading was due to passive resistance toward authority was probably incorrect and her resolve to avoid power struggles had proved ineffective. She had established a better relationship with him, and as a consequence he was more motivated to learn. Nevertheless, he could not syllabicate or read and spell phonetically. When he confronted a word, however simple, common, or phonetic, that was not in his sight vocabulary, he was unable to decipher it. He was unable to sound out or blend component letters and syllables of a word. He usually guessed at words from minimal cues such as the first or last letter or the word's length. He was a very poor speller, spelling correctly only those words in his sight vocabulary that he could revisualize.

Mrs. Jones recalled the method presented at Dick's conference where the psychologist analyzed the spelling errors Dick made in words in his sight vocabulary as well as in unknown words. She gave Jack ten words in his sight vocabulary and ten unknown words and showed the results to the psychologist. Jack had spelled correctly only three words. Jack's hodgepodge of misspellings were clearly dysphonetic since not even Jack himself could recognize the words he had attempted to spell. It appeared as if Jack tried to visualize each word and then copy down the image remembered. Consequently, he produced extraneous letter errors and omitted syllable errors and substituted parts of known words for words that were similar in appearance. When Jack was asked to spell words he could recognize on the WRAT, he spelled them from left to right as they appeared on the test form and correctly spelled the word *him,* which he missed on the WRAT spelling; it was as if he revisualized what he saw on the WRAT vocabulary. His drawing of his tutor revealed his excellent visual memory.

The psychologist decided to obtain additional information from formal testing. He commented, however, that the odds of Mrs. Jones's having two children in her classroom with a severe reading disability were quite low. In a study of 2767 school children (Myklebust & Boshes, 1969) approximately 7.5 percent were classified as having a learning disability. The severity ranged from moderate to severe disability, with 112 (4 percent) classified as having a severe disability. Of these 112, only a small number might be classified as having a primary reading disorder or as being dyslexic.

On the WISC Jack received an average IQ, but relative weaknesses were apparent in information, arithmetic, and digit span on the verbal scale and picture arrangement and coding on the performance scale.

Jack's answers to the WISC picture completion and vocabulary subtests revealed the substitution of words closely related conceptually but not phonetically. These errors, called *semantic substitution errors,* are typically overlooked by the untrained observer who views them as slips rather than as errors of recall. When labeling the missing parts of objects in the picture completion subtest, Jack substituted *aerial* for *antenna, screws* for *hinges,* and *horns* for *hoofs.* When defining *donkey* he said it was a *cattle* when he meant *animal.*

While visual-spatial skills were relatively well developed, letter order errors were present, for instance, *was* for *saw, flet* for *felt, limp* for *imply.* Jack's scores on the auditory-sequential memory and sound blending subtests of the ITPA were quite low (see Chapter 1).

Although Jack had difficulty with math, his functioning was considerably better than Dick's. Like Dick, he could do problems on paper better than in his head, but he could do considerably more problems than Dick. In fact, he could do multiplication on paper, although he could not add 8 + 7 in his head without counting on his fingers. Consequently, his WRAT arithmetic score was at grade level, while his WISC arithmetic subtest was at a retarded level.

Like Andrew in Chapter 1, Jack was considered a visile rather than audile learner (Boder, 1971; Wepman, 1962). Because Jack's primary deficit was in the auditory modality and because he could not analyze words phonetically, he was tentatively considered an *auditory dyslexic,* after Myklebust (1965). Children with this disorder are considered to have mild aphasias. The school staff, however, preferred not to label Jack, particularly since the learning of phonics requires considerable attentional skill and sustained motivation, both lacking in Jack's past efforts. While the evidence strongly suggested a specific auditory disorder, labeling Jack auditory dyslexic implied a degree of diagnostic certainty that was not present. The staff felt that Jack had a specific learning disorder but that the term dyslexia was applied loosely to many children with reading problems. They had labeled Dick as having a primary reading disorder because he displayed all the classic signs presented in the literature and came from a family with a history of reading failure (Critchley, 1970). Both Jack and Dick would be referred for neurological evaluation in the hope that the neurologist could clarify the exact nature of the disorders displayed by these two boys.

Jack's remediation Although reluctant to label Jack an auditory dyslexic, the staff did feel that the remedial procedures suggested for auditory dyslexics would be beneficial for him. The initial procedure focused on whole word techniques to develop a sufficient sight vocabulary (Johnson & Myklebust, 1967). Remedial phonics would be initiated only after an adequate sight vocabulary had been established. Tactile-kinesthetic procedures also would be employed. Initial remedial efforts to improve spelling were directed toward converting Jack from a dysphonetic to a phonetic speller (Boder, 1971). Emphasizing "good errors," that is, readable phonetic equivalents, helped motivate Jack to set realistic goals for himself.

Parental reactions   Explaining to Dick's parents that his problems resulted from a primary reading disorder was much easier than giving such an explanation to Jack's family. Dick's parents were both sophisticated individuals. Although Dick's father had become frustrated by Dick's response to his tutoring, this reaction was temporary. The father was aware that several members of his family were poor readers and had struggled through school. He was also aware that, although he was successful in business, he avoided reading and recalled early school difficulties.

Although visibly upset by the information received, both he and his wife resolved to use the help offered and to arrange for special tutoring for Dick. They also expressed interest in joining the local chapter of the Association for Children with Learning Disabilities. They seemed neither defensive about their child's disorder nor burdened with guilt. Their chief concern was to get as much help for Dick as possible and to ease pressures for reading achievement. Dick's father promised to spend more time with him in father-son activities and to stress his abilities in other areas. Fortunately, except for the problems in tutoring, Dick had had a good relation with his father before business pressures had temporarily separated them.

Jack's family was another story. The psychologist and teacher both felt that his parents would equate developmental disorder with mental disorder. They would equate defect in their child with defect in themselves and, therefore, deny its existance or distort information received. They would probably push Jack harder and be angry at him for displaying inefficiency and thereby embarrassing the family. The father was expected to be especially harsh. They could almost hear him say to Jack, "If I have to come to school again about this here reading nonsense, I'll whale the tar out of you." In addition, he would probably blame his wife for Jack's troubles. "I work two jobs, day and night for you two, and all I ask is a little cooperation. Is this the appreciation I get?" He would continue to forget that he had never read well, had hated school, and had run away from home because he always argued with his father. Hurt by his father's rejection of him, he would be equally hurt by the knowledge of his son's deficiency, knowledge he would not accept.

For these reasons, no family conference was held. Instead, Jack's mother was invited to witness some of the tutoring Jack would receive to improve his reading. Each week the tutor sent reports home stating that Jack had learned several new words and that he should be praised for this fine accomplishment. At no time was it mentioned that Jack had a disorder suspected to be the result of neurogenetic factors. The school agreed to let Jack be graded according to progress over his own base rate of performance.

Peer reactions   Most children who fail in school are subjected to teasing and ridicule from other students. If the teacher reacts in a matter-of-fact manner toward a disability and can explain it without anxiety, overelaboration, or solicitousness, children usually accept their classmate's problem without negative reaction. Several ways to demonstrate that a child who cannot read easily is not "dumb" is to duplicate the dyslexic's performance in the normal child. Children are asked to close their eyes and tattoo the word *you* on a piece of paper held to their forehead. When they take the card down most will have written *uoy*. A second demonstration involves having children trace a star pattern seen only through a mirror. The class is simply told that some children make the kinds of errors other children make when they trace the star pattern as seen in the mirror, that Jack and Dick are two such children, and that is why they require extra attention and tutoring. These same demonstrations can be used with parents. In addition, the teacher can criticize the parents while they perform the star-tracing task (Stover & Guerney, 1968).

Types of dyslexia   Boder (1971) presented evidence that some nonreaders can be classified as visual or visile learners, as was Jack, and others as auditory or audile learners. Visual learners lack phonetic skills and, therefore, learn words by sight. They can spell only those words in their sight vocabulary that they can revisualize. Auditory learners cannot remember what words look like and, therefore, learn to read by ear, by sounding out familiar and unfamiliar letter combinations.

The primary deficit in audile learners lies in the visual modality. They are unable to perceive whole words as visual Gestalts. They read laboriously, as if seeing each word for the first time, and even have difficulty remembering what letters look like. The term letter blind could be applied to children in this group. Although such children have good auditory memory and often can recite the alphabet, they may not be able to recognize or write letters until as late as the fourth grade. When no longer letter blind, they may still be word blind. Typically, they are analytic readers, reading by ear while sounding out familiar and unfamiliar letter combinations either to themselves or out loud. The sight vocabulary of such children is less than that of visile learners. However, they may be able to read word lists by phonetic analysis up to or near grade level, missing only words that cannot be decoded phonetically.

Audile learners spell poorly but not bizarrely. They spell as they read —phonetically. Consequently, misspellings are phonetic and usually can be identified. For example, they may spell *circle* as *sykel*, *house* as *hows*, *ready* as *redee*, or *funny* as *funee*. Simple nonphonetic words in their limited sight vocabulary are usually written incorrectly on a test of known words (words child can recognize in a word list), while long and unfamiliar phonetic words not part of their sight vocabulary may be written correctly on a test of unknown words.

On measures of intelligence, audile learners tend to do poorly on subtests measuring spatial organization and better on subtests measuring symbol manipulation (Smith, 1970).

Remediation of audile learners who cannot read, sometimes classified as *visual dyslexics,* focuses on developing letter recognition and an adequate sight vocabulary using tactile-kinesthetic techniques (Fernald, 1943). Since these children learn readily through phonics, remedial phonics after Orton-Gillingham is featured (Orton, 1966). Johnson and Myklebust (1967) note that visual dylexics rarely learn by an ideovisual approach and consequently need a phonetic or phonovisual approach during the initial phase of remediation.

Other investigators also have delineated auditory and visual dyslexia as specific syndromes (Myklebust, 1968; Quiros, 1964). On the basis of ITPA profiles Bateman (1968) identified three subgroups among children with reading disabilities: poor auditory but good visual memory, poor visual but good auditory memory, and deficits in both visual and auditory memory. The reading disability was the most severe and persistent in the subgroup with both visual and auditory memory deficits. Her findings suggest that, in terms of reading, auditory memory is the most important psycholinguistic ability measured by the ITPA. Ingram, Mason, and Blackburn (1970) identified two subgroups, children who made predominately visual-spatial errors and children who made predominately audiophonic errors. The majority of their sample, however, made both errors with equal frequency. Frostig, Lefever, and Whittlesey (1961) described poor readers who possess adequate auditory discrimination but inadequate development of prereading visual skills.

The concept of visile as opposed to audile learners is not new. Charcot (Freud, 1953) spoke of audile children as those whose learning is easiest in the auditory modality and who utilize the language functions dependent upon audition earlier than do children who are visile. In contrast, the visile child may have delayed oral language but does well in areas of language calling for visual skill.

In addition to clinical evidence in support of visual versus auditory strategies for approaching verbal learning, there is evidence from experimental studies (Mallory, 1972). Studies of normal children indicate that material presented only in the visual mode may be spontaneously labeled and orally rehearsed (Flavell, Beach, & Chinsky, 1966). Similarly, material presented only in the auditory mode may be visualized and the visual image of the word recalled rather than its sound (Paivio, 1970). Although the strategies differ, the research suggests that both auditory and visual learners perform equally well on auditory and visual tasks (Bruininks, 1969; Freer, 1971; Robinson, 1968; Waugh, 1973).

However, none of the children used in these studies were classified as dyslexic.

In spite of case typing, most investigators report that dyslexic children have both visual and auditory deficits. Some also have tactile-kinesthetic disorders. Boder would classify these children as having *mixed dyslexia*. Nevertheless, Boder (1971) stated that 63 percent of her sample could be classified as auditory dyslexics, 9 percent as visual dyslexics, and 22 percent as mixed dyslexics. She classified her sample on the basis of reading and spelling performance alone. She feels that traditional evaluative procedures, which have emphasized neurological concomitants, intellectual patterns, right-left disorientation, cerebral dominance, perceptual-motor dysfunction, and language delay, have tended to overemphasize associated disorders and obscure the differences between visual and auditory types. Even the direct diagnosis of errors in reading and spelling has created the illusion that dyslexic children are a homogeneous group. Dyslexic errors are considered to be static and kinetic reversals (first emphasized by Orton in 1937) and extraneous letter and omitted letter errors that persist beyond the age of 8. Boder observed these classic visual-spatial and letter-order errors in visile, audile, and mixed groups. Analysis of these errors, however, failed to reveal the distinct subtypes. She states (1971, p. 314), "Diagnosis of developmental dyslexia through reading-spelling patterns reflecting both functional assets and deficits, offers a fuller range of prognostic and therapeutic implications than traditional diagnosis through dyslexic errors, which reflect functional deficits alone." Unfortunately, Crinella's (1973) factor analytic studies of children with MBD failed to include adequate measures of actual academic deficiencies and stressed visual rather than auditory functioning. For this reason, there may be additional subtypes of children with MBD.

Boder's finding that the preponderance of children with reading difficulty have auditory deficiencies is supported by a number of other studies (Blank, Weider, & Bridger, 1968; McGrady, 1968; McGrady Olson, 1970; Sabatino, 1969). Nevertheless, Orton, were he alive today, would probably not consider some of the children classified into these two groups to have true dyslexia. He placed this label only on children with deficiencies in the secondary symbol system. Orton (1937) stressed impairment in directional sense as the reason for reading failure. The impairment was thought to affect only symbolic stimuli. Thus, the perceptual deficit was integrally connected with visual language functions, not visual functions in general. Orton made no mention of impaired directional sense in nonlanguage problems. In fact, he wrote that many of his dyslexic subjects had excellent visual-motor coordination and sense of direction and that their interpretation of pictorial and diagrammatic material was frequently quite good.

More recently, Benton (1962) has stated that nonsymbolic visual-perceptive deficits accounts for only a small proportion of cases of developmental dyslexia in older children. When the older dyslexic does show disturbed form perception and directional sense, it is usually when the tasks require implicit verbal mediation for optimal performance.

If one adheres to the original definition of dyslexia as a deficiency in the secondary symbol system, then Myklebust's (1968) and perhaps Boder's (1971) concepts of visual and auditory dyslexia are inappropriate, since both types of youngsters showed deficits in the primary symbol system. These deficits are delayed speech development, poor auditory discrimination, and poor sequencing skill in the auditory dyslexic and delayed visual-perceptive development and poor spatial orientation in the visual dyslexic. Perhaps future factor analytic studies of MBD children will reveal that the dyslexics described by Orton belong to a subgroup that has yet to be clearly delineated.

BARRY REMEMBERS

Barry remembers very clearly the long-awaited day when he entered first grade. He had looked forward to school and particularly to learning how to read. As a young child he had enjoyed listening to his mother read stories to him. It was reassuring to be told that after he started school he could learn to read and understand all those strange marks in the book.

Barry's first weeks in school were most satisfying to him. He liked to make friends, he liked his teachers, and he liked the things he was doing in class. During those beginning weeks, Barry spent a lot of time with activities such as matching pictures or telling the class about his trip on an airplane and others things he had done. Barry felt quite proud when he took some papers home which had gold stars on them.

Finally, Barry was placed with a group of children and they all were given little books to read. His teacher said that soon they would be reading the books all by themselves. And so Barry, eager to learn, launched upon his first real venture into reading.

However, as the weeks progressed, Barry found that he was unable to remember all the words like the other children in his group. He couldn't seem to keep straight in his mind how some of the letters looked, no matter how much the teacher or his mother worked with him. Soon Barry found himself with another group of children. The gold stars were a thing of the past now and Barry felt that the world was not as friendly as before.

The remainder of the first grade was spent with more of the papercover books and Barry was very much aware of the fact that the children in the group he had started with were reading from a big hardcover book. Toward the end of the first grade Barry overheard his parents talking about whether or not they should have him repeat first grade. Barry worried a lot about this and felt ashamed because he had not done better in school.

The next fall, Barry did go on to second grade and thought, "Maybe I'll really learn to read this year." He knew that learning to read was the thing he wanted to do most and so Barry started the new school year with some regained enthusiasm. But, this soon disappeared when his old friends the pre-primers made their appearance once more.

It was the same story all over again and Barry found himself making the same old mistakes. If he paid attention to the beginning part of the word, he would often be wrong about the rest of it. If he tried to remember the whole word, he would likely say *pony* for *penny* or *house* for *horse*. And what was worse, some of the other children would laugh at his mistakes. Barry found himself resenting the other children who could read and obviously enjoyed reading. Although Barry didn't know why, he began to tease some of the children and do things that seemed to annoy the teacher. Even though the attention he received wasn't the best kind (Barry often dreamed about being praised for doing some school work especially well), it was better than none.

Perhaps the worst part for Barry now was that he was beginning to have serious doubts about himself. It was not an illogical conclusion to think of himself as stupid when he compared himself to the other children in the class. By the end of the second grade, reading was a hated activity to Barry, who had been able to associate only failure and frustration with it. Just being called upon to read made him anxious because he did not want to expose his "stupidity" for all to see. To read orally to the group was an ordeal and usually Barry would find that the harder he tried to do a good job the more mistakes he would make.

From the third grade on, Barry has been defensive about reading. He feels left out of much of the classroom activities—particularly those which center around reading. There isn't much about school that he really likes, except perhaps playground where he makes up for many of his other frustrations by attempting to outdo the rest of the class in athletic feats. There is little doubt that Barry does find some compensation for his other failures by being an excellent ball player.

At the age of nine and a half, Barry has more than his share of problems. First, inexplicably, he finds that he cannot recognize or remember words as well as other children and he does not know why he should be so different. Barry also knows he has tried to learn to read even if the teacher and his parents sometimes act as though he were lazy or did not care. He is insecure partly because no matter how much he tries to please his parents or teacher they always seem to criticize his mistakes instead of noticing the things he can do well. At this point there seems to be little doubt that Barry will be added to the roll of school drop-outs in a few years if drastic changes do not occur in his education.

From R. L. Carner. Dyslexia—two points of view. *Academic Therapy Quarterly*, 1966, **1**, 134–138.

Dyslexia as a developmental-philological disorder Satz and Sparrow (1970) have advanced the theory that specific reading disorders result from a maturational lag in the lateralization (sidedness) and differentiation of motor, somatosensory (body sensations), and language functions subserved by the dominant left hemisphere. According to this theory, the pattern of deficits observed in dyslexic children, rather than representing a syndrome of disturbance, should resemble the behavioral patterns of chronologically younger children. In other words, the level of brain maturation in dyslexic children is lower and less differentiated than in normal children of the same age and is closer to the maturational level of younger normal children. The early delay in maturation displayed by the dyslexic child forecasts immaturity at each successive stage of hierarchical development. Thus, a child who lags in visual-motor development at age 7 or 8 may eventually "catch up" by age 11 or 12, but will then lag in skills that have a later ontogenetic development (e.g., symbolic language). Their research (Satz, Rardin, & Ross, 1971) and that of Benton (1962) support this maturational lag hypothesis.

The recent emphasis on auditory deficiencies suggests that insufficient development of memory also may be a critical factor in dyslexia. A number of authorities feel that reading, although a visual task, is dependent upon auditory learning, that the reading process involves a kind of perceptual learning in which visual symbols are perceived and related to already known auditory symbols of spoken language (Buswell, 1947). The child must associate his new visual learning with previously acquired auditory learning. If a child who is slow in auditory development is exposed to phonetic methods of reading, he would experience difficulty in learning to read. Wepman's (1960, 1961) studies demonstrated the relationship between poor auditory discrimination and poor reading skill. Children who had poor auditory perception were slower in beginning to talk and slower in acquiring speech accuracy. Some children did not develop adequate sound discrimination until the age of 8. Similarly, Cole and Walker (1966) report that delayed acquisition of speech occurs in the background of many dyslexics.

Delayed speech acquisition in some children may be a function of poor memory for orally presented material. Later, the child has to remember what particular sound goes with what visual symbol and then remember the sequences of sounds that make up a word. In this vein, errors in word recognition correlate positively with the word's orthographic complexity, that is, the number of graphemes that can represent a phoneme and vice versa (Shankweiler & Liberman, 1972). A *phoneme* is a single speech sound in any spoken word. Its written symbol is called a *grapheme*. Several graphemes can represent one specific phoneme in English.

For example, the phoneme /iy/ can be spelled seven ways: *e* as in recede, *ee* as in green, *ea* as in leaf, *ae* as in taenia, *ei* as in receive, *ie* as in field, and *i* as in fatigue. The child with short- or long-term memory problems would have considerable difficulty spelling words with this phoneme.

To complicate matters, many graphemes have several phonemes associated with them. This is particularly true for the vowels of our language. For example, the grapheme *ou* can be pronounced eight ways:

cough, rough, you, journey, four, loud, could, and *boulder.* There are innumerable examples of this phoneme-to-grapheme mix-up in the English language. This mix-up, called irregular orthography, is what many consider the heart of the language problem of dyslexic children (Bannatyne, 1972).

Children learn most easily words containing graphemes that almost always represent the same sound, or phonemes that are always represented by a single grapheme (Bridge, 1968; Coleman, 1970). Children with reading disorders are no exception (Shankweiler & Liberman, 1972).

If reading disabilities are accentuated by irregular orthography, the incidence of reading disorders should be lower in languages with less complex orthography. Makita (1968) cited cross-cultural data that supports this notion. For example, poor readers are extremely rare among Japanese children where kana, the script used in primary instruction, has a script-phonetic relationship that is almost a key-to-keyhole situation. Every sound in kana, like the i.t.a. (initial teaching alphabet) developed in this country, is represented by a specific letter. (In i.t.a., 22 augmented letters were added to the 26 Roman letters so that 48 notations were devised to correspond one to each sound.)

If the rarity of dyslexia among Japanese children is related to the orthographic simplicity of kana, there should be less dyslexia among children exposed to i.t.a. in this country. While Makita (1968) noted that dyslexics show considerable improvement when placed on i.t.a., there is no solid evidence to support this claim. Because i.t.a. is more effective than traditional orthography in teaching children to read and to spell (Downing 1967; Downing & Jones, 1967; Oliver, Nelson, & Downing, 1972; Peters, 1969), dyslexics should profit from instruction in i.t.a. In any case, Makita feels that the irregularity of the language used is the most potent contributing factor in reading disorder. Languages that are irregular or are characterized by unstable grapheme-phoneme relationships, as is English, cause those with poor memory to have the most difficulty reading.

Thus some reading disorders may be considered a developmental-philological rather than a neuropsychiatric problem. Developmental deficiency in memory and verbal coding tasks is a predisposing factor in reading difficulties (Bryden, 1972). The degree to which the deficiencies become manifest is determined by the orthography of the language to be learned.

PROBLEMS IN IDENTIFICATION OF MINIMAL BRAIN DYSFUNCTION

Neither Dick nor Jack was identified as having severe reading problems until third grade. Other children escape identification altogether. How can this be so? One would think that as the child got older his poor reading would stand out like a sore thumb! This would be true if the child was a static being. Most children react to their vague sense of imperfection in ways that conceal their weaknesses from others. Faced with a frustrating learning task, they hide their inability to complete it by leaving their seat, poking others, talking, or drifting off into fantasy. As they get older, they reject tasks they can master if the tasks are at a lower learning level than those being done by their peers; they do not want other children to see them doing "baby stuff."

If a child comes from a fairly stable family, evaluation can reveal these maladaptive behavior patterns for what they really are—patterns that are adaptive for the child because they hide his weaknesses but maladaptive since they prevent further learning. The child would be considered pseudoneurotic since his emotional reaction is a secondary response to a more basic problem. Treating the basic problem should clear up the secondary emotional reaction.

What about children from disorganized families? These children are the most difficult to identify since they suffer from many problems. In fact, the reading disorder may show up only after considerable therapeutic effort has been directed at other difficulties. The case of Angel, a youngster enrolled in a residential treatment center, illustrates this problem. The material presented is a transcription of a multidisciplinary staff conference concerning his difficulties. Although his teacher was aware of some of his academic problems, the questions posed at the end of the conference reveal that the staff did not conceive of his problem as a reading disorder stemming from brain dysfunction. As will be seen, this youngster was later identified as dyslexic.

ANGEL

Angel was placed in the center because of unmanageable behavior in school. He was disruptive, inattentive, and distractible, constantly wandering in school and crossing the street without caution. He did the opposite of what he was told, marked school walls, and destroyed school property. School staff also felt he had auditory hallucinations. Since outpatient treatment was not possible, he was admitted to a residential center at age 11.

Social history Angel was black and his alleged father was a "black-Puerto Rican." Angel was his mother's second out-of-wedlock child. He was born at a state farm where the mother was serving a two-year sentence for violation of parole. The mother had not seen Angel since infancy, when he was placed in a foundling hospital nursery at age 8 months. He remained there until 20 months and was then placed in a foster home where he lived until admission to the center.

Angel's birth was normal. At 9 months he was sitting, at 13 months he walked with support and drank from a cup. At 17 months he walked alone. He spoke simple sentences at 3 years. Angel's mother was epileptic, having seizures since the age of 7. Angel was troubled by a recurrent rash and has had asthmatic attacks, the last one reported when he was 7, some 4 years ago. He has also suffered from repeated injuries.

While in the foundling nursery, Angel was cheerful, happy, and played well with other children. Upon placement in the foster home, Angel had temper tantrums, displayed intense sibling rivalry, was aggressive, and demanded complete attention. The foster mother's guardedness and evasiveness made it difficult to obtain a clear picture of Angel's history. She said he rocked himself to sleep many nights.

Angel's foster parents are described as having both intrapersonal and interpersonal problems. In addition to Angel, they had two natural children and two other foster children, a 12-year old girl and Angel's natural half-sister, age 11. All the children had personality problems that the foster mother denied. She was rigid, demanding, and inconsistent, but at the same time related to the children as if they were siblings. The foster father left the family three years ago. He had been extremely passive, with little interest in being either a husband or father. The foster maternal grandmother had lived in the home for several years, but left because of the foster parents' marital conflict. She continued to visit regularly and was a warm person who related well to the children. Although there was some improvement in the home following the foster parents' separation, the problems there eliminated this home as a future placement for Angel.

Child care worker's report Angel was a friendly, outgoing, and appealing youngster of 11 years who adjusted quickly to our program. Nevertheless, he was hyperactive, impulsive, and reacted strongly to any teasing or interference from peers. These reactions seemed deliberate and controlled, yet were very explosive. Angel could turn off these reactions as quickly as he could turn them on. Angel was friendly with adults and enjoyed their exclusive attention when it was given. He manipulated adults in a joking, semiaggressive manner and then escalated his tactics if he met a favorable response. He tended to go too far and played on adults' feelings to get his way. When mad or upset, he threw objects at his offender; he would throw chairs to defend himself even when he was the provoker. He expressed feelings of physical inadequacy to explain his aggressiveness. Eating and sleeping habits were good, but he rocked and banged his head each night and morning.

Teacher's report Academically, Angel functioned on a third grade level. His reading was poor, his word attack skills limited, and his sight vocabulary small. Although his discrimination of letter sounds, including blends, diagrams, and diphthongs was excellent, he could not integrate them when confronted with an unfamiliar word. It took many repetitions of a new word for him to learn it. Angel occasionally demonstrated the *d-b* reversal, that is, reading *bay* for *day*.

In spelling Angel relied heavily on rote memory to learn new words. In writing he made reversal errors, *was* for *saw* and *on* for *no*, although these errors seldom occurred when reading. In math Angel relied on aids, such as his fingers or a times-table, and his number concepts were poor. He could add, subtract, borrow and carry, and multiply multiplace numbers with the aid of a times-table.

In general, Angel worked hard and had a positive attitude toward school. His interactions with his peers were his major source of difficulty. Angel teased the other boys but got upset if they teased back. He had little respect for their property, grabbed things, and then threw them back at the person who demanded their return. Angel was particularly hostile to Bill, who had the same therapist, and to Sam, who constantly challenged him.

Angel often violated one limit after another, getting more excited as he did so. Usually he could calm down if I insisted he just sit in his seat. I had to remove him from class on three occasions for about an hour. After each removal, he was extremely cooperative for two or three days, but the cycle would then repeat itself. In summary, Angel was an impulsive, quick-tempered boy, with poor social skills and an academic retardation of two years.

Therapist's report It has been difficult to establish a meaningful therapeutic relationship with Angel despite his occasional congeniality and good sense of humor. He expressed his resentment of the therapy hour by complaining that it took him away from art and religious instruction. Actually, this resentment was due to his dissatisfaction with what transpired during therapy. Angel was ambivalent about how to use therapy. He enjoyed testing limits and playing games, yet responded poorly to limitations placed on him and sulked if he did not win games. He was sometimes willing to engage in conversation, yet conversation made him uncomfortable.

Angel had a strong need to "be the pro" and control situations. When he felt threatened, he resorted to controlled loss of temper. As this continued, Angel actually would lose control. Consequently, he was handicapped by not having appropriate ways of expressing anger or frustration.

Summary of psychological testing On the WISC Angel obtained a full scale IQ of 96 (verbal IQ 94; performance IQ 99), placing him within the average range of intellectual functioning. Subtest performance was remarkably even for our population, all generally within an average range. Projective material was limited due to his extreme negativism and resistance to taking these tests. There were scattered indications of conflicts in the areas of aggression, dependency, and sexuality and a tremendous ambivalence toward the foster mother.

About six months after Angel's initial evaluation and after his transfer to a diagnostic teacher, the following disabilities were noted.

1. Confusion about sequences of days, months, and seasons.
2. Frequent loss of materials and frequent inability to find his place or the page itself.
3. Directional confusion.
4. Difficulty in discriminating between close gradations of sound (*pit, bit*).
5. Extreme difficulty following oral directions but no problem if directions demonstrated or given visually.
6. Poor self-monitoring behavior; shows anticipatory behaviors, answers without thinking, starts assignments hurriedly.
7. Literal-minded, often failing to see humor in cartoons and jokes.
8. Difficulty in comprehending the main idea from material given orally.
9. Difficulty with analogies, opposites, verbal or pictorial absurdities.
10. Difficulty in recalling exact words when talking.

These deficiencies were revealed only after Angel felt comfortable with his classmates and teacher. He no longer had to engage in behaviors which hid his failures from others.

Much of Angel's previous behavior could be reinterpreted in light of this knowledge. Angel probably resisted therapeutic efforts directed at verbal interchange because verbal expression was not easy for him. Not being able to recall words to express his ideas, he would avoid situations calling for this ability. His joking manner was perhaps a counterreaction to his literal-minded humor. Much of his hyperactive behavior was probably due to his poor self-monitoring skill and disorganization.

Because Angel's background was so pathological, stress was laid on those factors as causative agents. Fortunately, the divorce of his foster parents prevented undue attention on environmental psychopathology. Had they remained together, wasted effort might have been placed on clearing up family problems. While such a strategy would have helped Angel, it would have left his basic problem untouched. If a child has a primary reading disability, efforts should focus on the child regardless of the family situation. Once the child feels better about himself, he may be able to handle family problems better and contribute less to them. Had Angel remained in his home and had his family been treated on an outpatient basis without awareness of his disability, very little progress would have been made. As it was, valuable time had been lost which could have been devoted to providing the appropriate academic remediation.

Had Angel been properly diagnosed, his psychotherapist might have taken a different tack. Rather than attempting to uncover unconscious conflicts or to foster verbal interchange focusing on interpersonal problems, he would have designed a therapeutic approach to foster the building of a positive self-image. The child's disorder was the result of a disability; talking about it wouldn't make it go away. Directing therapy toward modification of self-image can break down resistance to trying the "baby stuff" the child needs to do to learn basic skills missed in the past.

Early identification

Certainly educators would like to avoid the kind of misidentification that took place in Angel's case and in other cases referred to the residential center. In fact, most would like to identify children with the potential for developing learning problems as soon as, or even before, they enter school. Both Dick and Jack were not discovered until third grade. Although it may not be possible to identify the "true" dyslexic before he attempts to learn to read (by definition his disorder is confined to the secondary symbol system), children whose problems stem from deficiencies in basic perceptual and conceptual processes could be identified earlier. In fact, studies of autonomic reactivity and early environmental factors suggest that identification of children might take place within the first year of life (Denhoff, Hainsworth, & Hainsworth, 1971; Korner, 1971; Smith, Flick, Ferris, & Sellmann, 1972; Thomas, Chess, & Birch, 1968).

Let us describe some of the behaviors that could be identified before formal reading instruction. Many children with MBD have difficulties in auditory perception. They cannot follow or retain temporal and pattern sequences. They sometimes comprehend short conversational units, but are confused by long detailed instructions. "They are word snatchers and inexpert guessers of context, and penalized by any situation that puts a premium on listening" (Hardy, 1967, p. 76). Since their initial auditory perception is "fuzzy," their stored memory patterns lack clarity. This in turn is reflected in their expressed language and speech. Their verbal output not only is immature and lacking in articulatory detail, but also is poorly organized.

Other children display poor memory for auditory stimuli or visual stimuli. One informal method a teacher can use to obtain a rough idea of a child's ability to recall visual and auditory stimuli, as well as to learn and recall auditory-visual associations, is to present several graphic symbols, each paired with a nonsense name. For example, Chalfant and Flathouse (1971) use those below in the following manner.

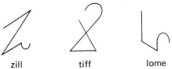

| zill | tiff | lome |

The teacher draws the three symbols on the blackboard and then gives the name for each symbol, "This is zill." "This is tiff." "This is lome." The child is asked to learn the names of the symbols. As soon as he indicates he knows the names, the teacher points to each symbol, both in and out of sequence, and asks the child to name it. After a 10-minute break, during which the blackboard is thoroughly erased, the child is asked to draw the three symbols first in and then out of sequence. Finally, the child is asked to name the graphic symbols both in and out of sequence on three presentations.

In this manner the teacher can watch how the child attempts to learn the symbols and their names and whether he can remember the names (immediate recall), remember the names when given the symbol (short-term memory for auditory-visual associations), and remember the symbols (short-term visual memory). Sometimes a child can remember the symbols or their names only when given in their original sequence. Other children can remember the symbols but cannot recall their names, although they can recognize the name and its symbol if the teachers says the name (that is, they establish correspondence between the symbol and name only at the level of recognition).

This procedure can be altered for use in small groups. The teacher can also test long-term memory by asking children to draw and name the symbols several days later. If the teacher feels she has identified a child with poor memory for symbols or poor sequencing, she can refer the child for more formal evaluation or she can have her aide attempt to drill the child in writing the symbols and saying their names. If the child displays any of the difficulties described above after considerable drill, his failure is probably symptomatic of a specific learning disability. The type depends upon whether his difficulty is in recalling the symbols or their names or in making the associations. Chalfant and Flathouse (1971) present a third grader who failed to name the graphic symbols even after 90 minutes of drill. They contrast his performance with a mildly retarded child (IQ of 75) of the same age who could name the symbols after 8 minutes of drill.

Teachers, as well as psychologists, need to be more specific than simply saying they think a child cannot perform tasks requiring auditory memory. When Dick was tested, memory for digits forward, digits backwards, related syllables, unrelated words, and sentences of increasing length were all presented. To make an adequate assessment of memory, it is necessary to study the tasks, how the tasks are presented, and the response required of the child.

Johnson and Myklebust (1967) pointed out that a memory dysfunction can occur either at the level of recognition or at the level of recall. One child may fail to recognize words visually and, therefore, have difficulty reading. A second may recognize words visually, but be unable to recall or revisualize the words and, therefore, have difficulty in spelling. A third may recognize words when he hears them, but be unable to recall the words when required to speak or write them. A fourth child, like Dick, may be deficient in all three skills.

As we have seen, poor visual discrimination and visual-motor coordination characterize some MBD children, while poor laterality, directionality, and body image characterize others. Some children have fine and gross motor incoordination, either alone or in combination with other deficiencies. Many of the tests previously mentioned can be employed to assess these areas, but the astute nursery school or kindergarten teacher can observe these problems or employ informal evaluation procedures to pinpoint deficiencies. Valett (1967) has developed a series of tasks that the teacher can use to evaluate a child's performance and compare it to developmental norms. He suggests remedial procedures to help a child accomplish the developmental tasks considered crucial prerequisites for future learning. Ahr (1967) has developed a group test for screening preschool children that can also be used by teachers.

In a study of first graders three diagnostic subgroups of children doing poorly in beginning reading were identified (Hagin, Silver, & Corwin, 1971). The first subgroup were children with a specific language disability. These children demonstrated problems in developing body image concepts and in establishing clear-cut cerebral dominance for language. They had difficulty in the orientation of figures in space and of sounds in time.

The second subgroup, called organics, demonstrated many of the behaviors of the specific language disabilities, but had, in addition, signs of abnormality on the classical neurological examination, primarily in muscle tone synergy, in cranial nerve functioning, and in both deep and superficial reflexes. There was evidence of hyperkinesis in some and hypokinesis in others. Choreiform movements, poor fine motor coordination, and apraxia were present. Rarely did findings point to focal brain damage, and rarely were specific etiologic factors found in the history.

The third subgroup were children with developmental immaturity. There was no clinical or historical evidence of CNS dysfunction in this group. Slowness in reaching developmental landmarks in all areas was the sole pattern. They were small in size and looked younger than their chronological ages. The only consistent finding to appear in their histories was low birth weight (see the discussion of prematurity in Chapter 3). Thirty percent of the 82 children studied in this inner city school fell into one of these three groups!

The findings that reading impairment most frequently occurs in association with a complex of deficits are widely supported. Rarely is a child's problem the result of one isolated deficit.

EDUCATION OF THE CHILD
WITH MINIMAL BRAIN DYSFUNCTION

The education of the child with MBD depends upon the type of academic difficulties the child shows and the deficit that results in these difficulties. We have said that most children with MBD are deficient readers, but that the deficits that lead to poor reading are different in different individuals. Some MBD children are poor readers because reading requires sustained attention and concentration, abilities lacking in several subgroups of MBD children. Others display difficulties in discriminating letter shapes because of basic deficiencies in visual-perceptual processes. Still others are poor in auditory discrimination.

Other MBD children display gross and fine motor incoordination, abilities frequently needed during latency when athletic prowess relates to peer group acceptance. Fine motor skill is needed for writing, model building, handicraft work, etc. The child with both gross and fine motor incoordination who also is a poor reader has very few assets upon which to build adequate self-esteem. As a result of his inability to master activities that his peers master, he is likely to feel helpless and eventually to become depressed.

Before we examine ways to educate MBD children, we must note that there are those who advocate an almost unitary approach to their education. We consider these approaches to be fads rather than sound practices. Let us examine several of them.

Unitary approaches

Changing eye dominance Recall that Nick's parents tried to "cure" his retardation by involving him in a patterning program (Chapter 3). Because of the large body of research demonstrating that many inadequate readers fail to exhibit a consistent preference for a dominant hand, foot, and eye (Chalfant & Scheffelin, 1969, p. 97), Delacato (1959, 1963, 1966) hypothesized that establishing dominance would improve reading performance. To establish unilateral dominance, Delacato recommends many of the same procedures employed to foster Nick's development. Patterning, therefore, as well as eye occlusion have been used to treat reading failure. More specifically, Delacato has postulated that lack of corresponding eye-hand dominance represents a neurological disorder of the cortex caused by injury to the brain. Treatment requires reversal of eye dominance before providing remedial reading.

Berner and Berner (1953), however, demonstrate that the dominant eye for monocular tasks (aiming a gun) is not always the controlling eye for binocular vision. While their procedure for determining the controlling eye may differ from Delacato's (they use the Keystone tests of visual skill and binocular skill), their treatment rests on the same theory —the shifting of eye control to the side of the dominant hand. This procedure has been used in several different settings (Benton, McCann, & Larson, 1965; Berner, Uhler, Berner, & Horn, 1963).

Since the span between the Berners's first publication of their theory and their most recent publication is nearly thirty years (Berner & Berner, 1938; Berner, Horn, Berner, & Uhler, 1967), the idea cannot be considered a passing one. Nevertheless, both Delacato's and the Berners's theories have been rejected by most workers in the field. Their research has been faulted for improper experimental procedures and the influence of bias, and their theories have been rejected because of incompatible scientific evidence (Money, 1962, p. 28).

Studies have demonstrated that there are individuals who have failed to establish cerebral dominance but are adequate readers and there are individuals who have established cerebral dominance but are poor readers (Bell, Lewis, & Bell, 1972; Bettman, Stern, Whitsell, & Gofman, 1967; Chalfant & Scheffelin, 1969). Most likely the presence of poor reading and poor lateralization in some children is due to a third factor— cerebral damage, structural disorder, or uneven maturation (Zangwill, 1962). To attempt to change eye dominance, then, is analogous to fixing the windshield in a car with a defective motor—you might see better but you can't go anywhere!

Reducing environmental stimulation   An approach to educating brain-impaired children, which has gained widespread popularity, involves limiting the stimulation present in the instructional environment. This is done because of the brain-impaired child's hyperactivity, distractibility, and poor attentional skills. Cruickshank (1967, p. 273) describes such a classroom.

In several experimental classrooms for brain-injured children, among other things the walls, furniture, and woodwork have been painted the same color; bulletin boards have been removed; windows have utilized translucent glass instead of transparent window lights; and all cupboards have been equipped with solid wooden doors. This alone will reduce stimuli significantly. Wall-to-wall carpeting and sound treatment of ceilings will reduce extraneous auditory stimuli a great deal more. From time to time in certain classrooms the pencil sharpener and the communication system have been removed or disconnected because for certain children they presented unnecessary auditory stimuli. The goal in preparing an adequate learning environment for the brain-injured child is reduction of stimuli, and from this writer's point of view, the reduction can be carried to the furthest extreme. For some children the furthest extreme is necessary. The child is unable to refrain from reacting to stimuli (a psychopathological need situation): education responds to that need by removing stimuli so that the child's energy can be directed toward those stimuli which are important in his learning and adjustment and through which he can achieve success experiences.

The second aspect of environmental structure pertains to space. As space increases, so stimuli increase; as space decreases, the stimulus value of space also decreases. With this in mind a room smaller than the standard sized classroom has been found to be more satisfactory for the brain-injured child. Furthermore, within the classroom, experience has demonstrated the value of small cubicles, either permanent or temporary, one for each child, in which the children's desks, firmly fixed to reduce motor disinhibition, are placed and in which all work which requires attention is done. Various modifications of the cubicles have been successfully employed. In some situations, the cubicle is as a minimum approximately $2\frac{1}{2} \times 3\frac{1}{2}$ feet in size, with the partitions between cubicles extending about 10 inches from the child when he is seated at this desk in order that he cannot be distracted visually by the child in the next cubicle. *(William M. Cruickshank. The education of the child with brain injury. In William M. Cruickshank and G. Orville Johnson (Eds.),* Education of exceptional children and youth *(2nd ed.)* © *1967. Reprinted by permission of Prentice-Hall, Inc., Englewood Cliffs, N.J.)*

Unfortunately, there is no solid research evidence to support the notion that brain-injured children learn better in such environments. Several studies reported no difference between those taught in cubicles and in more normal settings (Rost & Charles, 1967; Shores & Haubrich, 1969). In spite of the lack of empirical support, this procedure became almost standard practice in classrooms for the brain injured. The Pathway School, a private residential and day school for brain-injured children, designed their classrooms to meet the specifications described by Cruickshank. Over the years, however, Pathway staff began to realize that the blanket application of this procedure was a poor practice. Brain-impaired children, like others, want their work displayed in the room. The barren walls prevent the room from being a warm, pleasant place, and the staff felt this lack of warmth actually increased hyperactivity. (It might be predicted from Wender's theory of MBD that such stimulus deprivation would increase rather than decrease hyperactivity.)

Staff gradually returned the classroom to a more traditional environment, and employed other procedures to help the children develop control over distractibility and hyperactivity (Champion, 1970).

Movement training Although accepted in many quarters, movement training is considered another fad. As discussed in Chapter 2, Barsh (1966), Getman (1965), and Kephart (1971) postulate that children with learning problems have suffered breakdowns in perceptual-motor or visual-motor development at one of the earlier stages of development. They conclude, therefore, that a program in sensory-motor training should be basic to the education of children with perceptual-motor impairment. Cruickshank (1967, pp. 279–280) describes such training.

No educational program for brain-injured children is complete without daily motor training, usually accomplished on an individual basis, for approximately 30 minutes. This is an ideal place for the utilization of volunteers who have been oriented to the nature of the brain-injured child and to the type of motor activities which are to be followed. Motor training which serves to provide the child with an understanding and awareness of body parts, orientation to space and direction within space, practice in coordination of legs and arms and leg and arm, facility in activities which involve sighting followed by motor action, and other activities of this nature go far in helping the child to acquire a positive body image. They are the basis for the development of fine-motor movements involving fingers later to be utilized in handwriting and other forms of learning tasks. *(William M. Cruickshank. The education of the child with brain injury. In William M. Cruickshank and G. Orville Johnson (Eds.),* Education of exceptional children and youth *(2nd ed.)* © *1967. Reprinted by permission of Prentice-Hall, Inc., Englewood Cliffs, N.J.)*

As stated in Chapter 2, little evidence exists to support the notion that perceptual-motor training improves reading ability (Mordock & DeHaven, 1969; Reed, 1968). In fact, research does not even support Cruickshank's notion that the exercises he describes improve fine motor skills (DeHaven & Mordock, 1970; DeHaven, Bruce, & Bryan, 1971) and gross coordination improves as much after participation in regular games and sports as it does after participation in specially designed exercise programs (DeHaven, Bruce, & Bryan, 1971). The Pathway School also adopted many of the visual-motor exercises described by Getman (1967). Eventually, however, staff felt time spent in these activities could be better used in other ways and the wholesale adoption of these procedures was dropped (Champion, 1969, 1970). Perhaps this was just as well, since one of the exercises designed to achieve smooth eye movements while reading (watching a ball swinging on a string) contrasted with research indicating that in reading the eye moves in irregular stops and starts and is fixed about 90 percent of the time (Tinker, 1946). Other research indicates that many visual-perceptual aptitudes are independent of motor functioning (Cratty, 1967).

As to improving reading or behavior, current research suggests that movement training achieves no such effect. In Chapter 2 we emphasized that little is known about the functional links between the motor region of the brain and the other analyzers, but we suggested that adequate motor functioning was not a prerequisite for adequate reading. One familiar with brain-behavior relationships would not expect improved motor coordination to result in improved reading. Nevertheless, improved coordination may raise a child's self-esteem and thereby increase his motivation to read. These positive changes reinforce those who advocate movement training and, therefore, these programs continue.

Stimulant drugs The use of psychoactive drugs to modify the hyperactivity frequently associated with cerebral dysfunction has increased in recent years. The stimulant drugs seem to have a paradoxical effect when used in some hyperactive children; the stimulants reduce their motor activity and make them calmer and more compliant. Actually, the drug action in the hyperkinetic child is not a pharmacological paradoxical effect; the drugs have a direct stimulating effect that increases the ability to fix and focus attention, to shut out the irrelevant, and to organize body movements more purposefully. Since responses to interfering stimuli are decreased, the child is more receptive to stimuli presented by teachers and parents and more amenable to social control.

Research by MacKay and her colleagues (Beck, MacKay, & Taylor,

1970; MacKay, Beck, & Taylor, 1973) found that some children who showed improved behavior when placed on stimulant drugs also showed fewer slow waves on the electroencephalogram. In other children improvement on the electroencephalogram was not accompanied by changes in behavior, and in one child improved behavior was noted even when increases in slow wave activity occurred.

Wender (1971, 1972) hypothesized that the stimulant drugs stimulate functionally underactive neurotransmitters so that specific areas of the central nervous system function together more effectively. As a consequence, there is less need for self-stimulation and a better response to reinforcement.

The stimulant drugs have a positive effect on from 50 to 60 percent of properly diagnosed MBD children who are hyperactive. Unfortunately, stimulant drugs are often administered to children without undertaking a thorough investigation of the reasons for their hyperactivity. Recent estimates are that stimulant drugs are being prescribed for between 150,000 and 200,000 children (Lipman, 1970). Many of the children are given these drugs without being seen by a pediatric neurologist or clinical psychologist and many physicians do not adequately monitor the child's drug use (Solomons, 1973).

It would seem that some schools "have seized on the label 'hyperactive' as a catchall label for their problem children, and on psychoactive drugs as a simplistic method of restraint" (Krippner, Silverman, Cavallo, & Healy, 1973, p. 267). Instead of trying to help overly active children through special educational techniques, they attempt to calm them by the simplest method available. Fish (1971) cautions that a stimulant is the drug of choice for only *some* hyperactive children and concludes that some may need no medication. Similarly, Eisenberg (1971) remarks that if drugs are used indiscriminantly in response to symptoms rather than to the underlying medical disorder, abuses of the drug will occur.

The indiscriminant use of drugs can divert one's efforts away from a direct attack on the source of the symptoms, much as a prescription of aspirin for a headache caused by a tumor allows the tumor to grow unchecked by diminishing the signal that warns of its presence. For example, a child who always comes to school without breakfast can be restless as a result of hypoglycemia (low blood sugar); to give such a child a stimulant drug would be criminal. Similarly, to medicate a child who is hyperactive in response to an incompetent teacher or to an improper curriculum (hyperactivity as a learned avoidance reaction to achievement anxiety) would also be an irresponsible medical action. Unfortunately, many physicians prescribe medications without even inquiring about the child's classroom situation! Eisenberg (1971, p. 378) states:

Medication should not be used to relieve the physician of the responsibility for seeking to identify and eliminate factors causing or aggravating the underlying disorder. Stimulant drugs treat symptoms, not diseases. Symptomatic relief is not to be disparaged; often, it is the most the physician can offer. However, since symptom suppression can delay appropriate intervention, treatment should follow, not precede, thorough diagnostic evaluation.

Even when the drugs are given after diagnostic study and are effective in calming the child, the drugs do no more than make it possible for the child to learn. Because the child has failed to learn or to acquire correct learning habits, he will need remedial educational measures. Thus, drug administration constitutes only part of a total treatment program that should encompass appropriate educational plans, parent counseling, recreational activities, and other growth promoting activities. *(Copyright 1971, the American Orthopsychiatric Association, Inc. Reproduced by permission.)*

Stewart, an early pioneer in the use of stimulant drugs with hyperactive children, followed up his patients (Morrison & Stewart, 1971) and reported (Stewart, 1972, p. 8) that hyperactivity is

a cluster of personality traits that are with the person for good. Once you accept this, it's a completely different ball game. Any treatment you use as a holding action until the child outgrows his hyperactivity is ridiculous. Once you start this person on drugs, you would have to treat him the rest of his life. . . . By the time the child reaches puberty, he is a child who does not know what his undrugged personality is. And, worse, the child's family does not know how to accept this undrugged personality.

Stewart claims that medication "takes away the parent's and teacher's motivation to change their approach to the child." While Stewart's position may be extreme, it certainly deserves our consideration. More detailed information about his viewpoint is given in Sroufe and Stewart (1973) and in Stewart and Olds (1973).

Werry and his colleagues (Werry, Minde, Guzman, Weiss, Dogan, & Hoy, 1972, p. 449) also feel that educators should accommodate their approach to the child rather than vice versa. They state that the hyperactive syndrome is often "a biological variant made manifest by affluent society's insistance on universal literacy and its acquisition in a sedentary position."

In a study of a nonclinical population of children, mothers of highly active males were found to be critical, disapproving, unaffectionate, and severe in their punishment. The authors conclude (Battle & Lacey, 1972, p. 772):

With the present concern about the advisability of encouraging drug dependence as a desirable alternative to other forms of environmental intervention, it would seem wise to consider the possibility of changing the social context surrounding motor hyperactivity for young boys and for elementary school age girls. The consequent appearance of improved orientations toward achievement and social situations would be accomplished as the result of improved adult-child interactions rather than as the result of an impersonal external intervention.

Gordon's (1970, pp. 249, 252) statements serve as a cogent summary for this section.

Suddenly, brain injury is a learning or perceptual disability; and lo and behold, almost everybody has one. Then the witch doctors move in with one-shot solutions. Pushers-publishers of educational material follow, and the thick fog of optimism begins to obscure the essential dilemma: that most brain-injured children probably have cerebral damage, which means permanent disability requiring extensive rehabilitation and guidance; and that such children cannot be stereotyped, however carefully they are categorized and documented by research.

In any group of 100 brain-injured children, 15-20 teaching methods are required to meet varying academic needs. But too many people fail to recognize this need for diversity. They are like the remedial educators who force all students with disabilities into one or two categories and ignore underlying psychological blocks. . . .

There is no impressive evidence that brain-injured children learn better, or learn at all, when their educational environment is highly structured and free from extraneous stimulation. In fact, isolating, programmed routines reinforce dependence and feelings of inferiority. But somehow we find a simpler solution disconcerting. If a child is blocked in reading, we should not give him more reading; instead we should teach him swimming, photography, or any other ego-enhancing activity. Similarly, I have seen whole fifth-grade classes of children who could no longer be taught even simple arithmetic, but who grasped chess, checkers, or monopoly. Of course, part of life is coping with irrelevance and boredom. But children should be exposed to such experiences only in small doses. Certainly, some routines are good, but not too many, and only those designed for relatively unimportant areas of life. Yes, some exercises are necessary, but don't expect children to enjoy them.

Individualized approaches

Although restriction of environmental stimulation, medication, and sensory motor training may all be necessary in the education of some children, their blanket application in the instruction of children diagnosed as brain-impaired is uncalled for. Such application implies that MBD is a unitary syndrome. As we have seen, children with MBD display a variety of disorders. Researchers have described dysfunctions in the analysis of sensory information (auditory, visual, and tactual processing), dysfunctions in the synthesis of sensory information (integration and memory), and dysfunctions in symbolic operations (acquiring auditory language, decoding written language, encoding written language, and integrating language). Thorough evaluation of sensory and symbolic functions helps reveal the child's disabilities; study of these separate functions, therefore, is in keeping with the individual profile approach.

Children can be classified according to the actual problem they show —motor encoding problem, writing disorder (agraphia), auditory-receptive disorder. Nevertheless, children rarely show one isolated defect; the brain is not that simple. While damage to the peripheral nervous system (see Chapter 5) may result in a single deficiency (e.g., poor sight), we have seen that CNS damage affects how the different sensory modalities operate together. It would be unusual, therefore, for a child to have problems in visual stimulus processing (decoding act) and be a good writer (encoding act). While there are children who write poorly because of poor coordination, usually these children display other difficulties as well (DeHaven, Mordock, & Loykovich, 1969).

Each child's assets and liabilities should be profiled and educational procedures planned according to the needs dictated by the profile (Silver, & Hagin, 1967a, 1967b, 1971). Hewett (1964) has developed a hierarchy of educational tasks for children with learning disorders. If a child's profile reveals that his functioning is characteristic of children at a particular level of development, educational procedures are employed which are considered appropriate at that level. Chapter 12 includes a discussion of such an approach in greater detail.

Types of remedial reading programs with severe reading deficiencies

Dyslexia is not a simple unitary disorder calling for a uniform program of teaching. It is almost as if dyslexia is caused by short-circuits, but each child has shorted in different areas, in different degrees and in different combinations of circuits (Ellingson, 1967, p. 23).

In essence the dyslexic child may be likened to a special type of computer. The computer has a potential capacity for processing information. However, it will not function properly unless fed with a particular program which satisfies the necessary criteria for production. A program which fits one computer will not necessarily work for one of a different type. Furthermore, an incorrect program will be rejected by the computer, and under no circumstances will the processing of information occur with that program (International Reading Association, 1969, p. 102).

The manner in which one chooses to intervene in the case of reading disorders depends upon one's beliefs about the etiology of reading disability in general and the specific diagnostic picture of the child one is to teach (Silver & Hagin, 1967b). In many public schools children who are experiencing difficulty with prereading or reading and, as a consequence, are "failing" kindergarten or first grade are being placed in "junior firsts" or "transitional" classes. Often they go from the junior first to the junior second and then to the special class for the neurologically impaired. Analysis of the content of these programs reveals very little knowledge about reading problems and an inability to state educational or behavioral objectives for each child enrolled. Teachers lack special training and knowledge about the process of learning to read. Without knowledge of each step in the reading process and the steps that a child has already mastered, remediation is likely to be unsuccessful.

Silver and Hagin (1967b) describe a 5-year old boy with good auditory skill, but with numerous perceptual problems and a meager and inexact vocabulary, who was taught in i.t.a. (which depends on phonic regularity). When reevaluated at age 7, he scored at the seventh grade level on an oral reading test. Nevertheless, his comprehension was so poor that he could not explain what he had just read aloud, even if it was easy and interesting material. The approach had emphasized only one area and had neglected the more basic deficiency in comprehension.

It is popular in the transitional and even in special education classes to find material that is of interest to the child and use this material to increase motivation. The teacher, teacher aide, or tutor sits with the child while he tries to read this material. The tutor tries to give contextual cues, "Look at the picture on top," or "tells" the child words he doesn't know. If the tutor is slightly more sophisticated, he may try to develop a sight vocabulary through flash cards or use some of the perceptual-motor training aids available commercially.

Corrective reading programs in many schools address themselves to developing word recognition and comprehension skills. Practice material is presented in workbooks, drill pads, and books. The students read the material to themselves and demonstrate comprehension by answering multiple-choice questions. Silver and Hagin (1967b, p. 43) state that "this program, too, does not deal with the basic defects of specific reading disability." The research of Anderson and Stern (1972) supports this impression.

Specific remedial programs have emphasized word recognition skills. Two approaches predominate. One is the attempt to bombard the child with all types of sensory stimuli; the VAKT (visual-auditory-kinesthetic-tactile) and the Fernald training techniques are examples currently in use. The second identifies the child's intact perceptual channels and chooses a teaching approach utilizing these strengths, for example, audile learners are taught phonics and visile learners are taught a sight vocabulary. Findings from follow-up of children taught by the second approach, however, were disappointing (Silver & Hagin, 1964). Consequently, some investigators favor a direct assault on deficit areas (Silver, Hagin, & Hersch, 1967). They advocate improving perception through training in three stages: (1) a recognition-discrimination stage, (2) a copying stage, and (3) a recall stage. Techniques are directed toward only one perceptual modality at a time, before the child attempts intermodal tasks or attempts to relate language and perception.

This was the approach taken by the staff of the residential center where Angel was enrolled after their research revealed that many of the children studied displayed deficits in perceptual synthesis. Would discrimination training on similar perceptual synthesis tasks lead to improved performance on a retest of the perceptual synthesis task?

Six children were given 30-minute sessions once a week until they could correctly master six perceptual synthesis tasks. Following mastery, the children were retested with the initial perceptual synthesis task from Birch and Lefford (1964). Six other children served as controls. Five of the six experimental children successfully completed the training to criterion. All these five showed improvement on the initial perceptual synthesis materials, although the degree of improvement was less than anticipated. Only one child in the control group improved (Schiff, Talmadge, & Mora, 1968).

Simultaneous with this specialized tutoring the children showing perceptual impairments were grouped into two classes by age. Each child was taught according to recommendations similar to those in the brief sketches of the four children presented earlier. At the end of one year of perceptual training the younger group (about age 8) improved significantly in word discrimination, spelling, arithmetic computation, and overall grade level on the Metropolitian Achievement Tests. The older group (about age 10), although demonstrating a trend toward improvement, failed to improve significantly in any area of achievement. The younger group may have made greater progress, however, because they were initially more academically retarded (Hayden, Copsen, McKinstry, Ansari, & Talmadge, 1968).

Although the Frostig training procedures for visual-perceptual disorder were part of the remedial program offered in the residential center, more recent research suggests that improvements in children placed on Frostig exercises are due more to the personal attention given them than to the unique remedial powers of the program (Anderson & Stern, 1972; Jacobs, Wirthlin, & Miller, 1968; Pryzwansky, 1972). Anderson and Stern (1972) suggest that two Frostig training programs, for eye-motor coordination and for figure-ground difficulties, might be of value if used for an eight-week period but no longer. As we will see, training in one sense modality is unlikely to be of long-lasting benefit since reading is a task requiring adequate intersensory functioning.

Developers of the ITPA, while advocating remediation of deficits, recommend organizing an approach integrating sensory motor channels simultaneously, so that a channel of relative strength can be utilized to help develop a channel of weakness (Bateman, 1968). For example, if a child is high in manual expression and low in verbal expression, the child would carry out manual tasks and simultaneously try to explain verbally what he was doing. If a child is high in auditory reception and low in visual reception, he might profit from describing verbally the details and meanings of various pictures. For a child low in a visual association and high in auditory association, verbally classifying objects into categories by shape, composition, color, or function might prove beneficial. Although this approach would seem to make sense, research cited earlier in our discussion of visual and auditory learners suggests that children learn equally well under procedures that teach to their strengths or to their weaknesses.

These studies fail to support the notion that single sensory systems (visual or auditory) function independently of one another. There is more evidence that the functioning of one sensory system is affected or modified by the functioning of other sensory systems, whether the system functions independently or in coordination with other systems (Birch & Lefford, 1964). Reading is basically an intersensory task (relating the auditory word-name /kæt/ with the visual graphic word *cat*). Most remedial programs, therefore, rely on multisensory approaches regardless of the classification.

PSYCHOEDUCATIONAL EVALUATION: DAVID, AGE 9-7

David was observed being tutored by his paraprofessional. It became immediately noticeable that old learnings markedly interfered with new learnings. For example, any time the word *I* started a sentence, David would automatically say the word *want*. Cued by the teacher, he would make a second and more appropriate attempt. Things that should be automatically learned have not been, so that there is interference and confusion among various symbols. He still cannot recognize individual letters that start words, and when asked to look at a list of letters, he will find the one that visually matches the one in the reading book, and will then recite the alphabet to himself, counting on his fingers until he reaches the one on the list. This is a rather complex way to remember letters when he could be taught simpler ways.

David has a limited repertoire of sounds, and to any visual symbol he will respond with these sounds. When his error is brought to his attention, his second attempt is more often correct. David has no auditory-visual correspondence. When given a letter name, he usually cannot give its sound; when given the sound, he cannot give the letter name; when given just the visual image of the letter, he cannot do anything. I observed that David learns best by sight. For example, if given the word *hear*, he will learn it, although he will not remember that it begins with *h* sound nor will he remember the *h* sound.

Educational recommendations. The more sounds you try to teach David that aren't overlearned, the more they will interfere with his learning. If he is to be taught letter sounds, they should be taught by the use of flash cards until he can make automatic associations, such as *d-da, b-ba*.

Second, his sight vocabulary should be built up by flash cards and by tachistoscopic presentations. One should start with his present sight vocabulary, no matter how low, overlearn these materials, and then introduce several new words to this list at a time. He then should read only those words that are in his sight vocabulary so that there is no guess work.

In order to develop a sight vocabulary, a word-box should be employed, with David placing words in the box once he has learned them. He should then make sentences out of the words and write these sentences; this he could do by himself. David could also be taught dictionary skills in order to increase his attention to words. He should not be required to learn the meaning of the word but simply to find it in the dictionary. Once he knows where words that begin with *g* are in the dictionary, then he could be given all words beginning with *g* to look up by looking at the second letter; this will increase his attention to the entire word. Words which he has looked up can then be learned through flash card presentations and placing in his word-box. These visual training techniques should increase his sight vocabulary. Phonics training should be ignored until he has a sight vocabulary at least to the third grade level.

The word-box can be made into building blocks for a tower or some other device. The words presented should be easily illustrated ones.

Durrell Murphy practiced phonics using picture clues for word selection, and word family expansion might be useful here.

David should be read to and encouraged to choose subjects in which he is interested. Furthermore, he should be encouraged to write stories, using scribble writing when he does not know a word and, later, have it supplied by the teacher. This, then, could become a self-created reader.

Games can be created using sight words. For example, draw a winding path divided into blocks in which are written words from the child's vocabulary and a few penalties and bonuses. The child throws dice and moves along the path, saying each word and following directions. Card games like War can be played with flash cards; the child keeps the card when he says the word. Jeopardy is another game that can be played with the child's vocabulary.

The fact that reading is an intersensory task has important implications not only for remediation of reading disorders but also for reading instruction in general. Several investigations have revealed that good readers receive higher auditory-visual integration scores (material presented orally is discriminated from similar material when presented again visually) than poor readers (Birch & Belmount, 1964; Reilly, 1971). Furthermore, males do not develop this ability until the second grade and still display inefficiency at the fourth grade. In contrast, girls develop auditory-visual correspondence sometime between the first and third grade. If a child who is slow in developing these skills is pressured to read early, he might develop poor reading habits. The finding that reading disorders appear more often in males may be related to developmental differences between the sexes. In this vein, Ames (1968) feels that many children with learning disorders are those who were given reading instruction before they were ready. Several research studies support this impression (Koppitz, 1971; Satz et al., 1971).

In several of the cases presented in this chapter the approach was to present reading material initially through the stronger modality and then, in successive reading tasks, gradually fade out stimuli in this modality while introducing the modality in which the child is deficient. At the present time, however, limited knowledge exists about the effects of different types of remediation. There is evidence that changes can occur in perceptual-motor and spatial abilities (Painter, 1966), directionality (Hill, McCullum, & Sceau, 1967), and visual discrimination (Popp, 1967) and that such training sometimes results in improved reading ability (Lewis, 1968; Silver & Hagin, 1967b). The relative value of each different approach, that is, visual versus auditory training, one modality versus intermodal training, has yet to be determined.

Remediation by facilitating perception of linguistic structure Researchers who attribute reading disability primarily to the child's inability to handle the irregular orthography of the English language, attempt to remediate by facilitating the visual differentiation of graphemes within words or by making syllables the basic language unit.

The differentiation of graphemes sometimes involves color coding of graphemes that correspond to a particular phoneme. For example, graphemes for the phoneme /iy/ as in green, leaf, fatigue, receipt, etc., would be color coded green. This approach, described in detail by Bannatyne (1966b), is consistent with the finding that children can learn phoneme-grapheme correspondences better than they can grapheme-phoneme correspondences (Hardy, Smythe, Stennett, & Wilson, 1972).

Savin's (1972) approach makes the syllable the basic unit of language. The spelling of each syllable is taught without analyzing the spoken syllables into phonemes. For example, one would teach that the letter sequences doe, dow, and dough all are (sometimes) pronounced /dou/. There are several thousand syllable correspondences to be learned, but learning several thousand syllables may be far less formidable a task than learning irregular orthography or learning the tens of thousands of words from visual memory. Gleitman and Rozen (study in progress), of the University of Pennsylvania, are currently evaluating the effects of the syllabary method of teaching reading to normal children. Should this method prove effective, it could be adopted for use with dyslexic children.

HOW DO THEY FARE?

Because these handicaps are subtle, the impression may be that many children improve with age or following remedial efforts. This is not the case. Although perceptual-motor deficits as well as hyperactivity diminish somewhat by the time the MBD child reaches adolescence, other deficits remain. The MBD adolescent often fails to progress to the age-appropriate conflicts of adolescence; instead stresses stem from social isolation, differences from peers, and inability to integrate into the normal teenage world. Relationships with parents, siblings, and peers and involvement in jobs and hobbies are more like those of the latency-age child. Relationships with parents are markedly dependent, and siblings often regard the MBD child as a social liability. Greatest maladjustment is observed in peer relationships.

In addition to being isolated, MBD adolescents are often unable to respond to rudimentary social cues and seek companionship with children four or five years younger (Bauman & Green, 1970). Among exceptionally bright adolescents, difficulties in verbal fluency, visual sequencing, formulating abstractions, and organizing stimuli are characteristic (Cohen, 1969). Several investigations have revealed that CNS dysfunction is significantly higher in hospitalized adolescent psychiatric patients than in normals (Pollack, 1967), implying that these developmental difficulties foreshadow later maladjustment.

Follow-up of both dyslexic and hyperactive children with suspected MBD reveals that from 50 to 97 percent fail in school. Hinton and Knights (1971) followed children with learning problems over a three-year period. Approximately 50 percent had failed a grade in school. Out of 65 children, 41 did not maintain regular school progress, with 21 placed in a special class. Among hyperactive children, as high as 70 percent failed one or more grades in school (Weiss, Minde, Werry, Douglas, & Nemeth, 1971). Among disabled readers, 97 percent were retained (Hardy, 1968). Other studies have found one in four to be very antisocial, with a significant proportion of the total group disobedient and rebellious and suffering from chronically low self-esteem (Mendelson, Johnson, & Stewart, 1971).

Koppitz (1971, 1972–1973) followed children enrolled in special classes for the learning disabled (primarily MBDs) over a five-year period. She concluded that progress was positively correlated with the extent of the disability. For example, if the child had difficulty only in visual-motor perception, he made better progress than the child who had both visual-motor and auditory-perceptual difficulties. During the follow-up period, roughly one-fourth of the pupils studied returned to the regular classroom. Koppitz concluded that the majority of the children studied matured at a much slower rate than regular class children, supporting Ames's (1968) notion that allowances should be made for the inability of many MBD children to learn at an "average" rate.

Koppitz (1972–1973, pp. 137–138) emphasized that learning disabilities cannot be corrected or "cured" by any specific teaching method or technique:

Published articles and presentations often tell of the wonderful accomplishments of special education in a mere matter of weeks or months. Countless projects are reported that demonstrate the remarkable success of various teaching techniques or methods in helping youngsters with learning problems. Yet many or even most special class teachers find that they are less successful when they apply a given method in their own classrooms. A teaching method may work well for one child, but may not be suited for another child in the same class. Teachers also discover that it is often difficult to maintain the initial rate of progress that many new special class pupils tend to make. The follow-up study revealed that the special class pupils aged seven or older made their greatest academic gains during the first year after they were introduced to a new teacher and the special education program. This initial spurt in progress was often spurious and was rarely maintained in subsequent years. The pupils' rate of academic progress in the special classes usually leveled off or even hit a plateau after a while. Other investigators have found similar results. I have come to view, therefore, most short-term studies with caution. The initial, often impressive gains disappear too often or get "washed out" a year or two later. Many more long-term follow-up studies of children with learning disabilities and of teaching methods are needed in order to really assess the impact of special education.

There are two long-term follow-up studies of hyperactive children (Menkes, Rowe & Menkes, 1967; Weiss et al., 1971), both of which indicate that satisfactory personal and occupational adjustment occurs in less than 20 percent. Findings from a study of the families of hyperactives reveal a high prevalence of alcoholism, sociopathy, and hysteria among family members, suggesting that many parents were ex-hyperactives (Morrison & Stewart, 1971).

Long-term follow-up studies of children with severe reading disability show a great deal of variation in successful adult adjustment (Barlow & Blomquist, 1965; Hardy, 1968; Preston & Yarington, 1967; Rawson, 1968; Robinson & Smith, 1962; Silver & Hagin, 1964). Silver and Hagin (1964, p. 101) state that "with conventional teaching methods, the prognosis for the 'organic' is not favorable; therefore, it may be necessary to devise new teaching procedures appropriate to the pattern of his neurological and perceptual deficiencies."

Studies do show that children with high intellectual ability who have supportive families have a much more successful occupational career and better personal adjustment than those with low IQ and with nonsupportive families. Even the intelligent, however, still display difficulty reading.

CONCLUDING REMARKS

We have now seen how brain dysfunction handicaps a child. If it is severe, he usually is raised apart from the mainstream of society; if it is mild, he may remain in his community but usually is educated apart from his nonimpaired peers. There is no "cure" for brain dysfunction, only compensation. Unfortunately, society frequently prevents the child from compensating for his disorder. Communities demand that the child look and behave "normal." Schools require that all children enter at the same age and on a set date and that they progress at a given rate in a lock-step grade system. Efforts to correct specific disabilities, while neglecting general education, border on prejudice—a rejection of the child as he is and conveying to him that his acceptance depends upon his being more like others. Although some children will always be functionally illiterate, this does not mean that they cannot be educated. Schools should teach children what they can learn rather than expecting all children to learn the same thing. Until we do this, we will continue to hide rather than help our exceptional children.

References

Ahr, A. E. The development of a group preschool screening test of early school entrance potentiality. *Psychology in the Schools*, 1967, **4**, 59–63.

Ames, L. B. Learning disabilities: the developmental point of view. In H. R. Myklebust (Ed.), *Progress in learning disabilities*. Vol. 1. New York: Grune & Stratton, 1968.

Anderson, W. F., & Stern, D. The relative effects of the Frostig program, corrective reading instruction, and attention upon the reading skills of corrective readers with visual-perceptual deficiencies. *Journal of School Psychology*, 1972, **10**, 387–395.

Bannatyne, A. The color phonics system. In J. Money (Ed.), *The disabled reader*. Baltimore: Johns Hopkins Press, 1966a.

Bannatyne, A. A suggested classification of the causes of dyslexia. *Word Blind Bulletin*, 1966b, **1**, 5–13.

Bannatyne, A. *Language, reading and learning disabilities*. Springfield, Ill.: C. C Thomas, 1972.

Barlow, B., & Blomquist, M. Young adults ten to fifteen years after severe reading disability. *Elementary School Journal*, 1965, **66**, 44–48.

Barsh, R. H. Teacher needs—motor training. In W. M. Cruickshank (Ed.), *The teacher of brain-injured children: a discussion of the basis for competency*. Syracuse, N.Y.: Syracuse University Press, 1966.

Bateman, B. *Interpretation of the 1961 Illinois Test of Psycholinguistic Abilities*. Seattle: Special Child Publications, 1968.

Battle, E. S., & Lacey, B. A context for hyperactivity in children over time. *Child Development*, 1972, **43**, 757–773.

Bauman, S. S., & Green, S. K. Brain dysfunction in adolescence. II. Life styles. *American Journal of Orthopsychiatry*, 1970, **40**, 334–335.

Beck, L., MacKay, M. C., Taylor, R. Methylphenidate; results on children's psychiatric service. *New York State Journal of Medicine*, 1970, **70**, 2897–2902.

Bell, D. B., Lewis, F. D., & Bell, B. W. Is the Schilder Hand Test really an adequate measure of cerebral dominance. *Academic Therapy Quarterly*, 1972, **7**, 339–347.

Benton, A. L. *Right-left discrimination and finger localization*. New York: Harper & Row, 1959.

Benton, A. L. Dyslexia in relation to form perception and directional sense. In J. Money (Ed.), *Reading disability: progress and research needs in dyslexia*. Baltimore: Johns Hopkins Press, 1962.

Benton, C. D., Jr., McCann, J. W., & Larson, M. Dyslexia and dominance. *Journal of Pediatric Ophthalmology*, 1965, **2**, 53–57.

Berner, G. E., & Berner, D. E. Reading difficulties in children. *Archives of Ophthalmology*, 1938, **20**, 829–838.

Berner, G. E., & Berner, D. E. Relation of ocular dominance, handedness, and the controlling eye in binocular vision. *Archives of Ophthalmology*, 1953, **50**, 603–608.

Berner, G. E., Horn, M. B., Berner, D. E., & Uhler, W. M. *The treatment of visual and visual-motor problems: an interim report.* (The Devereux Monograph Series) Devon, Pa.: Devereux Foundation, 1967.

Berner, G. E., Uhler, W. M., Berner, D. E., & Horn, M. B. A clinical investigation of crossed control in a residential treatment center. *Southwestern Medicine*, 1963, **44**, 51–56.

Bettman, J. W., Stern, E. L., Whitsell, L. J., & Gofman, H. F. Cerebral dominance in developmental dyslexia. *Archives of Ophthalmology*, 1967, **78**, 722–729.

Betts, E. A. *Foundations of reading instruction.* New York: American Book, 1954.

Birch, H. G., & Belmount, L. Auditory-visual integration in normal and retarded readers. *American Journal of Orthopsychiatry*, 1964, **34**, 852–861.

Birch, H. G., & Lefford, A. Two strategies for studying perception in "brain-damaged" children. In H. G. Birch (Ed.), *Brain damage in children*. Baltimore: Williams & Wilkins, 1964.

Blank, M., Weider, S., & Bridger, W. H. Verbal deficiencies in abstract thinking in early reading retardation. *American Journal of Orthopsychiatry*, 1968, **38**, 823–834.

Boder, E. Developmental dyslexia: prevailing diagnostic concepts and a new diagnostic approach. In H. R. Myklebust (Ed.), *Progress in learning disabilities.* Vol. 2. New York: Grune & Stratton, 1971.

Bradway, K. P. Birth lesions in identical twins. *American Journal of Orthopsychiatry*, 1937, **7**, 194–203.

Bridge, J. T. Rank ordering of letters and letter combination according to ease of learning their sound associations. Unpublished master's thesis, University of Texas at El Paso, 1968.

Bruininks, R. H. Relationship of auditory and visual perceptual strengths to methods of teaching word recognition among disadvantaged Negro boys. *Dissertation Abstracts*, 1969, **30A**(1–3), 1010A.

Bryant, N. Some principles of remedial instruction for dyslexia. *Reading Teacher*, 1965, **18**, 567–572.

Bryden, M. P. Auditory-visual and sequential-spatial matching in relation to reading ability. *Child Development*, 1972, **43**, 824–832.

Buswell, G. T. The sub-vocalization factor in the improvement of reading. *Elementary School Journal*, 1947, **48**, 190–196.

Chalfant, J. C., & Flathouse, V. E. Auditory and visual learning. In H. R. Myklebust (Ed.), *Progress in learning disabilities.* Vol. 2. New York: Grune & Stratton, 1971.

Chalfant, J. C., & Scheffelin, M. A. *Central processing dysfunctions in children: a review of research.* (National Institute of Neurological Diseases and Blindness, Monograph No. 9) Washington, D.C.: U.S. Government Printing Office, 1969.

Champion, B. W. Movement: means or end? Paper presented at the annual international convention of the Council for Exceptional Children, Denver, April 1969.

Champion, B. W. Educating the child with minimal cerebral dysfunction. Paper presented at the annual conference of the American Physical Therapy Association, Washington, D.C., July 1970.

Clarkson, F. E., & Hayden, B. S. *A developmental study of perceptual, conceptual, motivational and self-concept differences between and within hyperactive and normal groups of preadolescent boys.* (Final Report Project No. 5-0414) Bureau of Education for the Handicapped, Washington, D.C.: U.S. Government Printing Office, 1971.

Clarkson, F. E., & Hayden, B. S. The relationship of family background and neurological status in a normal class setting. Paper presented at the annual convention of the American Psychological Association, Honolulu, September 1972.

Clements, S. D. *Minimal brain dysfunction in children: termination and identification, phase one of a three phase project.* (National Institute of Neurological Diseases and Blindness, Monograph No. 3, Public Health Service Publication No. 1415) Washington, D.C.: U.S. Government Printing Office, 1966.

Cohen, W. J. Thought organization of the learning disabled adolescent: some implications for the classroom. *Devereux Schools Forum*, 1969, **5**, 42–51.

Cole, E. M., & Walker, L. Reading and speech problems as expressions of a language disability. *Bulletin of the Orton Society*, 1966, **16**, 55–73.

Coleman, E. B. Data base for a reading technology. *Journal of Educational Psychology Monograph*, 1970, **61**(4, Part 2).

Conners, C. K. Psychological assessment of children with minimal brain dysfunction. In F. F. De La Cruz, B. H. Fox, & R. H. Roberts (Eds.), *Minimal brain dysfunction, Annals of the New York Academy of Sciences*, 1973, **205**, 283–302.

Cratty, B. J. The independence and interdependence of visual perception and movement in infants and children. Paper presented at the Child Achievement Center, Sherman Oaks, Calif., July 1967.

Crinella, F. M. Identification of brain dysfunction syndromes in children through profile analysis: patterns associated with so-called "minimal brain dysfunction." *Journal of Abnormal Psychology*, 1973, **82**, 33–45.

Crinella, F. M., & Dreger, R. M. Tentative identification of brain dysfunction syndromes in children through profile analysis. *Journal of Consulting and Clinical Psychology*, 1972, **38**, 251–260.

Critchley, M. *The dyslexic child.* (2nd ed.) Springfield, Ill.: C. C Thomas, 1971.

Cruickshank, W. M. The education of the child with brain injury. In W. M. Cruickshank & G. O. Johnson (Eds.), *Education of exceptional children and youth.* (2nd ed.) Englewood Cliffs, N.J.: Prentice-Hall, 1967.

Czudner, G., & Rourke, B. P. Age differences in visual reaction time of "brain-damaged" and normal children under regular and irregular preparatory interval conditions. Paper presented at the annual meeting of the Midwestern Psychological Association, Detroit, May 1971.

Daryn, E. Problem children with "diffuse brain damage." *Archives of General Psychiatry*, 1960, 4, 299–306.

DeHaven, G. E., Bruce, J. D., & Bryan, D. B. *Remediation of coordination deficits in youth with minimal cerebral dysfunction.* (Final Report, Research Grant 15-P-55120/3-02) Devon, Pa.: Social and Rehabilitation Service and the Devereaux Foundation Institute for Research and Training, 1971.

DeHaven, G. E., & Mordock, J. B. Coordination exercises for children with minimal cerebral dysfunction. *Physical Therapy*, 1970, **50**, 337–343.

DeHaven, G. E., Mordock, J. B., & Loykovich, J. M. Evaluation of coordination deficits in children with minimal cerebral dysfunction. *Physical Therapy*, 1969, **49**, 153–157.

Delacato, C. H. *The treatment and prevention of reading problems: the neuro-psychological approach.* Springfield, Ill.: C. C Thomas, 1959.

Delacato, C. H. *The diagnosis and treatment of speech and reading problems.* Springfield, Ill.: C. C Thomas, 1963.

Delacto, C. H. *Neurological organization and reading.* Springfield, Ill.: C. C Thomas, 1966.

Denhoff, E., Hainsworth, P., Hainsworth, M. Learning disabilities and early childhood education: an information-processing approach. In H. R. Myklebust (Ed.), *Progress in learning disabilities.* Vol. 2. New York: Grune & Stratton, 1971.

Downing, J. *Evaluating the initial teaching alphabet.* London: Cassell, 1967.

Downing, J. The perception of linguistic structure in learning to read. *British Journal of Educational Psychology,* 1969, **39,** 267–271.

Downing, J., & Jones, B. Some problems of evaluating i.t.a.: a second experiment. *Educational Research,* 1967, **8,** 100–114.

Dykman, R. A., Walls, R. L., Suzuki, B. S., Ackerman, P. T., & Peters, J. E. Children with learning disabilities: conditioning, differentiation, and the effect of distraction. *American Journal of Orthopsychiatry,* 1970, **40,** 766–782.

Eisenberg, L. Behavioral manifestations of cerebral damage in childhood. In H. G. Birch (Ed.), *Brain damage in children.* Baltimore: Williams & Wilkins, 1964.

Eisenberg, L. Principles of drug therapy in child psychiatry with special reference to stimulant drugs. *American Journal of Orthopsychiatry,* 1971, **41,** 371–379.

Ellingson, C. *The shadow child.* Chicago: Topaz, 1967.

Fernald, G. *Remedial techniques in basic school subjects.* New York: McGraw-Hill, 1943.

Fish, B. The "one child, one drug" myth of stimulants in hyperkinesis: importance of diagnostic categories in evaluating treatment. *Archives of General Psychiatry,* 1971, **25,** 193–203.

Flavell, J. H., Beach, D. R., & Chinsky, J. M. Spontaneous verbal rehearsal in a memory task as a function of age. *Child Development,* 1966, **37,** 283–289.

Freer, F. Visual and auditory perceptual modality as related to success in first grade reading word recognition. Unpublished doctoral dissertation, Rutgers, The State University, 1971.

Freud, S. *On aphasia.* New York: International Universities Press, 1953.

Frostig, M., Lefever, D. W., & Whittlesey, J. A developmental test of visual perception. *Perceptual and Motor Skills,* 1961, **12,** 383–394.

Getman, G. N. The visuomotor complex in the acquisition of learning skills. In J. Hellmuth (Ed.), *Learning disorders.* Vol. 1. Seattle: Special Child Publications, 1965.

Getman, G. N. *The Pathway School program of eye-hand coordination exercises.* Boston: Teaching Resources, 1967.

Goldfarb, W. *Childhood schizophrenia.* Cambridge, Mass.: Harvard University Press, 1961.

Gordon, S. Sense and nonsense about brain injury and learning disabilities. *Academic Therapy,* 1970, **5,** 249–254.

Hagin, R. A., Silver, A. A., & Corwin, C. J. Clinical-diagnostic use of the WPPSI in predicting learning disabilities in grade one. *Journal of Special Education,* 1971, **5,** 221–232.

Hardy, M., Smythe, P. C., Stennett, R. G., & Wilson, H. R. Developmental patterns in elemental reading skills: phoneme-grapheme and grapheme-phoneme correspondences. *Journal of Educational Psychology,* 1972, **63,** 433–436.

Hardy, M. I. Clinical follow-up study of disabled readers. Unpublished doctoral dissertation, University of Toronto, 1968.

Hardy, M. P. The evaluation of communication skills. In D. L. Newcomb (Ed.), *Proceedings: 1967 international convocation on children and young adults with learning disabilities.* Pittsburgh: Home for Crippled Children, 1967.

Hayden, B. S., Copsen, S. I., McKinstry, R., Ansari, M., & Talmadge, M. Interim evaluation of the Astor classes for perceptually impaired children. Unpublished paper, Astor Home, Rhinebeck, N.Y., 1968.

Hewett, F. M. A hierarchy of educational tasks for children with learning disorders. *Exceptional Children,* 1964, **31,** 207–214.

Hill, S. D., McCullum, A. H., & Sceau, A. G. Relation of training in motor activity to development of right-left directionality in mentally retarded children: exploratory study. *Perceptual and Motor Skills,* 1967, **24,** 363–366.

Hinton, G. G., & Knights, R. M. Children with learning problems: academic history, academic prediction, and adjustment three years after assessment. *Exceptional Children,* 1971, **37,** 513–519.

Ingram, T., Mason, A., & Blackburn, I. A. A retrospective study of 82 children with reading disability. *Developmental Medicine and Child Neurology,* 1970, **12,** 271–281.

International Reading Association, *Reading disability and perception.* Newark, Del.: International Reading Association, 1969.

Jacobs, J. N., Wirthlin, L. D., & Miller, C. B. A follow-up evaluation of the Frostig visual-perceptual training program. *Educational Leadership, Research Supplement,* 1968, **26,** 169–175.

Jenkins, R. L. Dissimilar identical twins: results of brain injury at birth. *American Journal of Orthopsychiatry,* 1935, **5,** 39–42.

Johnson, D., & Myklebust, H. R. *Learning disabilities: educational principles and practices.* New York: Grune & Stratton, 1967.

Kenny, T. J., & Clemmens, R. L. Medical and psychological correlates in children with learning disabilities. *Journal of Pediatrics,* 1971, **78,** 273–277.

Keogh, B. Hyperactivity and learning disorders. *Exceptional Children,* 1971, **38,** 101–110.

Kephart, N. C. *Slow learner in the classroom.* (2nd ed.) Columbus, Ohio: Merrill, 1971.

Kinsbourne, M., & Warrington, E. Developmental factors in reading and writing backwardness. In J. Money (Ed.), *The disabled reader: education of the dyslexic child.* Baltimore: Johns Hopkins Press, 1966.

Knights, R. M., Hyman, J. A., & Atkinson, B. R. The effects of verbal and tactual pretraining on a formboard task. *Canadian Psychologist,* 1967, **7a,** 384–390.

Knights, R. M., Hyman, J. A., & Wozny, M. A. Psycho-motor abilities of familial, brain-injured and Mongoloid retarded children. *American Journal of Mental Deficiency,* 1966, **70,** 454–457.

Koppitz, E. M. *Children with learning disabilities: a five-year follow-up study.* New York: Grune & Stratton, 1971.

Koppitz, E. M. Special class pupils with learning disabilities: a five-year follow-up study. *Academic Therapy,* 1972–1973, **8,** 133–139.

Korner, A. F. Individual differences at birth: implications for early experience and later development. *American Journal of Orthopsychiatry,* 1971, **41,** 608–619.

Krippner, S., Silverman, R. Cavallo, M., & Healy, M. A study of "hyperkinetic" children receiving stimulant drugs. *Academic Therapy,* 1973, **8,** 261–269.

Lewis, J. The improvement of reading ability through a developmental program in visual perception. *Journal of Learning Disabilities,* 1968, **1,** 652–653.

Lipman, R. Statement and testimony. In *Federal involvement in the use of behavior modification drugs in grammar school children: hearing before a subcommittee of the Committee on Government Operations.* Washington, D.C.: U.S. Government Printing Office, 1970.

Luria, A. R. *Human brain and psychological processes.* New York: Harper & Row, 1966.

Makita, K. The rarity of reading disability in Japanese children. *American Journal of Orthopsychiatry,* 1968, **38,** 599–614.

Mallory, W. A. Abilities and developmental changes in elaboration strategies in paired-associate learning of young children. *Journal of Educational Psychology,* 1972, **63,** 202–217.

Marwit, S. J., & Stenner, A. J. Hyperkinesis: delineation of two patterns. *Exceptional Children,* 1972, **38,** 401–406.

McGrady, H. J. Language pathology and learning disabilities. In H. R. Myklebust (Ed.), *Progress in learning disabilities.* Vol. 1. New York: Grune & Stratton, 1968.

McGrady, H. J., Jr., & Olson, D. A. Visual and auditory learning processes in normal children and children with specific learning disabilities. *Exceptional Children,* 1970, **36,** 581–589.

MacKay, M. C., Beck, L., & Taylor, R. Methylphenidate for adolescents with minimal cerebral dysfunction. *New York State Journal of Medicine,* 1973, **73,** 550–554.

Mendelson, W., Johnson, N., & Stewart, M. A. Hyperactive children as teenagers: a follow-up study. *Journal of Nervous and Mental Disease,* 1971, **153,** 273–279.

Menkes, M. M., Rowe, J. S., & Menkes, J. H. A twenty-five year follow-up study on the hyperkinetic child with minimal brain dysfunction. *Pediatrics,* 1967, **39,** 393–399.

Milman, D. Organic behavior disorder. *Journal of Diseases in Children,* 1956, **91,** 521–528.

Money, J. Dyslexia: a postconference review. In J. Money (Ed.), *Reading disability: progress and research needs in dyslexia.* Baltimore: Johns Hopkins Press, 1962.

Mora, G., Talmadge, M., Bryant, F., Amanat, E., Brown, E. M., & Schiff, D. Implications of neurological findings for residential education. *American Journal of Orthopsychiatry,* 1968, **38,** 643–646.

Mordock, J. B., Effect of stress on perceptual-motor functioning of adolescents with learning difficulties. *Perceptual and Motor Skills,* 1969, **29,** 883–886.

Mordock, J. B. Behavioral problems of the child with minimal cerebral dysfunction. *Physical Therapy,* 1971, **51,** 398–404.

Mordock, J. B., & DeHaven, G. E. Interrelationships among indexes of neurological "soft signs" in children with minimal cerebral dysfunction. *Proceedings of the 76th Annual Convention of the American Psychological Association,* 1968, **3,** 471–472.

Mordock, J. B., & DeHaven, G. E. Movement skills of children with minimal cerebral dysfunction: the role of the physical therapist. *Rehabilitation Literature,* 1969, **30,** 2–8.

Morrison, J. R., & Stewart, M. A. A family study of the hyperactive child syndrome. *Biological Psychiatry,* 1971, **3,** 189–197.

Myklebust, H. R. *Development and disorders of written language: Picture Story Language Test.* New York: Grune & Stratton, 1965.

Myklebust, H. R. Learning disabilities: definition and overview. In H. R. Myklebust (Ed.), *Progress in learning disabilities*. Vol. 1. New York: Grune & Stratton, 1968.

Myklebust, H. R., & Boshes, B. *Minimal brain damage in children*. U.S. Public Health Service. Washington, D.C.: U.S. Government Printing Office, 1969.

Oliver, P. R., Nelson, J. M., & Downing, J. Differentiation of grapheme-phoneme units as a function of orthography. *Journal of Educational Psychology*, 1972, **63**, 487–492.

Orton, J. L. The Orton-Gillingham approach. In J. Money (Ed.), *The disabled reader: education of the dyslexic child*. Baltimore: Johns Hopkins Press, 1966.

Orton, S. T. *Reading, writing, and speech problems in children*. New York: Norton, 1937.

Owen, F. W., Adams, P. A., Forrest, T., Stolz, L. M. & Fisher, S. Learning disorders in children: sibling studies. *Monographs of the Society for Research in Child Development*, 1971, **36**(4, Whole No. 144).

Painter, G. The effect of a rhythmic and sensory motor activity program on perceptual motor spatial abilities of kindergarten children. *Exceptional Children*, 1966, **33**, 113–116.

Paivio, A. On the functional significance of imagery. *Psychological Bulletin*, 1970, **73**, 385–392.

Patterson, G. R. A tentative approach to classification of children's behavior problems. Unpublished doctoral dissertation, University of Minnesota, 1955.

Peters, M. L. The influence of certain reading methods in the spelling ability of junior school subjects. *Bulletin of Psychology and Sociology*, 1969, **19**, 62. (Abstract)

Pollack, M. Suspected early minimal brain damage and severe psychopathology, in adolescence. Paper presented at the annual meeting of the American Orthopsychiatric Association, Washington, D.C., April 1967.

Pope, L. Motor activity in brain-injured children. *American Journal of Orthopsychiatry*, 1970, **40**, 783–794.

Popp, H. The measurement and training of visual discrimination skills prior to reading instruction. *Journal of Experimental Education*, 1967, **35**, 15–26.

Preston, R. C., & Yarington, D. J. Status of fifty retarded readers eight years after reading clinic diagnosis. *Journal of Reading*, 1967, **11**, 112–129.

Pryzwansky, W. B. Effects of perceptual-motor training and manuscript writing on reading readiness skills in kindergarten. *Journal of Educational Psychology*, 1972, **63**, 110–115.

Quiros, J. de. Dysphasia and dyslexia in school children. *Folia Phoniatrica*, 1964, **16**, 201–222.

Rabinovitch, R. Reading and learning difficulties. In S. Arietti (Ed.), *American handbook of psychiatry*. Vol. 2. New York: Basic Books, 1959.

Rawson, M. B. *Developmental language disability: adult accomplishment of dyslexic boys*. Baltimore: Johns Hopkins Press, 1968.

Reed, J. C. The ability deficit of good and poor readers. *Journal of Learning Disabilities*, 1968, **1**, 44–49.

Reilly, D. H. Auditory-visual integration, sex, and reading achievement. *Journal of Educational Psychology*, 1971, **62**, 482–486.

Robinson, H. H. Visual and auditory modalities related to two methods for beginning reading. In H. Hausdorff (Ed.), *AERA Paper Abstracts*. Washington, D.C.: American Educational Research Association, 1968.

Robinson, H. M., & Smith, H. K. Reading clinic clients—ten years after. *Elementary School Journal*, 1962, **63**, 22–27.

Rogers, M. E., Lilenfeld, A. M., & Pasamanick, B. Prenatal and perinatal factors in the development of childhood behavior disorders. *Acta Psychiatrica Scandinavica*, 1955, 1(Suppl. No. 102), 1–157.

Rost, K. J., & Charles, D. C. Academic achievement of brain injured and hyperactive children in isolation. *Exceptional Children*, 1967, **34**, 125–126.

Rutter, M., Graham, P., & Yule, W. *A neuropsychiatric study in childhood.* London: Spastics International Medical Publications, Heinemann, 1970.

Sabatino, D. A. Identifying neurologically impaired children through a test of auditory perception. *Journal of Consulting and Clinical Psychology*, 1969, **33**, 184–188.

Satterfield, J. H., & Dawson, M. E. Electrodermal correlates of hyperactivity in children. *Psychophysiology*, 1971, **8**, 191–197.

Satz, P., Rardin, D., & Ross, J. An evaluation of a theory of specific developmental dyslexia. *Child Development*, 1971, **42**, 2009–2021.

Satz, P., & Sparrow, S. Specific developmental dyslexia: a theoretical reformulation. In D. J. Bakker & P. Satz (Eds.), *Specific reading disability: advances in theory and method.* Rotterdam: University of Rotterdam Press, 1970.

Savin, H. B. What the child knows about speech when he starts to learn to read. In J. F. Kavanagh & I. G. Mattingly (Eds.), *The relationship between speech and reading.* Cambridge, Mass.: MIT Press, 1972.

Schiff, D., Talmadge, M., & Mora, G. Modification of perceptual responses in minimal brain-damaged children through discrimination training. Paper presented at the annual convention of the American Orthopsychiatric Association, Chicago, 1968.

Schulman, J., Kasper, J., & Thorn, F. *Brain damage and behavior.* Springfield, Ill.: C. C Thomas, 1965.

Shankeweiler, D., & Liberman, I. Y. Misreading: a search for causes. In J. F. Kavanagh & I. G. Mattingly (Eds.), *The relationship between speech and reading.* Cambridge, Mass.: MIT Press, 1972.

Shores, R. E., & Haubrich, P. A. Effect of cubicles in educating emotionally disturbed children. *Exceptional Children*, 1969, **36**, 21–24.

Silver, A. A., & Hagin, R. A. Specific reading disability: follow-up studies. *American Journal of Orthopsychiatry*, 1964, **34**, 95–102.

Silver, A. A., & Hagin, R. A. Specific reading disability: an approach to diagnosis and treatment. *Journal of Special Education*, 1967a, **1**, 109–118.

Silver, A. A., & Hagin, R. A. Strategies of intervention in the spectrum of defects in specific reading disability. *Bulletin of the Orton Society*, 1967b, **17**, 39–46.

Silver, A. A., Hagin, R. A., & Hersh, M. A. Reading disability: teaching through stimulation of deficit perceptual areas. *American Journal of Orthopsychiatry*, 1967, **37**, 744–752.

Smith, R. C., Flick, G. L., Ferriss, G. S., & Sellmann, A. H. Prediction of developmental outcome at seven years from prenatal, perinatal, and postnatal events. *Child Development*, 1972, **43**, 495–507.

Smith, M. Patterns of intellectual abilities in educationally handicapped children. Unpublished doctoral dissertation, Claremont College, Calif., 1970.

Solomons, G. Drug therapy: initiation and follow-up. In F. F. De La Cruz, B. H. Fox, & R. H. Roberts (Eds.), *Minimal brain dysfunction, Annals of the New York Academy of Science*, 1973, **205**, 335–344.

Sroufe, L. A., & Stewart, M. A. Treating problem children with stimulant drugs. *New England Journal of Medicine*, 1973, **289**, 407–413.

Stevens, J. R., Sachdev, K., & Milsein, V. Behavior disorders of chilhood and the electroencephalogram. *Archives of Neurology*, 1968, **18**, 160–177.

Stewart, M. A. Comments made at a seminar sponsored by the Missouri State

Medical Association, Kansas City, Mo., May 1972. Cited in: Drugs for hyperactivity said to endanger child and family. *Medical Tribune*, 1972, **22**(13), 8.

Stewart, M. A., & Olds, S. *Raising a hyperactive child*. New York: Harper & Row, 1973.

Stover, L., & Guerney, B. G. A demonstration technique for interpreting perceptual-motor neurological difficulties to parents and teachers. *Journal of School Psychology*, 1968, **6**, 275–278.

Talmadge, M., Hayden, B. S., & Schiff, D. Longitudinal analysis of intellectual and educational achievement changes in culturally-deprived, emotionally disturbed boys. *Perceptual and Motor Skills*, 1969, **29**, 435–440.

Thomas, A., Chess, S., & Birch, H. G. *Temperament and behavior disorders in children*. New York: New York University Press, 1968.

Tinker, M. A. The study of eye movements in reading. *Psychological Bulletin*, 1946, **43**, 93–120.

Valett, R. A. A developmental task approach to early childhood education. *Journal of School Psychology*, 1967, **5**, 136–147.

Waldrop, M. F., & Halverson, C. F., Jr. Minor physical abnormalities and hyperactive behavior in young children. In J. Hellmuth (Ed.), *The exceptional infant*. Vol. 2. New York: Brunner-Mazel, 1971.

Waugh, R. P. Relationship between modality preference and performance. *Exceptional Children*, 1973, **39**, 465–469.

Weiss, G., Minde, K., Werry, J. S., Douglas, V., & Nemeth, E. Studies on the hyperactive child. VIII. Five year follow-up. *Archives of General Psychiatry*, 1971, **24**, 409–414.

Wender, P. H. *Minimal brain dysfunction in children*. New York: Wiley, 1971.

Wender, P. H. The minimal brain dysfunction syndrome in children. I. The syndrome and its relevance for psychiatry. II. A psychological and biochemical model for the syndrome. *Journal of Nervous and Mental Disease*, 1972, **155**, 55–69.

Wepman, J. M. Auditory discrimination, speech and reading. *Elementary School Journal*, 1960, **60**, 325–333.

Wepman, J. M. The interrelationship of hearing, speech and reading. *The Reading Teacher*, 1961, **14**, 245–247.

Wepman, J. Dyslexia: its relation to language acquisition and concept formation. In J. Money (Ed.), *Reading disability: progress and research needs in dyslexia*. Baltimore: Johns Hopkins Press, 1962.

Werry, J. S. Developmental hyperactivity. *Pediatric Clinics of North America*, 1968, **15**, 581–599.

Werry, J. S., Minde, K., Guzman, A., Weiss, G., Dogan, K., & Hoy, E. Studies on the hyperactive child: neurologic status compared with neurotic and normal children. *American Journal of Orthopsychiatry*, 1972, **42**, 441–450.

Wikler, A. W., Dixon, J. F., & Parker, J. B., Jr. Brain function in problem children and controls: psychometric, neurological, and electroencephalographic comparisons. *American Journal of Psychiatry*, 1970, **127**, 634–645.

Zangwill, O. L. Dyslexia in relation to cerebral dominance. In J. Money (Ed.), *Reading disability: progress and research needs in dyslexia*. Baltimore: Johns Hopkins Press, 1962.

9
Learning difficulties: economic and ethnic factors

Mr. Fish and his consultant had just finished evaluating the effects of supplementary instruction for economically disadvantaged elementary school children. Over the year, 40 children left their regular classes for a particular period each day and went to the learning center where they received individualized instruction. Mr. Fish and a teacher aide concentrated on developing reading readiness in the kindergarten children and on improving reading skill in the older children. On the average the 40 children were one and a half years behind grade level when they entered the program.

The results of the evaluation indicated that, as a whole, the older children gained about a year on standardized reading achievement tests after nine months in the program. Both Mr. Fish and the consultant felt that the year's gain indicated that the center's program was a success. Prior to their participation in his program the children had gained only three-quarters of a year for each year in school and would have been expected to show similar gains had they not participated. Mr. Fish evaluated the effectiveness of his program by subtracting each child's actual gain from his expected gain; the expected gain was calculated by dividing the child's achievement score just prior to participating in the center's program by the number of years he had been in school. For example, if the child's reading achievement was at a third grade level and he had completed six years of school, then his expected gain over the next year would be 0.5 years. If his actual gain was 0.9 years, then 0.4 years of gain could be attributed to the center's program. A better way to evaluate the center's effectiveness would have been to compare the group of children who participated in the center's activities with a similar group who had not. Unfortunately, the funding stipulated that all 40 disadvantaged children in the school should participate in the program. Surveys of schools throughout the country, however, indicate that, on the average, children from economically disadvantaged families achieve about 0.7 of a month for every month of instruction. This figure, as well as the difference between the group's expected and actual gain, indicated that Mr. Fish's learning center significantly increased the reading skills of children in attendance.

Not every child gained more than his expected gain. About 40 percent of the children showed gains less than or equal to their expected gain. The total gains made were greater than the total losses, so the group average did show a gain. However, looking only at the average gain obscures the fact that the center made a substantial impact on some children, but little or no impact on others.

The finding that close to 30 percent did worse than was expected indicates that this method of calculating expected gain may have limited usefulness in assessing treatment effects. Some children from disadvantaged environments may show decreasing gains each year, rather than a gain equal to the gains of each previous year. Many underachieving children reach a third grade level in reading by fifth grade but achieve little more during their remaining years in school.

The learning center operated by Mr. Fish was funded by a federal grant (Title I) made to the state for use in improving the academic functioning of children from economically disadvantaged families. School systems that have a substantial number of disadvantaged children enrolled are eligible to apply for Title I funds. Some schools use the money to establish summer programs, to hire extra teachers, or to set up learning centers similar to the one administered by Mr. Fish. All the programs are directed at helping children whose background has not equipped them to function adequately in school settings.

Most people are by now aware that poor children are less often exposed to intellectually stimulating materials at home, have less varied recreational outlets, are less knowledgeable about the world outside their immediate neighborhood, and frequently attend inferior schools. Yet, that is all many teachers know about the poor who attend their schools. Part of the learning center's program was to acquaint classroom teachers with the reasons for federal support of special programs and with the differing life styles of students. Each month a seminar devoted to a particular topic was held for teachers within the school system.

The most frequent question put to the center's director at this seminar was "Poverty has been with us for some time and our country has always prided itself on 'poor boy makes good'; why are we now so concerned with a special group labeled 'the economically disadvantaged'?" This question is usually asked by the teacher who has come from poor parents and who has worked hard to obtain his education. Underlying his question is usually an attitude that people are poor because they lack initiative. Opinion surveys reveal that the vast majority of Americans hold this attitude (Feagin, 1972). Mr. Fish devoted his fall seminar for new teachers to an overview of factors that led up to the establishment of his program.

This chapter will provide such an overview. We will discuss learning difficulties that may be attributed to ethnic and economic factors. We will learn that living in impoverished environments affects children differently and that the term environment needs to be more precisely defined in order to be useful. It is not simply being poor that handicaps a child, but rather his exposure to particular child rearing practices, patterns of family attitudes and emotions and societal reactions that occur in conjunction with, but are not exclusive to, poverty. As part of our discussion of the poor, we also will examine how learning is affected by racial or ethnic group differences.

We will describe some of the intervention programs designed to offset the negative effects of impoverished environments and attempt to determine their overall effect, why some children are helped and not others, and how the programs might be improved.

EFFECTS OF POVERTY ON GROUP SCORES ON INTELLIGENCE AND ABILITY TESTS

Certain generalities apply to all poor people, regardless of the place where they live or their ethnic or racial background. For example, they often score low on both intelligence and achievement tests. Nevertheless, studies of the scores of disadvantaged children have revealed some group patterns related to place of residence, race, and ethnic group.

The rural poor

Rural schools have their share of disadvantaged pupils. The school system in which Mr. Fish taught was located in a rural area and by looking at some of his test results, we can see what group characteristics are revealed for the rural poor.

The forty children enrolled in Mr. Fish's learning center were from families whose income was at or below the 1971 government poverty line of $4137. (In 1971 there were 25.6 million people who had an income below that level). While some of these children were achieving at grade level, the large majority were well below grade level. Testing revealed that certain generalizations could be made regarding group characteristics. The majority were deficient in perceptual-motor functioning, as indicated by a group average of one and one-half years' retardation on the Berry Test of Visual-Motor Integration (the child is required to copy a series of geometric designs). The scores of the group were similarly deficient on the Peabody Picture Vocabulary Test (the child is asked to select from four pictures the one that shows an object or action named). The majority of children could neither define words adequately nor communicate ideas efficiently. If asked to make up a story about a picture presented to them, many could do little more than name the objects in the picture; verbal elaboration skills were minimal. Mr. Fish felt that these deficiencies contributed significantly to the academic retardation of the children.

The Peabody Picture Vocabulary Test is considered a measure of verbal intelligence. The fact that the majority of children in the center had low Peabody scores suggests either that they were less bright than children from advantaged families or that Peabody scores are not valid measures of intelligence for children in this group. Several teachers in Mr. Fish's seminar had no problem accounting for these findings. They proposed that in an open society the brighter and more ambitious move up in social status while the less able retain their lower class membership. Assuming that intelligence is largely hereditary, the children of those who moved up the social ladder would be brighter than those left behind. Rather than accept this conclusion, Mr. Fish turned to the research literature to help him answer this question.

Numerous studies have found lower class children to have lower intelligence test scores than middle class children (Deutsch & Brown, 1964; Hunt, 1961; Jensen, 1968, 1969a; John, 1963; Lesser, Fifer, & Clark, 1965) regardless of the geographical regions in which they live, but even lower scores are found among rural children (Lehmann, 1959). In addition, the more isolated the community in which the rural child lives the lower his measured intelligence (Sherman & Kay, 1965). The intelligence test scores of rural children, however, can be increased by both training (Boger, 1952) and improvement of educational conditions (Wheeler, 1942). Movement from rural to urban areas also is accompanied by increases in measured IQ. Intellectual quotients increase with length of city residence, but level off after five or six years (Klineberg, 1935; Lee, 1951). Blacks who are born in urban areas generally score higher than do those who arrive from rural areas after elementary school age (Moriber, 1961). Similarly, Indians living on remote Indian reserves show lower IQs than those living closer to the white urban culture, although the latter are still lower than the whites. The low IQ of isolated Indian groups is attributed to an underdevelopment of reflective verbal thought rather than to a biologically determined inadequacy (Schubert & Cropley, 1972).

The urban poor

Children in urban areas appear to suffer from overstimulation rather than understimulation. While more is known about the effects of sensory deprivation than sensory flooding, recent investigations suggest that children exposed continuously to random noises (buses, cars, sirens, etc.) tend to tune out these noises. Some investigators have conjectured that this tuning-out continues after school entrance (Glass & Singer, 1972). Partially for this reason, educational programs designed for urban children attempt to bombard the listener in order to attract and maintain his attention (witness the approach of "Sesame Street"). Glass and Singer (1972) report that children exposed to unpredictable and uncontrollable noise show decreased tolerance for frustration, loss of learning efficiency, and deficits in auditory discrimination. They suggest that these deficiencies partially account for the verbal deficits and lowered reading achievement noted among urban children.

Ethnic differences

Confusion of racial, ethnic, and class differences   In studies of the disadvantaged child attempts are often made to trace the source of deficiencies to ethnic, racial, or class characteristics. However, if a particular ethnic group occupies a marginal economic position, it is difficult to separate ethnic from economic or class influences on the development of its members. Also, there is sometimes some confusion in distinguishing between racial and ethnic differences.

Racial differences are those due to biophysiological factors, while ethnic differences can be attributed to the customs, values, and manners of a particular subgroup of humanity. There is considerable doubt, however, whether any nonsuperficial differences exist among different racial groups or, for that matter, among different ethnic groups (Cole & Bruner, 1971).

When we study ethnic factors in the United States, perhaps Lévi-Strauss's (1963, p. 295) definition of culture would be an appropriate definition of an ethnic group: "What is called 'culture' is a fragment of humanity which from the point of view of the research at hand . . . presents significant discontinuities in relation to the rest of humanity." The terms race, ethnic group, and class often are loosely applied to different groups. For example, comparisons of lower class blacks to middle class whites may not be racial comparisons but social class comparisons. Since race and social class are confounded in such comparisons, the results often are difficult to interpret. Even when poor blacks are compared to poor whites, the blacks may be poorer or may differ on some dimension other than race. For example, there may be more children in the household, the father may be absent from the home, or the ratio of children to rooms may be different. Even if all these variables were equated in both blacks and whites, differences between the two groups may be learned differences (ethnic group differences) rather than biophysiological differences (racial differences).

Further, scientists frequently lump all members of a racial group together and call them an ethnic group. The fact that two individuals are black does not mean they come from similar cultural backgrounds. Blacks originally came to America from widely different subcultures within Africa. Consequently, as much difference may exist among blacks as between blacks and whites. Similarly, Gross (1967) demonstrated that different abilities existed in two groups of Jewish children raised in the same neighborhood in Brooklyn. Although children from both groups attended the same schools and the same synagogues, spoke English at home, and had native-born mothers, those whose origin was Ashkenazic (middle and northern European) scored higher on several ability measures than those whose origin was Sephardic (Mediterranean and mideastern descendents of former Spanish and Portuguese Jews). This difference was attributed to subcultural rather than genetic influences.

Even those Afro-Americans who did come from similar cultures in Africa had little chance to maintain an ethnic identity, cultural heritage, or native language, since slaves brought from the same region in Africa were deliberately kept apart and gatherings among them were forbidden to prevent the possibility of unified resistance. Patterson (1972, p. 59), after careful study of black history, concluded that "the black masses no longer form an ethnic group but a redundant lumpenproletariat." Nevertheless, he does feel that some common aspects of the diverse African backgrounds have survived in musical forms and religion.

Some investigators think there is a universal black English language that serves to handicap the child when he enters schools directed by Anglo-Americans. One investigator has even written a dictionary of black slang that, he implies, is universal to all blacks (Foster, 1971). Yet, northern urban blacks, unless they have relatives in the South, may not be able to understand the slang of southern blacks any better than northern whites and vice versa.

Had this chapter been written several generations ago, it would have included a discussion of the poor Italians, the poor Irish, the poor Greeks, and other ethnic groups that at that time were marginal (not yet fully integrated into the mainstream of American culture). At the present time, the blacks, Spanish-speaking people (Mexican-Americans and Puerto Ricans), and native Americans (Indians) are the most prominant marginal groups within the general subculture of the disadvantaged classes. The integration of these groups into the larger society and their opportunity to improve their standard of living has been limited by several factors. Racial and linguistic differences have made them the objects of more prejudice than earlier marginal groups. Also, the economic climate and reduced mobility within the larger society operate to keep all the disadvantaged classes impoverished. For example, the poor Chinese in Hawaii acquired wealth by banding together and buying property jointly, marrying into Hawaiian royalty, and sending selected members of their group to law school in order to ensure fair representation in financial dealings. Eventually, the Chinese moved out of the sugar fields and were replaced by the newly arriving Japanese. The Japanese saved their money and became small businessmen. Eventually, they left the sugar fields to be replaced by the Filipinos. By the time the Filipinos came to Hawaii, the cost of living was quite high, land was no longer available, there was no Hawaiian royalty to marry, and greater emphasis was placed on higher education in hiring practices. Consequently, it was, and still is, very difficult for them to rise above their current standard of living. To some extent, blacks, Mexican-Americans and Puerto Ricans are in the same position on the mainland United States as are the Filipinos in Hawaii.

Cultural backgrounds of racial and ethnic groups   It is important for educators to have some knowledge of the backgrounds of the various ethnic groups that are represented in their schools. Unfortunately, many of the statements about different ethnic groups are not documented by research. In some cases, a group's cultural heritage contains features that conflict with the dominant American culture, features that make adjustment or acculturation difficult. We will simply mention briefly one or two features in the complex ethnic backgrounds to illustrate this point.

The black   The black family has been described as an unstable matriarchy (Benard, 1966), because black women often find jobs more easily than black men and therefore are listed as heads of the household. For example, the proportion of black families in which husband and wife were living together was 68.1 percent in 1970. The number of black families that were headed by a female was 28.3 percent in 1970 (U.S. Census Bureau and Bureau of Labor Statistics, 1970). However, Mack (1971) reports that investigators have failed to recognize social class differences among blacks. Among disadvantaged families black women often appear to run the household, but among advantaged black families this is not the case. In addition, Diggs (1973) reports that even among disadvantaged blacks the black man runs his family whether he is home or away. Interviews with various family members of both disadvantaged blacks and whites suggest that both the black mother and father are viewed as powerful. In white families the father is viewed as more dominant in his conjugal role than in his child rearing role (TeHoute, 1970).

We do know that the cultural roots of blacks were partially destroyed when they were brought to the United States as slaves (Patterson, 1972). Family members were deliberately separated, and slave status resulted in loss of self-esteem and change in sex-role behavior. The extent to which these role differences have remained is subject to debate. We know that twice as many black girls as black boys reach college; the exact opposite is true for whites (Silberman, 1967). The extent to which this greater academic achievement by girls is due to the mother's influence in the home has been inadequately researched.

The Puerto Rican   Many of the Puerto Ricans who first came to the United States came from an agricultural background. In addition to burdens caused by shifts from rural to urban living and by language difficulty, confusion exists regarding their racial identity. Puerto Rican racial characteristics range from Caucasoid to Negroid. Although intermingling of those with different racial features is common, social structure in Puerto Rico is divided into three categories: black, intermediate, and white. Puerto Ricans in the intermediate group are said to resent the black-white dichotomy prevalent in the United States (Bonilla, 1966).

In Puerto Rico men spend considerable time away from their families. They engage in group activities with friends or in gatherings of their family of origin. As a consequence, women have chief responsibility for child rearing. This responsibility, however, is shared with other mothers in the neighborhood. Children are passed among mothers when necessary, and women gather together in mutual company for social activities as well as for communal childcare. In the United States the cold weather and urban living conditions often prevent such shared activity. Isolated from social contact, deficient in the English language, untaught in the dominant social mores, and burdened with the sole responsibility for child care, Puerto Rican women frequently become depressed and withdrawn. As a result, many Puerto Rican children receive inadequate mothering.

SKETCH BOOK ENTRY, DECEMBER 28, 1839: LAWS

Spent an hour or two in the course of the day in examining the laws of this state in reference to slaves and free people of colour. A more inconsistent, unchristian bloody code never disgraced the statutes of the worst of tyrants. No wonder that free negroes are but little, if any, better off than slaves. The very laws guaranteeing freedom are oppressive and unjust. Place any people under a similar economy and it will be miserable and wretched. There are no inducements, no encouragements, no nothing held out to the free negro. Ignorance like a dark curtain is drawn about his mind and his only stimulants are those which man possesses in common with the brute. Yet even these precautions to crush the intellect does not in every case destroy the upward tendency of mans restless spirit. Some few there are who are intelligent and virtuous. Who acquire property and some standing in life. I believe in spite of the phrenologist that the mind of the negro is capable of expansion and cultivation. Give him a sphere to act in, and I see no reason why he may not fill it. As it is the present condition of the free people of colour is no argument against emancipation. It is only an additional reason for it. They in a sense, themselves need emancipating. But before these things are set at rights I believe there are to be convulsions and heavings in the public mind as yet but little anticipated.

From J. D. Adams. *Ephraim Adams' sketch book.* San Francisco: J. D. Adams (Sorg printing), 1968. P. 38.

The Mexican-American The first Mexican-Americans who came to the United States are said to have come from an agrarian, patron-peon economy. Knowlton (1966) states that when these peons moved to the United States to find employment, they brought with them cultural values that stressed dislike for personal competition, a present rather than future orientation, and a lack of initiative in problem solving. Although Knowlton's book has no bibliography, several studies suggest that Mexican-Americans do become more competitive as they move from rural to urban settings (Madsen, 1967; Madsen & Shapira, 1970). In any case, writers often overgeneralize about differences in values between advantaged and disadvantaged populations. For example, studies indicate not only that many poor, regardless of race, firmly believe in upward mobility based on individual initiative, thrift, and education (Safa, 1970), but also that children who display these characteristics are more popular among poor children (Brozowich, 1970).

The Indian-American Traditional American Indian society fostered a belief in supernatural determination of one's fate. Accumulation of individual wealth was considered greedy; sharing and generosity were esteemed characteristics. Consequently, Indian society was largely socialistic, and individual entrepreneurship was a foreign concept (Spindler & Spindler, 1966). The extent to which these values are present in the American Indian today could influence his response to our current educational programs.

Ethnic group scores on ability tests Because many of the racial groups mentioned are overly represented in the lower socioeconomic classes, they also do poorly on both intellectual and achievement measures. Puerto Rican and Mexican-American children are believed to be further handicapped by their bilingual status, and blacks are handicapped by cultural values conflicting with the dominant Anglo-American Culture. Prominent among comparisons of racial-ethnic factors and intelligence is the voluminous literature on black-white differences. Much of this research was reviewed by Dregor and Miller (1960), Farnham-Diggory (1970), Kennedy (1969), Kennedy, Van De Riet, and White (1963), Kleinberg (1963), Lesser et al., (1965), Pettigrew (1964), and Shuey (1958). In general, the numerous studies revealed that, on the average, blacks score about 10 points lower than whites on IQ tests regardless of social class.

Validity of the tests Some investigators attribute the low racial-ethnic group scores on measures of intelligence to the improper construction and interpretation of intelligence tests. They claim that existing tests are actually measures of a child's exposure to Anglo culture. For example, Mercer (1972, pp. 95–96) states, "The more Angloized a non-anglo child is, the better he does on the I.Q. test. In short, when we controlled for social background there were no differences in intelligence between Anglos and blacks, or between Anglos and Chicanos." Similarly, Garcia (1972, pp. 43, 74) remarks, "When Chicano children score lower than Anglos on a test made of Anglo items there's no need for debate about hereditary and environmental factors. . . . An Anglo IQ measured on a black person exists more on the psychometrist's score record than it does on the mind or brain of the black." Other investigators attribute differences in intelligence when social class is controlled to poor motivation, examiner influences, or other unknown factors. Pettigrew (1964) summarized factors other than innate differences that could explain black-white intelligence test differences.

Nevertheless, intelligence tests measure considerably more than just exposure to Anglo culture. In fact, children from some ethnic groups actually score higher on tests originally developed for use with Anglo children. For example, studies in Hawaii revealed that Japanese-American children exceed the norms of American white children on tests of visual perception, spatial orientation, and sustained attention, but fall below norms on arithmetic and verbal tests (Darsie, 1926). Darsie attributed the verbal deficit to bilingualism, and the assets to Oriental stress on art and handicraft.

Sioux, Hopi, Zuni, Zia, Navaho, and Papago Indian children do as well as whites on performance tests of intelligence but less well on tests involving language. On a drawing test of intelligence, they may do better than white children, with boys excelling girls. These differences are attributed to the traditional masculine interest among Indians in graphic art (Dennis, 1942; Havighurst, Gunther, & Pratt, 1946). Klineberg (1927) found Yakima Indian children to differ qualitatively from white children. On the Pinter-Patterson Scale of Performance white children were quicker, but the Indian children made fewer errors.

Lesser, Fifer, and Clark summarize their study of ethnic group differences in intelligence as follows. On verbal ability, Jewish children rank first, blacks second, Chinese third, and Puerto Ricans fourth; on spatial reasoning, Chinese rank first, Jews second, blacks third, and Puerto Ricans fourth; on numerical reasoning, Jews rank first, Chinese second, Puerto Ricans third, and blacks fourth. Differences in social class produced significant differences between groups in the absolute level of each mental ability, but they did not affect the patterns just described. Stodolsky and Lesser (1967) have replicated some of these findings.

The poor performance of Mexican-American, Puerto Rican, and Oriental children on verbal measures of intelligence are often attributed to their having learned English as a second language rather than to racial or ethnic differences in ability (Anastasi & Cordova, 1953; Cline & Dryer, 1968).

For example, about 5 percent of American school children score below 75 on IQ tests and are considered retarded, whereas 13 percent of Mexican-American youngsters fall below 75. The percentage of Mexican-American children receiving low IQs is two and a half times the percentage of Mexican-Americans in the population. Mexican-American children are over represented at all IQ levels below 100 (average) and underrepresented at all IQ levels above 100. In fact, only 12 percent of Mexican-Americans receive IQ scores above 100. Consequently, Mexican-American children are overrepresented in the lower tracks of most school systems (Ortego, 1970).

Additional support for the notion that unfamiliarity with the English language contributes to lowered test scores comes from studies of factors that contribute to the high verbal intelligence test scores displayed by some Puerto Rican and Mexican-American children. For example, studies of Puerto Rican children raised in foster care indicate that there is a negative correlation between a child's verbal intelligence and the number of visits by his natural parents; the less they visited the higher the child's intelligence quotient (Fanshel, 1972).

Comparisons among Mexican-American children show that those with superior language development come from families that manifest an "Anglo middle class" attitudinal structure (Stedman & McKenzie, 1971). Similarly, the intelligence test scores of American Indian children increase markedly after one year of schooling (Cundick, 1970). Nevertheless, some ethnic groups who are considerably removed from western culture show higher performance IQs than particular ethnic groups in the United States. For example, Eskimo children are as adept on performance tests of intelligence as are white Americans (Berry, 1971), while blacks as a whole score from 8 to 10 points lower than either group on these same tests.

In general, this brief review demonstrates that intelligence tests do measure skills that are influenced by exposure to Anglo culture, but that they also measure skills that other cultures hold in common. If this were not the case, all groups other than Anglo-Americans would do poorly on all measures of intelligence developed in the United States. The review also demonstrates that, in general, children who live in relatively poor families receive lower scores on measures of intelligence. While those in rural regions of the country score lower than those in urban areas, the poor in large cities still score lower than the national average regardless of race.

Nature versus nurture in test results   In recent years there has been a renewed debate between those who hold that intelligence tests measure largely innate abilities and those who feel the abilities measured are heavily influenced by environmental factors. Those who regard the intelligence test as a measure of innate factors attribute differences between the races that occur when socioeconomic factors are controlled to hereditary rather than to environment (Jensen, 1969a, 1969b).

Willerman (1972), who takes a middle-of-the-road position, notes the correlation of intelligence test scores with low birth weight (the lower the birth weight, the lower the IQ) and cites evidence revealing that, while birth weight increases with increasing social class, black infants weigh less than whites at all social class levels. Although there may be genetic factors producing both a low birth weight and low IQ, Willerman refers to research that demonstrates that children conceived within three months after the birth of an older sibling have the lowest birth weights (Holley, Rosenbawn, & Churchill, 1969). Since lower class blacks often have larger families than other ethnic groups, low birth weight rather than genetic factors may produce the intellectual differences found in comparisons between lower class blacks and whites.

In addition to its effect on lowered birth weight, the close spacing of children acts as an environmental factor related to the finding that verbal reasoning ability decreases as family size increases (Kellaghan & Macnamara, 1972; Rosenberg & Sutton-Smith, 1969). Because parents have less time to spend with each child as successive children are born, younger children receive less language stimulation. Increased spacing between children is said to reduce this decrement.

High household density, a natural result of large family size combined with low income, may also contribute to lowered intellectual functioning. For example, verbal facility is lower in children who cope with anxiety by withdrawal from stressful situations. Since household density is correlated with both anxiety (Richards & McCandless, 1972) and absence from school (Greenberg & Davidson, 1972), perhaps the anxiety kept the child from attending school. The more favorable the room-to-person ratio, the lower the child's anxiety and the less frequent his absence from school.

Other environmental factors may account for intellectual differences between the races. For example, many studies that equate roughly for socioeconomic status ignore the tendency of black families to fall near the low end of a broad division by income. Frequently, black families within one broad income level may have an average annual income substantially below the average of white families in that level (Herzog, Newcomb, & Cisin, 1972). Deutsch (1960) found 65 percent of lower class blacks to have never traveled more than twenty-five blocks from home, 50' percent reported having no pen or pencil at home, and the majority had no books. Many of the children in these families had to fix their own meals and came to school improperly clothed and fed. In addition, negative self-image was related to being black.

SKETCH BOOK ENTRY, OCTOBER 30, 1839:
NEITHER FOOLS NOR ASSES

Whether people live in actual fear of their slaves I know not. But true it is they dare not give them the means of being acquainted with the true relations of man to man. To learn them to read is a criminal offence. But some of them do learn to read and that too in a manner which shows them neither fools nor asses. Knowing a man's name they learn some of their letters by his sign. In this way getting the alphabet they spell their way along to plain reading. Upon such occasions as fires and when negroes are assembled together the military is called out. They are not allowed to assemble even to worship their maker unless a white person be present. At eight o'clock in the evening the vesper bell rings after which no negro is permitted to be abroad without a written pass from his master. Then too are let out those terrible blood hounds, taught to be around back doors, as much feared by the negro as the hyena by the wandering traveller. If a negro is found after this time he is locked up in jail for the night. In the morning if he is free he must pay 75 cents or be flogged: if he is a slave his master can save him 25 stripes by paying $1.00. Such are some of the expedients tried to dehumanize humanity. O when will the day come?

From J. D. Adams. *Ephraim Adams' sketch book*. San Francisco: J. D. Adams (Sorg printing), 1968. P. 17.

Because we are still learning about the effects of environment on intelligence test scores, we cannot yet conclude that there are quantitative differences between the races on general intellectual ability. Regarding the contribution of hereditary and environment to intelligence test scores in all racial groups, Jencks and his colleagues (Jencks, Smith, Acland, Bane, Cohen, Gintis, Heyns, & Michelson, 1972) estimate that 45 percent of the variance in Stanford-Binet IQ scores in this country relates to genetic variation, about 35 percent to environmental variation, and about 20 percent to genetic-environmental covariance. Those who hold a hereditary viewpoint assign this last element to genes, but genotypically bright individuals are usually raised in enriched environments, and thus their IQ scores cannot be allocated exclusively to either hereditary or environmental influences.

Regardless of how intelligence is determined, less than half the variation among individuals on academic achievement measures can be accounted for by intelligence test scores (Anastasi, 1968). This figure is considerably less when intelligence is correlated with success in occupational endeavors, particularly in skilled and semiskilled occupations (Super & Crites, 1962). Consequently, the differences demonstrated between racial groups probably have little bearing on how well these individuals will do in school or in life. We saw in Chapters 2 and 3 that even intelligence test scores between 50 and 89 are poor predictors of eventual economic achievement. When investigators talk about differences in intelligence test scores between whites and blacks, they are often talking about relatively small differences.

THE PSYCHOLOGIST'S CREED: DOING UNTO OTHERS WHAT IS BEING DONE UNTO US

"O.K., Suzie, In what kind of store do we buy sugar?"

"A grocery store."

"Now tell me: How many pennies make a nickel?"

"Five."

"How many days in a week?"

"Seven."

"Now think, Suzie, Who discovered America?"

"No one discovered it. It was just there, and people lived there."

"Yeh, that's true in a way, dear, but what man first found it that we know about?"

"I don't know. The Indians were there a long time ago."

"Of course, but remember 1492 and all that?"

"Oh, you want to know who the first white man to come to America was. Why didn't you say so. Christopher Columbus."

"Well, yeh, o.k. It was Columbus that discovered America."

"He didn't discover it. It was there all the time. How can someone discover something that was already there?"

"Well, assured, but that's just the way we . . . uh . . . put things."

"How come all my subjects and books get 'put' that way?"

"I guess its because . . ."

"And how come you can tell how smart I am by stupid questions?"

"And how come . . .

"And how come . . .

"And how come . . .

Adapted from material distributed by Psychologists for Social Action.

SOME SPECIFIC DEFICIENCIES IN DISADVANTAGED CHILDREN

We have said that academic retardation is common among disadvantaged children. Since intelligence is only a partial predictor of academic performance, let us examine some of the other deficits displayed by the disadvantaged children in the center. We will then examine factors that contribute to the development of these deficiencies.

Perceptual deficits

Many disadvantaged children score below age level on tests of perceptual-motor integration. Perceptual ability is a skill necessary to assign meaning to various undefined sensory experiences. Studies of auditory, visual, tactile, and kinesthetic abilities are considered efforts to define more precisely the basic processes underlying intellectual and conceptual ability. Several investigators have postulated that lower class children have special perceptual problems that contribute to their intellectual deficiency.

Inadequate auditory and visual discrimination has been associated with the academic and reading retardation of disadvantaged children (Deutsch, 1964; Gill & Herdtner, 1968; Katz, 1967), and poor auditory discrimination has been associated with articulation deficits (Christine & Christine, 1964). In addition to discrimination deficits, Farnham-Diggory (1970) has revealed visual synthesis errors in blacks. Lower class children also need more time to process visually presented information. Bosco (1972) reported that middle class children enter the first grade with a mean processing speed equal to lower class children who are in the sixth grade. This finding supports the impression that the average classroom moves too fast for disadvantaged children.

Deutsch (1965) put forward the cumulative deficit hypothesis to explain the deficits of disadvantaged children. This hypothesis proposes that exposure to inadequate environmental stimulation results in increased deficit with advancing age. Inadequate exposure to basic learning skills makes more difficult the transition from one learning level to the next; instead of cumulative learning, lower class children experience cumulative deficit.

According to this theory, longitudinal comparisons between advantaged and disadvantaged children should show an increasing gap between the two groups with increasing age. Studies have supported this hypothesis regarding academic achievement, but they have failed to do so regarding basic abilities. For example, the differences in information processing noted earlier are less with advancing age, and differences in intelligence test scores remain about the same (Hertzig & Birch, 1971; Kennedy, 1969). Sometimes the gap is narrowed by educational efforts but quickly reaches an asymptote. For example, the differences in intelligence test scores between Indian and Anglo-American children often decrease during the first two years of school, but the differences achieved by second grade remain the same thereafter (Cundick, 1970).

A theory more in keeping with the data than the cumulative deficit hypothesis has been put forward by both Jensen (1966) and Staats (1971). Their position is that all learning occurs in a hierarchical and cumulative fashion. For example, a child who has developed a good attentional repertoire, has learned to follow directions, and so forth, can be given training in other skills sooner than a child who has not learned these basic behaviors. Staats (1971, pp. 288–289) remarks, "The general statement here is that acceleration or the acquisition of one repertoire accelerates the acquisition of the next. Because of this cumulative effect, vast differences in the level of behavioral skill of different children can be produced."

Staats goes on to say that the child who has not acquired his basic behavioral repertoires in good quantity and quality will have considerable difficulty acquiring additional conceptual and language behaviors. When such a child enters school, he will display a lower level of skill than others his age and will learn new skills more slowly and laboriously. As a consequence, he will receive less reinforcement for his behavior than will other children. Plotting the rate of this child's acquisition of new learning over time would show a decelerated learning curve.

Several studies suggest that the perceptual deficiences noted in disadvantaged children sometimes occur because the children are not familiar with items used to measure perceptual abilities. For example, after direct familiarization with the test item content of one perceptual discrimination test, lower class children improved in discrimination performance more than upper class children (Covington, 1967). This result cannot be extrapolated to other types of functioning, however, since intelligence test scores of lower class children do not increase significantly more than scores of middle class children when children are familiarized with testers, test language, materials used, and test taking situations (Golden & Birns, 1971; Kinnie & Sternlof, 1971).

Conceptual ability

According to the hierarchical concept of learning, we would predict that children lacking the basic skills of attention, perception, and discrimination would show conceptual deficiencies at later stages in development.

Conceptual ability refers to "skill in organizing and reducing ambiguity and imprecision of the environment impinging upon the senses" (Boger & Ambron, 1969, p. 24). The ability to use symbols and classifications is viewed as the initial step in learning. Conceptual ability is essential for those aspects of school learning requiring generalization ability, including reading. The term conceptual style refers to individual performances in mode of perceptual organization and conceptual categorization that are stable across situations (Kagan, Moss, & Sigel, 1963).

In almost every study of social class differences in conceptual ability, both in the United States and abroad, children from lower socioeconomic groups score lower than middle class children. Let us examine the types of conceptual skill assessed in some of these studies.

Piaget has postulated that children's conceptual development moves through a series of stages. During one stage, the child is not able to appreciate that the weight of an object does not change when the shape of the object is altered (conservation of weight), that the quantity of liquid does not change when the liquid is poured into a container of a different size (conservation of quantity), or that the number of beans in a pile does not change when the beans are spread out over a larger area (conservation of number). At this stage the child's decision is influenced by variations along one dimension—the height of the liquid in a container determines the quantity of the liquid. At a later stage the child demonstrates the attainment of conservation concepts and he can examine two dimensions at once—the height of the liquid and the shape of the container determines the quantity. Piagetians maintain that instruction and practice on problems involving conservation will benefit only the child who is developmentally ready to enter the more advanced stage. However, if a child lacks the opportunity to manipulate materials and observe relationships between them, his progress to the succeeding stages of conceptual development can be delayed. Instruction that provides such opportunity is therefore beneficial.

Economically disadvantaged children usually lag behind other children in development of conservation concepts; in some cases as much as two years (Almy, 1966; Wasik & Wasik, 1971). Nevertheless, investigators occasionally find no significant socioeconomic class differences in conservation (Keller, 1971). Evidently, some lower class environments compel the child to organize his thinking more than others. Regarding training, lower class children sometimes require more practice than middle class children in order to acquire conservation concepts (Figurelli & Keller, 1972).

If learning proceeds in a hierarchical and cumulative fashion, then children with attentional deficiencies would be expected to show retarded conceptual development, since attending to two dimensions at once is one prerequisite for conservation. Lower class children, both black and white, often demonstrate an impulsive rather than reflective conceptual style (Harrison & Nadelman, 1972; Kagan, 1966a). Impulsivity, in contrast to reflectivity, is associated with errors in reading and in inductive reasoning tasks (Kagan, 1965; Kagan, Pearson, & Welch, 1966) and may affect the ability to acquire conservation principles at the normal time.

Lower class children also show other conceptual deficiencies. For example, they often classify objects on the basis of concrete, functional relationships as opposed to abstracted physical attributes and classify actual objects better than pictures, implying that they acquire inadequate representation of familiar objects (Sigel, Anderson, & Shapiro, 1966).

As we have already intimated, many of the conceptual deficiencies reported were revealed by methods requiring sustained attention and persistence. Factor analysis of the Binet intelligence test suggests that for young children, 2 to 4 years of age, the most important factor may be general persistence on the part of the child. Above age 4 this factor is supplanted by a general factor called symbol manipulation, or thinking with words (Hofstaetter, 1954). Perhaps this shift takes place later for disadvantaged children, and, therefore, a lack of persistence might contribute to the conceptual deficiencies reported in this group. Data suggesting that lower class children develop conceptual organization and task oriented communication one or more years later than their middle class peers support this notion (Kaplan & Mandel, 1969).

Reissman (1964) suggested that lower class children have a better understanding of events and objects than they can communicate with words, and he emphasized that their expressive abilities emerge in spontaneous rather than in demand contexts. Others also believe that these children are less able to enunciate their thinking in communicative language (Deutsch, 1965; Kaplan & Mandel, 1969). Deficiencies in conceptual skills, therefore, could be attributed to factors other than cognition, factors such as lack of persistence, poor language skill, impulsivity, or lack of motivation. Hopefully, future researchers will take a closer look at children who display conceptual deficiencies in order to determine if they also lack the prerequisite behaviors necessary to solve conceptual problems.

Language skill

"Language skill is a socially conditioned set of communication variables such as phonetic structure, syntactic structure, and complexity. In addition, it should be recognized that there is both a covert and overt dimension to language and that perceptual and conceptual abilities as well as intelligence are reflected in language skill" (Boger & Ambron, 1969, p. 22). Before we examine language skills in disadvantaged white and black children, we will first discuss the children who have obvious language handicaps, the Mexican-Americans and the Puerto Ricans.

Spanish-speaking children   We have already mentioned that children from Spanish-speaking families receive lower scores on verbal measures of intelligence. This finding is true even when the tests are administered in Spanish (Lesser et al., 1965). This suggests that the norms of these tests are not suitable for use with Spanish-speaking children. Simply because a Spanish word is substituted for an English equivalent does not make the test appropriate. The Spanish equivalent of an English word may appear less frequently in Spanish language use than it does in English. Consequently, vocabulary words ranked according to their frequency of usage in English might be ranked differently in Spanish. (The difficulty of a word is a function of both the frequency of its use and the extent of its association with other words.) Nevertheless, the verbal IQ scores of Spanish-speaking children are valid predictors of their ability to function in English-speaking schools, just as are the verbal IQ scores of deaf children. As we have seen, the Spanish-speaking child who does well on verbal IQ measures often comes from a family with a more Anglo, middle class attitude structure (Stedman & McKenzie, 1971).

Spanish-speaking children are not simply deficient on the output side of communication skills, but also are deficient on the input side, especially in understanding sentences and pictures placed in sequence (Killian, 1971). They also show delayed ability to decode verbal instructions and encode them in nonlanguage behaviors, even when the instructions are given in Spanish. They are even more handicaped when instructions are given in English (Van Duyne & Gutierrez, 1972).

Children whose parents speak both English and Spanish in the home do no better on tests of verbal skill administered in English than do those whose parents speak only Spanish (Killian, 1971; Spence, Mishra, & Ghizeil, 1971). Those who are instructed in both English and Spanish in school, however, perform better on verbal measures of intelligence (Spence et al., 1971).

The language of black Americans Reviews of the literature conclude that lower class black children demonstrate considerable language deficit. They use fewer words, speak shorter, less complex sentences, and sometimes use a nonstandard form of English (Deutsche, 1964; Figurel, 1964; Milner, 1951; Thomas, 1962). Their vocabulary development also is significantly less than the middle class child's (Figurel, 1964).

It has been suggested that the low intelligence scores of lower class black children result from these verbal deficiencies. However, specifying what is meant by verbal ability is not an easy task. Verbal production and verbal comprehension are not identical abilities. While production usually cannot occur without comprehension, comprehension can occur without production (Chomsky, 1967; Lenneberg, 1962). The confusion between the two abilities has resulted in some false conclusions. For example, conceptual deficits have been attributed to language deficits. Ausubel (1964) believed that delay in the acquisition of certain formal language codes makes difficult conceptual development from concrete to abstract thought. Bereiter and Engelmann's (1966) work, perhaps the best-known language intervention program, was based on the belief that language deficits of lower class children must be identified and remediated because they hinder conceptual development. This belief has been particularly predominant among those working with disadvantaged black children. In Chapter 5 we emphasized that deaf children perform adequately on a variety of measures of conceptual development. Yet considerable emphasis has been placed on the language deficiencies of black children and how these deficiencies contribute to conceptual inadequacy (Blank & Solomon, 1968, 1969; Bereiter & Engelmann, 1966).

Some of this confusion regarding language and cognition comes from the misapplication of the work of Bernstein, a well-known British linguist. Bernstein (1960, 1961, 1962a, 1962b, 1964, 1968) identified two linguistic codes, restricted and elaborated. He uses the word *code* to refer to the principles that regulate the selection and organization of speech events. *Restricted* and *elaborated* refer to a dimension along which speech may be placed. This continuum is defined by the relative predictability of grammatical units and word choice, with the restricted code more predictable in both cases. Speech events classified as restricted are more dependent upon the ongoing social context to be interpretable and, therefore, are more stimulus-bound, situation-specific, and concrete (e.g., communication within the context of games or sports).

Some American educators have employed Bernstein's concepts to explain school failure. They assert that lower class children use restricted codes, based upon the observation that their language is simple, short, condensed, and nonspecific. They conjecture that the lower class child is isolated linguistically and perhaps conceptually from the cultural mainstream (Boger & Ambron, 1969). Consequently, these educators emphasize language remediation for the disadvantaged. However, Bernstein never meant his restricted code to be equated with linguistic deficiency, and this erroneous equation has contributed to a misunderstanding about black dialects.

Linguists emphasize that the language used by poor blacks is not a deficient language but a dialect with its own structure and systematic differences from standard English (Dillard, 1972; Stewart, 1970). For example, Dillard claims that black English is completely different from standard textbook English, having its own syntax and rules. He says that the slaves invented black English according to the basic syntax of West African languages. When the slave traders separated the blacks who spoke the same tribal tongue, the slaves borrowed the vocabulary of their masters and wedded it to the rules of their own tongues so they could communicate with one another.

Other linguists reject the notion that black English is a different language. They emphasize that the structural differences between dialects spoken in this country are relatively superficial; differences that do exist can best be represented by rule differences of a minor, transformational nature (Bailey, 1967; Baratz, 1968; Houston, 1970, 1973). This group of linguists regard the language of the black child as a totally developed, but in some ways different, system from the standard English spoken by the middle class population. Instead of considering the black language a different language or a *sub*standard American English, they consider it a *non*standard American English. They point out that black language follows a consistent and predictable set of rules, which are different from those governing standard English.

Houston (1973) states that the chief difference between the language of the black and white child is in pronunciation, or phonology. This difference is not enough to establish black English as a totally different language. Each form is a variant of the same language, and they are, in principle, mutually intelligible.

All linguists agree, however, that the failure to appreciate differences between blacks and middle class whites in language usage have contributed to misunderstandings about black children's conceptual skills.

Perhaps Labov has been the most vocal opponent of the concept of linguistic deprivation and its accompanying assumption of cognitive incapacity. Labov (1970) provides a series of examples where black children, who would be assessed as linguistically retarded by standard test procedures, engage in conversations in a perfectly adequate manner and display very clever arguments in the process. Labov's chief target is Carl Bereiter (Bereiter & Engelmann, 1966), whose language remediation program will be presented later. Part of his attack is aimed at misinterpretations of such phrases as "They mine." Bereiter refers to these phrases as a "series of badly connected words" (Labov, 1970, p. 171), while Labov analyzes them in terms of rules of contraction.

Labov demonstrates the inadequacies of traditional language assessment procedures by evaluating language use under two conditions. First, an interview that is similar to those employed in standard psychological assessments is conducted. Then, the interviewer goes to the same child's apartment, brings some of the boy's friends with him, lies down on the floor, produces some potato chips, and begins talking about taboo subjects in black dialect. The differences in language use between the two evaluations is often remarkable. Labov (1970, p. 163) asserts that the typical getto child is

bathed in verbal stimulation from morning to night. We see many speech events which depend upon the competitive exhibition of verbal skills—sounding, singing, toasts, rifting, louding—a whole range of activities in which the individual gains status through the use of language. . . . We see no connection between the verbal skill in the speech events characteristic of the street culture and success in the school room.

Other researchers also have suggested that observed language deficits among uneducated speakers are due to their being observed in situations where their language use is different. Disadvantaged black children seem to have two styles of language, one for use at school, in formal and constrained situations or in the presence of authority figures, and the other for use in other settings. The one used in school is simplified, rather limited, and unrevealing of their attitudes, ideas, or feelings; the one used with friends and family, and with which they express themselves with ease, is similar to the expected syntactic patterns characteristic of middle class children, but different phonologically (Houston, 1969a, 1969b).

LANGUAGE

Language is an example. Excluding the use of various common epithets applied to Negroes in America, their language and accent was all just more or less Southern, ranging all the way from the "reckoning" and "commencing" kind of talk to just "ah" instead of "I" or "er." They didn't care for the "s" of the third person singular, and accentuated this by rarely using auxiliaries, so that you heard, He a good man, He fight all the time, She trying to get me in trouble. Even when they were reading aloud from a text, nothing would convince them that that "s" at the end of a verb was in decency pronounceable. But many Americans, I think, are attracted to Southernisms; almost all popular singers use some variation of a Southern accent (witness even such old, inappropriate guys as Woody Herman) so that where there were many more common outrages against proper usage than those mentioned, it very soon began to cease to matter. My own ear soon heard it as normal and my own tongue came to utter it too in the end.

From James Herndon. *The way it supozed to be.* New York: Bantam, 1969. Pp. 55–56.

Why does the black child use one language in school and another at home? Labov (1970) feels that the usual situations in which language competence is assessed elicit deliberate defensive behavior from the child who believes that to talk openly is to invite criticism. Houston (1970) states it more simply—they are not reinforced for the use of their natural language in schoollike situations. Nevertheless, the black ghetto child may be unable to utilize language of a decentered type, language taken out of the context of social interaction and used in an abstract way to deal with hypothetical possibilities and to spell out hypothetical plans (Cole & Bruner, 1971). If this is true, then the ghetto child may become locked into the life of his own ethnic group because he uses a form of language unsuitable for eventual success in the power and prestige endowing pursuits of middle class culture. Consequently, he must be trained to use the language of middle class society.

In any case, disadvantaged black children can understand standard English (Eisenberg, Berlin, Dill, & Sheldon, 1968; Hall & Turner, 1971; Labov & Cohen, 1967; Peisach, 1965; Quay, 1972; Weener, 1969). In fact, their recall of messages spoken in English is sometimes superior to their recall of those spoken in black dialect (Weener, 1969). These results do not support the notion of some linguists (Baratz, 1969; Stewart, 1969) that the language and achievement deficits of black children result from using white linguistic patterns in assessment and instruction, patterns they say the black child cannot understand.

Actual language deficiencies among lower class children Lower class children are not as efficient as middle class children in communication requiring the exchange of descriptive information (Baldwin, McFarlane, & Garvey, 1971; Heider, Cazden, & Brown, 1968). They also are less able to find labels for many of the action concepts they possess (Jeruchemowicz, Costello, & Bagur, 1971). A study by Baldwin and his colleagues (Baldwin et al., 1971), contrary to earlier research, did not disclose social class differences in speech productivity. In their study children talked to one another rather than to adults, suggesting either that group differences in verbal productivity are situation-specific or that lower class speech is more inhibited in the presence of authority figures.

Noncognitive correlates of success

We have reviewed the perceptual, conceptual, and language deficiencies displayed by lower class children, but these deficiencies are probably less important than motivational factors, although the two cannot be easily separated. The child who quickly falls behind in school because he lacks the necessary prerequisite skills is unlikely to receive the reinforcement necessary to maintain his motivation to achieve in school.

Kagan (1966b) has identified three broad classes of needs he believes motivate children to learn in school: (1) the desire for nurturance, praise, and recognition, (2) the desire to increase perceived similarity to a model individual, and (3) the desire for competence and self-worth.

A number of studies suggest that disadvantaged children have a poor academic self-concept; they see themselves as lacking the ability to achieve (Anderson & Evans, 1969; Epps, 1969; Williams & Byars, 1968). Self-confidence is viewed as a system of self-evaluative verbal responses that serve both as rewards for learning and motivation for performing the behavior to be evaluated. The lack of self-confidence leads to active avoidance of those situations that are likely to lead to negative evaluation and to an increase in anxiety (Marston, 1968). Part of the self-concept involves perception of success as self-determined (Weiner & Kukla, 1970). Studies have suggested that disadvantaged children, particularly black children, attribute success to external factors, such as luck or task difficulty, while middle class children judge ability and effort as more important in performance (Buck, 1971; Crandall, Katkovsky, & Crandall, 1965; Friend & Neale, 1972; Messer, 1972). While these findings are by no means universal (Entwisle & Greenberger, 1972) and may apply to boys more than to girls (Clifford & Cleary, 1972), they suggest that living in impoverished environments leads to attitudes that can interfere with learning—the child believes that he is unable to control his own fate.

One can draw an anology here to findings from animal experiments. Recall from Chapter 7 the studies that demonstrated that prior exposure to an unavoidable shock interfered with the acquisition of an escape response to avoidable shock. While there is always danger in reasoning too closely from animal to human psychology, it would seem that when an individual's initial efforts meet with failure he is predisposed to make minimal efforts in future learning situations. Although this effect was short lived in the animal studies cited, perhaps prolonged early exposure to failure leads to a belief that one's fate is controlled by external factors. Contrary to popular conceptions of the disadvantaged child as carefree and without anxiety, lower class children report greater school anxiety with increasing age (Dunn, 1968), perhaps because they feel they can do nothing about their failure.

Motivation to achieve also is a function of incentives. Early research on incentives suggested that lower class children perform better with material incentives, such as candy, tokens, etc. (Terrel, Durkni, & Wiesley, 1959). More recent research, however, indicates that tangible reinforcers may be unnecessary, particularly with children exposed to Project Head Start (Quay, 1971). In fact, material rewards may interfere with the performance of both lower and middle class children (Spence, 1971). Evidently, the phenomenon of performance enhancement through the use of response-contingent material reward is either highly fragile or dependent upon variables yet to be identified.

Personality traits also play a major role in success or failure in school. When asked to select the prerequisites they considered the most important for school success, both teachers and parents picked social skills, goal directedness, and emotional stability rather than IQ or aptitude (Getzels & Jackson, 1961). In studies of the disadvantaged these variables have been overshadowed by research on intellectual variables. Although studies have examined the high prevalence of psychiatric disorder and antisocial behavior among members of lower class families, relatively few comparisons have been made between actual personality traits of lower and middle class children.

Environmental factors related to these deficiencies?

While we have seen that children from disadvantaged families compare unfavorably with others on variables relating to school achievement, we have not discussed the aspects of lower class environments that result in these differences. The most important influence is the impact of different home atmospheres.

Family atmosphere Bloom (1964) interpreted data from 1000 longitudinal studies in an attempt to identify and explain stability of intelli-

gence, personality, achievement, and other behaviors and to determine the
conditions under which behaviors could be modified. Among his findings
was the tremendous influence of the home environment in the early
years; the home has its greatest impact on a characteristic during its
most rapid period of growth. Factors cited that influence conceptual
and intellectual development are: (1) stimulation of verbal development,
(2) reward for verbal reasoning accomplishment, and (3) encouragement
of problem solving skill. In general, Bloom found that children with
higher intelligence test scores come from homes where: (1) parents hold
high expectations for the child, (2) the mother is knowledgeable about
her child's intellectual behavior, (3) opportunities are provided for
enlarging vocabulary, (4) parents create learning situations at home, and
(5) parents assist the child in learning situations, both in school and
nonschool activities.

Hess (1969), in a similar review, related family characteristics to school
achievement. Factors correlating with high achievement fell into three
categories: (1) an intellectual atmosphere characterized by demands for
high achievement, maximization of verbal interaction, engagement with
and attentiveness to the child, maternal teaching behavior, and diffuse
intellectual stimulation; (2) an affective relationship characterized by
warm feelings for the child and high regard for child and self; and (3)
interaction patterns characterized by pressures for independence and
self-reliance, clarity, and severity of disciplinary rules and the use of
conceptual rather than arbitrary regulatory strategies. Many of these
characteristics were absent among lower class families.

More specifically, Hess and his colleagues (Hess & Shipman, 1965;
Hess, Shipman, Brophy, & Bear, 1968) have related three strategies of
maternal control to the child's cognitive efficiency: (1) imperative or
status-normative (commands based on norms or appeal to authority:
"Don't do that because I say so!"); (2) subjective-personal (based on consideration of one's own inner states or those of others: "Don't do that
because you'll hurt mommy's feelings!"); and (3) cognitive-rational (based
on explanation of the future consequences of a given behavior: "If you
do that, the wheels won't turn!"). Mothers from working class backgrounds tend to use more status-normative statements in interaction with
their children. Other investigators also have reported that lower class
mothers, in both black and white homes, rarely use explanations when
disciplining their children (Bradshaw, 1968; Kamii & Radin, 1967).

Observations in the home reveal that children in low income homes
receive less verbal input, more commands to inhibit behavior, and less
input directed toward specific behavioral acts. Middle class mothers are
more likely to provide their child with an orientation to tasks, to request
verbal responses rather than simple physical compliance, to be specific
in their instructions, to use motivational techniques that involve implicit
or explicit reward, and to provide information needed to complete tasks

or to monitor performance (Schoggen & Schoggen, 1971). It should be noted that, in all the studies cited, characteristics attributed to one class were displayed by some mothers in the other class, indicating that one should proceed with caution when attempting to apply findings to individual families.

The mother's language style has far-reaching implications. Mothers who use an elaborate and abstract style of language tend to have children who are superior on verbal concept sorting tasks (Olim, 1970). In fact, the mother's language style is a better predictor of her child's cognitive performance than either the child's or the mother's intelligence test score or the family's socioeconomic class. However, these factors are related, in the sense that mothers in the lower socioeconomic class do tend to use a less elaborate style.

We said earlier that lower class children often see achievement as resulting more from external events than from individual initiative. While this attitude can be learned from parents who believe they have little control over their own life (Gordon, 1969), child rearing practices also contribute to the development of this attitude. Parents who maintain a supportive, positive relationship with their child and who encourage early independence are more likely to foster a child's belief in internal control than are parents who are punitive, rejecting, and critical (Katkovsky, Crandall, & Good, 1967). In addition, the larger the family in which the child lives and the lower his ordinal position, the less he believes he can control his environment (Crandall, Katkovsky, & Crandall, 1965). This is probably because parents have less time to spend with children as the size of their family increases.

Some investigators have suggested that class differences in the use of parental authority are consistent with a general picture of middle class mothers as more democratic and lower class mothers as more authoritarian. Lower class parents more frequently use "unqualified power assertions," such as direct threats, deprivations, and physical force, as disciplinary techniques (Hoffman, 1960). Mothers in slum areas emphasize to their child that he should relate well to the school's authority figures rather than that he should learn something, e.g., "Be a good boy and don't get in trouble" (Hess, 1969). Disadvantaged children, therefore, are said to react toward school authorities as they do toward other authority figures—with passive compliance or disobedience and with either violent or evasive resistance (Cloward & Ohlin, 1960). There is, however, no empirical support for this statement. Children who are disobedient and violent in school are so for much more complex reasons. Some of these will be reviewed later in a section on conduct disorders.

Authoritarian child rearing attitudes do not always have a negative effect on the development of early independence and the belief in internal control. Baumrind (1972) found that the most self-assertive and independent lower class black girls had the most authoritarian mothers. She suggests that authoritarian child rearing practices may not always be accompanied by the authoritarian personality syndrome (see Chapter 7) and that black authoritarian parents are one example. Authoritarian practices may have as their objective the development of toughness and self-sufficiency and may be perceived not as rejecting, but as nurturant care.

Father absence The proportion of fatherless families is very high among the poor. For example, the 1970 census revealed that 25 percent (600,000) of the children in New York City under 18 reside with one or with neither parent. This figure represented a 72 percent increase over the 1960 census when 17 percent was the figure (Community Council of Greater New York, 1973).

Although sweeping generalizations often are made about the effects of father absence on children, at least three independent reviews have concluded that there is no firm evidence to support the notion that father absence contributes directly to delinquency, poor school achievement, or confused sex identity (Herzog & Sudia, 1970; Kadushin, 1968; Kohlberg, 1966). Research concerning poor school achievement of father-absent children often is confounded by inadequate control for socioeconomic status and suffers from insufficient differentiation between temporary and continuing father absence and between honorific and stigmatized reasons for the absence.

A well-designed study by Santrock (1972) revealed that father absence due to divorce, desertion, or separation has a negative influence when it occurs in the first two years of a child's life. This absence results in lowered academic achievement in the elementary grades, particularly among boys. In contrast, father absence due to death during this same period does not adversely affect academic achievement. In addition, the mother's remarriage during the first five years of the child's life has a positive effect on the cognitive development of boys, but not of girls. Future research should focus on the mediating processes involved in father separation since Santrock's results provide only descriptive data.

Other characteristics of the lower class environment Many other features of the cultural or socioeconomic environment undoubtedly contribute to different behavioral patterns among children. Direct study of these variables, however, is just beginning. Some of the variables characteristic of lower class environments are the vulnerability to disaster, the lack of prestige, and the limited availability of alternatives to action (Hess, 1969). Lower class life also is characterized by more work-related friendships and kinship contacts, mistrust of the unfamiliar, and rejection of intellectuality (Hess, 1969).

Aware of his lack of power, exploitation, low self-esteem, and limited opportunity, the lower class adult is said to feel deep rage as well as mistrust (Grier & Gobbs, 1968). In time, these feelings must affect the growing child's attitudes and disposition. For example, Aldous (1969) reported that lower class females of preschool age view males as less powerful and less competent than middle class youngsters. Thus, at an early age, lower class females see males as less apt to play the male role customarily assigned.

The school environment Just as there are myths about the disadvantaged, there are myths about the reactions of middle class professionals toward disadvantaged children. *Psychology Today,* a popular magazine that presents the scientific evidence bearing on social problems, recently published an article (Watson, 1972) that suggested that differential expectations for black disadvantaged children result in a self-fulfilling prophecy of lower achievement. The article stated that when black children are tested by white testers they achieve lower intelligence test scores than when they are tested by black testers. A review of the literature found no solid evidence to corroborate this report. One study did note that black children obtained significantly higher IQs when tested by black testers, but so did white students. The black testers gave significantly higher scores to all children regardless of race (Solkoff, 1972). Other studies suggest that children receive higher scores when they are evaluated by testers who use an optimizing rather than standarized testing technique and who establish a warm and concerned testing environment (Thomas, Hertzig, Dryman, & Fernandez, 1971; Zigler & Butterfield, 1968); the tester's race is less important. Since both middle and lower class children usually benefit equally from optimizing approaches (Golden & Birns, 1971; Kinnie & Sternlof, 1971), we cannot assume that the personality of the tester will decrease the gap between disadvantaged and advantaged children.

Similarly, a disadvantaged child's academic performance in the classroom may be influenced more by variations in the personality characteristics of the teachers than by their race (Yando, Zigler, & Gates, 1971).

Ethnic traits that may act as deficiencies

Some coping strategies of different ethnic groups, although unrelated to measured intelligence, may interfere with adequate achievement as defined by the dominant culture. For example, Hertzig and her colleagues (Hertzig, Birch, Thomas, & Mendec, 1968, p. 46) speculate that Puerto Ricans tend to encourage social interaction rather than task completion.

It may be that the Puerto Rican children come from a person-oriented culture and that they lack sufficient opportunity for the exercise of independence in advance of task mastery, which would permit the development of successful problem solving behavior under conventional educational conditions. The style of culture may be one in which verbalizations are heavily weighted to communicate affective and social contents rather than task-directed ones, with the result that the ability to engage in verbal behavior in response to cognitive demands fails to develop in the same way that it does in middle class children.

Some ethnic groups value cooperation more than competition and may therefore send the child to school unprepared for our competitively oriented school system. For example, several Indian and Polynesian cultures emphasize cooperation over competition (Miller & Thomas, 1972; Sloggett, 1968). A group of Hawaiian students who were potential dropouts from school were found to work harder for group rewards than for individual rewards (Rubano, 1972). Other studies have suggested that some marginal student groups show helping and friendship behaviors among their members, while achieving groups show deviant helping behavior, that is, helping only when it aids them in achieving good grades (Tricott, Kelly, & Todd, 1971). Madsen's research (Madsen, 1967; Madsen & Shapira, 1970) demonstrated that cooperative behavior decreases among Mexican-Americans as they integrate into Anglo-American culture.

The lower class southern black child, unlike both his middle class black peers and his white peers from both social classes, reacts differently to instructions to repeat a story to other children. Rather than trying to reproduce the story's details, the poor black child takes the original story as a base line from which to demonstrate his imagination and creativity by creating a somewhat different, original story. In addition, he interacts with his partners more often than the children in the other social class groupings and attends more to his partners than to the adults present. He also prompts his partners nearly twice as often as the others and makes greater use of nonverbal behavior and whole body gestures when doing so (Houston, 1973).

Torrance (1972), basing his conclusions on some formal research, but largely on informal observations of poor black children, listed 18 characteristics he calls "the creative positives of disadvantaged children": (1) ability to express feelings, (2) ability to improvise with everyday materials, (3) articulateness in storytelling and sociodramatic play, (4) enjoyment of and ability in the visual arts, (5) enjoyment of and ability in creative dance, (6) enjoyment of and ability in music, (7) expressive speech, (8) fluency and flexibility in nonverbal media, (9) enjoyment of and skill in group activities, (10) responsiveness to the concrete, (11) responsiveness to the kinesthetic, (12) expressiveness of gestures, (13) humor, (14) richness of imagery in informal language, (15) originality of ideas in problem solving, (16) problem centeredness, (17) emotional responsiveness, and (18) quickness of warm-up. Some of these are traits that Patterson (1972) feels have survived in black peoples from their African ethnic background. Labov's and Houston's research on black English, cited earlier (Labov, 1970; Houston, 1969a, 1969b, 1970), supports Torrance's observations. In addition, creativity dimensions studied in middle class children often appear with equal salience in lower class subjects (see Chapter 10).

These 18 characteristics do not necessarily correlate positively with academic achievement, and they might even interfere with adequate functioning in school settings where children are expected to work independently, memorize facts, and pay close attention to the teacher. It has also been found that many of these traits exist in greater degrees in gifted children. Follow-up studies of children identified as gifted sometimes reveal that many do not work up to their potential, particularly when curricula are not geared to their abilities (Meeker, 1968). These findings also may be true of some disadvantaged children.

Investigators sometimes interpret their findings as revealing deficits rather than differences and therefore minimize the value of their data. For example, in a study of associative style blacks give a high percentage of unique associations to descriptive adjectives and a low percentage to concrete and abstract nouns (Wilcox, 1971). Because whites respond in the opposite manner, blacks are said to have a developmental lag in language development. However, the differences may reflect the black's richness of imagery in informal language rather than a language deficiency.

EDUCATIONAL EFFORTS TO HELP THE DISADVANTAGED

The disadvantaged child enters school lacking the skills necessary to cope with the school curriculum. The two main approaches to this problem are busing to racially integrated schools and enrichment programs designed to offset the effects of poverty.

Busing

One method to upgrade the education of the city poor is to transport children from one school to another in order to make schools more heterogeneous with respect to socioeconomic background. This approach resulted from court rulings, but was supported by the research of some social scientists. For example, the Coleman report (Coleman, 1966) emphasized that a child's success in school depended more on the characteristics of his schoolmates than on any other factor. The 1967 report of the U.S. Commission on Civil Rights emphasized that disadvantaged children with the most academic gains had attended classes in which the majority of pupils came from white middle class families. The report concluded that: "Changes in the social class or racial composition of schools would have a greater effect on student achievement and attitude than changes in quality" (U.S. Commission on Civil Rights, 1967).

Achievement may improve not only because other class members serve as models and reinforcers of good performance but also because of the child's dependence upon and desire to belong to a group (Bronfenbrenner, 1969).

Bronfenbrenner cautioned, however, that modeling is a two-way phenomenon. Both Wilson (1959) and Pettigrew (1967) noted the poorer performance of middle class children enrolled in lower class schools. Pettigrew reported that white children in predominately lower class black schools who had close black friends scored significantly lower in verbal achievement than other white pupils in the same school. Another related phenomenon is the increased willingness of an entire class to engage in antisocial behavior in the presence of a small lower class minority (Bronfenbrenner, 1969).

In spite of these cautions, middle class children have maintained their former level of achievement in those schools to which lower class black children are transported in order to achieve interracial balance (Pettigrew, Useem, Normand, & Smith, 1973). In addition, black children show statistically significant academic gains in these desegregated settings. Pettigrew concluded that these results justify continued use of busing to desegregate schools. On the other hand, Armor (1972) concluded from his review of the same research that black achievement has not been helped in any significant way by busing. He found that, while some positive results have been demonstrated by forced integration, black students are often forced to compete for grades with children who are sometimes three years ahead of them in academic growth. While they may narrow the gap between themselves and middle class white students by two months, he asks if this gain is worth the possible harmful effects that the black child might experience when he still finds himself far behind his white, advantaged peers. Armor's review also suggests that race relations worsen as a result of induced school integration. In any case, busing has become increasingly unpopular; Gallup polls have revealed that nearly 75 percent of those polled were against busing.

Early enrichment

Many studies have been made to determine at what stage in the child's development ethnic group or class differences emerge and what type of intervention program would decrease the resulting deficiencies.

In nearly all the studies presented, academic or behavioral deficiencies attributed to ethnic group or social class membership appeared before school entrance. Some studies have reported that social class differences do not appear until about the third year of life. At this age a shift from sensorimotor to symbolic conceptual levels occurs. All children below age 3, regardless of social class, seem to have equal opportunity for gross motor development. In fact, studies suggest that lower class children sometimes display accelerated motor development (Ponthieux & Barker, 1965; Wallach & Martin, 1970; Williams & Scott, 1953). Disadvantaged children, however, have less opportunity to develop fine motor skills (Lillie, 1968). We have seen how they also have restricted opportunity for language and conceptual growth, growth which needs a particular parental role to develop and flourish.

Other investigators have observed social class differences as early as 1 year of age and have attributed these differences to child rearing patterns (Caldwell, 1970; Kagan, 1966a; Wachs, Uzgiris, & Hunt, 1967). Regardless of when class differences appear, initial school difficulty and progressive retardation are displayed by a considerable number of disadvantaged children.

With the passing of the Elementary and Secondary School Act of 1965 and the establishment of the Office of Economic Opportunity, American educators proceeded rapidly to establish preschool education programs designed to offset these deficiencies. Private foundations, most notably the Ford Foundation, helped develop programs for deprived children dwelling in urban areas. Almost overnight, Head Start and day care centers sprang up across the country. Unfortunately, under pressures to get started, little thought was given to the special needs of disadvantaged children. As a result, most programs patterned themselves after the traditional nursery schools operating in their area. The programs differed greatly in length, timing, objectives, and type of treatment. Very few programs included in their conception the means to evaluate the effects of intervention procedures or to follow up their children after the program's completion. The Westinghouse Learning Corporation (1969) independently investigated the effects of Head Start by gathering information on children who had completed Head Start programs (Cicirelli, Evans, & Schiller, 1970; Smith & Bissel, 1970). The Westinghouse survey revealed that Head Start had no predictable long-term effect on achievement or personal adequacy. Although the gap between lower and middle class children decreased after the Head Start program, many lower class children returned to their former standing as time passed.

While many educators became disillusioned by these results, others had expected them. If you put a highly trained swimmer in a race with a poorly trained one and give the trained one a head start, no amount of additional training will enable the second one to catch up. (The middle class child has the head start; the term Head Start means head start on school not on other children.) The first swimmer will continue to increase his lead while the second is being trained. Add to the second swimmer's handicap by making him race in an adjoining pool filled with dirt and obstacles and unless he's stupid or has been sold a bill of goods, he'll pull out of the race all together. He might not do so immediately, particularly if his coach keeps prodding him with incentives or forbids his looking at the adjoining pool, but eventually he'll see the futility of his efforts and, coach or no, he'll climb out.

Five specific programs for black children   A few of the many and varied programs that were initiated did make an effort to clearly state objectives and to assess the outcome of participation in the program. They asserted they were training the unskilled swimmer in a manner different from the skilled, enabling him to catch up quickly. Several of these programs had begun before 1965. One of the first, initiated in 1959, was the Early Training Project for Disadvantaged Children at George Peabody College for Teachers in Nashville (Gray & Klaus, 1970). The goal of the program was to develop aptitudes and attitudes that correlated with academic achievement, as well as to foster socialization for competence by development of cognitive skills necessary for environmental mastery. More specifically, the curriculum was based on an information processing model. Three types of skills were emphasized—sensory skills, abstracting and mediating skills, and response skills. Sequences of specific behavioral expectations were developed by further subdivision of each of the three general areas. Lesson plans and activities are described in detail in Gray, Klaus, Miller, and Forrester (1966). The differences between the program and a more traditional nursery school environment were given as: (1) the use of toys for learning, (2) the high ratio of adults to children, and (3) the amount of time devoted to the use of different kinds of materials and equipment.

Probably the best known intervention program was conceived by Bereiter and Engelmann (1966), a program that primarily stressed language development. Prescribed drills, teacher behavior, and classroom management procedures were laid out in sequence. Emphasis was placed on preparing the child for the regular classroom, rather than accommodating the school to the child. Students "chanted" replies to the teacher as part of the language mastery program. The child was made to use articles, prepositions, conjunctions, and short verbs and to use *not* in sentences. For example, "This is a ball" instead of "Dis' ball" or "He is sitting on the chair" instead of "He sittin' chair." Tables 9.1 and 9.2 outline the format and content of this program.

A third program, developed by Karnes (1969), was called the ameliorative curriculum because it was defined as an approach that "improves or makes better." The format and content of the program is also outlined in Tables 9.1 and 9.2.

A fourth major language intervention program was developed by Weikart (1967). This program, originally called the Perry Preschool Project, was initiated in 1962 and longitudinal data was gathered for each succeeding year. Several different curricula were employed over the years, including those based on Bereiter and Piaget. In addition, weekly home visits were made to encourage parent participation in the child's

Table 9.1   IMPLEMENTATION OF TWO ACADEMIC PRESCHOOLS

	Ameliorative curriculum (Karnes)	Bereiter-Engelmann program
Instructional format	Daily schedule centered around 3 20 min. structured learning periods in each content area (math, science, social studies) Music period and directed play period; children form own peer groupings Structured game format	20 min. structured learning periods in each content area Teacher-directed instruction, clearly specified, fast moving alternating statement, question, and response pattern Seatwork activity, music, art, and less structured activity
Grouping	15 children in each class divided into 3 subgroups on basis of Binet IQ 1 teacher to each subgroup (1 to 5 teacher-pupil ratio) Instruction in small cubicles off main room Each cubicle equipped for one content area	15 children in each class divided by ability into 3 groups for work in 3 subject areas 3 teachers per class (1 to 5 ratio)
Sequencing of content	Concrete to abstract Hierarchical order (previous knowledge used to learn new knowledge) Guide lines provided by ITPA and Guilford's Structure of the Intellect model Individual diagnostic testing and prescription	Sequenced so that each skill forms base for later tasks Regular testing to insure that each child in group is ready to move on to more complex material

education. During the first three years children experienced an instructional method that Weikart described as "verbal bombardment." The teacher attempted to draw the child's attention to important stimuli through a constant series of questions and comments. Weikart thought this method would make the child more aware of various uses of language. In later years Weikart shifted the emphasis from language to cognition; he developed one program emphasizing training in concept formation and a second based on Piaget (see Table 9.3).

A fifth program was developed by Blank and Solomon (1968). The curriculum was based on the assumption that language deficiencies were related primarily to a lack of a symbol system for thinking. Specifically, the curriculum included: (1) training in selective attention, (2) learning categories of exclusion, (3) developing imagery of future events, (4) developing relevant inner verbalization, (5) separating words from referent models for cause-effect reasoning, (6) developing the ability to categorize, (7) developing an awareness of language, and (8) sus-

Table 9.2 CONTENT OF TWO ACADEMIC PRESCHOOLS

	Ameliorative curriculum (Karnes)	Engelmann-Becker program (based on Bereiter-Engelmann program)

Reading	(Within language program) Primarily readiness activities (e.g., holding book, turning pages, associating pictures with stories, left-to-right progression, associating printed symbol with meaning)	Phase I
		  letters as sounds
		  sequencing
		  blending and unblending
		  sound sliding
		  reading sounds and words
		Phase II
		  alphabet
		  reading instructions and more difficult stories
		  vocabulary
		  comprehension

Mathematics	Sets
	Numerals
	  basic number concepts
	  counting as a functional concept
	  numbers as visual symbols
	Geometry
	  identification of 5 geometric shapes
	Measurement
	  matching quantity
	  addition and subtraction with objects (sticks, peg boards)
		Phase I
		  counting operations
		  symbol identification
		  equality and equal sign
		  addition and subtraction
		
		Phase II
		  counting by 2s and 5s
		  algebra addition and subtraction
		  multiplication
		  negative numbers
		  fractions
		  fact derivation
		  area

Science	Useful vocabulary Classification skills Sensory discrimination Observation (One unit on "time")	Measurement Telling time Direction Solar system Geological time
Other	Language (includes reading readiness) Social science Music Directed play Body awareness Unit on family members	Language Social science (principles that influence man's behavior) Art Music

taining sequential thinking. The instructional format consisted of daily 15-minute periods of individual instruction for each child in addition to regular group work.

Evaluation of the programs   Karnes (1969) evaluated five preschool programs arranged on a theoretical continuum from nondirective to direc-

Table 9.3   CONTENT AREAS OF PRESCHOOL CURRICULA BASED ON PIAGET'S THEORY

Classification	Uniting, disuniting, reuniting Grouping things that are identical/similar Inventing one's own criteria and using them consistently Shifting the criteria to group and regroup objects in different ways Thinking independently rather than judging the correctness of the conclusion
Seriation	Ordering objects on the basis of size, quantity, or quality Arranging a series of graduated cups, dolls, etc. from biggest to smallest or vice versa by perceptual configuration
Number	Arranging, disarranging, and rearranging Establishing numerical equivalence by one-to-one correspondence Foster conservation
Spatial Reasoning	Development of child's structuring of space from topological space to geometric space Development of static space into more dynamic transformations Reconstruction of sensorimotor space on representational level
Temporal Reasoning	Structuring time into sequence, but not intervals Developing sense of speed (slow or fast) Dealing with time in terms of periods having a beginning and an end Learning that events can be chronologically ordered and time periods can have variable lengths

Other	Physical knowledge
	Representation
	  Index
	    part of object
	    marks causally related to object
	  Symbol
	    imitation
	    make-believe
	    onomatopoeia
	    three-dimensional mode
	    pictures
	  Sign
	    words and other signs

tive. Programs considered directive were the Bereiter program and the ameliorative program. The nondirective end of the continuum was represented by two traditional programs: one given to disadvantaged youngsters as a group and the other a community integrated program in which from two to four lower class children were enrolled in each of several classes in a traditional middle class nursery school. In the middle of the continuum was a Montessori program. In general, children in the two directive programs demonstrated the most gains at the end of the preschool year. During the second year the two nondirective groups, the Montessori group, and the ameliorative group went to regular kindergarten, while the Bereiter group continued class sessions. The ameliorative group also attended a one hour per day supportive program. At the end of the second year the Bereiter group was superior to the others. However, after first grade there were no significant differences among the groups. Considering, the low teacher-pupil ratio in the Bereiter group (1 to 5) the entire effort hardly seems worth it (Hall & Mery, 1970).

Weikart (1969) compared the results of three highly structured experimental curricula. All three experimental groups differed on achievement test scores from a traditional preschool group, but none differed from each other. This finding is consistent with other reports suggesting that the amount of teacher direction and the degree of structure in an intervention program are crucial variables.

There also is some evidence that the highly programmed, skill-focused preschool may be sacrificing later learning potential for immediate outcome (Miller et al., 1971; Weikart, 1971). Miller's findings indicate that when children taught by the Bereiter-Engelmann method entered regular classrooms, they performed at the lowest level of any group studied.

Follow-up of children in the Early Training Project (Gray & Klaus, 1970) revealed that three years after all intervention had ceased (intensive work for three summers, followed by weekly home visits) the experimental group remained superior to control children on intelligence tests. This trend was maintained on measures of achievement and language, but differences were no longer significant by the end of fourth grade. Unfortunately, specific aspects of the program, such as home visits, were not evaluated separately, making impossible statements about the value of the program's separate facets.

Evaluation of Blank and Solomon's (1968) tutorial methods revealed that experimental groups were significantly superior to controls, but adequate follow-up data were not provided.

Although these five programs were relatively successful, their replication in a standard public school setting may not be possible. The standard school usually does not have enough highly trained and supervised teachers to provide highly individualized instruction, a research staff, special equipment, and a commitment to a particular philosophical or theoretical approach. Perhaps a more important question is whether these programs should be replicated. It has been found that a little intervention is not significantly beneficial; programs must be "total push" programs, taking place throughout the day over a four- or five-year period (Karnes, 1969). Also as we have noted, there is a question as to whether the immediate gains derived from such highly programmed approaches are outweighed by diminished potential for later learning.

Weikart (1971, p. 9) concluded that "as far as various preschool curricula are concerned, children profit intellectually and socio-emotionally from any curriculum that is based on a wide range of experiences."

Considering only those programs reporting positive results, how do the theoretical notions on which they were based fit the data reviewed earlier? The Bereiter and the Blank and Solomon programs assumed that language deficiencies were primarily responsible for the poor academic functioning of disadvantaged children. Research by both Labov and Houston suggests that language use is deficient only in school situations. Labov asserts that the disadvantaged child should learn to use standard English, but that it should be taught in a "quasi-foreign language situation." In addition, teachers should be familiarized with the various forms of nonstandard English.

Houston advocates that augmentation of language of the disadvantaged, if it is necessary, should be done through conversation; classification of colored blocks and objects is merely an exercise and not a learning activity. Citing Joos (1964, p. 207), she emphasizes that most disadvantaged children see school as unrelated to any real situations encountered elsewhere; students follow school commands only because they are supposed to, never knowing there is a geography of their hometown or a rhetoric of persuasion within their circle of friends.

PILGRIMS

One day we were looking at a picturebook of the Pilgrims. José understood that they had crossed the Atlantic, but something in the way he said it made me doubt his understanding. I asked him where the Atlantic was. I thought he might point out the window, since it lay not very far away. But his face took on an abject look, and he asked me weakly, "Where?" I asked him if he had ever gone swimming at Coney Island. He said, "Sure, man!" I told him that he had been swimming in the Atlantic, the same ocean the Pilgrims had crossed. His face lit up with pleasure and he threw back his head and laughed. There was a note of release in his laughter. It was clear that he had gained something more than information. He had discovered something. He and the Atlantic belonged to the same world! The Pilgrims were a fact of life.

From G. Dennison. *The lives of children: the story of the First Street School.* New York: Vintage, 1969. Pp. 171–172.

The Early Training Project (Gray & Klaus, 1970) emphasized language production rather than comprehension. The data we have reviewed suggest that language production is situation-specific and that disadvantaged children understand more than they can or will convey. There also was no evidence that lower class children cannot use language to attain self-defined goals or that their behavior is not under verbal control.

Hall and Mery (1970, p. 36) remark, "Anyone who has taught for long periods of time knows that there is wide variation in attending behavior within and between classes. When there are only one or two teachers involved in the intervention being evaluated, it may well be that the teacher's ability to elicit attending behavior is more important than the treatment itself." Perhaps a 1:5 teacher-pupil ratio also enables better control of attention. Weikart's (1969) finding that there were no differences between three differently structured curricula supports this assumption.

Working through parents These follow-up studies suggest that gains associated with carefully planned and well-executed preschool and early elementary school programs cannot be maintained unless subsequent educational endeavors are equally well planned and executed. In addition, although efforts can be directed at improving education at all levels, Lucco (1972) suggests that a child will be at a cognitive disadvantage when individuals in his home environment function at a lower level of conceptualization than is required of him in school. Consequently, several programs have attempted to help disadvantaged parents take an active role in the cognitive development of their child. These programs have met with varying degrees of success.

The toy demonstrators Perhaps the most interesting project is the Mother-Child Home Program developed by the Family Service Association of Nassau County, New York, in 1965 (Levenstein, Kochman, & Roth, 1973). The program consists of regular home visits by interviewers, called toy demonstrators. These visits begin when the child is 2 and continue on a semiweekly basis until the child is 4. The main activity of the home sessions is a structured, yet fun-oriented "curriculum" of verbalized play with the child, designed to foster his verbal and conceptual development. The goal of the toy demonstrator is to involve the mother in each play session with the child and thereby transfer the main responsibility for promoting verbal interaction from himself to the mother. The interviewers are called toy demonstrators to deemphasize the didactic aspects of their interaction with mothers, since direct teaching of the mother often is perceived as demeaning (Hess, 1969).

Children who participate in the Mother-Child Program demonstrate an average IQ gain of about 17 points after two years in the program. Initial gains in IQ, however, are less important than the possibility that parents who participate in this program come to view themselves as "educators" of their children. In a similar program, Radin (1972) reported that parental involvement in a preschool program appeared to have no affect on the child's intellectual performance if IQ changes were examined immediately following the preschool experience. However, if tested one year later, children of participating parents had higher IQs than those whose parents did not participate.

Programs for older children Although parental training programs at preschool levels are undoubtedly important, it is unlikely that their effects will be long lived unless further programs are provided. It is unreasonable to expect that parents given specific training in verbal interaction skills can provide the proper stimulation needed for their child's academic success at all educational levels. It is one thing to converse with a child and another to support him in endeavors well beyond the ability of the parent. Consequently, programs need to be developed at all educational levels.

One interesting notion is the community school. In this view the school is the center of community activity and the institution most able to bring together a community's resources. The community is viewed as the "school" and the school as the "community"; planning for the one includes planning for the other. One example is the community school developed in Flint, Michigan. The entire community educational program for Flint was placed under one budget. The school program, therefore, included adult education, job training, sports, remedial programs for underachievers, industrial arts, etc., and facilities were open both day and night. Perhaps this kind of program will draw school and community closer together and result in more meaningful learning activities.

Special programs also have been initiated for older children within traditional school systems. One such program, funded as a demonstration project in 1956, was called New York's Higher Horizons Program (Havighurst, 1961). An inner city junior high school received special funds to develop a program designed to increase the achievement of the students identified as the most gifted. Trips were made to various cultural centers, remedial and enrichment services were provided, and individual counseling was included when requested. Teachers were given lighter instructional loads to allow time for in-service education designed to upgrade both their skill and salary. Students responded to this effort with better school achievement. Although some critics attributed the changes to increased attention or morale rather than to the specific procedures, the program was received favorably and expanded to include 65 slum schools. Detroit's Great Cities Improvement Project achieved similar ends (Marburger, 1961). Similarly, predominantly middle class schools have developed special programs for the "alienated" junior high school student (Hayden, Talmadge, Mordock, & Kulla, 1970).

Programs for Spanish-Americans Often the Mexican-American or Puerto Rican child comes to school speaking Spanish. In addition, his proficiency in Spanish often is limited. Nedler and Sebera (1971) have demonstrated that a sequenced curriculum beginning with a low order of language skill and proceeding to high level skills is more effective than a traditional day care preschool program. Concepts are first presented in Spanish; when these concepts are mastered, they are introduced in English, an approach in keeping with the knowledge that Spanish-speaking children do better when instructed in both Spanish and English. This program has been successfully replicated in a number of settings (Randall, 1972).

General recommendations for intervention

Hall and Mery (1970) suggest that teachers learn the relevant differences between dialects and not expect children to modify their dialect substantially when the only time such modification is needed is during school hours. They stress the following order of priorities: (1) ability to understand the spoken English of the teacher, (2) ability to read and comprehend, (3) ability to communicate (to the teacher) in spoken English, (4) ability to communicate in writing, (5) ability to write in standard English grammar, (6) ability to spell correctly, (7) ability to use standard English grammar in speech, and (8) ability to speak with a prestige pattern of pronunciation. Note that speech production comes after comprehension and that pattern of pronunciation is last on the list. Implementation of the above list would require a long-term effort rather than a "one-shot" program.

More direct involvement of parents is also recommended in order to integrate the school with the larger community. Parental training should be attempted on a wider scale, since several programs in addition to the toy demonstrators have reported promising results (Karnes, Tesha, Hodgins, & Badger, 1970). However, if only immediate academic proficiency is considered, direct tutoring in the home is sometimes more effective than training mothers to tutor their children (Barbrack, 1970).

The learning center directed by Mr. Fish was an attempt to provide extra help for disadvantaged children throughout their school experience. In addition to the help given to the children, attempts were made to involve parents in the center's program in a manner that would facilitate their positive interaction with their children. The primary thrust of the center's program was directed at the development of prereading skills and the improvement of reading. Verbal elaboration training and vocabulary development were featured. A sequential lesson plan was developed for each student and the parent was asked to participate in particular phases of the plan. Efforts were made to improve the child's self-esteem, using procedures modified from those found successful elsewhere (Barcai, Umbarger, Pierce, & Chamberlain, 1973; Flowers & Marston, 1972).

Nevertheless, nearly 40 percent of the children made no substantial progress during the first two years of the center's program. The children included those whose parents never visited the center and those whose families experienced considerable disruption while the children were enrolled. Still others were found to have minimal brain dysfunction, a syndrome that appears more frequently among lower class populations (Amante, Margules, Hartman, Storey, & Weeber, 1970), probably because conditions such as prematurity, complications of pregnancy and delivery, neonatal distress, poor prenatal care, and malnutrition associated with MBD also occur more frequently among this population (Hertzig et al., 1968; Pearson, 1970).

The center staff planned to initiate a formal study to try to determine the differences between children who were helped by the program and those who were not. Several studies indicate that children who gain the most from programs for the disadvantaged are those who make more realistic demands for help from teachers, who cope more effectively with failure to receive help by working independently, and who are more autonomous in learning under conditions of intrinsic reinforcement (Bellar, 1969; Jacobson & Greeson, 1972). Children who display these behaviors are probably those whose parents support and encourage achievement behavior even though the parents may have not lived up to their own ambitions.

CONDUCT DISORDERS

Many of the children enrolled in special intervention programs will drop out of school and some may become problems for their community. Although children with severe behavior problems appear in all social classes, a disproportionate number come from the lower socioeconomic classes, particularily from families on welfare (Langner, Greene, Herson, Jameson, Goff, Rostkowski, & Zykorie, 1969). Unlike the neurotic child (described in Chapter 7), the unsocialized, aggressive, and disruptive child, often labeled predelinquent if he is pre-teen or delinquent if in his teens, comes into major conflict with society, rather than with himself or with his family. Since the delinquent is overrepresented in lower class families, we have chosen to present him in this chapter.

GRACE

Grace was born in Metropolitan Hospital. Little was known about her early life other than that she lived with her mother in Manhattan until she was 4 years of age. Her mother was the only female of five children born to a minister and his wife. The mother's father died while a patient in a county mental hospital. Grace's mother left her family and came to New York where she became pregnant with Grace. For a time, mother and child were supported by the father; later they received public assistance. The welfare center demanded a psychiatric evaluation, stating that the mother was secretive and belligerent. The evaluation did reveal marked hostility and suspiciousness, but hospitalization was not recommended. Later, without provocation, the mother attacked a neighbor with a meat cleaver. She received a suspended sentence and was committed to a state hospital.

Grace, then 4 years old, was placed in a temporary shelter. After the mother's release from the hospital, she visited Grace regularly but either beat her or ignored her. The visits upset Grace so much that regular contact was discouraged.

When Grace was 5, she was referred to the Children's Aid Society for foster home placement. The mother was strongly against this plan and became extremely hostile. She developed the delusion that she had gotten sick because Grace was not with her. Nevertheless, Grace was placed, and with time her mother became less negativistic.

When Grace was 8, her mother was readmitted to the state hospital, where she delivered a second child who was immediately placed for adoption. Grace was unaware of this half-sibling since communication with her mother ended before the birth of the child. The mother was believed to be back in the state hospital.

The foster home in which Grace was placed was a lower middle class family with upward mobile strivings. The foster father was a quiet, passive man who did not communicate readily. The foster mother was more verbal and firmer with Grace. Grace made heavy demands on her time. The foster mother recounted that Grace compulsively sought candy, jumped and hopped constantly, spoke rapidly and moved in a jerky, uncoordinated manner. She also destroyed toys and clothing. Her relationship with her foster sibling broke down as Grace's demands increased.

In school Grace was in the most advanced second grade and she kept up easily in academic achievement. Nevertheless, her behavior was so erratic that the school suspended her. For eight months after suspension Grace was treated by chemotherapy, but none of the various medications administered produced any change. Grace was referred to a residential treatment center when her relationship with her foster family deteriorated (we will discuss Grace's treatment later.)

Types of delinquents

Grace displayed behaviors that her community could not tolerate; she responded with aggressive and disruptive behavior to tensions and conflict in her environment. Grace was considered a high risk to become a delinquent when she got older. According to the Federal Bureau of Investigation's Annual Uniform Crime Reports for 1967 more than two million arrests were made of persons under 21 years of age. Those arrested who are under 18 are considered juvenile delinquents.

The term juvenile delinquency often conveys disparate meanings. Some professionals see delinquency as aggressive acting out in response to frustration; others consider it the result of conflict between the individual's internalized values and the values of the larger society. Because the term is so broadly used, it has no precision as a behavioral concept.

Delinquency is actually a legal category. A girl, for example, may be declared delinquent by a court for sexual promiscuity, truancy, running away, serious physical aggression, or theft. She usually is brought to court by her mother or the police or referred by the school or a social agency. Following the adjudication of delinquency, she may be placed on probation or sent either to an institution for delinquents or to a mental hospital. A girl committing delinquent acts is more likely to be brought to court and institutionalized if she is from the lower socioeconomic classes (Kovar, 1968). More than half of those girls who run away, are incorrigible, or commit sexual offenses are adjudged delinquent. Sexual promiscuity is not an offense for boys, and similar behavior usually is tolerated from girls of more socially favored families.

Approximately 350 institutions in the United States are set aside for children declared delinquent by the courts. Most are state or county operated agencies (Mac Iver, 1967). In 1965 the 220 state operated juvenile facilities had a total daily population of 42,389, and the cost to operate these facilities was $144,596,618. Of the 220 state facilities, 56 were exclusively for girls and 13 were coed. The ratio of institutionalized boys to girls will probably change since arrests are increasing at a faster rate for girls than for boys.

Within these institutions are children with diverse backgrounds and different personality characteristics, yet the term delinquent is applied to them all. Without some form of differential diagnosis, study of these children is less precise.

Recently, investigators have developed personality and behavioral classification systems for delinquency in an effort to reduce its heterogeneity. Quay (1965) has delineated four types: (1) the psychopathic, (2) the anxious and conflicted neurotic, (3) the deviant value oriented, but not maladjusted subcultural, and (4) the inadequate immatures.

Psychopathic delinquents exhibit antisocial behavior that is usually unaccompanied by anxiety. They are insensitive and callous toward others, using people only to satisfy their own needs. The psychopath's lack of social responsiveness and opposition to compliance with societal laws appear as a long-standing deficit, possibly resulting from a history of poor socialization, which may include a lack of parental reinforcement for dependency, approval seeking, and other prosocial behaviors (McCord & McCord, 1964). Patterson (1969) proposed that this type of delinquent is raised by parents who rarely use positive reinforcements. Failing to gain positive reinforcements from parents, the child resorts to more extreme forms of behavior to receive reinforcement. Eventually, he finds peers who reward him for such behavior. This acceptance makes him less responsive to other adults who may be potentially reinforcing.

Neurotic delinquents act out impulsively, but anxiety, guilt, and depression usually accompany their antisocial behavior. They are more socialized and more likely to form dependent, affectional relationships with others.

Subcultural or gang delinquents behave antisocially as a result of their acceptance of the deviant values of peer groups who pride themselves on social defiance, aggression, and bravado. Subcultural delinquents are somewhat socialized, but because of a history of parental neglect and indifference are more responsive to their peer group.

The immature delinquent is one who gets into difficulty because of poor judgment and impulsivity. He is usually not acceptable to his peers because of his immature behaviors and may engage in antisocial behavior in order to gain their acceptance. Some minimally brain injured children may fall into this category.

Common factors in the development of the delinquent personality

Disturbed family relationships   When Quay formulated his categories, he cited evidence suggesting that psychopathic delinquents were generally unresponsive to social rewards, in contrast to neurotic and subcultural delinquents who were highly susceptible to social rewards. A recent review of the literature (Hedlund, 1971) presents contrary evidence that sometimes the psychopath is more responsive to social reinforcement than the neurotic delinquent. Research does support other components of the different personality pictures and has identified some common factors in their development. For example, extreme neglect and punitiveness combined with deviant-aggressive behavior characterize the parents of the psychopathic delinquent. In contrast, the neurotic or subcultural delinquent more often comes from a family characterized by young parents, large size, neglect, frequent parental absence, and delegation of parental responsibility (Jenkins, 1968; Koller, 1971; Mc-Cord, McCord & Howard, 1963).

Common to three of Quay's subtypes is a background of disturbed family relationships and a negative self-concept fostered primarily by nonnurturant parents. In addition, marked early affectional or maternal deprivation, overstimulation in sexual and aggressive spheres, promiscuity and bodily exposure by parents, violent abuse of the child or the child's mother by the father, inconsistent discipline or irrational limits, and indifference alternating with unpredictable, irrational, and violent punishment are common features in the backgrounds of many delinquents (Scharfman & Clark, 1967). The outstanding feature of the delinquent's life history is "abandonment" by the family, either physical or emotional.

Poor self-concept   As a result of parental rejection, the child comes to reject himself. He also rejects those he feels have rejected him (Deitz, 1969; Gold & Mann, 1972). Unable to tolerate this derogated self-image, the child engages in acts designed to refurbish this image, and, in the process, anesthetizes himself from the anxiety generated by the realization that he feels unworthy (Gold & Mann, 1972). Boys are likely to engage in daring acts they consider highly masculine. Girls may enhance their self-image by engaging in behaviors they consider more feminine (sexual acting out) or more exciting. Many delinquent girls become involved sexually in order to be accepted or to feel needed, either by their sexual partner or by the unborn child, who they feel will give them undemanding love. Sexual activity itself often is aversive to them (Niklason, 1967–1968). Many take a great deal of abuse in heterosexual relationships because they prefer abuse to loneliness (Konopka, 1966). Even those who prefer homosexual relationships do so usually because they either consider themselves ugly and undesirable, feel sex is disgusting, see males as brutal and threatening, or seek neurotic revenge against boyfriends who have jilted them. Girls most likely to form homosexual attachments in institutional settings are those who have little contact with their family (Lamberti, 1963).

Inadequate self-control   Also common to the different delinquent subtypes is inadequate development of self-control. Self-control may be defined as the inhibition of socially prohibited behavior in the absence of explicit or threatened external punishment. This definition implies resistance to temptation or deviation, the curbing of culturally disapproved urges, and the application of moral judgments and standards of right and wrong. Self-control also includes postponement of culturally approved, immediate reinforcements in favor of some potentially more rewarding long-term goal. The capacity to delay gratification can explain a person's "responsibility" to an endeavor and his persistence in the face of its dull aspects.

Another aspect of self-control is the self-administration and self-regulation of rewards and punishments. Children learn to evaluate their own performance and frequently set standards that determine, in part, the conditions under which they administer or withhold numerous readily available self-gratifications and self-punishments. Failure to meet widely varying self-imposed performance standards often results in self-denial or even harsher self-punishments, whereas attainment of difficult criteria more typically leads to liberal self-reward and a variety of self-congratulatory responses.

Basically, self-control involves not only self-restraint, but self-criticism. It may be associated with concepts such as conscience or morality, the individual's internalization of cultural rules of social action. Rules are internalized if they are conformed to in the absence of external, situational incentives or sanctions.

Current research findings, though far from consistent, suggest that children who experience relatively early socialization pressures tend to exhibit greater self-control than children who are leniently or inconsistently trained (Aronfreed, 1964, 1968, 1969; Bandura & Walters, 1959). Assuming that socialization efforts reflect the extent to which parents reward conformity and punish noncompliance, these findings provide evidence that patterns of parental reinforcement are important determinants of the habit strength of self-control responses in children.

The differential effects of reward and punishment are extremely complex and depend on timing, intensity, nature, status of the punishing agent, and learning history of the individual. In addition, the type of self-control training that is most effective may vary with the sex and age of the child. At an early age, the effects of certain disciplinary practices may have different effects on boys than on girls. Punishment and reward may be most effective, while at a later stage in the development of moral judgment the use of reasoning and self-punitive responses may assume greater importance because of the maturation of the child's language and cognitive functioning.

Because the learning of self-control occurs in a number of ways, and because self-control, while not totally random, is not uniformly exhibited across all stimulus situations that might require its application, we cannot say that delinquents necessarily have no "conscience." It is doubtful if a unified concept of conscience exists. Rather, conscience might be conceptualized as a number of sets of partially independent specific behaviors that govern resistance to temptation, feelings of guilt after transgression, and means for making amends.

While we can generalize from clinical and observational data that parental neglect and indiscriminate use of severe punishment result in delinquent acts by their children, we cannot easily predict the conditions under which the delinquent child will display a lack of self-control nor can we always say that lack of self-control is a factor in delinquent acts. Perhaps future research into relationships between delinquency and child rearing practices, self-esteem, and self-control will increase our understanding in this area.

Environmental pressures Although parents often are blamed for their child's delinquent behavior, many delinquents come from economically deprived families where the parents themselves live with frustration. Ignorance, fear, and degradation often accompany poverty. It is not difficult to understand why communication, essential in parent-child relations, breaks down in poor families.

If a community is alienated from the larger society in which it exists, its younger members are likely to act out the aggressive feelings shared by those confined to that community. The experience of growing up as a member of a disadvantaged minority makes it difficult for the adolescent to identify with the values the larger society favors. Discriminated against for religious, ethnic, or economic reasons, the child or adolescent may strike out against those he feels are responsible for his disfavored position. Family pathology, therefore, is closely related to social structure. Being poor often erodes the family structure and causes family members to relate to one another in destructive ways (Eisenberg, 1965).

In New York State alone, 45,000 children live away from their families (U.S. Department of Health, Education, and Welfare, 1972). For most, the placement away from home follows family strife brought about by impoverished conditions, marital conflict, parental abandonment, or institutionalization of one or both parents. Approximately 70 agencies near New York City provide childcare for youngsters from eastern New York State either on a short- or long-term basis.

Growing up in a relatively stable family environment is preferable to growing up in large, impersonal institutions where frequent staff turnover is the rule rather than the exception. It costs over \$30 a day to keep a child in such an institution, and in many instances a number of children from the same family are under care. Simply turning this money over to families and providing them with additional training might enable many children to remain home. Our pattern of service delivery seems to be aimed at separating families rather than keeping them together (Billingsley & Giovannoni, 1972). While no adequate follow-up of children raised in child care institutions has been reported, informal observation suggests that a high percentage of these children eventually become delinquent.

Physiological deficiencies Any sample of delinquents contains children whose behavior seems to be relatively independent of family factors. Recall that in Chapter 4 we indicated that borderline schizophrenics often become delinquents. Some electroencephalographic surveys of delinquents have found abnormal or borderline EEG tracings in close to 55 percent of their samples (Arthurs & Cahoon, 1964). Perhaps these tracings are the result of prolonged environmental stress upon body chemistry rather than a neurological disorder. Norland (1969) found that EEG patterns change as a function of stress. Nevertheless, there is a high incidence of minimal brain dysfunction among delinquents (Tarnopol, 1970), suggesting that some mildly retarded and learning disabled children respond to their frustration and failure by committing antisocial acts. We have already stated that a significantly greater proportion of children with minimal brain dysfunction are found in disadvantaged than in advantaged populations.

Other research suggests that some delinquents seek a high level of varied stimulus input in response to a physiological arousal defect. The delinquents with low levels of autonomic activity engage in more fighting and make more escape attempts while institutionalized than children with normal levels of arousal response (Farley & Farley, 1972). Recall from Chapter 7 that Wender postulated an arousal defect in some children displaying the MBD syndrome. Perhaps additional study of the subjects in Farley's sample would reveal the presence of this syndrome in the low arousal group.

Treatment

Treatment for conduct disorders varies depending on the severity. The first step is to try to effect changes in the child's home situation through cooperation with community agencies and through family counseling. Often community services are unavailable or parents are uncooperative. Consequently, the child ends up in a day or residential center if classified as emotionally disturbed. If he is older and the offense is serious, the child goes either to a state or to a voluntary residential center for delinquents.

Treatment, however, is by no means easy. Let us examine in more detail the kinds of problems Grace presented after her enrollment in the residential center.

GRACE AFTER ADMISSION TO THE RESIDENTIAL CENTER

Group mother's report

Grace was admitted to her living group on May of 1971. Being the youngest member, she was initially accepted by the girls, but this acceptance soon diminished due to her extreme hyperactivity, impulsivity, distractibility, and low frustration tolerance. She became and remained the scapegoat of the group.

Grace was always in constant motion, verbally and physically, and this erratic movement irritated the other girls. Her extremely low self-concept was often verbalized by such phrases as "nobody likes me," "you hate me," and "everybody is against me." For some time, Grace had no friends and was the target of the other girls' hostility. Interventions to reverse this process proved futile.

The real problem began prior to the Thanksgiving holidays. Her anxiety mounted as she saw all the others "going home" and she exhibited a complete inability to control herself. Her hyperactivity and impulsivity markedly increased and she lost her hold on reality in a great many situations. She increased her "no one likes me" behavior and spoke, quite frequently, of killing herself—the threats primarily centering on putting metal objects into light sockets. During one temper, she broke a picture that was in her room, cutting her finger on the glass.

Grace became completely uncontrollable within the group. She went through a period where she physically attacked me. Blow-ups became daily occurrences, with Grace screaming or banging on her door. She was taken to the quiet room on numerous occasions. She accepted no responsibility for her actions and was unable to realize that she was disliked because of them. She had many psychosomatic problems (primarily stomach) and would go to bed "sick." She also claimed that the girls always talked about her, stole from her, or went through her drawers. She verbalized the reality of the foster home situation ("they were mean to me," "they don't want me") and at the same time declared her real mother was dying of lung cancer from smoking and consequently couldn't visit her.

Grace remains in this uncontrollable, uncommunicative, hyperactive state, with an occasional "good" day. Her frustration tolerance is low and she has no patience for her own uncoordination. She will, however, play fairly well with one or two girls when they are able to tolerate her. She is able to occupy herself quite well, loves to read, and will do so for fairly long stretches of time. She will participate in group activities, but unless she is "captain" or "first" she creates a fuss.

At times there is a masochistic flavor to much of her behavior. Just as things are going well (e.g., someone is playing with her, I choose her for something special, etc.), she will deliberately do something to bring discipline and punishment (stronger limits) upon herself. At these times she derives more pleasure from being scapegoated than from being a positive group member.

The blow-ups have lessened over the past two weeks, yet there seems to be no way to work with Grace, no place to start. She remains picked on by the majority of girls and ignored by the rest.

Teacher's report

Grace is a bright girl who works when given individual attention. Her frustration level is low and lately she has been saying she is stupid. When told this isn't so she maintains "everyone says so." To counteract this attitude, she is given immediate verbal praise and rewards when she does well in class. She enjoys reading, which she does well on a fourth grade level. She is weakest in mathematics.

Initially staff disagreed about this case. The therapist felt Grace's extreme hyperactivity was a defense against overwhelming depression. "If I keep moving, I won't have time to notice how sad I am" was her nonverbal communication. The child care staff felt she was brain-damaged and pressured for neurological evaluation in the hopes that a positive diagnosis of organicity would result in a medication program that would control her behavior. The neurologist, however, found no such evidence; in fact he was impressed by what he considered were depressive features.

Eventually, Grace revealed her depression to the therapist and a video tape of the session was shown to child care staff. The tape revealed a different Grace, a child who dragged her feet and stooped her shoulders when with the therapist whom she trusted. While the eventual changes in Grace were attributable to all phases of the program, the reports of her therapist reflect her change in attitude.

Therapist's reports

THERAPY SUMMARY, OCTOBER 1970: Grace's behavior in therapy is difficult to describe. Initially she was hyperactive, but this is now subsiding and she is becoming more organized in her play. She accepts limits well, but occasionally becomes bossy toward me when limited in ways she cannot accept. She seeks and accepts interpersonal closeness but becomes afraid of it and runs away. She takes great pleasure in hurting me physically for no apparent reason, perhaps letting me know what she experienced as a child. She certainly sees herself as considerably younger than she is and responds emotionally like an infant.

THERAPY SUMMARY, NOVEMBER, 1970: I have seen Grace about eighteen times. Grace went through a period of being quite fearful of me but is now relaxed and comfortable during the time we spend together. She is less hyperactive and has less need to test limits. She is now able to verbalize both her fear of and anger towards me.

Grace is often depressed. She fears her sad states and defends against them by pretending to be happy. She is confused about her emotional reactions and asks for reassurance as to their validity. "This is fun, right?" Grace is extremely immature emotionally and looks on herself as younger than her years. So far the main theme to emerge in play is one of loneliness and hopelessness. Grace has a tendency to make all stories end unhappily in fighting or aggression.

Grace continues to deny responsibility for her own actions. She is actively rejected by all of the children in her group. My immediate goal is to focus more on these realities and help her to develop ways of coping with them.

THERAPY SUMMARY, MARCH, 1971: Grace continues to move toward expressing her independence. She now routinely provides the structure for the therapy hour, decides what we are going to do, and directs the activity. Activities are usually safe, highly structured games, such as checkers, mechanical basketball, etc. Grace has a strong need to win in such competition.

The important tasks in therapy: to give to Grace freely in a nurturant way in order to meet her need to be dependent; to encourage and support efforts at self-direction; to label affect so that feelings can be talked about and expressed verbally rather than acted out.

THERAPY SUMMARY, APRIL, 1971: Grace is still playing very structured games during the therapy hour. Winning seems to be less important now than formerly. She values the personal interaction of a game, not caring who wins.

In relation to me, Grace is more trusting and dependent. She is more willing to expose her babyish needs. She seems to have idealized notions about how parental figures should relate to her and tries very hard to manipulate people into meeting these expectations. Grace wants our relationship to be very exclusive and protests when I take other children for therapy or testing.

THERAPY SUMMARY, JUNE, 1971: Grace recently heard from an uncle and now feels she has a family. The extent of the uncle's involvement is not yet certain, but in Grace's mind she will soon be going to live with him.

Grace is beginning to talk about her problems with peers. I now refuse to participate in structured games, such as checkers, and Grace is consequently less able to conceal from me the things which are concerning her. She has talked about other girls using her and being her friend when she has something they want. She has decided that she will no longer permit this to happen. She has also talked about some of the girls' going out of their way to make her life miserable, but is still unaware that she invites this kind of attack.

We have talked about how Grace's happy states inevitably lead to sad states; in her exuberance to get close to people she bugs them and puts them in the position of driving her away. We have talked about how she uses hyperactivity and disruptiveness to keep others from seeing her sadness.

On one occasion Grace climbed into my lap and sat there comfortably, obviously enjoying being held. There has been no repetition of this, in spite of my receptiveness to it.

Grace eventually went to live with her uncle and his wife and did reasonably well, attending public school without incident and satisfactorily engaging in community activities.

Behavior shaping programs Within some institutional settings for delinquents, various specific reinforcement procedures have been tried in order to change the delinquent's attitudes and behavior. Some of these procedures are based upon operant conditioning principles. The delinquent is concretely rewarded for displaying socially adaptive rather than socially maladaptive behaviors. Unfortunately, the majority of studies published prior to 1968 failed to report any subsequent follow-up of their subjects (Stumphauzer, 1968). While the results of these behavior modification programs appear promising, they are unlikely to have a long lasting effect unless the total institutional environment is programmed according to behavioral principles and the behaviors shaped can be maintained outside the institution. The main reason why a total effort is needed lies in the "other behavior modification" program that exists in most institutions for the delinquent. Study of the peer group pressures within these settings indicates that the reinforcements dispensed by other inmates are more powerful than those dispensed by staff; peers reward delinquent behaviors and punish moves toward socially acceptable behavior more consistently and more frequently than institutional staff alternatively punish and reward the inmates for the same acts (Buehler, Patterson, & Furniss, 1966; Patterson, 1963).

Other studies reveal that institutional life seems to maximize the opportunity to participate in abnormal interpersonal relationships. The pseudofamily is a phenomenon well known to staff in institutions for delinquent girls. Girls who assume the roles of parents are the more aggressive members of a group. The father role is played by masculine-appearing girls who are the most verbally aggressive. The mother role is played by the most attractive. The pseudofamily represents the seeking of a father's protection, a mother's care, and the befriending of siblings, situations that never existed in their own families. Even in pseudofamilies, however, roles are tenuous and uncertain and "disowning" is an habitual occurrence, a reflection of the impermanence and uncertainty in their own families (Kovar, 1968). In addition, if relationships became too intense (overtly homosexual), the girls often become anxiety-ridden (Lamberti, 1963). The family fantasy helps maintain deviant behavior and prevents the development of adequate feminine identification.

From both these sets of studies, it would seem that institutions for delinquents are actually places to learn delinquent behaviors rather than places to be rehabilitated!

Attempts to change moral attitudes   In addition to operant approaches to altering behavior, several investigations of nondelinquent children have suggested that combinations of modeling and reinforcing procedures can result in shifts from one stage of moral development to another (Cowan, Langer, Heavenrich, & Nathanson, 1969; Bandura & McDonald, 1963). These findings led to efforts to apply similar techniques to modify the behavior of delinquents whose moral behavior was demonstrably deficient and whose moral concepts appeared to be retarded. The results of these studies suggest that the level of the delinquent's moral concepts can be raised but that their moral behavior does not change, implying a lack of isomorphism between level of moral judgment and significant moral behaviors (Prentice, 1972). Obviously, many internal as well as external factors influence whether or not delinquent attitudes are translated into behavior.

Hopefully, designers of the future will develop ways to rehabilitate the delinquent and prevent institutionalization. Better services for the families of the delinquent would go a long way toward preventing future delinquent acts. Schools also might redesign their academic programs so that success replaces failure. Perhaps success in school can help the child replace his poor self-image with a better one. Only time will tell.

How do they fare?

Robins (1966) followed a large number of child guidance clinic patients who were classified as antisocial (presociopathic) and compared them with neurotic children referred to the same clinic and with normal children.

At the time of initial referral, the children had a median age of 13. Most of them were a year or more behind in school and the majority had IQs between 80 and 99. More than a third had already appeared in juvenile court and 5 percent had already been in a public correctional institution. Theft and incorrigibility were the most common reasons for referral.

Half of the boys and a third of the girls were official juvenile delinquents by the time they were 18 and half had been institutionalized. Almost half did not complete elementary school and only 14 percent were high school graduates.

Diagnosis at follow-up 30 years after initial referral found the antisocial children more often psychiatrically ill, with more than half diagnosed as psychopathic personalities. The majority had a high number of arrests and displayed alcoholism, poor work histories, child neglect, and dependency on social agencies. More specifically, 78 percent of the first marriages had ended in divorce. Among both control groups only 25 percent of first marriages had ended in divorce. Ninety-four percent of the psychopathic group had adult non-traffic arrests, compared with 48 percent of the neurotic group and 17 percent of the normal group. Twenty-one percent of the psychiatric group had been hospitalized for mental illness, compared to only one of the normal subjects and one of the neurotics.

In regard to family factors, more than two-thirds of the presociopathics had a sociopathic or alcoholic father. Antisocial behavior in the father was associated not only with juvenile antisocial behavior in the patients but also with the display of antisocial behavior in adulthood by children who had been minimally antisocial in childhood. Robins concluded that antisocial behavior predicts class status more efficiently than class status predicts antisocial behavior. He found that sociopathic men gravitated to the bottom of the social ladder and passed on their behavior patterns to their children. Of children living in the same community those whose parents were not antisocial were more likely to

rise out of the lowest social stratum. All children in the sample, however, were white Americans. Whether this finding would occur with
black Americans, more often subjected to prejudice and discrimination,
remains to be seen.

Robins suggests that social agencies should take over more of the child
rearing responsibilities from parents. Residential centers do just that.
How do children fare who have been placed in residential centers? The
findings of those who have traced children after their discharge suggest
that the effectiveness of residential care depends on a number of factors.
In studying centers that admit predelinquent children between the ages
of 6 and 13 and discharge them approximately two years later, the age
of the child at the time of follow-up is a significant factor. The youngest
group, those under 13, had the highest adjustment ratings; the ratings
then progressively decreased until age 19, at which time there was a
significant increase in maladjustment. The lowest ratings went to the
group between 16 and 19 years of age, those in the storm center of
adolescence (Astor Home, 1963).

Adjustment of children who returned to their own homes was related to the extent of family pathology. In addition, those with higher
intelligence test scores were doing better. Children with the poorest adjustment were those originally classified as having inadequate personalities, the so-called empty children, raised from infancy in institutions,
whose basic inability to form meaningful relationships with others constitutes a barrier to effective treatment.

In general, intensive treatment can change the life course of many
children considered high risk youngsters, that is, children considered
likely to commit serious antisocial acts in the future. Out of 130 children
followed by the Astor Home over an average period of 5 years (range
2 to 10 years), only 9 were in state reformatories and 19 were in state
hospitals. The finding that over 10 percent were in state hospitals supports the notion that many children who show unsocialized aggression
are actually psychotic. Many psychotics have such vulnerable egos that
they experience minor frustrations as severe personal insults. They
therefore react with extreme hostility and attempt to change the external world to suit their special needs. Defiance and hostile behavior
serve as attempts to defend against internal collapse and thus prevent
psychotic breakdown. These aggressive defenses are tolerated less as the
child grows older (Watt, Stolorow, Lubensky, & McClelland, 1970).

Follow-up studies point out the need for more extensive support and
help for children after they leave a treatment program. Aftercare facilities, such as group and foster homes, are necessary. One study compared children who were placed in aftercare facilities with children
who returned to their own home, to the home of relatives, or to former
foster homes. Aftercare facilities were most helpful to the following:
those discharged at adolescence, those who had been in institutions prior

to residential treatment, those with minimal brain dysfunction or with passive-dependent personalities, and those with low intellectual functioning (IQ less than 89). Children with schizoid personalities did poorly whether in an aftercare facility or in an unsupervised setting (Chan, 1970).

CONCLUDING REMARKS

Although development is determined by the actions and interactions of heredity and environment, environment takes on greater importance when certain conditions conducive to normal and socially acceptable development are absent. It has been clearly established that family interaction patterns, reward conditions, intellectual climate, and impoverished living relate to school failure and to antisocial behavior.

The parental behaviors necessary to prepare a child to function adequately in school and community are absent among many lower class families. Parental behavior has a functional-cognitive dimension, a dimension extremely important when considering children's development. The degree to which poverty and powerlessness affect this dimension is still being evaluated. In any case, a large percentage of lower class children enter school poorly prepared for academic learning. With advancing age, they fall farther behind other children and eventually leave school. Some strike back at the society they feel cheated them. They become parents and the cycle begins again.

To interrupt this cycle, schools can make an effort to increase the involvement of parents with the school-community. Perhaps the first step in helping both the disadvantaged and the delinquent child should be to increase parent power.

Many parents, as Gordon (1969) pointed out, never experienced competence in their own lives; to expect them to foster competence in their child is unrealistic. Until intervention programs include involving the parents, and until these efforts have the support of the entire school-community, their effect on the children is likely to be only minimal and short-lived.

References

Aldous, J. Children's perceptions of adult roles as affected by class, father-absence and race. *Demonstration and Research Center for Early Education Papers and Reports*, 1969, **3**(4).

Almy, M. *Young children's thinking: studies of some aspects of Piaget's theory.* New York: Teachers College, Columbia University, 1966.

Amante, D., Margules, P. H., Hartman, D. M., Storey, D. B., & Weeber, L. J. The epidemiological distribution of CNS dysfunction. *Journal of Social Issues*, 1970, **26**, 105–136.

Anastasi, A. *Psychological testing.* (3rd ed.) New York: Macmillan, 1968.

Anastasi, A., & Cordova, F. A. Some effects of bilingualism upon the intelligence test performance of Puerto Rican children in New York City. *Journal of Educational Psychology,* 1953, **44,** 1–19.

Anderson, J. G., & Evans, F. B. Achievement and the achievement syndrome among Mexican-American youth. In P. Kutsche (Ed.), *Measuring sociocultural change.* Boulder, Colo.: Associated University Press, 1969.

Armor, D. J. The evidence on busing. *The Public Interest,* 1972, **28,** 90–126.

Aronfreed, J. The origin of self-criticism. *Psychological Review,* 1964, **71,** 193–218.

Aronfreed, J. *Conduct and conscience.* New York: Academic Press, 1968.

Aronfreed, J. The concept of internalization. In D. A. Goslin (Ed.), *Handbook of socialization theory and research.* Skokie, Ill.: Rand McNally, 1969.

Arthurs, R. G. S., & Cahoon, E. B. A clinical and electroencephalographic survey of psychopathic personality. *American Journal of Psychiatry,* 1964, **120,** 875–877.

Astor Home. What we have learned: A report of the first 10 years of the Astor Home, a residential treatment center for emotionally disturbed children. Unpublished paper, Astor Home, Rhinebeck, N.Y., 1963.

Ausubel, D. P. How reversible are the cognitive and motivational effects of cultural deprivation? *Urban Education,* 1964, **1,** 16–38.

Bailey, B. L. Concern for special curriculum aspects: bilingualism. In A. Jallonsky (Ed.), *Imperatives for change: proceedings of the New York State Education Department conferences on college and university programs for teachers of the disadvantaged.* New York: Yeshiva University, 1967.

Baldwin, T. L., McFarlane, P. T., & Garvey, C. J. Children's communication accuracy related to race and socioeconomic status. *Child Devleopment,* 1971, **42,** 345–358.

Bandura, A., & McDonald, F. J. Influence of social reinforcement and the behavior of models in shaping children's moral judgments. *Journal of Abnormal and Social Psychology,* 1963, **67,** 274–281.

Bandura, A., & Walters, R. H. *Adolescent aggression.* New York: Ronald, 1959.

Baratz, J. C. Language in the economically disadvantaged child: a perspective. *Journal of the American Speech and Hearing Association,* 1968, **10,** 143–145.

Baratz, J. C. Teaching reading in an urban Negro school system. In J. C. Baratz & R. W. Shuy (Eds.), *Teaching black children to read.* Washington, D.C.: Center for Applied Linguistics, 1969.

Barbrack, C. R. The effects of three home visiting strategies upon measures of children's academic aptitude and maternal teaching behaviors. *Demonstration and Research Center for Early Education Papers and Reports,* 1970, 4(1).

Barcai, A., Umbarger, C., Pierce, T. W., & Chamberlain, P. A comparison of three group approaches to underachieving children. *American Journal of Orthopsychiatry,* 1973, **43,** 133–141.

Baumrind, D. An exploratory study of socialization effects on black children: some black-white comparisons. *Child Development,* 1972, **43,** 261–267.

Bellar, E. K. The evaluation of early educational intervention of intellectual and social development of lower-class disadvantaged children. In E. Grotberg (Ed.), *Critical issues in research related to disadvantaged children.* Princeton, N.J.: Educational Testing Service, 1969.

Benard, J. *Marriage and family among Negroes.* Englewood Cliffs, N.J.: Prentice-Hall, 1966.

Bereiter, C., & Engelmann, S. *Teaching disadvantaged preschool children.* Englewood Cliffs, N.J.: Prentice-Hall, 1966.

Bernstein, B. Language and social class: a research note. *British Journal of Sociology*, 1960, **11**, 271–276.

Bernstein, B. Social structure, language, and learning. *Educational Research*, 1961, **3**, 163–178.

Bernstein, B. Social class, linguistic codes and grammatical elements. *Language and Speech*, 1962a, **5**, 221–240.

Bernstein, B. Linguistic codes, hesitation phenomena and intelligence. *Language and Speech*, 1962b, **5**, 31–46.

Bernstein, B. Elaborated and restricted codes: their social origins and some consequences. In J. J. Gumperz & D. Hymes (Eds.), The ethnography of communication. *American Anthropologist Special Publication*, 1964, **66**, 55–69.

Bernstein, B. A socio-linguistic approach to socialization with some reference to educability. Unpublished paper. University College, London, England, 1968.

Berry, J. W. Psychological research in the North. *Anthropologica*, 1971, **13**, 143–157.

Biber, B. Preschool education. In R. Ulich (Ed.), *Education and the idea of mankind*. New York: Harcourt Brace Jovanovich, 1964.

Billingsley, A., & Giovannoni, J. M. *Children of the storm: black children and American child welfare*. New York: Harcourt Brace Jovanovich, 1972.

Blank, M., & Solomon, F. A tutorial language program to develop abstract thinking in socially disadvantaged pre-school children. *Child Development*, 1968, **39**, 379–390.

Blank, M., & Solomon, F. How shall the disadvantaged child be taught? *Child Development*, 1969, **40**, 47–61.

Bloom, B. *Stability and change in human characteristics*. New York: Wiley, 1964.

Boger, J. H. An experimental study of the effects of perceptual training on group IQ scores of elementary pupils in rural upgraded schools. *Journal of Educational Research*, 1952, **46**, 43–53.

Boger, R. P., & Ambron, S. R. Subpopulation profiling of the psychoeducational dimensions of disadvantaged preschool children. In E. Grotberg (Ed.), *Critical issues in research related to disadvantaged children*. Princeton, N.J.: Educational Testing Service, 1969.

Bonilla, E. S. Social structure and race relations. In S. W. Webster (Ed.), *The disadvantaged learner: knowing, understanding and educating*. San Francisco: Chandler, 1966.

Bosco, J. The visual information processing speed of lower- and middle-class children. *Child Development*, 1972, **43**, 1418–1422.

Bradshaw, C. E. Relationship between maternal behavior and infant performance in environmentally disadvantaged homes. Unpublished doctoral dissertation, University of Florida, 1968.

Bronfenbrenner, U. Motivational and social components in compensatory education programs: suggested principles, practices, and research designs. In E. Grotberg (ed.), *Critical issues in research related to disadvantaged children*. Princeton, N.J.: Educational Testing Service, 1969.

Brozowich, R. W. Characteristics associated with popularity among different racial and sociometric groups of children. *Journal of Educational Research*, 1970, **63**, 441–444.

Buck, M. R. Factors related to school achievement in an economically disadvantaged group. *Child Development*, 1971, **42**, 1813–1826.

Buehler, R. E., Patterson, G. R., & Furniss, J. M. The reinforcement of behavior in institutional settings. *Behavior Research and Therapy*, 1966, **4**, 157–167.

Caldwell, B. The effects of psychosocial deprivation on human development in infancy. *Merrill-Palmer Quarterly*, 1970, **16**, 260–277.

Chan, D. F. An evaluation of an agency-operated after-care program: a follow-up study. Unpublished master's thesis, Fordham University School of Social Services, 1970.

Chomsky, N. The formal nature of language. In E. Lenneberg (Ed.), *Biological foundations of language*. New York: Wiley, 1967.

Christine, D., & Christine, C. The relationship of auditory discrimination to articulatory defects and reading retardation. *Elementary School Journal*, 1964, 65, 97–100.

Cicirelli, V. G., Evans, J. W., & Schiller, J. S. The impact of Head Start: a reply to the report analysis. *Harvard Educational Review*, 1970, 40, 105–129.

Clifford, M. M., & Cleary, T. A. The relationship between children's academic performance and achievement accountability. *Child Development*, 1972, 43, 647–655.

Cline, M. G., & Dryer, A. S. *Establishment of regional Head Start research and evaluation centers—a descriptive report of the evaluation design, population and program characteristics and pre-test data of the full year 1967 evaluation of Project Head Start*. Washington, D.C.: Office of Economic Opportunity, 1968.

Cloward, R. A., & Ohlin, L. E. *Delinquency and opportunity*. New York: Free Press, 1960.

Cole, M., & Bruner, J. S. Culture differences and inferences about psychological processes. *American Psychologist*, 1971, 26, 867–876.

Coleman, J. S. *Equality of educational opportunity*. Washington, D.C.: U.S. Office of Education, 1966.

Community Council of Greater New York. *Census Bulletin, Research and Program Planning Information*, 1973, No. 18.

Covington, M. V. Stimulus discrimination as a function of social class membership. *Child Development*, 1967, 38, 607–613.

Cowan, P. A., Langer, J., Heavenrich, J., & Nathanson, M. Social learning and Piaget's cognitive theory of moral development. *Journal of Personality and Social Psychology*, 1969, 11, 261–274.

Crandall, V. C., Katkovsky, W., & Crandall, V. J. Children's beliefs in their own control of reinforcements in intellectual-academic achievement situations. *Child Development*, 1965, 36, 91–109.

Cundick, B. P. Measures of intelligence on Southwest Indian students. *Journal of Social Psychology*, 1970, 81, 151–156.

Darsie, M. L. Mental capacity of American-born Japanese children. *Comparative Psychology Monographs*, 1926, 15(3).

Deitz, G. E. A comparison of delinquents with nondelinquents on self-concept, self-acceptance, and parental identification. *Journal of Genetic Psychology*, 1969, 115, 285–295.

Dennis, W. The performance of Hopi children on the Goodenough Draw-a-Man Test. *Journal of Comparative Psychology*, 1942, 34, 341–348.

Deutsch, C. P. Auditory discrimination and learning: social factors. *Merrill-Palmer Quarterly*, 1964, 10, 277–296.

Deutsch, M. Minority group and class status as related to social and personality factors in scholastic achievement. (Monograph No. 2) Unpublished paper, Society for Applied Anthropology, Ithaca, N.Y., 1960.

Deutsch, M. The role of social class in language development and cognition. *American Journal of Orthopsychiatry*, 1965, 35, 78–88.

Deutsch, M., & Brown, B. Social influences in Negro-white intelligence difference. *Journal of Social Issues*, 1964, 20, 24–35.

Diggs, I. Comments made during a symposium on Culture and the Black Struggle, Queens College, New York, March 1973.

Dillard, J. L. *Black English: its history and usage in the United States.* New York: Random House, 1972.

Dregor, R. M., & Miller, K. S. Comparative psychological studies of Negroes and whites in the United States. *Psychological Bulletin*, 1960, **57**, 361–402.

Dunn, J. A. The approach-avoidance paradigm as a model for the analysis of school anxiety. *Journal of Educational Psychology*, 1968, **59**, 388–394.

Eisenberg, L. Developmental approach to adolescence. *Children*, 1965, **12**, 131–135.

Eisenberg, L., Berlin, C., Dill, A., & Sheldon, F. Class and race effects on the intelligibility of monosyllables. *Child Development*, 1968, **39**, 1077–1089.

Entwisle, D. R., & Greenberger, E. Questions about social class, internality-externality, and text anxiety. *Developmental Psychology*, 1972, **7**, 218.

Epps, E. G. Correlates of academic achievement among Northern and Southern urban Negro students. *Journal of Social Issues*, 1969, **25**, 55–70.

Fanshel, D. Findings of the Child Welfare Research Program. Unpublished paper, Columbia University School of Social Work, New York, 1972.

Farley, F. H., & Farley, S. V. Stimulus-seeking motivation and delinquent behavior among institutionalized delinquent girls. *Journal of Consulting and Clinical Psychology*, 1972, **39**, 94–97.

Farnham-Diggory, S. Cognitive synthesis in Negro and white children. *Monographs of the Society for Research in Child Development*, 1970, **35**(2, Serial No. 135).

Feagin, J. R. Poverty: we still believe that God helps those who help themselves. *Psychology Today*, 1972, **6**, 101–110, 129.

Federal Bureau of Investigation. *Uniform crime reports, 1966.* Washington, D.C.: U.S. Department of Justice, 1967.

Figurel, J. A. Limitations in the vocabulary of disadvantaged children: a cause of poor reading. In *Improvement of reading through classroom practice.* (Monograph No. 9) Newark, Del.: International Reading Association, 1964.

Figurelli, J. C., & Keller, H. R. The effects of training and socioeconomic class upon the acquisition of conservation concepts. *Child Development*, 1972, **43**, 293–298.

Flowers, J., & Marston, A. Modification of low self-confidence in elementary school children. *Journal of Educational Research*, 1972, **66**, 30–34.

Foster, H. L. A lexicon of words with standard meanings. Unpublished paper, Faculty of Educational Studies, State University of New York at Buffalo, 1971.

Friend, R. M., & Neale, J. M. Children's perceptions of success and failure: an attributional analysis of the effects of race and social class. *Developmental Psychology*, 1972, **7**, 123–128.

Garcia, J. I.Q.: the conspiracy. *Psychology Today*, 1972, **6**, 40–43, 92–94.

Getzels, J. W., & Jackson, P. W. *Creativity and intelligence.* New York: Wiley, 1961.

Gill, N., & Herdtner, L. L. Perceptual and socioeconomic variables, instruction in body-orientation, and predicted academic success in young children. *Perceptual and Motor Skills*, 1968, **26**, 1175–1184.

Glass, D. C., & Singer, J. *Urban Stress.* New York: Academic Press, 1972.

Gold, M., & Mann, D. Delinquency as defense. *American Journal of Orthopsychiatry*, 1972, **42**, 463–479.

Golden, M., & Birns, B. Social class, intelligence, and cognitive style in infancy. *Child Development*, 1971, **42**, 2114–2116.

Golden, M., Birns, B., Bridger, W., & Moss, A. Social-class differentiation in cognitive development among black preschool children. *Child Development*, 1971, **42**, 37–45.

Gordon, I. J. Developing parent power. In E. Grotberg (Ed.), *Critical issues in research related to disadvantaged children.* Princeton, N.J.: Educational Testing Service, 1969.

Gray, S. W., & Klaus, R. A. The early training project: a seventh-year report. *Child Development,* 1970, **41,** 909–924.

Gray, S. W., Klaus, R. A. Miller, J. O., & Forrester, B. J. *Before first grade.* New York: Teachers College, Columbia University, 1966.

Greenberg, J. W., & Davidson, H. H. Home background and school achievement of black urban ghetto children. *American Journal of Orthopsychiatry,* 1972, **42,** 803–810.

Grier, W. H., & Gobbs, P. M. *Black rage.* New York: Basic Books, 1968.

Gross, M. Learning readiness in two Jewish groups: a study in cultural deprivation. Unpublished paper, Center for Urban Education, New York, 1967.

Hall, V. C., & Mery, M. Language intervention research: rationale, results and recommendations. Unpublished paper, Syracuse University Center for Research and Development in Early Childhood Education, Syracuse, N.Y., 1970.

Hall, V. C., & Turner, R. R. Comparison of imitation and comprehension scores between two lower-class groups and the effects of two warm-up conditions on imitation of the same groups. *Child Development,* 1971, **42,** 1735–1750.

Harrison, A., & Nadelman, L. Conceptual tempo and inhibition of movement in black preschool children. *Child Development,* 1972, **43,** 657–688.

Havighurst, R. J. Metropolitan development and the educational system. *School Review,* 1961, **69,** 251–269.

Havighurst, R. J., Gunther, M. K., & Pratt, I. E. Environment and the Draw-a-Man Test: the performance of Indian children. *Journal of Abnormal and Social Psychology,* 1946, **41,** 50–63.

Hayden, B. S., Talmadge, M., Mordock, J. B., & Kulla, M. The alienated student: an effort to motivate at the junior high level. *Journal of School Psychology,* 1970, **8,** 237–241.

Hedlund, C. S. Relationship of positive social reinforcement to delinquency and subtypes of delinquent behavior: a test of Patterson's etiological model. Unpublished doctoral dissertation, West Virginia University, 1971.

Heider, E. R., Cazden, C. B., & Brown, R. *Social class differences in the effectiveness and style of children's coding ability.* (Project Literacy Reports, No. 9) Ithaca, N.Y.: Cornell University, 1968.

Hertzig, M. E., & Birch, H. G. Longitudinal course of measured intelligence in preschool children of different social and ethnic background. *American Journal of Orthopsychiatry,* 1971, **41,** 416–426.

Hertzig, M. E., Birch, H., Thomas, A., & Mendec, O. Class and ethnic differences in the responsiveness of preschool children to cognitive demands. *Monographs of the Society for Research in Child Development,* 1968, **33**(1, Serial No. 117).

Herzog, E., Newcomb, C., & Cisin, I. H. But some are more poor than others: SES differences in a preschool program. *American Journal of Orthopsychiatry,* 1972, **42,** 4–22.

Herzog, E., & Sudia, C. Children in fatherless families. In B. Caldwell & H. Ricciutti (Eds.), *Review of child development research.* Vol. 3. Chicago: Society for Research in Child Development, University of Chicago Press, 1970.

Hess, R. D. Parental behavior and children's school achievement: implications for Head Start. In E. Grotberg (Ed.), *Critical issues in research related to disadvantaged children.* Princeton, N.J.: Educational Testing Service, 1969.

Hess, R. D., & Shipman, V. C. Early experience and the socialization of cognitive modes in children. *Child Development,* 1965, **36,** 869–886.

Hess, R. D., Shipman, V., Brophy, J. E., & Bear, R. M. *The cognitive environ-*

ment of urban preschool children. Chicago: School of Education, University of Chicago, 1968.

Hoffman, M. L. Power assertion by the parent and its impact on the child. *Child Development,* 1960, **31,** 129–143.

Hofstaetter, P. R. The changing composition of intelligence: a study of T technique. *Journal of Genetic Psychology,* 1954, **85,** 159–164.

Holley, W., Rosenbaum, A., & Churchill, J. Effects of rapid succession of pregnancy. In *Perinatal factors affecting human development.* Washington, D.C.: Paho Science Publications, 1969.

Houston, S. H. A sociolinguistic consideration of the black English of children in northern Florida. *Language,* 1969a, **45,** 599–607.

Houston, S. H. Child Black English: the school register. Paper presented at the annual meeting of the Linguistic Society of America, San Francisco, 1969b.

Houston, S. H. A reexamination of some assumptions about the language of the disadvantaged child. *Child Development,* 1970, **41,** 947–963.

Houston, S. H. Black English. *Psychology Today,* 1973, **6,** 45–48.

Hunt, J. McV. *Intelligence and experience.* New York: Ronald, 1961.

Jacobson, L. I., & Greeson, L. E. Effects of systematic conceptual learning on the intellectual development of preschool children from poverty backgrounds: a follow-up study. *Child Development,* 1972, **43,** 1111–1115.

Jencks, C., Smith, M., Acland, H., Bane, M. J., Cohen, D., Gintis, H., Heyns, B., & Michelson, S. *Inequality: a reassessment of the effect of family and schooling.* New York: Basic Books, 1972.

Jenkins, R. The varieties of children's behavioral problems and family dynamics. *American Journal of Psychiatry,* 1968, **124,** 1440–1445.

Jensen, A. R. Social class and perceptual learning. *Mental Hygiene,* 1966, **50,** 226–239.

Jensen, A. R. Patterns of mental ability and socioeconomic status. *Proceedings of the National Academy of Sciences,* 1968, **60,** 1330–1337.

Jensen, A. R. How much can we boost IQ and scholastic achievement? *Harvard Educational Review,* 1969a, **39,** 1–123.

Jensen, A. R. Reducing the heredity-environment uncertainty: a reply. *Harvard Educational Review,* 1969b, **39,** 449–483.

Jeruchemowicz, R., Costello, J., & Bagur, S. Knowledge of action and object words: a comparison of lower- and middle-class preschoolers. *Child Development,* 1971, **42,** 455–464.

John, V. P. The intellectual development of slum children: some preliminary findings. *American Journal of Orthopsychiatry,* 1963, **3,** 813–822.

Joos, M. Language and the school child. *Harvard Educational Review,* 1964, **34,** 203–210.

Kadushin, A. Single parent adoptions—an overview and some relevant research. Paper presented at the northwest regional conference, Child Welfare League of America, Portland, Ore., April 1968.

Kagan, J. Reflection-impulsivity and reading ability in primary grade children. *Child Development,* 1965, **36,** 309–328.

Kagan, J. Developmental studies in reflection and analysis. In A. H. Kidd & J. L. Rivoire (Eds.), *Perceptual development in children.* New York: International Universities, 1966a.

Kagan, J. A developmental approach to conceptual growth. In H. J. Klausmeier & C. W. Harris (Eds.), *Analysis of concept learning.* New York: Academic Press, 1966b.

Kagan, J., Moss, H. A. & Sigel, I. E. Psychological significance of styles of conceptualization. *Monographs of the Society for Research in Child Development,* 1963, **28**(2, Serial No. 86), 73–112.

Kagan, J., Pearson, L., & Welch, L. Conceptual impulsivity and inductive reasoning. *Child Development,* 1966, **37,** 584–594.

Kamii, C. K., & Radin, N. L. Class differences in the socialization practices of Negro mothers. *Journal of Marriage and the Family,* 1967, **29,** 302–310.

Kaplan, M. L., & Mandel, S. Class differences in the effects of impulsivity, goal orientation and verbal expression on an object sorting task. *Child Development,* 1969, **40,** 491–502.

Karnes, M. B. *Research and development program on preschool disadvantaged children.* Vol. 1. Urbana, Ill.: Institute for Research on Exceptional Children, 1969.

Karnes, M. B., Teska, J. A., Hodgins, A. S., & Badger, E. D. Educational intervention at home by mothers of disadvantaged infants. *Child Development,* 1970, **41,** 925–935.

Katkovsky, W., Crandall, V. C., & Good, S. Parental antecedents of children's beliefs in internal-external control of reinforcements in intellectual achievement situations. *Child Development,* 1967, **38,** 766–776.

Katz, P. A. Verbal discrimination performance of disadvantaged children: stimulus and response variables. *Child Development,* 1967, **38,** 288–342.

Kellaghan, T., & Macnamara, J. Family correlates of verbal reasoning ability. *Developmental Psychology,* 1972, **7,** 49–53.

Keller, H. R. The lack of generality of middle- and lower-class children's performance on conservation and transitivity tasks. Paper presented at the annual meeting of the Society for Research in Child Development, Minneapolis, 1971.

Kennedy, W. A. A follow-up normative study of Negro intelligence and achievement. *Monographs of the Society for Research in Child Development,* 1969, **34**(2, Serial No. 126).

Kennedy, W. A., Van De Riet, V., & White, J. C., Jr. A normative sample of intelligence and achievement of Negro elementary school children in the Southeastern United States. *Monographs of the Society for Research in Child Development,* 1963, **28**(6, Serial No. 90).

Killian, L. R. WISC, Illinois Test of Psycholinguistic Abilities, and Bender Visual-Motor Gestalt Test performance of Spanish-American kindergarten and first-grade school children. *Journal of Consulting and Clinical Psychology,* 1971, **37,** 38–43.

Kinnie, E. J., & Sternlof, R. E. The influence of nonintellective factors on the IQ scores of middle- and lower-class children. *Child Development,* 1971, **42,** 1989–1995.

Klineberg, O. Racial differences in speed and accuracy. *Journal of Abnormal Social Psychology,* 1927, **22,** 273–277.

Klineberg, O. *Negro intelligence and selective migration.* New York: Columbia University Press, 1935.

Klineberg, O. Negro-white differences in intelligence test performance: a new look at an old problem. *American Psychologist,* 1963, **18,** 198–203.

Knowlton, C. Patron-peon pattern among the Spanish Americans of New Mexico. In S. W. Webster (Ed.), *The disadvantaged child: knowing, understanding and educating.* San Francisco: Chandler, 1966.

Kohlberg, J. A cognitive-developmental analysis of children's sex-role concepts and attitudes. In E. Maccoby (Ed.), *The development of sex differences.* Berkeley, Calif.: Stanford University Press, 1966.

Koller, K. M. Parental deprivation, family background and female delinquency. *British Journal of Psychiatry,* 1971, **118,** 319–327.

Konopka, G. *The adolescent girl in conflict.* Englewood Cliffs, N.J.: Prentice-Hall, 1966.

Kovar, L. *Faces of the adolescent girl.* Englewood Cliffs, N.J.: Prentice-Hall, 1968.

Labov, W. The logical non-standard English. In F. Williams (Ed.), *Language and poverty: perspectives on a theme.* Chicago: Markham, 1970.

Labov, W., & Cohen, P. *Systematic relations of standard and non-standard rules in the grammar of Negro speakers.* (Project Literacy Reports, No. 8) Ithaca, N.Y.: Cornell University, 1967.

Lamberti, A. A. A type of peer relationship in a girl's training school. *Bulletin of the Menninger Clinic*, 1963, **27**, 200–204.

Langner, T. S., Greene, E. L., Herson, J. H., Jameson, J. D., Goff, J. A., Rostkowski, J., & Zykorie, D. Psychiatric impairment in welfare and nonwelfare children. *Welfare in Review*, 1969, **7**, 10–21.

Lee, E. S. Negro intelligence and selective migration. *American Sociological Review*, 1951, **16**, 227–233.

Lehmann, I. J. Rural-urban differences in intelligence. *Journal of Educational Research*, 1959, **53**, 62–68.

Lenneberg, E. H. Understanding language without the ability to speak: a case report. *Journal of Abnormal and Social Psychology*, 1962, **65**, 419–425.

Lesser, G. S., Fifer, G., & Clark, D. H. Mental abilities of children from different social-class and cultural groups. *Monographs of the Society for Research in Child Development*, 1965, **30**(4, Serial No. 102).

Levenstein, P., Kochman, A., & Roth, H. A. From laboratory to real world: service delivery of the mother-child home program. *American Journal of Orthopsychiatry*, 1973, **43**, 72–78.

Lévi-Strauss, C. *Structural anthropology.* New York: Basic Books, 1963.

Lillie, D. L. The effects of motor development lessons on mentally retarded children. *American Journal of Mental Deficiency*, 1968, **72**, 803–808.

Lucco, A. A. Cognitive development after age five: a future factor in the failure of early intervention with the urban child. *American Journal of Orthopsychiatry*, 1972, **42**, 847–856.

Mac Iver, R. *The prevention and control of delinquency.* New York: Atherton, 1967.

Mack, D. Where the black-matriarchy theorists went wrong. *Psychology Today*, 1971, **4**, 24, 86–87.

Madsen, M. C. Cooperative and competitive motivation of children in three Mexican sub-cultures. *Psychological Reports*, 1967, **20**, 1307–1320.

Madsen, M. C., & Shapira, A. Cooperative and competitive behavior of urban Afro-American, Anglo-American, Mexican-American, and Mexican village children. *Developmental Psychology*, 1970, **3**, 16–20.

Marburger, C. L. Working toward more effective education for culturally deprived children. *Detroit Schools*, 1961, **22**, 31, 35.

Marston, A. R. Dealing with low self-confidence. *Educational Research* (Great Britain), 1968, **10**, 134–138.

McCord, W., & McCord, J. *The Psychopath.* Princeton, N.J.: Van Nostrand, 1964.

McCord, J., McCord, W., & Howard, A. Family interaction as antecedent to the direction of male aggressiveness. *Journal of Abnormal and Social Psychology*, 1963, **66**, 239–242.

Meeker, M. Differential syndromes of giftedness and curriculum planning: a four-year follow-up. *Journal of Special Education*, 1968, **2**, 185–196.

Mercer, J. R. I.Q.: the lethal label. *Psychology Today*, 1972, **6**, 44–47, 95–97.

Messer, S. The relation of internal-external control to academic performance. *Child Development*, 1972, **43**, 1456–1462.

Miller, A. G., & Thomas, R. Cooperation and competition among Blackfoot

Indian and urban Canadian children. *Child Development*, 1972, **43**, 1104–1110.

Miller, L. B., et al. Experimental variation of Head Start curricula: a comparison of current approaches. (Progress Report No. 9) Unpublished paper, Psychology Department, University of Louisville, Louisville, Ky., 1971.

Milner, E. A study of the relationship between reading readiness in grade one school children and patterns of parent child interaction. *Child Development*, 1951, **22**, 96–112.

Moriber, L. *School functioning of pupils born in other areas and in New York City.* (Pamphlet No. 168) New York: Bureau of Educational Program Research and Statistics, Board of Education of the City of New York, 1961.

Nedler, S., & Sebera, P. Intervention strategies for Spanish-speaking preschool children. *Child Development*, 1971, **42**, 259–267.

Niklason, L. V. Factors affecting status within a group of delinquent girls. *Adolescence*, 1967–1968, **2**, 503–523.

Norland, E. Conflict state and abnormal EEG: a study of boys with behavior disturbances and abnormal EEG. *Scandinavian Journal of Educational Research*, 1969, **4**, 199–221.

Olim, E. G. Maternal language styles and cognitive behavior. *Journal of Special Education*, 1970, **4**, 53–68.

Ortego, P. D. Montezuma's children. *The Center Magazine*, 1970, **3**, 23–31.

Patterson, G. R. The reinforcement of delinquent behavior by the delinquent peer culture. Unpublished paper, University of Oregon, Eugene, 1963.

Patterson, G. R. Behavioral techniques based upon social learning: an additional base for developing behavior modification technologies. In C. Franks (Ed.), *Behavior therapy*, New York: McGraw-Hill, 1969.

Patterson, O. Toward a future that has no past—reflections on the fate of blacks in the Americas. *The Public Interest*, 1972, **27**, 25–62.

Pearson, P. H. Relationship of biologic, psychologic, and social deprivation to learning and adaptive behavior. In M. J. Giannini (Ed.), *Proceedings of two-day institute on the pre-school retardate: comprehensive programming in disadvantaged communities.* New York: New York Medical College, 1970.

Peisach, C. E. Children's comprehension of teacher and peer speech. *Child Development*, 1965, **36**, 481–490.

Pettigrew, T. F. *A profile of the Negro American.* Princeton, N.J.: Van Nostrand, 1964.

Pettigrew, T. F. Race and equal educational opportunity. Paper presented at the symposium on the Implications of the Colman Report on Equality of Educational Opportunity at the annual convention of the American Psychological Association, Washington, D.C., September 1967.

Pettigrew, T. F., Useem, E. L., Normand, C., & Smith, M. Busing: a review of the evidence. *The Public Interest*, 1973, **29**, 88–118.

Ponthieux, N. A., & Barker, D. G. Relationships between race and physical fitness. *Research Quarterly*, 1965, **36**, 468–472.

Prentice, N. M. The influence of live and symbolic modeling on promoting moral judgments of adolescent delinquents. *Journal of Abnormal Psychology*, 1972, **80**, 157–161.

President's Committee on Mental Retardation. *The six hour retarded child.* Washington, D.C.: U.S. Department of Health, Education, and Welfare, 1970.

Quay, H. C. Personality and delinquency. In H. C. Quay (Ed.), *Juvenile delinquency.* Princeton, N.J.: Van Nostrand, 1965.

Quay, L. C. Language dialect, reinforcement, and the intelligence test performance of Negro children. *Child Development*, 1971, **42**, 5–15.

Quay, L. C. Negro dialect and Binet performance in severely disadvantaged black four-year-olds. *Child Development,* 1972, **43,** 245–250.

Radin, N. Three degrees of maternal involvement in a preschool program: impact on mothers and children. *Child Development,* 1972, **43,** 1355–1364.

Randall, R. S. A response to Gillmore and Stallings regarding a paper by Nedler and Sebera [1971]. *Child Development,* 1972, **43,** 1039–1040.

Richards, H. C., & McCandless, B. R. Socialization dimensions among five-year-old slum children. *Journal of Educational Psychology,* 1972, **63,** 44–55.

Riessman, F. Are the deprived non-verbal? In F. Riessman, J. Cohen, & A. Pearl (Eds.), *Mental health of the poor.* New York: Free Press, 1964.

Robins, L. N. *Deviant children grow up.* Baltimore: Williams & Wilkins, 1966.

Rosenberg, B. Q., & Sutton-Smith, B. Sibling age spacing effects upon cognition. *Developmental Psychology,* 1969, **1,** 661–665.

Rubano, J. *Culture and behavior in Hawaii.* (Hawaii Series 3) Honolulu: Social Science Research Institute, University of Hawaii, 1972.

Safa, H. I. The poor are like everyone else, Oscar. *Psychology Today,* 1970, **4,** 26, 28, 29, 32.

Santrock, J. W. Relation of type and onset of father absence to cognitive development. *Child Development,* 1972, **43,** 455–469.

Scharfman, M., & Clark, R. Delinquent adolescent girls: residential treatment in a municipal hospital setting. *Archives of General Psychiatry,* 1967, **17,** 441–447.

Schoggen, M., & Schoggen, P. Environmental forces in the home lives of three-year-old children in three population subgroups. *Demonstration and Research Center for Early Education Papers and Reports,* 1971, 5(2).

Schubert, J., & Cropley, A. J. Verbal regulation of behavior and IQ in Canadian Indian and white children. *Child Development,* 1972, **7,** 293–301.

Sherman, M., & Kay, C. B. The intelligence of isolated mountain children. In A. Anastasi (Ed.), *Perspectives in psychology,* New York: Wiley, 1965.

Shuey, A. M. *The testing of Negro intelligence.* Lynchburg, Va.: Bell, 1958.

Sigel, I. E., Anderson, L. M., & Shapiro, H. Categorization behavior of lower and middle class Negro preschool children: differences dealing with representation of familiar objects. *Journal of Negro Education,* 1966, **35,** 218–229.

Silberman, C. E. The city and the Negro. In A. H. Passow, M. Goldberg, & A. J. Tannenbaum (Eds.), *Education of the disadvantaged.* New York: Holt, Rinehart & Winston, 1967.

Sloggett, B. B. Classroom behavior modification of the rural Hawaiian adolescent as a function of group activities and reinforcement techniques. Unpublished master's thesis, University of Hawaii, 1968.

Smith, M. S., & Bissell, J. S. Report analysis: the impact of Head Start. *Harvard Educational Review,* 1970, **40,** 51–104.

Solkoff, N. Race of experimenter as a variable in research with children. *Developmental Psychology,* 1972, **7,** 70–75.

Spence, A. G., Mishra, S. P., & Ghizeil, S. Home language and performance on standardized tests. *Elementary School Journal,* 1971, **71,** 309–313.

Spence, J. T. Do material rewards enhance the performance of lower-class children? *Child Development,* 1971, **42,** 1461–1470.

Spindler, G. D., & Spindler, L. S. American Indian personality types and their sociocultural roots. In S. W. Webster (Ed.), *The disadvantaged learner: knowing, understanding and educating.* San Francisco: Chandler, 1966.

Staats, A. W. *Child learning intelligence, and personality: principles of a behavioral interaction approach.* New York: Harper & Row, 1971.

Stedman, J. M., & McKenzie, R. E. Family factors related to competence in young disadvantaged Mexican-American children. *Child Development,* 1971, **42,** 1602–1607.

Stewart, W. A. On the use of Negro dialect in the teaching of reading. In J. C. Baratz & R. W. Shuy (Eds.), *Teaching black children to read.* Washington, D.C.: Center for Applied Linguistics, 1969.

Stewart, W. A. Toward a history of American Negro dialect. In F. Williams (Ed.), *Language and poverty: perspectives on a theme.* Chicago: Markham, 1970.

Stodolsky, S. S., & Lesser, G. Learning patterns in the disadvantaged. *Harvard Educational Review,* 1967, **37,** 546–593.

Stumphauzer, J. S. Behavior modification with juvenile delinquents: a critical review. FCI Technical and Treatment Notes, Warden's Advisory Committee on Research of the Federal Correctional Institution, Tallahassee, Fla., 1968.

Super, D. E., & Crites, J. O. *Appraising vocational fitness.* (Rev. ed.) New York: Harper & Row, 1962.

Tarnopol, L. Delinquency and minimal brain dysfunction. *Journal of Learning Disabilities,* 1970, **3,** 200–207.

TenHouten, W. D. The black family: myth or reality. *Psychiatry,* 1970, **33,** 145–173.

Terrel, G., Jr., Durkin, K., & Wiesley, M. Social class and the nature of the incentive in discrimination learning. *Journal of Abnormal Social Psychology,* 1959, **59,** 270–272.

Thomas, A., Hertzig, M. E., Dryman, I., & Fernandez, P. Examiner effects in IQ testing of Puerto Rican working-class children. *American Journal of Orthopsychiatry,* 1971, **41,** 809–821.

Thomas, D. R. Oral language, sentence structure and vocabulary of kindergarten children living in low-socio-economic urban areas. *Dissertation Abstracts,* 1962, **23**(3), 104.

Torrance, E. P. Training teachers and leaders to recognize and acknowledge creative behavior among disadvantaged children. *Gifted Child Quarterly,* 1972, **16,** 3–10.

Tricott, E. J., Kelly, J. G., & Todd, D. M. Social environment of the high school: guidelines for individual change and organizational re-development. In S. Golann & C. Eisendorfer (Eds.), *Handbook of community psychology.* New York: Appleton, 1971.

Van Duyne, H. J., & Gutierrez, G. The regulatory function of language in bilingual children. *Journal of Educational Research,* 1972, **66,** 122–124.

U.S. Census Bureau and the Bureau of Labor Statistics. *The social and economic status of Negroes in the United States, 1970.* Washington, D.C.: U.S. Government Printing Office, 1970.

U.S. Commission on Civil Rights. *Racial isolation in the public schools.* Washington, D.C.: U.S. Government Printing Office, 1967.

U.S. Department of Health, Education, and Welfare. *Children served by public welfare agencies and voluntary child welfare agencies and institutions.* March, 1970. (Department of Health, Education, and Welfare Publication No. (SRS) 72-03258) Washington, D.C.: Center for Social Statistics, 1972.

Wachs, T. D., Uzgiris, I., & Hunt, J. McV. Cognitive development of infants of different age levels and from different environmental backgrounds. Paper presented at the biennial meeting of the Society for Research in Child Development, New York, 1967.

Wallach, M. A., & Martin, M. L. Effects of social class on children's motoric expression. *Developmental Psychology,* 1970, **3,** 106–113.

Wasik, B. H., & Wasik, J. L. Performance of culturally deprived children on the Concept Assessment Kit—Conservation. *Child Development*, 1971, **42**, 1586–1590.

Watson, P. I.Q.: the racial gap. *Psychology Today*, 1972, **6**, 48, 50, 97, 99.

Watt, N. F., Stolorow, R. D., Lubensky, A. W., & McClelland, D. C. School adjustment and behavior of children hospitalized for schizophrenia as adults. *American Journal of Orthopsychiatry*, 1970, **40**, 637–657.

Weener, P. D. Social dialect differences and the recall of spoken messages. *Journal of Educational Psychology*, 1969, **60**, 194–199.

Weikart, D. P. Preliminary results from a longitudinal study of disadvantaged preschool children. Paper presented at the annual international convention of the Council for Exceptional Children, St. Louis, Mo., 1967.

Weikart, D. P. Comparative study of three preschool curricula. Paper presented at the biennial meeting of the Society for Research in Child Development, Santa Monica, Calif., March 1969.

Weikart, D. P. Early childhood special education for intellectually subnormal and/or culturally different children. Paper presented at the National Leadership Institute in Early Childhood Development, Washington, D.C., October 1971.

Weiner, B., & Kukla, A. An attributional analysis of achievement motivation. *Journal of Personality and Social Psychology*, 1970, **15**, 1–20.

Westinghouse Learning Corporation. *The impact of Head Start: an evaluation of the Head Start experience on children's cognitive and affective development.* Athens: Westinghouse Learning Corporation, Ohio University, 1969.

Wheeler, L. R. A comparative study of the intelligence of East Tennessee mountain children. *Journal of Educational Psychology*, 1942, **33**, 321–334.

Wilcox, R. Racial differences in associative style. *Language and Speech*, 1971, **14**, 251–255.

Willerman, L. Biosocial influences on human development. *American Journal of Orthopsychiatry*, 1972, **42**, 452–462.

Williams, J. R., & Scott, R. B. Growth and development of Negro infants: IV. Motor development and its relationship to child rearing practices in two groups of Negro infants. *Child Development*, 1953, **24**, 103–131.

Williams, R. L., & Byars, H. Negro self-esteem in a transitional society. *Personnel and Guidance Journal*, 1968, **47**, 120–125.

Wilson, A. B. Class segregation and aspirations of youth. *American Sociological Review*, 1959, **24**, 836–845.

Yando, R., Zigler, E., & Gates, M. The influence of Negro and white teachers rated as effective or noneffective on the performance of Negro and white lower-class children. *Developmental Psychology*, 1971, **5**, 290–299.

Zigler, E., & Butterfield, E. Motivational aspects of changes in I.Q. test performance of culturally deprived nursery school children. *Child Development*, 1968, **39**, 1–14.

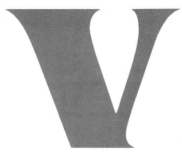

The intellectual extremes

When Sir Cyril Burt served as a consultant to the London County Council, he made a study of orphanage children. He found to his astonishment that, even when children had been admitted in early infancy and subjected to a uniform environment, individual differences in intelligence varied over an unusually wide range. In most cases differences were correlated with differences in the intelligence of one or both parents (Burt, 1954). Orphanage children of high intellectual ability turned out to be the illegitimate offspring of fathers of superior social or mental status who never acknowledged or cared for them.

A large literature on monozygotic twins reared apart reveals the influence which hereditary exerts on intelligence. Dobzhansky's (1964) review of 52 twin studies showed mean IQ intrapair correlations of 0.75 for identical twins reared apart, 0.53 for fraternal twins, and 0.23 for unrelated children brought up in the same foster homes or orphanages. The mean IQ correlation between foster children and foster parents was 0.12.

While there has been criticism of both Burt's and Dobzhansky's research methodology (Kamin, 1973) even if their figures are correct a correlation of 0.75 accounts for only 56 percent of the variability of differences in children's IQs. Other factors, therefore, account for a portion of these differences. In Chapter 9 we discussed environmental influences that influence IQ and in Part II the handicapping effect of brain disorders. In this part, we will discuss the extremes of intellect; these extremes, however, are the result of normal manifestations of the genetic pool in our population.

References

Burt, C. The inheritance of mental ability. *American Psychologist*, 1958, **13**, 1–15.

Dobzhanasky, T. *Heredity and the nature of man.* New York: Harcourt Brace Jovanovich, 1964.

Kamin, L. Intelligence, heredity, politics, and psychology. Paper presented at the annual meeting of the Eastern Psychological Association, Washington, D.C., May, 1973.

A dozen factors, among them genes, may enter into the making of a gifted child, but certainly appreciation is not to be overlooked. Traits and gifts that may wane or remain obscure under routine treatment will wax like the moon under perceptive recognition and kindness. It follows for all parents that a presumption of great ability could start a child toward the discovery of it in himself.

—Charles W. Ferguson

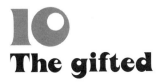

The gifted

Laymen usually use the word *gifted* to refer to especially talented individuals or to those who possess superior mental ability. Although some professionals use the word in much the same manner as the layman, others apply the term only to those who are creative thinkers, such as inventors scientists, or philosophers. It makes little difference to the layman which term is used because most would agree that individuals who make significant and original contributions to society possess unusual abilities. To the scientist, precise terms are more important because he seeks to identify abilities that are unique to the original thinker. Typically he administers a battery of tests to adults who have made original contributions in various fields in the hope of isolating the abilities possessed by these individuals. Do they display quantitative or qualitative differences from the average individual? Do they score higher on specially constructed tests or on intelligence tests? Experts in the field answer these questions differently.

As we will learn in this chapter, those who make significant and original contributions in their chosen field typically score high both on specially constructed tests and on intelligence tests, but there are exceptions. Intellectually superior adults often make insignificant contributions in their chosen vocations. Consequently, several investigators have chosen to ignore intellectual abilities. They concentrate their efforts instead on developing tests to identify the potentially creative individual, claiming that such efforts are necessary in order to identify early potentially creative children and provide them with every opportunity to develop their talents. These researchers use the term creative to denote those who possess particular thinking abilities. These abilities will be discussed later. As we will learn, however, the distinction between creative thinking abilities and those measured by intelligence tests is by no means clear.

In the present chapter we use the term *gifted* to mean the intellectually superior child, but will focus our discussion on the creative thinker because such individuals often are one and the same. We will introduce this topic by presenting the case of Peter.

TWO APPROACHES TO THE GIFTED CHILD

PETER

Mrs. Head was experiencing difficulty in refraining from acting upon her impulse to pick Peter up and give him a good shake. He was the most irritating child she'd ever had. "Been teaching fourth grade for ten years and never had one like him; he must come from some family!" Frequently, Peter just left his seat to avoid doing assignments. He would wander around the room until he found something that interested him. Interested him! Class was a place to learn and not a place to play. She'd be damned if she'd let Peter disrupt her class. "You sit down, young man, and do your lessons like the other children." Peter would protest feebly, but would eventually comply, at least for a while. "Young man, your writing needs considerable improvement and I suggest you get to it."

Sometimes Peter became so absorbed in tasks of his own choosing that nothing could distract him. This irritated Mrs. Head, and she considered taking away his free time. Why wouldn't he work as hard on projects that she assigned? She recalled a child evaluated by the school psychologist earlier in the year for whom contingency management had been recommended. Contingency management was a fancy name for an old gimmick of rewarding the child with a period of free play for his successful completion of a certain amount of assigned work. She guessed she'd better try this method with Peter; after all, the other children did their work, and she couldn't let Peter have free play without working or all the children might follow suit.

While contingency management was relatively successful, Mrs. Head still wasn't satisfied with Peter's progress. Perhaps she'd been too hard on him. After all, he was immature, perhaps even developmentally behind the other third grade children. Maybe his poor writing was the result of perceptual-motor immaturity and his high activity level the result of poor self-control. To validate these hunches, Mrs. Head referred Peter for psychological evaluation. She listed the behaviors leading to referral as wild ideas, immaturity, disobedience, inattention, and poor handwriting. She stated she had tried firmness and extra attention, followed by contingency management. She had not contacted Peter's parents nor could she judge Peter's relative standing among his peers. He enjoyed the attention he got from his antics, perhaps because he thought he'd make more friends by making them laugh. She had difficulty listing things Peter was good at. She finally put down his interest in nature and his curiosity. (She actually considered his questions a nuisance but felt she had to list several good traits or she might appear as if she really didn't know the boy.)

The psychologist didn't learn much from observing Peter in class, other than that Peter passively, and sometimes actively, avoided doing class assignments. One observation, however, did cause raised eyebrows. Under Peter's third grade workbook, hidden from Mrs. Head's view, was a book on science for children. Perhaps he simply looked at the pictures, but this observation certainly was worth mentioning. He asked Mrs. Head about the science book. Yes, she realized that Peter was excessively interested in science; she had confiscated several such books that he had been "reading" when supposed to be doing class work. She returned the books to him after he'd done a particular amount of schoolwork. If she let him, he'd read about science all day long and would fall behind in his other work. "Could he understand what he reads in the books?" asked the psychologist. "I suppose so," replied Mrs. Head. "Whenever we do have a science lesson, Peter seems to know a great deal." She went on to say that she considered intense interest in one thing as unhealthy. She'd read in Freud that intense interest in biology or science was disguised sexual curiosity. Maybe Peter was troubled and needed psychotherapy, but whatever the reason Peter didn't do his workbook exercises and often didn't read assigned materials.

The psychologist asked if she'd ever talked with Peter's previous teachers. She had not, primarily because his second grade teacher had left the system, his first grade teacher was in another building, and he had attended kindergarten in another school. In any case, his cumulative record revealed nothing outstanding, except that his first grade teacher considered him a sensitive and verbally skilled youngster. Mrs. Head responded to this judgment by claiming that she considered verbosity simply excessive talk, perhaps out of anxiety or need for attention.

The next day the psychologist gave Peter the Wide Range Achievement Test (WRAT) and the Weschler Intelligence Test for Children (WISC). On the WRAT Peter's spelling and mathematics scores were both at a fifth grade level. His reading was at a ninth grade level. The reading score was probably inflated because the test actually measures word pronunciation skills rather than reading per se. Peter was able to pronounce rapidly words he didn't know by sounding them out. The psychologist had several graded readers in his office and Peter read those at the sixth grade level without too much difficulty. On the WISC Peter received a verbal IQ of 140, a performance IQ of 130, and a full scale IQ of 137. His knowledge of abstract relationships among words was at a superior level, as was his word defining skill. The psychologist arranged for a conference with Mrs. Head and Peter's parents.

Both parents were aware that Peter was bright. They knew his vocabulary was large, that he could quickly master and recall factual material, and that he was a keen and alert observer. They felt his only problem was boredom in school. Peter told them that he was not interested in school because he already knew the material presented but had to do it anyway. The parents had seen his workbook and text material and agreed with him. Consequently, they attempted to make up for what they felt were the school's deficiencies. They took Peter to cultural events in the area and provided him with stimulating reading materials. Other parents of bright children had advised them not to pressure the teacher to tailor special programs for Peter unless the teacher first expressed an interest in doing so.

Throughout the conference Mrs. Head tried to impress upon Peter's parents that Peter was not completing his classroom assignments. There would be no "tailoring of programs" in her class until the child did his assigned work! She became annoyed when the psychologist reminded her that Peter was achieving at least three grade levels above his current grade placement and must be learning in spite of not completing assignments. Her last words at the conference were, "Make sure Peter does his homework assignments. Perhaps you can check them before he goes to bed."

Alone in his office, the psychologist recalled the week's events. First, Peter was referred for immature behavior and poor handwriting; second, he turned out to have an IQ higher than 99 percent of his peers, information that should have pleased his teacher since not many get the chance to tackle the challenge of an intellectually gifted child; third, the parent conference seemed to have ended in a stalemate, the teacher requiring Peter's participation in existing classroom activities before she would individualize his instruction and the parents insisting that the classroom activities were not meeting Peter's needs. The whole situation hadn't gone well; perhaps everyone would have been better off if Peter had not been tested at all.

Things went from bad to worse. Mrs. Head put more pressure on Peter to do the work assigned and seemed to take delight when he did not do well. She stopped the psychologist in the hall one day and said, "The results of the Iowa achievement scores just came in and Peter was only at the fifth grade level in reading, not ninth!" She seemed pleased that Peter might not be as bright as the psychologist and his parents thought he was. It was obvious that she would make no effort to devise an educational program commensurate with Peter's needs.

Since the school principal received copies of all psychoeducational reports, he knew of Peter's dilemma. In his periodic conferences with the psychologist, he inquired about Peter's current progress. After hearing the full story, he was annoyed but felt his hands were tied. He'd speak to Mrs. Head, but he believed in allowing his teachers the freedom to operate as they saw fit and felt pressure from him was uncalled for. The psychologist commented that outside pressure at this stage would only make it worse for Peter, and he suggested that the principal let the matter die. Perhaps he could transfer Peter to another class? The principal said he would not do so. If he did, parents would be on his back continually to transfer children simply because they didn't see eye-to-eye with their child's teacher. Children needed to learn to adjust to all sorts of people in their life rather than feel that people should adjust to them. No, Peter would remain where he was.

Negative teacher response to the gifted child

The psychologist was extremely frustrated and angered by the school's unwillingness to program for Peter, but he also wondered if he hadn't somehow contributed to this situation. In discussion with his supervisor they reviewed some of the basic principles of consultation. The first major principle was "taking the consultee" where he was at," and then, in small steps, leading him to "where he needed to go." Informing the teacher that Peter was gifted when she'd seen him as immature and maybe even a little backward, only served to create in her what some theorists would describe as a state of cognitive dissonance (Festinger, 1957).

Cognitive dissonance theory postulates that tension arises in an individual when a discrepancy exists between two or more cognitions that are in a relevant relation to each other and of equal importance. In this instance Mrs. Head believed herself to be a good teacher and knowledgeable about children. Yet, other data (Peter's behavior and the psychologist's findings) implied that both her teaching ability and judgment were poor. Cognitive dissonance can most easily be reduced by changing the original perception ("I guess I need more training in how to identify giftedness" or "Maybe it's not so important for Peter to be taught exactly the way I teach other children") or by denying the conflicting information (rejecting the findings that he is gifted or that he needs individualized instruction) and maximizing exposure in the future to information that agrees with the original position. When anxiety is extremely high, certain individuals are more likely to strengthen their original attitude rather than alter it (see Chapter 12).

The psychologist's supervisor felt that if the teacher had been informed gradually or had been helped to discover for herself Peter's giftedness, she might have been more willing to adapt her instruction to Peter's needs. Now it was too late. The only thing left was to help Peter's parents realize that their feelings about the school were jeopardizing Peter's adjustment. If they would encourage Peter to do his class assignments and reward him for doing so, his teacher might relate better to him.

Unlike Peter, the school psychologist would get another chance. Before the year's end, a number of underachieving children would be referred to him for evaluation. In some cases the teacher would realize the child was bright and would want to help to provide an appropriate educational program. In others the teacher would not be aware and would need help in recognizing the traits that accompany giftedness. What were the traits associated with giftedness that Peter displayed? Rereading the description of Peter reveals this list of behaviors: (1) marked absorption in tasks, (2) disinterest in the routine, for instance, practicing his handwriting, (3) high activity level, (4) unusual ideas, (5) marked curiosity, (6) intense interest in particular subjects, (7) large speaking vocabulary, (8) facile recall, (9) superior observational skill, and (10) marked sensitivity. Although all children display some of these behaviors, the presence of all of them in one individual identifies him as gifted (Arasteh, 1968).

CAN HE BELONG?

As far as a lot of public school teachers and administrators feel, the mentally gifted student is a big headache. I mean, little Johnny might be a nice little kid, but who wants to take the time to give him assignments he can really sink his teeth into? Or who wants to spend the time and money helping him with a project—or giving him the space and facilities to carry on his own independent study? There are also many people I know who would want to, but I've had a great deal of experience with the first type of people, whose opinions I've just described for them. Even the sincere teacher or administrator who wants to help Johnny usually can't do so because of the lack of funds, space, or facilities. We're all aware of the mental power of mentally gifted students, and also how lessons planned for average students don't seem to do much for them. Many a teacher is mystified at the student who seems instinctively to rebel against written assignments in favor of those he can think about or create with. The gifted student just doesn't belong in your average public school class. In all the schools I've attended and the many I've heard and read about, little Johnny can't create or try to be academically individual in many subjects because he might be chastised for it—for going against the grain, so to speak. Education ought be made fun and stimulating for little Johnny, but it is not. Johnny wants to do many worthy things, but is continually being held back by the inadequacy of the school he attends. What can we, as citizens and concerned sympathizers, do for Johnny and other gifted children like him with the same problems?

From J. A. Merritt. Project Discovery: educating the gifted. Paper presented at the U.S. Office of Education Western Regional Conference—Hearing for the Educational Needs of the Mentally Gifted, Los Angeles, December 1970. (Merritt is a preteen youngster.)

Peter had learned a great deal from his family and from his own astute observations, and, regardless of Mrs. Head's objections to his behavior, he achieved above grade level. Some children receive high IQ scores, but achieve below grade level (Fine, 1967). Teachers may feel more favorably disposed toward the underachiever since it is obvious he cannot learn without their help. Peter learned, but through his own methods rather than through his teacher's. The insecure teacher is threatened by learning independent of her efforts; because she is unsure of herself, the bright child offers a challenge with which she feels unable to cope. Jacobs (1971b) lists the traits displayed by the gifted, which he feels often cause the child to appear stubborn or immature: (1) less reliance on adults for approval, (2) less rigidity about absolute good and bad, (3) greater reliance on the self as an approver of actions, (4) greater capacity for emotional reactions and greater awareness of emotional interplays, and (5) greater sensitivity. Because of his keen sensitivity, the gifted child is often more aware than are other children of the negative and unjust reactions of adults. If the child points these out, the adult often reacts negatively to the child, a reaction that can lead to decreased utilization of the child's abilities.

The traits listed as characteristic of the gifted are those characterizing the abstract thinker. Creative children might be described as having an expansive learning style. As we will see when we discuss teacher personality traits and classroom atmosphere (Chapter 12), our traditional educational approach may not be suitable for gifted children.

Although Peter's teacher was made anxious by his presence in her classroom, other teachers are challenged by the gifted child and attempt to modify their instruction to suit his needs. Mrs. Miller is such a teacher.

STEVE

Mrs. Miller suspected that Steve was bright. He was not an underachiever for he enjoyed school and participated willingly in almost all classroom activity. While he was bored by many of the class assignments, he finished them quickly in order to pursue his own interests. Steve possessed a storehouse of information about a variety of topics and was interested in many adult topics, such as politics and religion. Sometimes his assertiveness and his tendency to dominate other children got him into trouble with his classmates, but, in general, he was well liked because he could be counted on to keep his promises and because he disliked bickering.

Nevertheless, Steve was hard for Mrs. Miller to teach. He displayed a high level of curiosity about many things, constantly asking questions about anything and everything. He offered unusual or unique solutions to problems, but solutions that usually could not be carried out in class.

He was very self-critical and would berate himself for a performance that other children could easily see was far superior to their own. In class discussions he frequently passed evaluative judgments on events when other children had not yet grasped the event's significance. If Steve had been in a sixth grade class, perhaps such behavior wouldn't matter, but in her third grade many of his actions confused or sidetracked the other children from their own tasks. While Steve was socially advanced for his age, he was already at a grade level one year above his chronological age. For this reason, further grade skipping was discouraged. Mrs. Miller asked the school psychologist if he could help her to tailor a more individualized program for Steve.

Evaluation

Formal tests to construct an individual profile   The psychologist did not need to test Steve's IQ to find out if he was bright; that was obvious. Steve displayed some of the behaviors observed in Peter and also others which are characteristic of gifted children: (1) rapid completion of assignments, (2) interest in topics which are usually the concern of older individuals, (3) tendency to dominate others, (4) trustworthiness, (5) distaste for dissension, (6) popularity, (7) high self-standards, (8) questioning attitude, and (9) judgmental attitude about information received (Arasteh, 1968; Gowan, 1971a; Kurtzman, 1967; MacKinnon, 1965; Weisberg & Springer, 1961).

In order to tailor an educational program for Steve, the psychologist needed more specific information about Steve's mental functioning. He decided to administer tests designed to measure performance on both intellectual and creative tasks. Mrs. Miller agreed to perform a number of informal evaluations in the classrooms, following the suggestions of Taylor (1964a). The formal and informal evaluations would give the psychologist and teacher the opportunity to see the interrelations between test performances as well as the relationship of test scores to classroom behavior.

From among the various tests designed to measure creativity, the psychologist selected the Torrance Tests of Creative Thinking (Torrance, 1966). These tests include items designed to measure sensitivity to problems, ability to redefine and restructure, fluency, flexibility, originality, and elaboration. The current test, the product of several revisions, consists of three nonverbal figural tasks (picture construction, picture completion, and repeated figures) and seven verbal tasks (ask questions, guess causes, guess consequences, product improvement, unusual uses, unusual questions, and imagine consequences.) Tests in the verbal battery are scored for fluency, flexibility, and originality, and those in the figural battery are scored for these qualities plus elaboration.

The nonverbal tests require the child to construct pictures from given materials, finish incomplete pictures, and reconstruct materials in novel ways. In the ask questions, guess causes, and guess consequences tests the child is shown a picture from a story (e.g., Tom the Piper's Son or other Mother Goose story) and asked to think of all the questions he can about what he sees in the picture, to guess as much as possible about the possible causes of the events depicted, and to give as many consequences, both immediate and long range, of the events depicted.

The unusual uses test includes items such as asking the child to think of as many uses as he can in a five-minute period for a tin can or toy dog, other than as a plaything (measure of ideational fluency and flexibility). Product improvement involves asking the child to think of ways to improve toys so as to make them more fun to play with.

Test results: Steve's abilities From the test results the psychologist was able to construct a profile of Steve's abilities. (The profile is determined by summing the subtest scores to obtain a total test score and then dividing the total by the number of subtests to obtain an average subtest score. Each subtest score is then compared to the average score and marked plus if greater than the average and minus if less.)

On the Torrance tests, Steve received the following scores:

Verbal tasks		**Figural tasks**	
verbal fluency	+	nonverbal fluency	−
flexibility	+	flexibility	+
originality	+	originality	−
		elaboration	−

On the Weschler tests:

Verbal tasks		**Performance tasks**	
information	+	picture completion	−
comprehension	+	picture arrangement	+
arithmetic	−	object assembly	−
similarities	+	block design	−
vocabulary	+	coding	−
digit span	−	mazes	+

Steve scored well above average on both intellectual and creative measures. The profile clearly revealed his greater ease and facility with verbal than with figural or perceptual-motor (performance IQ) materials. He also displayed relative inability in working out the details of an idea or planning the steps (elaboration). Compared with normative data, Steve's elaboration score was not much better than average. An educational enrichment program would, therefore, focus on developing creativity with figural materials as well as encouraging elaboration in all areas.

Informal evaluation procedures to identify the creative child After consultation with both the school psychologist and curriculum coordinator, Mrs. Miller agreed to incorporate certain exercises into her curriculum and to closely observe Steve's responses. She was excited about instituting these procedures, not only to help Steve, but because abilities of other children might also be revealed. It also meant the school approved of departure from standard curriculum and would support her in what she hoped would be a creative endeavor for her.

Over a two-week period Mrs. Miller provided her class with the following opportunities (after Taylor, 1964a).

1. They did more planning on their own and made most of their own decisions. She observed which children were the most independent and which had the most needs for training and experience in self-guidance.
2. They did exercises that required reporting of inner feelings and impulses as well as anticipation of correct courses of action.
3. They answered questions about issues the teacher considered too complex for most of her children to handle. She observed which students took a hopeful attitude and which felt solutions were impossible and that nothing can be done about them.
4. They had idea-generating sessions to see who had the most ideas, whose ideas brought out strong negative reactions in others, and who expressed the strongest negative reactions to others' ideas. She observed who had the most courage to maintain his views in the face of opposition and perhaps influence others to adopt his position.
5. They performed tasks done before but with most of the facilities previously available removed. She observed who was the most resourceful in accomplishing tasks without resource to the usual facilities.
6. Problems that required tolerance for ambiguity and uncertainty were presented.
7. Exercises from the idea books developed by Myers and Torrance (1965) and from the Image/Craft materials (Cunnington & Torrance, 1965, 1966) were given to all children and subjective impressions made regarding each child's approach to the materials.

Mrs. Miller was quite pleased with the results of these informal evaluation procedures because they uncovered several creative children. One youngster, Julie, did rather unusual work with figural materials. Mrs. Miller showed her work to a friend who taught art at a neighboring school. (She bypassed her school's art teacher because she felt that any art teacher whose major emphasis was on pasting different colored shapes on black paper or on coloring-in already prepared forms wouldn't know creativity if she saw it!) Her friend was particularly impressed by Mrs. Miller's description of the youngster's influence over other children.

Julie was markedly adept at discriminating among textures and colors. She could make abstract judgments about other children's art (not simple yes-no or good-bad statements) and could express how art objects made her feel. She would develop drawings around a single theme, for example, drawing a tree in a storm, a lonely tree surrounded by buildings, the same tree in a forest, a tree by a lake, a tree on a mountain, and even a tree growing up through a house. She would show each tree to other children and ask them how the tree felt about its existence. Eventually, the other children were expressing similar themes in their drawings. When a child became frustrated, "I have the picture in my mind, but I can't get it on the paper," Julie would try to get the child to realize that images in the mind are created in a different medium than those created by paints or brush. She would say, "The way it looks in your mind is not the way it will ever look on paper. Paintings are 'your invention.' If you want it to look just like in real life, you might just as well take its picture with a camera!" Yet Julie's verbal skills were not remarkable. Her grasp of the social significance of events was less than Steve's, as was her vocabulary usage. Her ability to elaborate in visual areas, however, was quite superior to Steve's.

IDEAS DEVELOPMENT

Q: How would you explain the approach you are using?

A: I think for one thing . . . our title indicates this by "Ideas Development Laboratory." We're interested in the kids' ideas and in their developing their own ideas. . . . We're always trying to find a nice balance between structure and the lack of structure. . . . The idea of coming in and saying you can do anything usually leads to chaos. And I think the other kind of thing leads to the children's disliking it and saying, "Why can't I do what I want to do." So we're always trying to strike a balance between these. We try to use an approach which allows for . . . psychological safety.

Q: Can you explain that?

A: Well, number one, that ideas can be spoken about and written about and you're not necessarily responsible to use these ideas. And, number two, we're not trying to—there isn't anything the child can say that the teacher is after. The only thing you can possibly do wrong here is *not* to have any ideas. Then we try to teach the idea that to get a few good ideas you have to have a great fluency of ideas. And we try to encourage this by mainly relying upon the students or getting the students involved rather than a lot of telling in this class. We use more discussion and stimulating and guiding the students.

From Ernest R. House, Joe M. Steele, and Thomas Kerins. *The gifted classroom.* Center for Instructional Research and Curriculum Evaluation. Urbana: University of Illinois, June 1971.

In addition to Julie and Steve, one other child was judged to be more creative than would have been predicted from his achievement. His strengths were revealed in figural and visual activities rather than in verbal activities. Mrs. Miller wondered whether his extreme shyness was responsible for his reluctance to participate in verbal activities; perhaps he was equally skilled verbally if she could "find the key to unlock" hidden skills.

Curriculum changes to enhance creativity

In consultation with the psychologist and curriculum coordinator, Mrs. Miller agreed to group children on the basis of similar profiles and then utilize some of the ideas presented in the Purdue Creative Thinking Program (Feldhusen, Treffinger, & Bahlke, 1970). Although the Purdue program is globally effective in fostering creative thinking (Covington, 1967; Olton, 1969; Thomas & Feldhusen, 1971), certain parts of the program are more effective than others in achieving particular ends (Thomas & Feldhusen, 1971).

The Purdue program was developed by the Purdue School of the Air. The series consists of a set of 28 audio tapes, each of which involves three or four activities. Each tape begins with the presentation of a principle that, if followed, would improve creative thinking. A story about a famous American is then presented. Activities concerning the story are designed so that the particular principle can be put into practice. For example, after listening to the presentation and the story, the children are asked questions such as, "Suppose you were George Washington. What would you have done when . . . ? How would you solve the problem which faced George?" If the principle is production of ideas, the children would be asked to write as many solutions as possible rather than looking for a correct one, since they are told it is good to produce a lot of ideas. In other instances, the children are asked to draw a picture of a scene from the story, to draw as many ideas as possible, to use colors, to draw with imagination, and then to title the picture drawn.

The school's curriculum library had the Purdue materials as well as several other canned programs. There was the Cunnington-Torrance (1966) Sounds and Images series on record, the Crutchfield-Covington (1965) and David-Houtman (1968) programmed materials, and the Myers-Torrance idea books (1965). Mrs. Miller listened to the various records. Although she could have borrowed these materials for use in her class, she preferred not to because of her personal distaste for canned programs. She felt she learned from having read and listened to the audio materials, but could easily incorporate the same principles into teacher-developed lessons. She therefore made up several stories about current figures known to most of the children and used this material in a fashion similar to the Purdue material. She did not bother presenting the principles or the brief lectures describing the various methods to think creatively, not only because of their relative ineffectiveness (Thomas & Feldhusen, 1971), but also because several children already displayed these behaviors and could be used as models to shape similar behaviors in others. Both she and the psychologist felt behavior shaping was a better method for behavior change than lectured persuasion. Very few unassertive and shy children change following a lecture on the merits of assertiveness; why should a lecture on creativity produce creative children?

Mrs. Miller also tried to adapt the activities for individual children in terms of their specific needs. For example, with Steve and others who were less developed in figural thinking, she emphasized activities that involved translating their verbal ideas into drawings. In order to strengthen Steve's elaboration ability, she impressed upon him the importance of carefully planning each step involved in the solution of problems.

Emphasis on reading   Reading is considered essential in any program for the gifted; it not only extends and satisfies interests but also may help the child in building an appropriate ideal of self (Witty, 1969). The teacher can direct the child to material that is relevant to his interests, needs, and personal situation. Steve was the oldest in his family and had two middle names. Mrs. Miller, therefore, asked him to read *Tikki Tikki Tembo* (Mosel, 1968), the story of what happened to a first-born child, first named by his father "Tikki tikki tembo-no sa rembo-cheri bari ruchi-pip peri pembo," that changed the old Chinese custom of giving first-born children long names.

For Julie, Mrs. Miller structured a program to develop verbal thinking and to increase vocabulary. She encouraged Julie to read books such as *My Tree* (Stark, 1969), a book which relates the remembered relationship of a child and her tree; *Fireflies* (Bollinger, 1970), a story of a large and beautiful firefly named Prosper; *Under a Mushroom* (Lobel, 1970), about a family who live under a mushroom; and *What Shall We Do and Allee Gallool* (Winn, 1970), which includes word-play songs. Mrs. Miller felt these books would have an immediate appeal for Julie because of their fine illustrations and would stimulate her interest and increase her vocabulary.

In class she encouraged Julie to respond more to "what happened pictures," a technique she used to get the children to express feelings (Aukerman, 1966). In this procedure a child is asked to guess what happened to cause an event depicted in pictures the child selected from magazines or drew himself.

Mrs. Miller felt she should concentrate on Julie's vocabulary development through formal instruction as well as through exposure to words in reading materials. However, her examination of materials designed to develop vocabulary led her to the same conclusions reached in the systematic survey of Petty, Harold, and Stoll (1968). Many of the materials they examined had one unfortunate characteristic in common; they were exceedingly dull and unimaginative. Very few provided even the crudest means of "creating in the pupil the capacity to react with enthusiasm, sensitivity and perception in all aspects of language" (Petty et al., 1968, p. 6).

Teachers surveyed by Petty and his colleagues were found to use a disproportionate amount of time having children look up words in the school dictionary. Using dictionaries is not only boring but frustrating to the child whose phonetic skills are limited or who speaks a nonstandard dialect. Looking up the word as he pronounces it only results in despair, as the word is never where he looks for it (Petty et al., 1968). A survey of superior readers revealed that they rarely look up unknown words in dictionaries; such interruptions spoil the pleasure in reading and result in loss of valuable time. Instead, these readers get a vague sense of the word from the context of the sentence and assume they will get a clearer understanding when they confront the word again in a slightly different context.

Mrs. Miller asked several of her colleagues if they knew of any direct ways to stimulate vocabulary development and yet maintain interest. From one teacher she learned about *Fun with Words* (Nurnberg, 1970), *Webster's Unafraid Dictionary* (Levinson, 1967), *The Left Handed Dictionary* (Levinson, 1968), *Perplexing Puzzles and Tantalizing Teasers* (Gardner, 1969), *Noah Riddle* (Bishop, 1970), *The Cat in the Hat Beginner Book Dictionary* (Eastman, 1964), and *Storybook Dictionary* (Scarry, 1969). She also learned that *The Gifted Child Quarterly*, a publication of the National Association of Gifted Children, frequently includes evaluative reviews of materials designed to stimulate vocabulary development as well as other academic skills (Pilon, 1971).

TESTING TO IDENTIFY THE GIFTED CHILD

Peter was viewed not only as an irritating child but also as rather backward, while Steve was immediately recognized as gifted. Julie and one other boy were not seen as gifted until after informal teacher evaluation.

If all teachers were as unperceptive as Mrs. Head, gifted children would go unrecognized. Mrs. Head considered a child gifted only when he achieved at above average levels on materials she assigned. Such achievement may or may not be an indication that a child is gifted. Children of average intellectual ability who have high needs for achievement can be overachievers, that is, they obtain high grades through diligent effort, particularly if the teacher emphasizes convergent thinking. And, as we have seen in Peter's case, gifted children may be underachievers. Emphasis on convergent thinking can obliterate differences between gifted and average children.

How perceptive are teachers in recognizing gifted children? Pegnato and Birch (1959) estimated that teachers are able to identify less than half of the gifted children in their classrooms. Other studies demonstrate even less ability (Baldwin, 1962; Holland, 1959; Jacobs, 1970, 1971a). In a sample of 654 kindergarten children, parents and teachers were asked to nominate children they believed to be gifted. Twenty-six parents felt their children were gifted, while the teachers nominated 44. The parents were correct in 16 cases (IQ >120); and the teachers were correct in only 2 (Jacobs, 1971a). Among the 654 children 19 had full scale IQs greater than 125 on the Wechsler Preschool-Primary Scale of Intelligence. Not one of these youngsters was identified by teachers as gifted (Jacobs, 1970).

Baldwin (1962) had teachers judge giftedness after six weeks and again after seven months of enrollment in kindergarten. After six weeks the teachers identified only 26 percent of the children who had Binet IQs greater than 130; after seven months 38 percent of these children were identified. Scores on the California Test of Mental Maturity, which agreed with Binet scores in 39 percent of the cases, were probably available prior to the second judgment and might account for the improvement.

The possibility that a child may develop a predisposition to underachieve is believed to be present when he enters school. The encouragement, approval, and guidance a child receives in his initial year of schooling may be the most critical prerequisite for future academic success. "The [kindergarten] teacher who identifies the gifted child easily is the teacher who observes children primarily in terms of their own purposes rather than in terms of the purposes of others. The gifted child in a teacher-centered kindergarten may appear to be a discipline problem" (Heffernan & Todd, 1960, p. 352).

Dissatisfaction with intelligence tests as measures of creativity

Because of the inability of teachers to identify creative children, a number of investigators have attempted to design tests that will identify these youngsters. Why didn't these investigators simply advocate greater use of individual intelligence tests to identify gifted children rather than developing new tests? Mainly because these particular investigators were dissatisfied with the notion that giftedness or creativity (the two terms are often used interchangeably) are synonymous with intellectual superiority. For a number of years, creativity was equated with intellectual giftedness. To be gifted meant to possess superior mental ability (Terman, 1925).

In 1921 Terman initiated a longitudinal study of 1528 children whose IQs ranged from 135 to 200. Children with an IQ in this range represent the top 1 percent of all school age children. Much of our knowledge about gifted individuals derives from studies of this group.

Witty (1953, 1971) took exception to equating giftedness with high IQ because he felt such a definition excludes children who are obviously talented in specific creative areas but are of only average intelligence.

THE DISBELIEVER

I am a staunch disbeliever in intelligence tests, and believe that intelligence cannot be accurately measured by using them. I am then advocating that new tests should and could be devised to accurately (or more so than now) measure intelligence. Supposing a lazy, listless, but very, very intelligent boy or girl lives in Watts, East Los Angeles, Harlem, or any ghetto area in any large city in the country. Due to the lack of testing, or of proper testing, maybe because of cultural barriers, this boy or girl who should be immediately brought to a Project Discovery campus (if such a thing existed), and would do quite well there, is thought to be of subaverage intelligence. Proper testing could show that this individual may be a genius, with his or her potential untapped. So you see that proper and effective testing is very important. I cannot, of course, suggest on improving tests or devising new ones, as I know very little about psychological and outright intelligence testing, but I do know that intelligence tests are often wrong about people and their intelligences, and for the Project Discovery program to function effectively, it needs an efficient and accurate testing system.

From J. A. Merritt. Project Discovery: educating the gifted. Paper presented at the U.S. Office of Education Western Regional Conference—Hearing for the Educational Needs of the Mentally Gifted, Los Angeles, December 1970.

In addition to Witty's dissatisfaction with the IQ, there are five other main reasons why investigators felt intellectual measures were not sufficient measures of creativity. Some are based more on opinion than on fact, while others have considerable empirical support. We shall examine the credibility of these five points later in the chapter.

1. Early studies of the gifted were limited to those whose measured IQ was in the superior range (Terman, 1925). Limiting the selection of the gifted to those with superior intelligence would result in failure to include approximately 70 percent of gifted children (Torrance, 1960, 1964).
2. Intelligence is only a partial predictor of later outstanding success (Cattell & Butcher, 1968).
3. Standard intelligence tests measure convergent thinking. The creative individual views things divergently (Isaacs, 1971d; Guilford, 1968).
4. Within groups of gifted children with IQs 130 and over, there are large differences in creativity.
5. Intelligence tests are not correlated with talented achievement outside of the classroom.

These five reasons, then, led the dissatisfied to develop tests to tap specifically creative abilities. However, to measure creativity, it first has to be defined. In what ways does it differ from intelligence, imagination, originality, curiosity, giftedness, and fantasy?

Creativity as process

Whether creativity is to be defined as a process or product constitutes a major issue in current research (Arasteh, 1968). Golann (1963) and Taylor (1964b) discuss this issue in depth. In general, studies of creativity in children have dealt with the process of creative development primarily because of difficulties in determining the degree of creativity expressed in a child's product. Products of adolescents and adults, however, have been studied and will be referred to in an effort to clarify findings with children. The emphasis on process also results from interests in identifying the potentially creative child in order to enhance his education.

The individual who has had the greatest influence on the study of creative process is Guilford. Guilford studied creative adults and is most noted for research on the structure of the intellect (Guilford, 1967). Guilford identified several abilities he considered essential to the creative process. Fluency is the ability to retrieve from memory storage in a short period of time a great many ideas relevant to a problem. The ideas do not need to be original or even workable; the ability to retrieve is the essential factor. Flexibility, the ability to shift direction and to change set when necessary, also was considered characteristic of the creative person. Originality, the ability to produce novel ideas, and the ability to analyze and synthesize were considered essential to the creative process. The ability to redefine tasks and the ability to understand at deeper levels were also considered basic skills.

Factor analytic (intercorrelational) studies of a variety of tests refined Guilford's initial impressions. The studies suggested that creative ability included sensitivity to problems and ability for elaborative thinking in addition to fluency, flexibility, originality, and redefinition ability, but did not necessarily include analyzing or synthesizing ability (Guilford, 1968). A redefinition ability was found in a test called Gestalt transformation. An item from this test is: Which of the following objects could most easily be adapted to making a needle? (a) rope, (b) onion, (c) fish, (d) cabbage, or (e) coin. The answer is (c) fish because the bone from a fish, given an eye, could serve as a needle. To answer correctly, the individual must redefine a fish, a swimming animal, into a source for needle-like objects.

Not one but four fluency factors were found: (1) recall of words to satisfy a spelling requirement, such as in a crossword puzzle; (2) recall of words or ideas to meet specifications of meaning, for example, thinking of substances that are solid yet flexible; (3) recall of words that bear some relation to another word, such as synonyms; and (4) ease of forming phrases or sentences (Guilford, 1968).*

Two factors of flexibility were found. One was called spontaneous flexibility, shifting from one class of ideas to another when test instructions could be satisfied without such a shift. The other was called adaptive flexibility, shifting to another class of ideas when such a shift is necessary in order to solve the problem (Guilford, 1968).

No factors identified as analyzing or synthesizing abilities were found. While analyzing and synthesizing abilities are involved in thinking, evidently they are situation-specific rather than generalized skills.

A factor involving the ability to understand at deeper levels was isolated, but was considered a cognitive rather than creative factor.

Because of the existence of separate factors within tests of creativity, Guilford (1968) believes that creativity is not a general trait and suspects that an individual who is creative in one area will not necessarily be creative in another. Nevertheless, considerable evidence exists that demonstrates that a child who is extremely talented in one area has the potential for development in other areas. Terman (1925), from among a population of over a quarter of a million, found only 20 specially talented children who did not have superior mental ability.

Tests to measure creativity

The Torrance tests   The Torrance Tests of Creativity follow Guilford's model of creativity. The tests were developed because of dissatisfaction with intelligence tests as measures of creativity, but do the Torrance tests actually measure traits that are independent of intelligence?

In some instances children who score high on the Torrance tests have IQs considerably below the average for their peers (some investigators use the term average loosely, however, sometimes labeling children with IQs of 120 as average). Torrance (1964) reported correlations ranging from 0.16 to 0.32 between creativity, as measured by the early versions of his tests, called the Minnesota Tests of Creative Thinking (MTCT), and intelligence as measured by group intelligence tests. The correlations were lower for girls than for boys and lower for selected (talented) groups. However, high scores on the Torrance tests were usually obtained by children with IQs of 115 or above. These findings support the idea that a substantial degree of intelligence is a necessary foundation for creativity but beyond that appears to be of no consequence. In addition, the creativity measures actually correlated higher with intelligence than with each other. While some studies support the notion that creativity

---

* Of incidental interest is the parallel between these four fluency factors and the hypotheses regarding various basic deficits in aphasia presented in Chapter 4. In fact, Head (1926) employed a system of classifying adult aphasics which included distinct disabilities not unlike the descriptions of the factors above.

scores do not correlate substantially with measured intelligence, other studies have reported rather substantial correlations between the MTCT and intelligence (Arasteh, 1968).

A second question is do the Torrance tests actually identify children who are creative better than intellectual measures do? Wodtke (1964, p. 408) states "In general, intelligence test scores predict performance on creativity and problem solving tests as well as, if not better than, the creative tests. There is no convincing evidence of independence and no evidence that intellectual measures do not contribute substantially to such predictions in unselected groups." A similar conclusion was reached by Yamamoto (1965).

In 1959 Torrance administered his test to 392 students in the University of Minnesota High School. The mean IQ of this group on the Lorge-Thorndike group intelligence test was 118 and their mean percentile mark on the Iowa Tests of Educational Development was 84 on national norms. A 12-year follow-up of 251 children from this group revealed that the creativity measures of fluency, flexibility, and originality were slightly better predictors of creative accomplishment than the group IQ score or achievement in high school. Creative achievement in writing, science, medicine, and leadership were better predicted by the creativity tests than were creative achievements in the arts, business, and industry (Torrance, 1972b).

Unfortunately, Torrance did not mention whether the 251 individuals who were followed could be considered representative of the total group of 392. For example, those who completed the questionnaire that revealed their creative accomplishments might have been a more highly motivated group. Those who failed to return the questionnaires or who could not be located may have been unmotivated. Equating for motivation would tend to increase the power of both intellectual and creativity measures to predict creative accomplishment.

The Wallach and Kogan tests   Wallach and Kogan (1965) developed a creative test battery based on Mednick's (1962) concept of associative flow. These investigators defined creativity as "the child's ability to generate unique and plentiful associations in a generally task appropriate manner and in a relatively playful context" (1965, p. 292). Their battery includes both verbal and visual tasks. Two of their subtests, alternative uses and instances and pattern meanings and line meanings, are quite similar to the Torrance test of unusual uses. In the alternative uses and instances test, a verbal task, the child is asked to give as many possible uses as he can for an object, such as a chair and a shoe, or to name as many things as he can that share a common feature, such as things with wheels. The pattern meanings and line meanings test, a visual task, requires the child to give as many alternative interpretations as possible to a series of abstract designs. The test responses are scored for number of associates only and not for uniqueness, since the number of ideas produced correlates higher with creative production than do the number of unique ideas.

Wallach and Kogan report high intercorrelations between their creativity measures and a low correlation between overall creativity and intelligence. Their tests have been used in the original and modified versions in studies with college students (Cropley & Maslany, 1968), with fifth graders (Pankove & Kogan, 1968), with second and third graders (Ward, 1968, 1969a), with kindergarteners (Biller, Singer, & Fullerton, 1969; Ward, 1968), and with nursery school children (Ward, 1969b). The tests correlated significantly with talented achievements outside the classroom in the areas of creative writing, science, art, and leadership (Wallach & Wing, 1969; Rotter, Langland, & Berger, 1972). (Table 10.1 gives correlations found in a group of 7-year old children.

While several other tests have been developed to measure creativity (Khatena, 1969; Schaefer, 1970b) and special scoring procedures have been used to analyze creativity in children's drawings (Griffiths, 1945) and on projective tests (Barron, 1963), the Torrance and the Wallach and Kogan tests appear to be the most promosing. The Torrance tests seem to be well suited to profiling differential strengths and weaknesses; Wallach and Kogan's test items, or similar tasks modeled on them, can be administered informally by the teacher.

Table 10.1 CORRELATIONS AMONG CREATIVE ABILITY, IQ TESTS, AND CREATIVE ACTIVITIES (N = 61)

Variable	1	2	3	4	5	6
1. Verbal creativity		.66†		—.14	—.12	—.14
2. Nonverbal creativity				—.03	.06	.02
3. Total creativity						
4. Language IQ					.53†	.84†
5. Nonlanguage IQ						.91†
6. Total IQ						
Creative writing and composition	.37†	.19	.28*	.02	—.09	—.04
Writing and reading	.29*	.26*	.30*	.11	.04	.08
Dramatics	.36†	.20	.29*	—.11	—.22	—.18
Life sciences	.28*	.15	.22	—.16	—.12	—.17
Games	.20	.06	.12	.22	.07	.15
Social studies	.07	.08	.08	.06	.13	.12
Physical science	.13	.03	.03	.11	—.01	.06
Arts and crafts	.14	.04	.08	.13	—.03	.05

* .05 level of significance.
† .01 level of significance.
From D. M. Rotter, L. Langland, & D. Berger. The validity of tests of creative thinking in seven-year-old children. *Gifted Child Quarterly*, 1971, **15**, 273–278, 296.

Which tests predict creative products?

We can now examine the evidence that bears on the validity of each of the five reasons given for rejecting intelligence tests as measures of creativity. Although Torrance claims that 70 percent of gifted children would be misclassified on the basis of IQ measures (point 1), there is no solid evidence to support this claim. Many children score high on the Torrance Tests of Creativity and low on IQ measures, but their high score on the Torrance tests does not necessarily mean they are all gifted. It simply means they score high on the test. Simply because Torrance defines his test as one that measures creativity does not mean *ipso facto* that it does so. There is a correlation between high scores on his test and creative acts, but the correlation is modest. More research is needed to substantiate that individuals who score high on Torrance's tests or on other tests of creativity, are potentially creative individuals.

Just as high IQ scores are only partial predictions of outstanding success (point 2), so are high scores on creativity tests.

Regarding point 3, that standard intelligence tests measure convergent thinking and that creative individuals think divergently, factor analytic studies of intellectual measures have not supported the notion that intelligence tests require primarily convergent thinking for successful performance. In addition, it is doubtful that individuals high in divergent thinking would be low in convergent thinking. More likely, intellectually gifted children are superior in both skills.

Isaacs (1971d) claimed that Terman's group included only a small number of creative people, primarily because of the measure of giftedness he employed. Bias rears its ugly head. No creative people in Terman's sample! Members of Terman's group have made outstanding contributions in the fields of science, music, literature, business, and the fine arts. Perhaps Isaacs based her statement on the finding that no truly great artist has yet to appear in Terman's group by midlife. Sample size alone could account for this occurrence. Terman studied only 1528 individuals drawn from a population of around a quarter of a million. Terman felt his findings demonstrated how rare real creativity is even in bright individuals, not that his tools were inappropriate.

There is substantial evidence that above certain IQ levels there are wide differences in creativity (Getzels & Jackson, 1962). Point 4 can, therefore, be accepted as valid.

Wallach and Wing's (1969) research supports the notion that creativity tests are better predictors of talented achievements outside the classroom than are intellectual measures, suggesting that point 5 can be tentatively accepted.

Although future refinements of creativity measures may establish them as entities independent from intellectual measures, their ultimate value depends not upon whether they correlate with intelligence, but upon the degree to which they predict actual creative achievements or products. Whether they predict as well as or better than intellectual measures remains to be determined. In all probability, future researchers will employ both intellectual and creativity measures in predictive studies. Differential weights can then be assigned to each measure and multiple correlation coefficients determined. (For example, IQ scores alone might correlate 0.50 with creative achievements and creativity tests alone correlate 0.30; together, however, they may correlate 0.60 with a criterion of creative achievement.)

EMOTIONAL ADJUSTMENT OF THE GIFTED CHILD

While every school psychologist could describe teachers like Mrs. Head who react negatively to gifted children, he could also describe many with Mrs. Miller's enthusiasm for the gifted. Nevertheless, a number of experts in the field of creativity state that the gifted child is subjected to considerable pressure to conform, resentment, and ridicule and is, therefore, likely to become emotionally maladjusted. Because the gifted child displays marked curiosity, persistence, purposefulness, and originality in ideas, he sometimes irritates adults. Some view him as disobedient or inattentive and often accuse him of being interested in all the wrong things (Ketcham, 1967).

Because the gifted child develops internal standards relatively early, he is less reliant upon teachers for approval. His greater capacity for emotional reactions, greater awareness of emotional interplay, and greater sensitivity can also act to his disadvantage. As we have seen, these traits may be perceived by some adults as stubborn or immature behavior and they respond to him in terms of this perception. Because the gifted child is sensitive to these unjustified and negative reactions, even when he knows his judgment is correct, he may respond by making less use of his ability or by developing a self-image that corresponds to the image of him held by others. In either case, the result can be a decrement in his performance.

Self-concept theorists postulate that a person acts in accordance with his concept of himself (Kelly, 1955; Rogers, 1961; Snygg & Combs, 1949). How will the student act if he is branded slow, lazy, or a behavior problem? He will behave as he sees himself, and if he is forced to see himself in this way because of ridicule from others or lack of intellectual challenge, then both the child and society suffer the consequences.

Torrance (1961, p. 18), states, "In no group thus far studied have we failed to find relatively clear evidence of the operation of pressures against the most creative members of the group, though they are far more severe in some classes than others." Isaacs (1971d) has even culled the Bible to support her notion that the gifted are frequently subjected to a great deal of hostility from others. From her experience as a consultant to schools, she cites cases where children have been mistreated because they are bright. She feels that hostility may even cause some gifted children to become intellectually retarded (Isaacs, 1971b). She stated that in some cases, if parents suggested to the school that their child was gifted, ways were discovered to "cut the child down to size" (Isaacs, 1971c).

Retrospective studies of gifted individuals seem to support the impressions of Torrance and Isaacs. Gibson (1962) wrote of the suffering that befell gifted men of medicine. Their scientific communities expressed hostility toward new ideas by rejecting the discoveries of these scientists and the scientists themselves. Staff positions were withdrawn and private practices boycotted. Maladjustment and loneliness are frequently portrayed in the retrospective description of creative individuals (Goertzel & Goertzel, 1962; Greenacre, 1958; MacKinnon, 1965; Rosner & Abt, 1970). In fact, Goertzel and Goertzel reported that three out of five in their study had serious school problems and that the majority were rejected by their classmates. Nevertheless, bias has a lot to do with the interpretation of findings. Careful examination of the writings published by the National Association for Gifted Children in *The Gifted Child Quarterly* reveals this bias. The articles published imply that our schools not only are unresponsive to the needs of creative children, but frequently hinder their growth through pressures toward conformity. Writers, as long ago as Plato, have often portrayed creative discoverers as alienated from a conformist culture. A number of current writers have portrayed classroom settings as places where children's natural creativity is transformed into group conformity and compliance to adult standards. In fact, teachers are said to prefer the intellectually gifted but rather conventional child over the gifted but creative one (Getzels & Jackson, 1962).

However, empirical studies of creative children contradict the subjective impressions of experts and the retrospective reports of creative adults. A review of these studies indicates that, compared to other children, the gifted display less maladjustment, less anxiety, less attitudinal rigidity, greater self-confidence and task persistence, stronger self-image, and more spontaneity and joy (Arasteh, 1968). Numerous studies relating creativity to self-actualization and mental health have reported positive correlations; Barron (1963) made such findings for writers; Blatt (1964) for scientists; and Drevdahl and Cattell (1958) for artists and writers.

Arasteh's (1968) review indicates the presence of a negative correlation between age and sociometric status of creative children, that is, they achieve high sociometric status in nursery school, but receive successively lower ratings as they get older. These studies, however, were cross-sectional rather than longitudinal, and their results may have reflected sampling error rather than real differences.

Creative adolescent boys are better accepted by their classmates than are creative girls (Kurtzman, 1967). Girls tend to perceive themselves as less acceptable to others even when the data does not support this self-concept (Schaefer, 1970a).

Walberg's (1969, 1971) research revealed that creative adolescents, identified by the winning of prizes and awards in the arts and sciences, were happily integrated into the social hierarchy of the school. In fact, they were even more deeply involved in school and other social activities than were other students. Other studies reveal the gifted's intense involvement in school and the influence of outstanding teachers upon their growth (Roe, 1953; Schaefer, 1970a).

Terman's 35-year follow-up of intellectually gifted individuals revealed that about 20 percent of the men did not attain the level of achievement he had predicted (Terman & Oden, 1959). After examining the family and childhood environments, Terman concluded that personality factors were largely responsible for the low achievement. Since 80 percent of those studied had achieved at levels commensurate with their ability, their school experience could not have been that harmful. Perhaps factors other than school are much more important in determining the life course of gifted children. In this vein, there is Bloom's (1964) review of longitudinal studies of the stability of human characteristics, which shows that half the variance of adult measured intelligence is predictable by age 4.

How do we reconcile the empirical findings with the retrospective reports of creative individuals who said that school had been a stifling experience for them or who recalled having school problems. One conjecture is that creative individuals may look back upon their school experience from an adult frame of reference and make judgments based on their current developmental needs rather than on those appropriate for children. For example, they may feel that structure and adherence to rules would be disadvantageous to them in their current role and, therefore, must have stifled them as children. Nevertheless, structure at that time may have been appropriate.

Another explanation is the possibility of a curvilinear relationship between creativity and social adjustment (Walberg, 1969). Individuals with moderate-to-high capacity for creativity may make a more favorable adjustment than those with the very lowest and very highest creative potential. Intensive study of children with IQs above 180 lends some support to this hypothesis. Because they play solitary games involving intellectual skills beyond those of their peers, they suffer a certain amount of isolation and are apt to be intolerant of others (Hollingworth, 1942).

Perhaps investigators have confused sensitivity with maladjustment.

Exceptionally bright and creative individuals may be more disturbed about the sufferings of others and may feel frustrated by their inability to make necessary changes in society. The level of aspiration of gifted children is also very high, leaving them dissatisfied with what they consider to be minor achievements. Their intense drives to achieve may leave them somewhat anxious and insecure, particularly in girls where conflict exists in autonomy-dependency and masculinity-feminity needs (Schaefer, 1970a).

The gifted are also believed to have greater difficulty in establishing their identity (Torrance, 1971c). Their greater reliance on internal standards may make them more reluctant than their less creative peers to accept externally imposed standards of values and life style. They seem to need time to wander and to obtain a variety of experiences in order to find themselves. The findings that creative adolescents have more post-high school job changes than their less creative peers (Torrance, 1971d) is not necessarily an indication of maladjustment, but perhaps more a reflection of this need to explore. Torrance equates their restless search with that portrayed in Alexander's (1967) fantasy, *Taran Wanderer*, the story of a youth who goes forth to come to grips with the truth about himself and to reshape his life out of his own inner resources.

Walberg's (1971, pp. 115-116) statement, which summarizes his findings regarding creativity and adjustment, aptly serves to conclude the present review.

Perhaps the incongruous image of the creator happily integrated into an institution of mass culture might be resolved by recognizing the genius of American society and institutions—their diversity and capacity to provide satisfying environments or subenvironments for high brows, middle brows, and low brows in many areas. . . . But society and the school have made places for its creative members. And while alienation and eccentricity, withdrawal and persecution, and poverty and suffering are sometimes realistically or romantically associated with creativity, they are apparently neither necessary nor sufficient conditions for its fruition.

FACTORS AFFECTING THE DEVELOPMENT OF CREATIVITY

Most researchers agree that at least above average intelligence (IQ >115) is a necessary prerequisite for creativity, but that increases in IQ beyond this level do not result in corresponding increases in creativity. What, then, accounts for differences in creativity among intellectually gifted children?

Family factors

In Chapter 7 we discussed how an autocratic child rearing approach could result in a rigid-inhibited learning style. Children with this style acquire factual information, but are considered poor problem solvers. In Chapter 9 we categorized parent-child interactions into those fostering cognitive development and those hindering such development. Although a preponderance of inhibiting styles was found among lower socioeconomic groups, all the styles were found within each socioeconomic group.

CAROL: AN EARLY READER

Caucasian girl; UM socioeconomic status; CA = 6.6; IQ = 161; initial reading grade = 2.8; terminal reading grade = 11.8.

Answers to interview questions indicated that Carol had been read to, by both mother and father, "since about the age of two." Carol's only sibling, a brother, had been four at that time. The mother commented that both children "loved to be read to," and that when she herself did the reading, she always tried to hold the book in such a way that the children could see the pictures. Carol, unlike her brother, was also interested in the words, and often asked her mother, "Where are you reading?" or "What word says that?"

The mother also recalled Carol's very special interest in *The Cat in the Hat*, a book both parents read to the children so often that "Carol practically memorized the whole thing." The mother believed this book in particular had done much to encourage her daughter's already great interest in the sounds of words. The mother mentioned that Carol could often be heard around the house "playing with sounds, and making up things that weren't even words."

Interview responses indicated it was not only while being read to by their parents that Carol and her brother spent time together. The mother said there were no children living on their block who were Carol's age, and so Carol often played with her brother and his friends. On days when the weather was inclement, the two children generally spent their time in a playroom. And, after the brother started first grade, the mother recalled, the playroom became a kind of classroom in which the six-year-old brother was the teacher and his four-year-old sister was the student.

From D. Durkin. *Children who read early.* New York: Teachers College, Columbia University Press, 1966, pp. 61–62.

The kind of home atmosphere, then, is probably as instrumental in fostering or hindering creative talents as it is in fostering intellectual development. Considering the current definition of creativity as the ability to produce and elaborate upon ideas, the type of home necessary to foster such skill would not be difficult to envision.

Witness the interchanges that took place in a store between mother and child and decide which interaction is conducive to the development of creativity.

Interchange one
MOTHER: Don't touch anything.
CHILD: Look at that thing over there!
MOTHER: Don't do anything. Just sit on this box.
CHILD: What's that, Mommy?
MOTHER: Don't ask so many questions!

Interchange two
CHILD: Mom, what's that?
MOTHER: A clothes pin.
CHILD: What's it for?
MOTHER: Some people don't have clothes dryers and hang their clothes on a line to dry in the sun.
CHILD: Suppose it's raining?
MOTHER: They hang them inside.
CHILD: Oh.

Interchange three
MOTHER: What do you suppose that is, son?
CHILD: I don't know.
MOTHER: Pick it up and examine it.
CHILD: Looks like some kind of a clip. It must hold something to something else.
MOTHER: Do you think its being made out of wood is an important clue to what it could hold?

In the first interaction the mother asked her child to eliminate his data gathering. She not only banned curiosity but inhibited capacity for communication. Other implications are that the child has nothing to communicate that would be of interest to the adult.

In the second interaction the mother is the source of all knowledge. When the child grows older and finds out his mother does not have all the answers, it may be too late for him to develop skills in problem solving. Perhaps he will look to others in authority for his answers, older peers, teachers, or soothsayers, but it is not likely that he will see himself as a source of knowledge.

In the third interaction the mother encouraged the child to develop his own powers of observation, inference, and logic so he can find solutions for himself. As the child grows older, his self-sufficiency may make him more difficult to manage than the child reared in the first or second home, but his contribution to society may be greater.

Turning to the research literature, parents of creative adolescents have been found to stress openness to experience, enthusiasm, and democratic decision making among family members. In contrast, parents of highly intellectual but not especially creative youth foster conformity, studiousness, and "good" behavior (Getzels & Jackson, 1961; Holland, 1961; Nichols, 1964).

Children with high scores on creativity tests come from families where parents fully express themselves, neither parent dominates the other, periodic regression in the child is tolerated, and the father functioned relatively independently in his chosen occupation. The parents stress individual divergence and expression of feelings more than parents of low scorers, and they involve children more in family activities. In addition, they use less coercive discipline, particularly of a physical nature, than do parents of low scorers (Dreyer & Wells, 1966; Ellenger, 1964; Weisberg & Springer, 1961).

The mother   Boys judged creative have mothers who encourage their interests and help them to assume varied responsibilities and to seek mature goals (Dyk & Witkin, 1965). Boys whose mothers are compulsive and who stress conformity have limited curiosity and are less creative (Dyk & Witkin, 1965; Weisberg & Springer, 1961).

Mothers of curious boys display more positive feeling, fewer restrictions, and less nonattention than do mothers of less curious boys. The mother's positive feelings correlate with the child's attentiveness and manipulation and with their own offering of information. The child's curiosity toward novel stimuli is also related to the mother's curiosity toward novel stimuli (Saxe & Stollack, 1971).

Retrospective reports of creative adults indicate that as children they had an unusual amount of freedom in making decisions and in exploring their environment, yet this freedom was in the context of definite standards of conduct and values (MacKinnon, 1965; Roe, 1953).

The father   While little research exists on the role of the father in the development of creativity, biographical sketches of eminent people suggest that the father is of decisive influence (Arasteh, 1968). Several experimental studies report a substantial relationship between the integrity of the father-child relationship and creative ability (Singer, 1961; Weisberg & Springer, 1961) and between identification with the father and problem solving ability (Milton, 1957).

In contrast, other clinical as well as retrospective studies suggest the presence of unresolved Oedipal conflicts in creative children and problems of identification with the father (Arasteh, 1968). Gifted architects (MacKinnon, 1965), as well as scientists, reported a distant relationship with their father. The scientists respected their fathers, but felt closer to their mothers (Roe, 1953). The girls in Schaefer's (1970a) study identified more with their fathers than mothers, but were emotionally independent of both parents.

In one stage of his thinking Gowan (1965) felt that Oedipal anxiety was of significant influence on later creativity. Closeness to the opposite-sex parent during this period, which corresponds to Erikson's initiative period, develops and strengthens the channel between the preconscious and conscious, a channel considered more open in creative adults (Kubie, 1958).

At this time, however, it is not clear whether the Oedipal conflicts are resolved by stronger identification or by increased competitive rivalry. In either case, the child could show more creativity. While future research may shed light on this question, psychoanalytic interpretations have a way of never being proved wrong since they always include the polar opposites of everything described (e.g. creativity is not only a product of the unconscious but also a product of synthetic organizing ego functions; a product not only of identification with the father but also of an effort to establish a unique identity).

Birth order Giftedness occurs more often in only or in first-born children than in younger siblings (Arasteh, 1968; Cutts & Moseley, 1954). Three-person families produce more winners in the annual Westinghouse Talent Search than any other size family.

Cutts and Moseley summarize the various hypotheses put forward to explain the higher incidence of giftedness and creativity among only children. If a sufficient interval occurs between the birth of children, these hypotheses could also apply to first-born children. First, IQ tests are based on the premise that language skills are a shorthand for higher thought processes. Since only children have more contact with adults than those in sibling groups, they acquire language more rapidly. Second, when there is a single child, parents have more time to encourage and give support to the child's activities. Third, in the absence of siblings the only child must invent ways to entertain himself. Such self-sufficiency and ingenuity become a strength throughout life. Fourth, being alone more, the only child learns to tolerate loneliness, a prerequisite for many solitary creative and intellectual ventures.

Lichtenwalner and Maxwell (1969) demonstrated the birth order effect across social classes, although middle class children are more creative than lower class regardless of birth position. In addition, parents of later-born children often are less concerned about their development, particularly those in lower class groups (Waldrop & Bell, 1964). Of incidental interest is the finding that the first-born child tends to adopt adult norms and values more readily than do his siblings. The child, therefore, may have strong drives to achieve irrespective of parental pressure. When only or first-born children display behavioral difficulties, they usually display those classified as neurotic disorders. In contrast, younger siblings tend to display impulse control disorders (Harris, 1961). When pressures become too great or levels of aspiration are placed too high, emotional distress is displayed in similar ways by children experiencing similar developmental patterns.

Cultural factors

Many writers believe that an authoritarian approach toward child raising adversely affects creativity. There is a great deal of evidence to support this assumption, evidence accumulated across different cultural and religious groups (Weyl, 1966; Weyl & Possony, 1963). Authoritarianism is often accompanied by limited environmental opportunity. In Chapter 9 data were presented suggesting that a large percentage of lower class mothers use appeal to authority as a disciplinary technique ("Do it this way because I say so!"). Exposed to such commands, lower class children would be expected to do poorly on measures of creativity. However, Torrance (1971b) reviewed twelve studies that examined racial and social class influences on creativity test scores and reported no differences due to social class or race. In fact, several studies found lower class children to exceed middle class children on figural measures of creativity. Torrance concluded that the life experiences of disadvantaged children better prepared them for creative achievement. Without expensive toys and play materials, the disadvantaged child learns to improvise with common materials. Torrance also believes that the large size and the life styles of disadvantaged families prepare children to participate more fully in group activities and to be more efficient problem solvers. In an indirect reference to black disadvantaged children, Torrance (1971b, p. 79) states, "The positive values placed by their families on music, rhythm, dance, body expressiveness, and humor keep alive abilities and sensibilities that tend to perish in more advantaged families."

There is no evidence that lower class families place greater emphasis on the values Torrance mentions. Although the popular cultural stereotype of the lower class black American conveys this image, little research exists to support such a stereotype. While study of the positive aspects of black American culture is certainly called for, there is no evidence to demonstrate racial differences in the values related to humor, music, and body expressiveness. The use of an unproven stereotype to explain racial differences in creativity seems unjustified. Iscoe and Pierce-Jones (1964, p. 796), in remarking about the apparent black superiority in divergent thinking tasks, conclude more sensibly, "The search for the types of experiences that foster originality in children, in a formal educational setting as well as in the environment at large, is a challenge that cannot be ignored."

Torrance's hypothesis regarding large families and creativity is directly contrary to the greater incidence of giftedness in first-born and only children. He implies that children from large families engage in more group play and, therefore, have a greater variety of children present upon whom to model their behavior. Only one published study reports that a significantly greater number of creative children have older siblings (Gowan, 1971a). Nevertheless, the high and low creative subjects used in this study were all selected from a large sample of intellectually gifted children, the majority of whom were from advantaged families where the relationship between birth order and creativity is less pronounced.

For a child to profit from play with other children, the other children must model creative behavior. If parents do not engage in creative or curious behavior or reinforce it in their children, the children are unlikely to display such behavior. The number of siblings a child has, therefore, is of no advantage if none display creative behavior and a disadvantage if they display behavior incompatible with creativity.

Children from large families who reside in urban areas often demand extra attention and affection from teachers. This seeking of extra attention to make up for emotional deprivation at home leaves less energy available for school activities and creative pursuits. These observations are consistent with Maslow's need hierarchy theory (Maslow, 1954, 1962). According to Maslow, man's needs are arranged in a hierarchy of priority. As those at one level are satisfied, those on the next level take precedence. Before one can satisfy needs for self-actualization or aesthetic experience, one must first have satisfied needs for belongingness, love, and self-esteem. The work of Barron (1963), Damm (1970), and others reviewed earlier supports this theory.

Although it is perhaps romantic to postulate the positives of ghetto living, the postulations don't square with current information. Nevertheless, Torrance does a great service by demonstrating that the potential for creativity is present in many children regardless of social class. That the disadvantaged rarely actualize this creativity is the real tragedy. Renzulli (1973) and Jordan (1974) suggest several strategies for identifying and maximizing the development of this understimulated segment of our school population.

Simplistic notions

Torrance (1971b) stated that the lack of expensive toys and play materials among disadvantaged children contributed to skill development in improvisation. While Torrance himself is aware of the multiplicity of factors that foster creativity, less sophisticated individuals often champion the cause of one uncritically accepted influence. Consequently, many people have said that mechanical toys destroy creativity. In actuality, the presence or absence of particular play materials in the home is probably insignificant. Children with a high predisposition toward fantasy elicit many fantasy themes from toys; children with a low predisposition elicit few. The amount of structure inherent in the toys makes little difference (Pulaski, 1970). Observation of children reveals that some make up a variety of ways to play with toys that were built for a singular purpose. The predisposition to use a variety of fantasy themes in play undoubtedly results from environmental factors previously reviewed.

Simplistic notions have always been popular in both lay and scientific circles. Research eventually dispels such notions. People once felt that comic books would produce a nation of delinquents or pornography a nation of sex perverts. The current interest in violence and television viewing falls into this category as do some of the treatment models mentioned throughout this text.

The idea that any one variable is all-important for creativity is exemplified by Lowenfeld's notion of the detrimental effects of coloring books. Lowenfeld (1956) stated, "A child, once conditioned to coloring books, will have difficulties in enjoying the freedom of creating. The dependency that such methods creates is devastating." His reasoning was as follows. As soon as a child is confronted with coloring a predetermined shape, he has been prevented from solving his own relationships creatively. In filling in the drawings, he is regimented into activity, that makes no provision for individual differences. "There is no opportunity for him to express his relationship and thus relieve himself of tensions of joy, hatred, or fear. There is no place in coloring books to express anxieties" (Lowenfeld, 1956). Lowenfeld goes on to explain that some children "by nature somewhat lazy" enjoy coloring books, but as they color they realize they could never draw the object colored as well as the one in the book. When asked to draw the object, they refuse to do so.

Ignoring the unscientific phrase "lazy by nature" and examining the implication of the second half of the paraphrased statement, we are led to believe that the child learns his relationships to reality only through comparisons of his products with those in coloring books. Observations of young children reveal that they try to draw what they see in both real life and in picture books and quickly learn that their drawings cannot duplicate reality—they don't need a coloring book to acquire that fact. More likely, coloring in coloring books has little relationship to artistic creation, and, even if some connection exists, its influence would be extremely minor compared to other variables.

Lowenfeld, like Torrance, probably would not put as much stress on a single variable as his article might imply. Nevertheless, the manner in which the article was written could result in uncritical acceptance by many readers. Parental attitudes, guidance, support, and example greatly outweigh any detrimental effects of mechanical toys or coloring books, no matter how intriguing such simplistic notions may sound.

Lowenfeld's notion of growth, however, parallels some currently popular ideas. This notion is that if children are left alone to shift for themselves, some kind of unfolding maturational process will occur that will automatically result in mastery and cultural achievement. There is no term to label this notion adequately, although terms associated with approaches based on it are permissive, unstructured, or child-centered.

These terms are often considered the polar opposites of structured, authoritarian, or adult-centered. However, structured, child-centered programs and unstructured, adult-centered programs are both possible. We have already mentioned that brain-injured, psychotic, and disadvantaged children do poorly in unstructured or child-directed activities. Although further discussion in Chapter 12 will help clarify these terms and relate them to empirical findings, the terms are still used unwisely.

This writer holds the view that the word structured should not be confused with the word authoritarian. Highly structured activities can be beneficial learning experiences depending upon the degree to which the child can create in such an atmosphere. For example, a teacher who places a piece of orange and black paper in front of each member of a fifth grade class and instructs them to draw a pumpkin for Halloween is not likely to develop individual creativity. On the other hand, the teacher who tells her first grade class to make anything they want for Halloween and then ignores them when they start running around the room is also not likely to foster creativity. In contrast, the teacher who places a variety of art supplies in front of each child, reminds them not to poke their neighbor but to work alone, and then circulates among them to encourage ideas is allowing for the actualization of individuality within a secure atmosphere. In addition, a child has to have certain basic skills before he can create. The teacher who required her class to make pumpkins might have been developing creativity had she been a kindergarten teacher.

CHILD DEVELOPMENT THEORY AND GIFTEDNESS

After reviewing the literature relating intellectual achievement and creativity to home atmosphere, creativity can be explained most readily within a social-learning theory that emphasizes imitation and social reinforcement. Research shows that creativity not only can be taught (Parnes & Brunelle, 1967) but can also be programmed (Reese & Parnes, 1970). These findings strengthen the social-learning theory's position. Until recently, social-learning explanations of creativity were overshadowed by Freudian explanations. The Freudian interpretation views creativity as the outcome of phallic thrust and mastery stemming from the narcissistic stage of psychosexual development; it is the product of repressed sexual or aggressive impulses and controlled regression to infantile modes of thought or experience, to thinking ungoverned by logical considerations (Schactel, 1959; Schneider, 1950).

However, psychoanalytic and social-learning theories are not mutually exclusive. In fact, one can complement the other. To explain creativity Gowan (1971b, 1972) presented an interesting theory that can be considered an integration of social-learning theory with the developmental theories of Erikson, Piaget, and Freud. He believes that creativity develops in Erikson's initiative stage (Piaget's intuitive, Freud's phallic) as a result of control over the environment facilitated through the affectional approach of the opposite-sex parent. During the initiative stage of child development (age 3½ to 6) the child is confronted with four interrelated tasks: (1) to learn whether to cope or defend (Bruner, 1966), (2) to learn the symbolic representation of experience (Bruner, 1966; Piaget, 1951), (3) to move along a continuum from adaptive to creative (Rank, 1932), and (4) to establish his preconscious (Kubie, 1958) or reorient his ego to reality (Piaget, 1951).

Although each of the four developmental tasks of the initiative stage is important, the learning of symbolic representation of experience is perhaps the most critical. When the child reaches symbolic representation, he can make his experience intellectually negotiable; he can describe and communicate it to others. By communciating his experience, he finds out that his experience is not unique but common to others and thus can be incorporated without fear into the "me" (Sullivan, 1953). This process is an important factor in how the child handles the first task. Reduction of fear and anxiety about his experience enable the child to continue learning; he can now cope and reach out for new experience rather than withdraw and defend against imaginary dangers. In addition, the child can now become involved in creative fantasy.

Mastery of symbolic representation of experience while still in the initiative period exposes the child to the creative possibilities of his preconscious at the same time that he has gained the ability to communicate experiences verbally. The intellectually gifted child reaches the level of symbolic representation earlier than the average. Therefore, a great deal of time in the initiative stage is devoted to the production and communication of verbal concepts that are highly influenced by fantasy. Such production is theorized to enhance the development of verbal creativity. Since the average child does not reach the stage of verbal fluency until he has passed through the stage of fantasy, his verbal production is more limited to concrete and activity-oriented concepts.

The bright child moves into the stage of industry or concrete operations (an object-oriented, affectively latent stage characterized by immersion in the world of the senses and busy activity) with a background of rich fantasy that can be used for better control over his environment and for more precise discriminations.* Such a background serves to enhance functioning at this stage and all subsequent stages. The average child, because of his later attainment of verbal fluency, lacks this background.

---

* The finding that creativity decreases during the last six months of kindergarten (age 5½ to 6½) lends some support to the notion that the stage of industry brings about more concern with external reality (Torrance, 1964).

Figure 10.1 graphically represents this theory. Chronological and mental age are represented by the horizontal and vertical axes respectively. Erikson's first four developmental stages are indicated in terms of the average chronological age at which they are achieved. The horizontal line in the graph represents the mental level of symbolic representation, which approximates reading readiness and is reached by the average child at about 6 years of age.

The diagonal representing the growth of the average child (IQ 100) intersects the horizontal at a mental age of 6 (IQ = MA/CA × 100). The diagonal representing the growth of the child with an IQ of 120 progresses at a sharper slope and reaches the level of symbolic representation at a chronological age of 5. (The child whose mental age is 6 when his chronological age is 5 would have an IQ of 120 (6/5 × 100). Such a child would gain 1.2 years of mental age for each chronological year.)

Parental encouragement, particularly by the opposite-sex parent, and an enriched environment is considered crucial during the initiative stage. If the child is reprimanded or discouraged by parental prohibitions, he may become docile and avoid behaviors that could bring negative consequences. Pankove and Kogan (1968) found a positive relationship between risk taking and creative ability in elementary school children, a finding that strengthens Gowan's position. Gowan's theory is

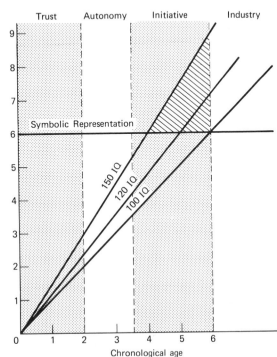

Figure 10.1 *Erikson's stages and creativity. (Adapted from J. C. Cowan. The development of the creative individual.* Gifted Child Quarterly, *1971,* **15,** *156-174.)*

explicitly stated in his latest book, *The Development of the Creative Individual* (Gowan, 1972).

SPECIAL PROVISIONS FOR THE GIFTED

Detailed discussion of individualization of instruction for gifted children is beyond the scope of this chapter. However the reader should get some idea of how the curricula can be enriched from the sketches and gifted briefs that appear throughout the chapter. Obviously, enrichment of the standard curriculum is the essence of such programs. Whether such enrichment is provided through individualized instruction within the regular classroom, in independent study, by acceleration, or through placement in special classes is left to the discretion of local school authorities. If no special provisions are made for the gifted, then frequently the classroom teacher has sole responsibility for the gifted child. His learning and perhaps his attitude toward school rest in her hands.

A variety of school programs have been tried to provide for the needs of the gifted. We will now turn to a discussion of the extent of these programs and their relative merits.

Throughout this text we have discussed the effect bias has upon the interpretation of data. Laird (1971) presented the results of a survey of the 50 states and concluded that very few provide for the gifted child. Questionnaires were sent to each state. If the state failed to reply to the questionnaire, Laird considered the state to have no programs for the gifted. Also, states reporting no legislative provisions for the gifted were classified in the same category. Nevertheless, articles have been written describing programs for the gifted in four of the twelve states that failed to reply to Laird's questionnaire. These states are California, Indiana, Kansas, and Tennessee. At least a dozen articles since 1960 have described programs in California (California State Department of Education, 1961; Durate Unified School District, 1964; Garlock, 1968; Hill, 1969; Martinson, 1960; Oakland Unified School District, 1963; Plowman, 1969; Plowman & Rice, 1967; Rice, 1970; Shore, 1962; Womack, 1963. Authors in Indiana (Gilfoy, 1958), Kansas (Ackerman, 1965), and Tennessee (Barbe, 1961) have published at least one paper during the same period.

Laird classified Colorado, Massachusetts, Minnesota, New Mexico, New York, North Dakota, Ohio, and Texas as having no programs for the gifted because there were no legislative provisions at the state level. Yet staff from various school districts within each of these states have written papers describing programs for the gifted: Roth (1967) in Colorado; Fredrickson and Rothney (1968) in Massachusetts; Hamm (1963) and the Twin City Institute for Talented Youth (1969) in Minnesota; Keeham and Mayhon (1963) in New Mexico; Mathisen and Smaltz (1961) and York (1961) in North Dakota; New York State Education Department

(1964) in New York; Barbe (1961), Gloss (1969), Horn (1963), and Scarvelis (1969) in Ohio; and Hall (1961) and Herring (1962) in Texas.

GIFTED BRIEF: PLANS AND PRODUCTS

Activity objectives. To encourage imaginative speculation; to foster appreciation for the value of problem solving and a methodological approach to it.

Major skills employed. Evaluation, convergent thinking, divergent thinking, hypothesis generation and testing.

Materials and/or equipment. Library resources, appropriate resource experts.

Procedures. After studying and discussing a variety of inventions and plans developed to aid man, the teacher encourages students to speculate upon the many undeveloped but needed products and ideas. There may be no imposed limits or the speculation might center around a single parameter only, e.g., environment improvers, field games, productive employment of waste materials, etc. Pupils work individually and/or in groups determining priorities of need, present potential for a solution, and interest in solving a particular problem. When a needed product or plan is decided upon, students prepare specific plans of attack, and where possible test them.

Activity modes

Individual   Students work independently on same problem. Analysis is made of the several approaches.

Small group   Hold competition among groups to determine best problem solving plans. Where appropriate invite an outside expert to serve as judge.

Class   A community need is determined. Class develops a plan of solution, seeks community and official endorsement, and implements plan of action.

Illustration. Class decides that senior citizens are generally ignored in their community. Ways of involving them in more activities and a plan for more complete utilization of their skills is developed.

Variation. Using a science fiction approach, students describe the development of a very exotic product or plan. Either a dramatic or literary format may be employed in making presentation.

From M. J. Gold. Introducing the gifted brief. *Exceptional Children*, 1971, **37**, 593–596. Reprinted with permission of The Council for Exceptional Children.

Two of the oldest special class programs for the gifted began in Ohio and in New York, the Major Work Program in Cleveland in 1922 and the Speyer School (Public School 500) in New York City. Hollingworth's (1938) early research with Speyer School students formed the basis for many decisions regarding the gifted. New York not only provides special enrichment classes in many public schools but also has special programs in separate schools for the gifted. Although these programs are not extensive, Laird's (1971, p. 216) conclusion that "it is evident that academically gifted students are now being grossly neglected" must be accepted with caution. Laird supports the idea of special classes for gifted children and interprets his data in light of this bias. It does not follow that lack of state support for special classes or failure to respond to his questionnaire means that there are no programs for the gifted in those states. While many people are in sympathy with the view that more should be done for the gifted, they would question the value of surveys that distort facts to make a point. If the point is worth making, perhaps a better approach would be to emphasize the successful programs within the various states and to emphasize the development of more of these programs. A recent report to the U.S. Congress (U.S. Office of Education, 1972) has taken that tack. Grouping the gifted in self-contained classes may not be the best approach. Research, not opinion, is needed to answer that question. As we have seen throughout this book, education is inundated with opinion rather than fact and to base educational programs on opinion can result in considerable waste of time and money, not to mention talent. We will now examine various approaches to educating gifted children: acceleration, early school entrance, enriched instruction in the regular classroom, and special grouping.

Acceleration

In the past the majority of identified gifted children whose initial school achievement was outstanding were advanced through school faster by skipping grades. This procedure has certain drawbacks; the differences in social, emotional, and physical status between the gifted child and his chronologically older classmates may make his adjustment in class more difficult. In addition, he may miss certain basic fundamentals, the lack of which go unnoticed.

GIFTED BRIEF: CHARACTER SWITCH

Activity objectives. To understand the interdependency of literary plot and characters; also among characters.

Major skills employed. Evaluation, convergent thinking.

Materials and/or equipment. Appropriate reading materials.

Procedures. This exercise attempts to assess the possible effects of replacing the personality of one character in literature with the personality of another. The effects may include likely variations in story line and resultant changes in other characters' personalities and actions. The pupils are assigned two readings. After determining that they are quite familiar with both plots and with the basic personalities of the major characters in both readings—novels, short stories, plays, poems may all be employed—the teacher suggests a character substitution. The students then speculate on changes that might come about.

Activity modes

Individual   Rewrite appropriate passage of a given piece of literature in light of the character switch.

Small group   Dramatize one section of the original story; then improvise the same scene as affected by character switch.

Class   Critique the accuracy of the several individual and small group activities.

Illustration. Substitute Kipling's *Elephant Child* for Dr. Seuss' *Horton.*

Variations

1. What would happen if a particular character were eliminated from a story?
2. Imagine that a character chose an alternate action to the one he actually followed.

From M. J. Gold. Introducing the gifted brief. *Exceptional Children*, 1971, **37**, 593–596. Reprinted with permission of The Council for Exceptional Children.

Perhaps the major disadvantage of grade acceleration is that advanced grades may place no more emphasis on developing divergent thinking skills and problem solving abilities than the earlier grades, perhaps even less. For example, accelerating a child from the second to the fourth grade could result in his being in a less creative atmosphere. Torrance (1963, 1968, 1969a) demonstrated what he called a "fourth grade slump" in creativity. He initially attributed this decrease to the school environment. Gifted children themselves pointed out that in the fourth grade they began to sit in straight rows with their feet on the floor and that classroom activity became more organized with papers expected to be neat. Teachers also relate to them in a more controlling fashion at the fourth grade level (Giammatteo, 1963).

Children entering fourth grade are emerging from the juvenile era to preadolescence, a stage where there is growing concern for consensual validation by one's peers and suppression of individuality (Sullivan, 1953). Evidence suggests that the slump is perhaps also due to the increasing concerns by fourth graders for consensual validation of their ideas. Concern about what others think is likely to reduce originality of expression and decrease the output of ideas and questions (Torrance, 1971a).*

* An interesting phenomenon that coincides with this slump is an upsurge in the proportion of children receiving psychological services in the fourth grade (Hosford, 1967). Torrance attributes these referrals to both classroom climate and peer pressures. A more likely explanation, however, is that the demands for independent reading skill increase markedly at this time and that children are referred because of reading difficulties that exacerbate behavioral problems.

There is also a definite shift in responsibility for arousing interest in school from the student to the teacher as higher educational levels are reached. Younger students display greater personal initiative and inherent motivation, while older students assume the teacher's duty is to make them learn (Frymier, 1964).

Although carefully planned grade skipping has proved beneficial, most educators would concede that it is the least desirable method of enriching the gifted child's educational experience (Gallagher, 1967). When acceleration is employed, boys seem to experience more difficulties in adjustment (Weinstein, 1966), and, if done at the secondary level, acceleration runs the risk of student attrition. In one study accelerated high school students performed no better than matched controls and a greater number dropped out of school (Adler, Pass, & Wright, 1963).

Researchers have been publishing studies of accelerated children since 1936 (Witkins, 1936), but there are still no answers to many questions regarding acceleration. For example, would there be better achievement by a nonaccelerated group placed in a special class than in an accelerated group?

One of the advantages of acceleration is that the child can enter college earlier. Other more specialized forms of acceleration, which require grouping of accelerated students, allow students to complete five years of curriculum in four or even two years in one. College credits can be obtained in high school, allowing the student to enter college with advanced standing. Nevertheless, acceleration implies that there exists some delineated body of knowledge that a child needs to acquire, and that the bright child should be allowed to acquire that knowledge faster so he can enter the world of work at an earlier date. In contrast, if school is considered a place where children can explore interests, develop talents, learn problem solving skills, and become more effective thinkers, acceleration may be less important.

Early school entrance

A second alternative is to allow the gifted child to enter school a year early, particularly since research indicates that the arbitrary chronological age limits now used by school systems do not coincide with new teaching techniques nor with the wide range of individual differences in children of 5.

Many favor early school entrance over grade skipping. Gifted children who start school early have higher achievement and better social acceptance at the end of the primary grades than nongifted children in the same class. Early school entrance, however, requires psychoeducational screening of preschool children in order to identify the gifted, and individual screening adds to the cost of the educational program. Ahr (1967a, 1967b) has developed a testing procedure to reduce this cost. He uses a preschool group test to identify potential candidates for early admission.

From these candidates children are selected for early admission who perform at a superior level (IQ > 120) on the Stanford-Binet Intelligence Scale and who perform at a kindergarten level on the Wide Range Achievement Test and the Goodenough Draw-a-Man Test. Ahr estimates that the cost of group screening combined with individual testing is about half the cost of individual testing alone and is equally effective.

GIFTED BRIEF: CHANCE-A-DATE

Activity objectives. To develop research skills; to develop the ability to make "educated guesses."

Major skills employed. Convergent thinking, evaluation, extrapolation.

Materials and/or equipment. Pair of dice, library resources.

Procedures. The pupil is given a pair of dice which he employs to determine a date that he will either research or speculate on, depending on whether it is pre- or post-1971. First roll one die to determine the number of digits in the dates. Then the student rolls both dice the number of times that there are digits in the date. (When 6 appears on one die it equals 0; 5 + 5 = 0). After the date is developed, a final roll of a single die determines whether it is B.C. or A.D.: An even value is B.C., an odd, A.D. The child is then assigned or chooses topic on which he works. Topics may include food, war, democracy, disease, homes, population distribution, etc.

Activity modes

Individual	Pre-1971—research paper; post-1971—creative writing exercise.
Small group	Pre-1971—dramatization; post-1971—panel of "experts" discuss topic.
Class	Develop a one day newspaper covering a variety of topics appropriate for the date chosen.

Illustration. First roll of one die (4) signifies 4-digit number; next roll 5 and 1; then 2 and 6; then add 3 and 3; finally 5 and 5. Date is 6260. One more roll of die produces even number. Therefore the date of the topic is 6260 B.C.

Variation. By developing a master topic list of subjects appropriate for a particular group, chance selection of a topic in addition to chance selection of a date can add to the "game" quality of the activity.

From M. J. Gold. Introducing the gifted brief. *Exceptional Children*, 1971, **37**, 593–596. Reprinted with permission of The Council for Exceptional Children.

His expenditures for selecting 17 children for early school entrance from among 90 applicants were only $559. Follow-up of 77 children selected over a seven-year period indicated that the academic achievement scores of these early entrants surpassed those of their older classmates. Teacher ratings of their social, emotional, and physical and motor development were average when compared with similar ratings of their classmates. Nevertheless, unless research is done to compare children entering school early with those entering at the normal time and then accelerated, many schools are unlikely to develop screening procedures.

Enriched instruction in the regular classroom

Enrichment of the regular class experience is the most widely accepted approach to educating the gifted. Unfortunately, it is probably the easiest to give lip service to. The classroom teacher has the major responsibility to supplement and enrich the educational experience of the gifted and creative children in her class. Since many teachers feel their efforts are judged by their class's scores on achievements tests, they may have no incentive to individualize instruction. To provide enriched experiences means departure from standardized materials and grade level workbooks, as well as special preparation; most teachers have little time for their regular preparation. Even if motivated, teachers often do not have a curriculum library to give them guidance in teaching exceptional children, nor are there resource personnel available to provide them with motivation, materials, and ideas.

The classroom teacher must be able to identify gifted children in order to provide for them; failure to identify automatically means failure to modify instruction. We have already seen that teachers are not always capable of identifying gifted children. Even more discouraging than studies of teachers' skills at identification was the finding of the U.S. Office of Education's 1969–1970 survey where 57.5 percent of schools surveyed reported having no gifted pupils (U.S. Office of Education, 1972)!

GIFTED BRIEF: PROVERBS

Activity objectives. To develop an ability to analyze proverbs; to appreciate the effectiveness of nondirect statements; to add to a feel for language.

Major skills employed. Analysis, translation, synthesis.

Materials and/or equipment. Dictionary, thesaurus.

Procedures. Following an analysis of standard proverbs, stimulus statements are presented to students. Utilizing a dictionary and/or thesaurus, the students attempt to generate their own proverbs from such stimulus phrases as: Love is better than hate; It pays to cooperate; Certain things should not be tolerated; There are many worthwhile things to do in life.

Activity modes
Individual   Develop as many proverbs from stimulus statements as possible within 30-minute period.

Small group	Groups compete attempting to develop many proverbs from a single stimulus.
Class	Teacher offers a stimulus statement. The student who generates the first proverb offers the next one. Continue for 30 minutes. The class attempts to compete with itself over time by keeping track of the number of quality proverbs generated each session.

Illustration. Stimulus: "There are differences among people that should be respected"; Generated proverb: "Bread is baked in all manner of ovens."

Variations
1. Pupil develops his own stimulus statement and matching proverb.
2. Students are asked to translate common proverbs.
3. Students translate each other's proverbs to determine how near the proverbs come to the stimulus statements.

From M. J. Gold. Introducing the gifted brief. *Exceptional Children*, 1971, **37**, 593–596. Reprinted with permission of The Council for Exceptional Children.

The appropriateness of regular kindergarten curricula for the gifted has also been questioned by experts in giftedness. For example, New Jersey's ban against teaching reading in kindergarten is cited as an example of a questionable practice (Laird, 1968). A survey of 180 kindergarten teachers judged by their school superintendents to be superior teachers revealed that over half reported they were not teaching reading (How top teachers teach, 1967). Yet, in Terman's studies, nearly half of the gifted learned to read before starting school (Terman & Oden, 1947). Some kindergarten age children even read at a fourth grade level (Durkin, 1966).

What does a teacher do in a kindergarten where children vary tremendously in ability? Pretend they're all equal! The National Education Association (1963) made a rather absurd statement when they stated that the spread of average achievement in an elementary school class slightly exceeds the number of the grade level, that is, the spread is more than three years in the third grade, four in the fourth grade, etc. By backward extension, then, the spread must be two in the second grade, one in the first, and zero in kindergarten!

Enrichment in the regular classroom has a nice democratic appeal. Educators stress that, "This procedure permits children of varying abilities to work and play together, to share goals and plans, and to experience achievement through the utilization of each individual's particular abilities" (Scheifele, 1953, p. 45). "Both gifted and average children profit from being in the same class, so studies have shown" (Henry, 1958, p. 202). What studies? A survey of the literature failed to turn up any well-designed study that demonstrated positive gains displayed by normal and gifted children when grouped together as opposed to their being grouped separately. In addition, published reports of enrichment in heterogeneous classes are relatively few (Dunlap, 1967). Studies have described gifted independent study after school (Witt, 1971) or during school hours (Bennett, Blanning, Boissiere, Chang, & Collins, 1971), but these special programs are not usually taught by the child's regular class teacher.

Enrichment that is not enrichment but is merely extra work can actually be a hazard. Isaacs (1971a) cites a case where the so-called enrichment program for one gifted child included helping the art teacher, doing library research for the English teacher, being the contact person for the teacher and the audiovisual aids department, teaching a second grade class when their regular teacher was absent and the substitute had not yet arrived, giving extra science reports, and coming to school early to study French. These activities, as unrelated to real enrichment as they were, might have been more bearable had the student at least been told she was doing these things because she was gifted.

GIFTED BRIEF: PROXIMITY

Activity objectives. To see verbal relationships; to work cooperatively and competitively.

Major skills employed. Convergent thinking, divergent thinking, evaluation.

Materials and/or equipment. Paper, pencils, stopwatch.

Procedures. "Proximity" is an exercise that fosters the relating of one place and/or person and/or thing and/or fact to another. Starting with only one cue term, the student, individually or in a group, adds a related term. Working against a specified amount of time, additional terms are added singly. This continues until time is exhausted. "Proximity" is effective with bright children from grade 3 through high school. (Older students will find it most intriguing when played around a particular theme, e.g., Spanish vocabulary, chemical relationships, ancient Greece.)

Activity modes
Individual   Child builds his own "chain," keeps record to compete with himself over time.
Small group   Competing teams have 5 minutes to prepare lists. Longest without error wins.
Class   Children called at random add items to list.

Illustration. "New York" (cue), "New Amsterdam," "Holland," "Edam cheese," "milk," "cow," "jersey," "sweater," etc.

Variations
1. Go in as few steps possible from the cue to an unrelated terminus word.
2. Work from the cue term back to itself without repeating any item.

From M. J. Gold. Introducing the gifted brief. *Exceptional Children*, 1971, **37**, 593–596 Reprinted with permission of The Council for Exceptional Children.

Special grouping

Merritt (1970), the preteen youngster quoted in Sketches 1 and 3 in this chapter, has designed what he considers the ultimate in grouping for the gifted. Merritt presented his ideas at the U.S. Office of Education Western Regional Conference—Hearing for the Educational Needs of the Mentally Gifted. He advocated that a special school should be built for the gifted. This school would operate as a public institution supported by public funds contributed by school systems throughout the United States, and all gifted students, up to the school's capacity, would be enrolled regardless of socioeconomic background. Merritt, aware that this undertaking is an unlikely possibility, has drafted several other plans for special grouping of the gifted.

Merritt reflects the opinion of many gifted youngsters as well as the thinking of the National Association of Gifted Children. Dunlap (1967) remarked that bright children often recognize their own needs to be in special classes with children like themselves and to "study the things they need to know." Several school systems do have "honor schools" for the gifted within the school system, but these are currently limited to students at the high school level. If special grouping takes place at the elementary level, such grouping occurs in the regular school setting.

NO ONE TELLS YOU!

If you are gifted, hardly anyone ever tells it to you outright. You have to figure it out on your own. And maybe you are coming up with a conclusion, that even those in authority and/or superior teachers have not stopped to realize applies to you. Often it is a seemingly minor, side remark which is most important for you to grasp and hold dear. It is an insight that can be terribly revealing. Yet given in so casual a manner that it can be easily overlooked. The remark may even be one which the speaker did not intend as a compliment or of particular value, and may instead have even been said as a joke.

Statement by a gifted child. Cited in A. F. Isaacs. Being gifted is a bed of roses, with the thorns included. *Gifted Child Quarterly*, 1971, **15**, 54–56.

Grouping can vary from a few hours a week to five full days each week. The most popular type is part-time grouping, where students are grouped homogeneously for academic subjects and regrouped heterogeneously for special subjects such as art, music, home economics, and physical education. Many such programs are described in the references cited during the discussion of Laird's (1971) survey. Dunlap (1967) and the U.S. Office of Education (1972) describe the type of content emphasized in many of these classes.

Studies on the effectiveness of grouping give contradictory results.

Dunlap (1967) concluded from his survey that unless ability grouping is accompanied by substantial changes in program content, it is of little value. However, when appropriate curriculum modifications are introduced, the gifted can profit from ability grouping (Martinson, 1960). Table 10.2 compares a sample of classes for the gifted child with classes for the average.

In Chapter 9 we discussed how ability grouping handicaps the child from disadvantaged communities and in Chapter 11 how special classes may handicap the retarded. What is beneficial to some, therefore, is harmful to others, leading to considerable criticism of ability grouping (Bjork, 1968). Considering the needs of all children, exceptional and

Table 10.2 COMPARISON OF CLASSES FOR THE GIFTED AND THE AVERAGE

Average	Gifted
1. Most classes emphasize few (two or less) thought processes.*	Most classes emphasize many (three or more) thought processes.
2. Most classes emphasize only one (if any) of the higher thought processes.	Most classes emphasize two or more of the higher thought processes.
3. As a total group, classes emphasize three of the seven levels of thinking: translation, interpretation, analysis.	As a total group, classes emphasize six of the seven levels of thinking: translation, interpretation, application, analysis, synthesis, evaluation (memory was not emphasized)
4. The teacher talks almost all the time in over half the classes; few teachers talk less than half the time.	The teacher talks almost all the time in two out of five classes; in one out of five classes, however, the teacher talks less than half the time.
5. Students in two out of five classes have the opportunity for and participate in discussion.	Students in almost all classes have the opportunity for and participate in discussion.
6. Students in one out of four classes feel a heavy stress on tests and grades.	Students in one out of five classes feel a heavy stress on tests and grades; however, another fifth of the classes feel no pressure of this kind.
7. There is an absence of enthusiasm in over half of the classes.	The presence of enthusiasm characterizes two out of three classes.
8. There is opportunity for independence in one out of four classes.	There is opportunity for independence in almost three out of four classes.
9. Students in most classes spend between one and two hours per week preparing for class.	Students in most classes spend more than two hours per week preparing for class.

* Lower thought processes: memory, translation, interpretation; higher thought processes: application, analysis, synthesis, evaluation.

Adapted from Ernest R. House, Joe M. Steele, and Thomas Kerins. *The gifted classroom.* Center for Instructional Research and Curriculum Evaluation. Urbana: University of Illinois, June 1971.

GIFTED BRIEF: TIME MACHINE

Activity objectives. To gain appreciation of the effect of individual personalities on history; to gain insights into the complexity and possible solutions of modern problems.

Major skills employed. Analysis, evaluation, synthesis.

Materials and/or equipment. Supportive source material.

Procedures. The "Time Machine" transports a figure of the past to the present in an attempt to solve a particularly disturbing modern problem. Generally this figure should be someone whose work, background, and attitudes have prepared him to solve the specified problem. After analyzing the character's experiences related to the topic itself, the student is encouraged to draw inferences as to how a figure of the past might handle a modern problem.

Activity modes

Individual   Researching a character and topic; writing a report, play, or diary entry.

Small group   Panel discussion; dramatization of steps leading to a solution.

Class   In committees, children explore the appropriateness of one of several historical figures who could handle the problem. Class makes a decision as to the most appropriate character.

Illustration. Theodore Roosevelt is charged with solving modern ecological problems.

Variations

1. Have a leading figure of the present transported back in time.
2. Have this same character sent into the future.

From M. J. Gold. Introducing the gifted brief. *Exceptional Children*, 1971, **37**, 593–596. Reprinted with permission of The Council for Exceptional Children.

average, many educators are currently advocating individualized instruction within a nongraded curriculum (Brown, 1965). In any case, it is safe to say that the gifted are being neglected in the vast majority of school systems (U.S. Office of Education, 1972). Such neglect can mean that many are not functioning up to their potential and could be classified as underachievers.

THEY TEACH EACH OTHER

Usually at the beginning of the year you will see a group of anywhere from five to ten being taught by a group of two to three other students who have previously investigated topics that center around books and pamphlets used as prime resource materials in the Amherst Series. Last week we were in the library doing research on topics which we are now presenting. You might have seen a tape or two in one of the other small groups, although usually I get them out of the room into another area where they can listen to a tape that fits in with their discussion. Aside from that and debates that might occur in the small groups you might see individual reading or individual research by some students. Some students may be in the library doing research or on independent study, although it's really not independent study because they will have their own aim in mind. It's independent for the group; it's not independent for the individual. You might see anything that goes on in a gifted classroom aside from anything that's teacher directed or teacher dominated.

From Ernest R. House, Joe M. Steele, and Thomas Kerins. *The gifted classroom.* Center for Instructional Research and Curriculum Evaluation. Urbana: University of Illinois, June, 1971.

UNDERACHIEVEMENT IN GIFTED CHILDREN

Estimates concerning the number of underachieving children are high; one of every four youngsters is reportedly a year and a half below grade level (Fine, 1967). Approximately 50 percent of boys and 25 percent of girls of above average ability could be classified as underachievers. The underachievement of boys becomes manifest in the early grades, while in girls not until junior or senior high school (Zilli, 1971). However, "years below grade level" may not be a good index of underachievement because the formula: (1) operates in an irregular manner, (2) gives a picture difficult to distinguish from normal variation, and (3) causes under-achievement to become larger as years of school increase (Ullmann, 1969).

A statewide survey of Iowa high school students with IQs of 120 or above indicated that 17.6 percent of this group had dropped out of school (Green, 1962). This figure probably represents a better estimate of under-achievement than those provided by others. However, a drop-out is not necessarily an underachiever. One youngster who dropped out of the Philadelphia school system did so to make a submarine for exploration. Clearly, he had not achieved in school, but his eventual achievement was greater than that of the entire faculty of his school—his submarine actually worked!

Although the National Association for Gifted Children implies that improper education is responsible for underachievement, other influences are probably much more important. Both Chapter 7 and 9 discuss environmental influences that contribute substantially to underachievement.

HOW DO THEY FARE?

There was a time when people believed that gifted and creative children developed into peculiar or alienated adults, but Terman's longitudinal studies showed clearly that gifted children fared better in society than did children with average ability. Some were relatively unsuccessful, but the unsuccessful had revealed at the time of the original study personality characteristics related to lack of success independent of mental ability—emotional instability, lack of perseverance, lack of self-confidence, and social maladjustment.

What about children who score high on specific tests of creativity? Do they differ in adulthood from those with similar IQ scores but low scores on measures of creativity? Torrance (1972a, 1972b) presented data from a 12-year follow-up of 116 women and 135 men tested with the Minnesota Tests of Creative Thinking in 1959 when they were between the ages of 13 and 18. The correlation between total MTCT scores and a combination of creative achievement criteria was 0.59 for boys and 0.46 for girls, giving some credence to the belief that women are less predictable than men. One reason for the lower correlation is that, among women, number of children is negatively related both to quantity and quality of creative achievements, as well as creativeness of aspirations. Among men, number of children is negatively related only to quality of creative achievement and creativeness of aspirations.

Of interest was a near zero correlation between IQ and quantity of creative achievements for women in contrast to the low but positive correlation between these two variables for men. Among women with above

GOALS

Q. What kinds of things do you do in class?

Diane: We write stories and just creative things . . . like say we were just having an assignment given to us—which is crisper: winter or celery? —you have to do things like that. We do Junior Great Books. We read them and he asks us questions. And if somebody objects to one of the answers, then they can just butt in and say anything about it—if they don't agree.

Paul: We write poetry, and right now I'm writing a book, an autobiography. Not everybody is doing this—we picked what we wanted to write. We're giving reports to the class. We pick a subject and we give five minute reports. And we're just having fun. We brainstorm.

Q: Are the activities different from regular classroom activities?

Paul: Yes, sure. For instance, I was in our reading class before IDL [Ideas Development Laboratory] and in reading we were told to read stories and answer questions, do work sheets, and it's different in IDL. . . . There's freedom of speech; you don't have to be as formal as you would usually be in the classroom. . . . I think we learn a lot from all of these things that I know we wouldn't learn if we were in reading. When we write compositions, I'm more inclined to use more imagination than I do in other classes. The teacher in other classes will say, "All right, write a story or poem about fish," and you have 15 minutes to write it and you don't get much done. But in IDL you can make your own choice. . . . We can think about what we're going to do and get ideas from our teacher.

From Ernest R. House, Joe M. Steele, and Thomas Kerins. *The gifted classroom.* Center for Instructional Research and Curriculum Evaluation. Urbana: University of Illinois, June, 1971.

---

average intelligence (mean for this sample was 122), measured IQ was a poor predictor of quantity of creative achievement. For quality of creative achievement, IQ was as good a predictor for men as were creativity scores; for women creativity scores were slightly better predictors of quality than were IQ scores. Unfortunately, Torrance did not present a multiple correlation of IQ and creativity scores with the creativity criteria. The extent to which predictability is increased by employing creativity scores in addition to intelligence scores is still unanswered!

The total sample was divided at the median on the combined MTCT scores obtained in 1959 to form a high- and low-creative group. The higher creative individuals more frequently reported their highest attainments in writing, creating educational materials, medical and surgical discovery, dissertation research, human relations and organization, and musical composition. The lower creative group more frequently reported their highest achievements in family, child rearing, and marriage accomplishments. Civic projects, editorial and advertising, writing, teaching, visual arts, and fashion and costume design were reported with equal frequency by the two groups (Torrance, 1972a, 1972b).

An earlier follow-up study (Torrance, 1969b) of high and low scorers on the MTCT revealed that a major difference between the two groups lay in their degree of satisfaction with present accomplishments. The high scores expressed significantly greater creative aspiration than the low scorers, who seemed satisfied with their present achievements and personal functioning. Torrance expects, therefore, that the differences between high and low MTCT scorers will become increasingly greater with passing years. While most of us don't look forward to getting older, perhaps the creative may be the exception!

CONCLUDING REMARKS

Merritt, the gifted youngster whose statements have appeared throughout this chapter, makes the following remark about public school education for the gifted (Merritt, 1970).

Most schools today offer little challenge to the demanding minds of the mentally gifted. Insofar as the elementary and secondary schools are concerned, there is little time for expression of creativity or for expanding one's knowledge past the curriculum. This certainly does not help the gifted, as they soon realize that what may be challenging and sometimes entertaining for the average in intelligence is far too easy and grossly boring to them. The gifted mind, once stimulated, usually has an unquenchable thirst for knowledge and, I'm sorry to say, the average school cannot aid these students, and even worse doesn't provide the stimuli that gets a mind to wondering, questioning and voluntarily learning. Thus, many of the gifted are virtually untapped as far as intellectual potential and achievement. Those who wish to expand their knowledge cannot rely on the public schools to aid them, as these institutions are curriculum-geared to serve mainly the average (although there are many remedial programs for the mentally and culturally deprived).

In general, Merritt's conclusions concur with those of the U.S. Office of Education (1972, p. 23).

Research studies of special needs of the gifted and talented demonstrate the need for special programs. Contrary to widespread belief, these students cannot ordinarily excel without assistance. . . . A good program for the gifted increases their involvement and interest in learning through the reduction of the irrelevant and redundant. These statements do not imply in any way a "track system" for the gifted and talented.

Nevertheless, long-term follow-up of gifted individuals, with perhaps women and the economically disadvantaged being the exceptions, indicate that the majority actualize their potential. Although a number of studies suggest that perhaps 25 percent fail to do so, this failure may be due to reasons other than poor educational programs. In addition, the researchers of this generation often hold the opinion that failure to complete college implies underdeveloped talent. The next generation may not feel that college attendance is a necessary prerequisite for creative development. Future studies may cast more light on these questions.

References

Ackerman, P. R. *Demonstration of the significance of a consultant-teacher for the gifted to a small rural secondary school.* Topeka: Kansas State Department of Public Instruction, 1965.

Adler, M. J., Pass, L. E., & Wright, E. N. A study of the effects of an acceleration programme in Toronto Secondary Schools. *Ontario Journal of Educational Research*, 1963, **6**, 1–22.

Ahr, A. E. The development of a group preschool screening test for early school entrance potentiality. *Psychology in the Schools*, 1967a, **4**, 59–63.

Ahr, A. E. Early school admission: one district's experience. *Elementary School Journal*, 1967b, **67**, 231–236.

Alexander, L. *Taran wanderer.* New York: Holt, Rinehart & Winston, 1967.

Arasteh, J. D. Creativity and related processes in the young child. *Journal of Genetic Psychology*, 1968, **112**, 77–108.

Aukerman, R. C. A dynamic new approach to developing thinking, speaking and writing. *Journal of the Reading Specialist*, 1966, **2**, 64–69.

Baldwin, J. W. The relationship between teacher-judged giftedness, a group intelligence test and an individual intelligence test with possible gifted kindergarten pupils. *Gifted Child Quarterly*, 1962, **6**, 153–156.

Barbe, W. B. *Educating tomorrow's leaders.* Columbus, Ohio: State Board of Education, 1961.

Barron, F. *Creativity and psychological health.* New York: Van Nostrand, 1963.

Bennett, F., Blanning, J., Boissiere, M., Chang, S., & Collins, W. Potentially gifted and talented high school youth benefit from independent study. *Gifted Child Quarterly*, 1971, **15**, 96–108.

Biller, H. B., Singer, D. L., & Fullerton, M. Sex-role development and creative potential in kindergarten-age boys. *Developmental Psychology*, 1969, **3**, 291–296.

Bishop, A. H. *Noah riddle?* Pictures by J. Warshaw. Chicago: Whitman, 1970.

Bjork, V. B. Down with ability grouping. *Grade Teacher*, 1968, **85**, 128–130.

Blatt, S. J. An attempt to define mental health. *Journal of Consulting Psychology*, 1964, **28**, 146–153.

Bloom, B. S. *Stability and change in human characteristics.* New York: Wiley, 1964.

Bollinger, M. *The fireflies.* Pictures by Jiri Trnka. New York: Atheneum, 1970.

Brown, B. F. *The appropriate placement school: a sophisticated nongraded curriculum.* West Nyack, N.Y.: Parker, 1965.

Bruner, J. S. *Toward a theory of instruction.* Cambridge, Mass.: Harvard University Press, 1966.

California State Department of Education. *Educational program for gifted pupils. A report to the California Legislature.* Sacramento: California State Printing Office, 1961.

Cattell, R. B., & Butcher, H. J. *The prediction of achievement and creativity.* New York: Bobbs-Merrill, 1968,

Covington, M. V. Some experimental evidence on teaching for creative understanding. *The Reading Teacher*, 1967, **20**, 390–396.

Cropley, A. J., & Maslany, G. W. Reliability and factorial validity of the Wallach-Kogan Creativity Tests. *British Journal of Psychology*, 1968, **60**, 395–398.

Crutchfield, R. S., & Covington, M. V. Programmed instruction and creativity. *Programmed Instruction*, 1965, **4**, 1–2, 8–10.

Cunnington, B. F., & Torrance, E. P. *Image/Craft Production.* Boston: Ginn, 1965.

Cunnington, B. F., & Torrance, E. P. *Sounds and images.* Boston: Ginn, 1966.

Cutts, N. E., & Moseley, N. *The only child: a guide for parents and teachers.* New York: Putnam, 1954.

Damm, V. J. Creativity and intelligence: research implications for equal emphasis in high school. *Exceptional Children*, 1970, **36**, 565–569.

David, G. S., & Houtman, S. E. *Thinking creatively.* Madison: Center for Cognitive Learning, University of Wisconsin, 1968.

Drevdahl, J. E., & Cattell, R. B. Personality and creativity in artists and writers. *Journal of Clinical Psychology*, 1958, **14**, 107–111.

Dreyer, A. S., & Wells, M. B. Parental values, parental control, and creativity in young children. *Journal of Marriage and Family*, 1966, **28**, 83–88.

Dunlap, J. M. The education of children with high mental ability. In W. M.

Cruickshank & G. O. Johnson (Eds.), *Education of exceptional children and youth*, Englewood Cliffs, N.J.: Prentice-Hall, 1967.

Durate United School District. *Program for children with high achievement potential.* Durate, Calif.: Durate Unified School District, 1964.

Durkin, D. *Children who read early.* New York: Teachers College, Columbia University Press, 1966.

Dyk, R. B., & Witkin, H. A. Family experiences related to the development of differentiation in children. *Child Development*, 1965, **36**, 21–56.

Eastman, P. D. *The cat in the hat beginner book dictionary.* New York: Random House, 1964.

Ellenger, B. The home environment and the creative thinking abilities of children. Unpublished doctoral dissertation, Ohio State University, 1964.

Feldhusen, J. F., Treffinger, D. J., & Bahlke, S. J. Developing creative thinking: the Purdue Creative Thinking Program. *Journal of Creative Behavior*, 1970, **4**, 85–90.

Festinger, L. *A theory of cognitive dissonance.* Stanford: Stanford University Press, 1957.

Fine, B. *Underachievers.* New York: Dutton, 1967.

Fredrickson, R. H., & Rothney, J. W. Statewide implementation of classroom practices for superior students. *Exceptional Children*, 1968, **35**, 135–140.

Frymier, J. Study of students' motivation to do good work in school. *Journal of Educational Research*, 1964, **57**, 239–244.

Gallagher, J. J. *The gifted child in the elementary school.* Washington, D.C.: National Education Association, 1967.

Gardner, M. *Perplexing puzzles and tantalizing teasers.* Illustrated by L. Kubinyi. New York: Simon & Schuster, 1969.

Garlock, J. C. Multiple criterion for including pupils in a gifted program based on trivariate distribution. *California Journal of Educational Research*, 1968, **19**, 87–94.

Getzels, J. W., & Jackson, P. W. Family environment and cognitive style: a study of the sources of highly intelligent and of highly creative adolescents. *American Sociological Review*, 1961, **26**, 351–359.

Getzels, J. W., & Jackson, P. W. *Creativity and intelligence.* New York: Wiley, 1962.

Giammatteo, M. C. Interaction patterns of elementary teachers, using the Minnesota categories of interaction analysis. Unpublished doctoral dissertation, University of Pittsburgh, 1963.

Gibson, W. C. Contributions of the gifted to scientific medicine. *Gifted Child Quarterly*, 1962, **6**, 130–138.

Gilfoy, L. W. Educating the most able high school students at Indianapolis. *Education*, 1958, **79**, 25–27.

Gloss, G. G., et al., *Sputnik plus ten; Ohio's program for the gifted 1957–1967.* Columbus: Ohio State Department of Education, 1969.

Goertzel, V., & Goertzel, M. G. *Cradles of eminence.* Boston: Little, Brown, 1962.

Golann, S. E. Psychological study of creativity. *Psychological Bulletin*, 1963, **60**, 548–565.

Gowan, J. C. What makes a gifted child creative? *Gifted Child Quarterly*, 1965, **9**, 3–6.

Gowan, J. C. Why some gifted children become creative. *Gifted Child Quarterly*, 1971a, **15**, 13–18, 35.

Gowan, J. C. The development of the creative individual. *Gifted Child Quarterly*, 1971b, **15**, 156–174.

Gowan, J. C. *The development of the creative individual.* San Diego, Calif.: Knapp, 1972.

Green, D. A. A study of talented high school drop-outs. *Vocational Guidance Quarterly,* 1962, **10,** 171–172.

Greenacre, P. The family romance of the artist. *Psychoanalytic Study of the Child,* 1958, **13,** 9–43.

Griffiths, R. *A study of imagination in early childhood.* London: Routledge & Kegan Paul, 1945.

Guilford, J. P. *The nature of human intelligence.* New York: McGraw-Hill, 1967.

Guilford, J. P. *Intelligence, creativity, and their educational implications.* San Diego, Calif.: Knapp, 1968.

Hall, B. New motivation for the gifted; superior and talented student project. *The Texas Outlook,* 1961, **45,** 42–44.

Hamm, R. L. Integrated program for the gifted. *Minnesota Journal of Education,* 1963, **44,** 8–10.

Harris, I. D. *Emotional blocks to learning.* New York: Free Press, 1961.

Head, H. *Aphasia and kindred disorders of speech.* Cambridge: Cambridge University Press, 1926.

Heffernan, H., & Todd, V. E. *The kindergarten teacher.* Boston: Heath, 1960.

Henry, N. B. (Ed.) *Education for the gifted.* Chicago: National Society for the Study of Education, 1958.

Herring, L. H. *Provisions and procedures for the rapid learning in selected Texas junior high schools.* Austin: Texas Study of Secondary Education, 1962.

Hess, R. D., & Shipman, V. C. Early experience and the socialization of cognitive modes in children. *Child Development,* 1965, **36,** 869–886.

Hill, M. B. *Enrichment programs for intellectually gifted pupils.* Sacramento: California State Department of Education, 1969.

Holland, J. L. Some limitations of teacher ratings as predictors of creativity. *Journal of Educational Psychology,* 1959, **50,** 219–223.

Holland, J. L. Creative and academic performance among talented adolescents. *Journal of Educational Psychology,* 1961, **52,** 136–147.

Hollingworth, L. S. An enrichment curriculum for rapid learners in Public School 500: Speyer School. *Teachers College Record,* 1938, **39,** 296–306.

Hollingworth, L. A. *Children above 180 I.Q.: origin and development.* New York: Harcourt Brace Jovanovich, 1942.

Horn, R. A. *Seventh grade mathematics for the academically talented, teachers guide.* Columbus: Ohio State Department of Education, 1963.

Hosford, P. M. *Atlanta Public Schools psychological services, 1966–1967.* Atlanta, Ga.: Psychological Services, Atlanta Public Schools, 1967.

How top teachers teach. *Grade Teacher,* 1967, **85,** 63–65.

Isaacs, A. F. Being gifted is a bed of roses, with the thorns included. *Gifted Child Quarterly,* 1971a, **15,** 54–56.

Isaacs, A. F. Do the gifted ever become retarded? *Gifted Child Quarterly,* 1971b, **15,** 66–68.

Isaacs, A. F. The gifted and parent-school relationships or parents of the gifted and schools. *Gifted Child Quarterly,* 1971c, **15,** 136–138.

Isaacs, A. F. Biblical research IV: perspectives on the problems of the gifted, and possible solutions as revealed in the Pentateuch. *Gifted Child Quarterly,* 1971d, **15,** 175–194.

Iscoe, I., & Pierce-Jones, J. Divergent thinking, age and intelligence in white and Negro children. *Child Development,* 1964, **35,** 785–797.

Jacobs, J. C. Are we being misled by 50 years of research on our gifted children? *Gifted Child Quarterly,* 1970, **14,** 120–123.

Jacobs, J. C. Effectiveness of teacher and parent identification of gifted children as a function of school level. *Psychology in the schools,* 1971a, **8,** 140–142.

Jacobs, J. C. Rorschach studies reveal possible misinterpretations of personality traits in the gifted. *Gifted Child Quarterly,* 1971b, **15,** 195–200.

Jordan, J. B. Foundation for exceptional children addresses the needs of the culturally different gifted child. *Exceptional Children,* 1974, **40,** 279–281.

Keeham, V. R., & Mayhon, W. G. *Operational future: a report of research through service to academically superior high school students in New Mexico.* Santa Fe: New Mexico State Department of Education, 1963.

Kelly, G. A. *The psychology of personal constructs.* Vol. 1. New York: Norton, 1955.

Ketcham, W. What research says about the education of gifted children. *The University of Michigan School of Education Bulletin,* 1967, **28,** 1–5.

Khatena, J. Onomatopoeia and images: preliminary validity study of a test of originality. *Perceptual and Motor Skills,* 1969, **28,** 335–338.

Kubie, S. L. *Neurotic distortion in the creative process.* Lawrence: University of Kansas Press, 1958.

Kurtzman, K. A study of school attitudes, peer acceptance and personality of the creative adolescent. *Exceptional Children,* 1967, **34,** 157–162.

Laird, A. W. Are we really educating the gifted child? *Gifted Child Quarterly,* 1968, **12,** 205–214.

Laird, A. W. The fifty states' educational provisions for gifted children. *Gifted Child Quarterly,* 1971, **15,** 205–216.

Levinson, L. L. *Webster's unafraid dictionary.* New York: Collier, 1967.

Levinson, L. L. *The left-handed dictionary.* New York: Collier, 1968.

Lichtenwalner, J. S., & Maxwell, J. W. The relationship of birth order and socioeconomic status to the creativity of preschool children. *Child Development,* 1969, **40,** 1241–1247.

Lobel, A. *Under a mushroom.* New York: Harper & Row, 1970.

Lowenfeld, V. The meaning of creative expression for the child. In *Imagination in education.* New York: Bank Street College of Education, 1956.

MacKinnon, D. W. Personality and the realization of creative potential. *American Psychologist,* 1965, **20,** 273–281.

Martinson, R. A. The California study of programs for gifted pupils. *Exceptional Children,* 1960, **26,** 339–343.

Maslow, A. H. *Motivation and personality.* New York: Harper & Row, 1954.

Maslow, A. H. *Toward a psychology of being.* New York: Van Nostrand, 1962.

Mathisen, J. D., & Smaltz, J. M. *Guides to special education in North Dakota, IX, the gifted child.* Bismarck: North Dakota State Department of Public Instruction, 1961.

Mednick, S. A. The associative basis of the creative process. *Psychological Review,* 1962, **69,** 220–232.

Merritt, J. A. Project discovery: educating the gifted. Paper presented at the U.S. Office of Education Western Regional Conference—Hearing for the Educational Needs of the Mentally Gifted, Los Angeles, December 1970.

Milton, G. A. The effect of sex-role identification in the formation of problem-solving skill. *Journal of Abnormal and Social Psychology,* 1957, **55,** 208–212.

Mosel, A. *Tikki tikki tembo.* Illustrated by B. Lent. New York: Holt, Rinehart & Winston, 1968.

Myers, R. E., & Torrance, E. P. *Ideabooks.* Boston: Ginn, 1965.

National Education Association Project on Instruction. *Planning and organizing for teaching.* Washington, D.C.: National Education Association, 1963.

New York State Education Department. *Education for the gifted in New York State.* Albany: New York State Education Department, 1964.

Nichols, R. C. Parental attitudes of mothers of intelligent adolescents and creativity of their mothers. *Child Development*, 1964, **35**, 1041–1050.

Nurnberg, M. *Fun with words*. Drawings by T. Schroeder. Englewood Cliffs, N.J.: Prentice-Hall, 1970.

Oakland Unified School District. *Program for gifted, grade six*. Oakland, Calif.: Oakland Unified School District, 1963.

Olton, R. M. A self-instructional program for developing productive thinking skills in fifth- and sixth-grade children. *Journal of Creative Behavior*, 1969, **3**, 16–25.

Pankove, E., & Kogan, N. Creative ability and risk-taking in elementary school children. *Journal of Personality*, 1968, **36**, 420–439.

Parnes, S. J., & Brunelle, E. A. The literature of creativity. Part I. *Journal of Creative Behavior*, 1967, **1**, 52–109.

Pegnato, C. V., & Birch, J. W. Locating gifted children in junior high schools: a comparison of methods. *Exceptional Children*, 1959, **25**, 300–304.

Petty, W. T., Harold, C. P., & Stoll, E. *The state of knowledge about the teaching of vocabulary*. Champaign, Ill.: National Council of Teachers of English, 1968.

Piaget, J. *Play, dreams and imitation in children*. (Translated by C. Gattegno & F. M. Hodgson) London: Heinemann, 1951.

Pilon, B. A. Come hither, come hither, come hither: word's worth. *Gifted Child Quarterly*, 1971, **15**, 23–31.

Plowman, P. D. Programming for the gifted child. *Exceptional Children*, 1969, **35**, 547–551.

Plowman, P. D., & Rice, J. P. *Demonstration of differential programming in enrichment, acceleration, counseling and special classes for gifted pupils in grades 1–9. Final report*. Sacramento: California State Department of Education, 1967.

Pulaski, M. A. S. Play as a function of toy structure and fantasy predisposition. *Child Development*, 1970, **41**, 531–537.

Rank, O. *Art and the artist*. New York: Tudor, 1932.

Reese, H. W., & Parnes, S. J. Programming creative behavior. *Child Development*, 1970, **41**, 413–423.

Renzulli, J. S. Talent potential in minority group students. *Exceptional Children*, 1973, **39**, 437–445.

Rice, J. P. *The gifted: developing total talent*. Springfield, Ill.: C. C Thomas, 1970.

Roe, A. A psychological study of eminent psychologists and anthropologists, and a comparison with biological and physiological scientists. *Psychological Monographs*, 1953, **67**(2, Whole No. 352).

Rogers, C. R. *Client-centered therapy*. Boston: Houghton Mifflin, 1961.

Rosner, S., & Abt, L. E. *The creative experience*. New York: Grossman, 1970.

Roth, L. H., et al., *Design for developing Colorado reading programs*. Denver: Colorado State Department of Education, 1967.

Rotter, D. M., Langland, L., & Berger, D. The validity of tests of creative thinking in seven-year-old children. *Gifted Child Quarterly*, 1971, **15**, 273–278, 296.

Saxe, R. M., & Stollack, G. E. The relationship of birth order and socioeconomic status to the creativity of preschool children. *Child Development*, 1971, **40**, 1241–1247.

Scarry, R. *Storybook dictionary*. New York: Golden, 1969.

Scarvelis, S. M. Guidance procedures supported by elementary school counselors and counselor educators of Ohio for the identification and guidance of the gifted. *Dissertation Abstracts International*, 1969, **30**(6-A), 2341–2343.

Schactel, E. G. *Metamorphosis*. New York: Basic Books, 1959.

Schaefer, C. E. A psychological study of 10 exceptionally creative adolescent girls. *Exceptional Children*, 1970a, **36**, 431–441.

Schaefer, C. E. The similes test: a new measure of metaphorical thinking. *Proceedings of the 78th annual convention of the American Psychological Association*, 1970b, **5**, 169–170.

Scheifele, M. *Gifted child in the regular classroom*. New York: Teachers College Press, Columbia University, 1953.

Schneider, D. E. *The psychoanalyst and the artist*. New York: Farrar, Straus & Giroux, 1950.

Shore, R. E. *Description of the San Rafael program for more able learners as prescribed in the California Administrative Code*. San Raphael, Calif.: San Raphael City Schools, 1962.

Singer, J. L. Imagination and writing ability in young children. *Journal of Personality*, 1961, **29**, 396–413.

Snygg, D., & Combs, A. W. *Individual behavior*. New York: Harper & Row, 1949.

Stark, S. K. *My tree*. Illustrations by F. Hori. Minneapolis, Minn.: Carolrhoda, 1969.

Sullivan, H. S. *Interpersonal theory of psychiatry*. New York: Norton, 1953.

Taylor, C. W. Developing creative characteristics. *The Instructor*, 1964a, **73**, 5, 99–100.

Taylor, C. W. (Ed.) *Creativity: progress and potential*. New York: McGraw-Hill, 1964b.

Terman, L. M. *Genetic studies of genius: Mental and physical traits of a thousand gifted children*. Stanford, Calif.: Stanford University Press, 1925.

Terman, L. M., & Oden, M. H. *Genetic studies of genius. Vol. 4. The gifted child grows up: twenty-five years' follow-up of the superior child*. Stanford, Calif.: Stanford University Press, 1947.

Terman, L. M., & Oden, M. H. *Genetic studies of genius. Vol. 5. The gifted group at mid-life: thirty-five years' follow-up of the superior child*. Stanford, Calif.: Stanford University Press, 1959.

Thomas, S. J. B., & Feldhusen, J. F. To spark an interest: think creatively. *Gifted Child Quarterly*, 1971, **15**, 36–41.

Torrance, E. P. Explorations in creative thinking. *Education*, 1960, **81**, 216–220.

Torrance, E. P. Problems of highly creative children. *Gifted Child Quarterly*, 1961, **5**, 31–34.

Torrance, E. P. *Education and the creative potential*. Minneapolis: University of Minnesota Press, 1963.

Torrance, E. P. Education and creativity. In C. W. Taylor (Ed.), *Creativity: progress and potential*. New York: McGraw-Hill, 1964.

Torrance, E. P. *The Torrance Tests of Creative Thinking: norms and technical manual*. Princeton, N.J.: Personnel Press, 1966.

Torrance, E. P. A longitudinal examination of the fourth grade slump in creativity. *Gifted Child Quarterly*, 1968, **12**, 195–199.

Torrance, E. P. Discontinuities in creative development. In E. P. Torrance & W. F. White (Eds.), *Issues and advances in educational psychology*. Itasca, Ill.: Peacock, 1969a.

Torrance, E. P. Prediction of adult creative achievement among high school seniors. *Gifted Child Quarterly*, 1969b, **13**, 223–229.

Torrance, E. P. Developmental changes in sources of consensual validation in preadolescence. *Gifted Child Quarterly*, 1971a, **15**, 3–10.

Torrance, E. P. Are the Torrance Tests of Creative Thinking biased against or in favor of disadvantaged groups? *Gifted Child Quarterly*, 1971b, **15**, 75–80.

Torrance, E. P. Identity: the gifted child's major problem. *Gifted Child Quarterly*, 1971c, **15**, 147–155.

Torrance, E. P. Is bias against job changing bias against giftedness. *Gifted Child Quarterly*, 1971d, **15**, 244–248.

Torrance, E. P. Creative young women in today's world. *Exceptional Children*, 1972a, **39**, 597–603.

Torrance, E. P. Career patterns and peak creative achievements of creative high school students twelve years later. *Gifted Child Quarterly*, 1972b, **16**, 75–88.

Twin City Institute for Talented Youth. *Annual Report*. St. Paul, Minn.: Twin City Institute for Talented Youth, 1969.

Ullmann, C. A. Prevalence of reading disability as a function of the measures used. *Journal of Learning Disabilities*, 1969, **2**, 556–558.

U.S. Office of Education. *Education of the gifted and talented. Report to the Congress of the United States*. Washington, D.C.: U.S. Government Printing Office, 1972.

Walberg, H. J. A portrait of the artist and scientist as young men. *Exceptional Children*, 1969, **36**, 5–11.

Walberg, H. J. Varieties of adolescent creativity and the high school environment. *Exceptional Children*, 1971, **38**, 115–116.

Waldrop, M. F., & Bell, R. Q. Relation of preschool dependency behavior to family size and density. *Child Development*, 1964, **35**, 1187–1195.

Wallach, M. A., & Kogan, N. *Modes of thinking in young children: a study of the creativity-intelligence distribution*. New York: Holt, Rinehart & Winston, 1965.

Wallach, M. A., & Wing, C. W., Jr. *The talented student*. New York: Holt, Rinehart & Winston, 1969.

Ward, W. C. Creativity in young children. *Child Development*, 1968, **39**, 737–754.

Ward, W. C. Rate and uniqueness in children's creative responding. *Child Development*, 1969a, **40**, 869–878.

Ward, W. C. Creativity and environmental cues in nursery school children. *Developmental Psychology*, 1969b, **1**, 543–547.

Weinstein, B. The adjustment of children in a suburban community who were accelerated in elementary school. *Journal of School Psychology*, 1966, **5**, 60–63.

Weisberg, P. S., & Springer, K. J. Environmental factors in creative function. A study of gifted children. *Archives of General Psychiatry*, 1961, **5**, 554–564.

Weyl, N. *The creative elite in America*. Washington, D.C.: Public Affairs Press, 1966.

Weyl, N., & Possony, S. T. *The geography of intellect*. Chicago: Regnery, 1963.

Winn, M. (Ed.) *What shall we do and Allee Galool*. Pictures by K. Kuskin. Musical arrangements by A. Miller. New York: Harper & Row, 1970.

Witkins, W. L. The social adjustment of accelerated pupils. *School Review*, 1936, **154**, 445–455.

Witt, G. The Life Enrichment Activity Program, Inc.: a continuing program for creative, disadvantaged children. *Journal of Research and Development in Education*, 1971, **4**, 67–73.

Witty, P. A. How to identify the gifted. *Childhood Education*, 1953, **29**, 312–316.

Witty, P. A. Reading for the gifted. In J. A. Figurel (Ed.), *Reading and realism, proceedings of the 13th annual convention of the International Reading Association*. Newark, Del.: International Reading Association, 1969.

Witty, P. A. The education of the gifted and the creative in the U.S.A. *Gifted Child Quarterly*, 1971, **15**, 109–116, 122.

Wodtke, K. H. Some data on the reliability and validity of creative tests at the elementary school level. *Educational and Psychological Measurement*, 1964, **24**, 399–408.

Womack, M., et al., *Academically talented program.* .Oxnard, Calif.: Oxnard School District, 1963.

Yamamoto, K. Effects of restriction of range and test unreliability on correlation between measures of intelligence and creative thinking. *British Journal of Educational Psychology,* 1965, **35**, 300–305.

York, G. L., et al., *The rapid learner.* Grand Forks, N.D.: Grand Forks Public Schools, 1961.

Zilli, M. G. Reasons why the gifted adolescent underachieves and some of the implications of guidance and counseling to this problem. *Gifted Child Quarterly,* 1971, **15**, 279–291.

In people there is no difference in kind, only in degree, and so the handicapped child must be regarded as a human being with the same emotions of love, hate, and fear.

—Helena T. Devereux

The mildly retarded

This chapter is very short; it is short for two reasons. First, the mildly retarded are not much different from their normal peers and, second, the disadvantaged often are wrongly included in samples of children considered retarded. In Chapter 3 we promised to discuss those children at the lower end of the polygenic distribution of intelligence—the "familial" retarded child. These are children whose intelligence test scores fall between 50 and 80 and who would be considered mildly retarded. While children can be mildly retarded for reasons other than hereditary influences (e.g., minimal brain dysfunction, economic deprivation), our remarks in this chapter are confined to children who are low in measured intelligence due to hereditary influences and whose IQ score would not increase substantially in response to environmental enrichment. Nevertheless, many children classified as mildly retarded do come from lower socioeconomic populations. The duller individual often does earn a substandard wage, but low income status may reflect a lack of opportunity to advance. In Chapter 9 we emphasized that both socioeconomic factors and culturally biased tests lower the intelligence test scores of children. If a child's only deficit is a low IQ score, then it is an error to classify him as mildly retarded because of genetic factors.

MISAPPLICATION OF THE RETARDED LABEL

Who classifies children as retarded? In most cases it is the schools. Out of a sample of 812 persons identified by one community as retarded, the majority were school-age children whose label had been affixed only by the school; after leaving high school, the retarded label was rarely applied (Mercer, 1972).

To diagnose a child as retarded, the schools rely primarily on intelligence tests administered by school staff. Most of the children they diagnose are not seen by other agencies. Consequently, their diagnosis is made without the support of more clinically sophisticated professionals. In addition, the schools use less stringent criteria for classification than do other agencies. In Mercer's study, 46 percent of those labeled retarded had intelligence test scores above 70, and 62 percent had no apparent physical disabilities.

The Mexican-Americans and blacks are overrepresented in most surveys of classes for the mildly retarded, primarily because the combination of measured low intelligence and language inefficiency is strongly associated with educational placement. In Mercer's California study 300 percent more Mexican-Americans and 50 percent more blacks were included in special classes than would have been expected from their proportion in the community.

The American Association on Mental Deficiency (1973) defines mental retardation as "subaverage general intellectual functioning . . . associated with impairment in adaptive behavior." Adaptive behavior is the key to this definition; many children score below normal on intelligence tests but display behavior adaptive to the situations in which they find themselves. Many schools and other social agencies have assumed that impaired social skill accompanies low measured intelligence.

The inability to select a correct cut-off score for subnormal intelligence further complicates the picture. The American Association of Mental Deficiency (AAMD) suggests the lowest 16 percent of the population, those with IQs below 84, should be considered subnormal. The schools usually designate an IQ of 75 to 79 or lower, the lowest 9 percent, as qualifying a child for special class placement. The test designers themselves suggest a much lower cut-off, the lowest 3 percent or those with IQs of 70 or lower.

Mercer and her colleagues (Mercer, 1972) administered a measure of social adaptability to 664 individuals who had been given an IQ test. The majority of adults whose IQs were between 70 and 84 were competent in the social roles usual for persons their age: 84 percent had completed eight or more grades in schools, 83 percent were employed, 65 percent held semiskilled or skilled jobs, 80 percent were financially independent, and almost all were able to manage their own affairs. Adults with IQs below 70 were less able to function adequately.

Mercer also compared those who scored at the third percentile level in both the adaptability and intelligence tests with those considered quasiretarded because they scored at the third percentile level (IQ below 70) on the intelligence test only. Those low on both measures had more trouble learning, were more often a grade or two behind their age-mates, and were more often in special education classes as children. As adults, the quasiretarded got along better in the community, with 80 percent graduating from high school and all reading books, holding jobs, and having adequate social relationships. Mercer (1972, p. 47) concluded, "When we added the behavior test to the IQ test, we found the rates of supposedly retarded persons fell to about half of what they were when the intelligence test was the only base."

Adding the behavior test scores to the IQ scores made little difference for Anglo-Americans; every Anglo with an IQ below 70 was also in the lowest 3 percent on the behavior scales. In contrast, 91 percent of blacks and 60 percent of Mexican-Americans with IQs below 70 scored above the third percentile on the behavior test. Mercer (1972, p. 47) stated, "This means that ethnic groups, and in general those of low socioeconomic status, are the most likely to be penalized by the current IQ only definition of retardation. As the cut off is raised, the proportion of minorities who get the retarded label increases." Mercer's findings support the notion that intelligence tests in current use are culture-specific, since the more "Anglocized" a non-Anglo child was in his study the higher was his IQ.

Jastak, MacPhee, and Whitman (1963, p. 139), after administering a four-hour test battery to a large sample of children in special classes, concluded that "As many as 80 percent of the individuals diagnosed as retarded by a single criterion may be found to be nonretarded if all . . . criteria are brought into play." More recently, Garrison and Hammill (1971) reached a similar conclusion. In their study 11-year old children in educable ($n = 378$) and regular classes ($n = 319$) were compared on five tests: the Slosson Intelligence Test for Children and Adults, an adaptation of the Test of Social Inference, an adaptation of the Temple Informal Reading Inventory, and the auditory reception and verbal expression subtests from the ITPA. To allow comparisons across these different measures, the distributions for the whole sample, that is, for retarded and nonretarded children, were converted into T scores (statistical method of normalizing test scores). A T score of 45 (equivalent in this data to an IQ of 75) was set as a pass-fail cut-off point on each test. The percentage of children scoring above and below this point in each of the two types of classes is shown in Figure 11.1. Immediately evident is the large number of special class children who score above the cut-off point on the various measures: 25 percent of special class children fell above the cut-off point on at least four of the five measures, while only 31 percent fell below the point on four or more measures. Children in the latter group were considered the "best" candidates for special education. The placement of the others in educable mentally retarded (EMR) classrooms was viewed as untenable.

When we talk about the mildly retarded, therefore, keep in mind that

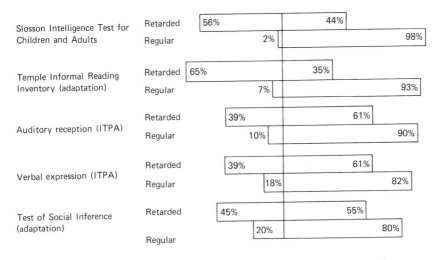

Figure 11.1 *Percentage of pupils in retarded and regular classes who pass (T score = 45) criterion measures. (Adapted from M. Garrison & D. D. Hammill. Who are the retarded?* Exceptional Children, *1971,* **38,** *13-20. Reprinted with permission of The Council for Exceptional Children.)*

a high percentage of those included in past studies of this group were probably quasiretarded and, therefore, not retarded because of genetic inferiority in intellectual ability.

DEFICIT VERSUS DEVELOPMENTAL VIEW OF RETARDATION

Those who are mildly retarded usually have difficulty in school. They quickly fall behind and eventually are placed in classes for the educable retarded child. For many years educators of the mildly retarded recommended teaching techniques implying that the retarded were deficient in rate of learning, retention, incidental learning, and the ability to transfer or generalize, to make new associations, to form abstractions, and to see relationships. The teaching recommendations stressed slow presentation of material, much repetition, a great deal of structure and guidance, use of concrete materials, teaching of specific responses to specific situations, and sequential presentation of new material (Cegelka & Cegelka, 1970; DeProspo, 1956; Garrison, 1956; Kirk & Johnson, 1951).

For example, when discussing the teaching of reading, Johnson (1967) stated that because the mildly retarded will never read much beyond the high third or low fourth grade reading level, they should be instructed similarly to normal children at the elementary level. We have no objection to this statement. But, Johnson adds that instruction at this level emphasizes the reading of whole words, an awareness of details within words, and development of word-attack skills, with little done in reading for content. These remarks suggest that the mildly retarded child should be given reading readiness skills for a considerably longer period of time than the normal. Jordon's (1962) statements have the same implication. The problem is that only the very skilled teacher can undertake such instruction and still maintain the interest of her students.

These same educators often emphasize social over academic education; that is, education to prepare the child for adult life. In programs of this kind the tool subjects of reading, writing, and arithmetic are considered of subordinate value "because the mentally handicapped has only a limited ability to understand and to make use of these skills, even though he is capable of mastering them to a fairly high level of competence in a purely mechanical manner" (Gunzburg, 1972, p. 364). Jordon (1962, p. 160) remarked that there is a deemphasis on academics in classrooms for the mildly retarded, that extra time is given to crafts and social development, after which a "Teacher may attempt to move the youngster towards some simple occupation."

Robbin (1970) suggested that mildly retarded children be given progress awards just like normal children. She described a program where retarded children were awarded for achieving the following criteria: doing good work, being nice people, and being good citizens. Similarily, Wettingfeld (1970) reported that the educable mentally retarded have proven to be eager, responsive, and reliable children when handling library materials and enthusiastic about carrying out simple library tasks. The demeaning nature of these well-intended remarks is obvious.

Implicit in all these recommendations is the assumption that the mildly retarded actually are deficient in learning. For example, in a review of studies on learning in the retarded, Denny (1964, p. 100) stated, "One problem which demands its share of speculation is untangling the data so as to identify the fundamental deficits in the retarded person's behavior." Research has not clearly established that mildly retarded subjects display learning deficiency. Most of the comparative learning studies conducted over the last twenty years have found that the retarded perform more poorly than normal subjects of equal chronological age, but similarly to those of equal mental age (Iano, 1971; Zigler, 1967, 1969). In addition, a number of studies of special areas of learning have found no differences between retarded and equal-age normal subjects, for example, Mordock's (1968a) review of paired-associate learning in the mildly retarded.

If the mildly retarded is viewed as a normal individual of low intelligence rather than as defective, then the findings from comparative learning studies begin to make sense. According to the developmental approach, the mildly retarded's intellectual development differs from the normal's only with respect to rate and the upper limit achieved. When rates of development are matched, as is grossly the case when retarded and normal children are matched on mental age, there should be no difference in the perceptual or conceptual processes relating to IQ. In other words, a child with an IQ of 70, a CA of 10, and thus an MA of 7, is viewed as equivalent intellectually to a child with an IQ of 100 and CA of 7 (Zigler, 1967). After maturity is reached, the retardate is viewed as capable of learning at normal rates.

Those holding the developmental view reject the notion that intellectual growth is primarily a quantitative accumulation of knowledge. Progressive levels, or age-stages, are viewed as not simply quantitatively different, but as qualitatively different. The significance of this view, espoused principally by Piaget and his colleagues abroad and by Kohlberg (1968) in America, is that a higher level of intelligence is not simply acquisition of more knowledge, but is the ability to organize and utilize knowledge differently, the ability to respond to the environment in new ways.

According to the defect approach, the retarded suffer from physiological or cognitive defects that permanently arrest development (Ellis, 1963; Luria, 1963). This view implies that the retarded will perform more poorly than normals regardless of age groups compared. Some studies have been reported that appear to support this notion. The developmentalist, however, attributes these differences to motivational and personality factors that are not inherent in retardation but are the result of the children's particular histories (Zigler, 1967). Support for this view comes from studies where younger retarded children are found to perform similarly to normals, while older retarded perform more poorly (Mordock, 1968b, 1968c). Although the deficit position is a legitimate and popular one, findings related to this position are equivocal. Let us examine in more detail, therefore, the developmentalist's view of the retarded.

KATHY

Kathy was 16 and her IQ was 68. She had spent the better part of her school years in a class for the educable retarded. When she was little, she had a number of friends, but she was now a social isolate. When her friends' parents found out she was "retarded," the friends were discouraged from playing with her. Other friends fell by the wayside after Kathy was transferred from the regular to the special class. Even when in the regular class, her deficiencies were so apparent that her classmates first teased and then ignored her. She enjoyed playing with the younger children in the neighborhood, but many parents, fearing she would set a bad example, cautioned their children not to play with her. In addition, her mother spent all of her free time with her, fearful that she would get into trouble, perhaps be attacked or led into sexual behavior. Consequently, Kathy developed phobic fears of being touched and avoided crowds. This behavior made her seem even stranger and alienated her even from children in her special class. Neighbors attributed these behaviors to her retardation, a common misconception about the maladaptive behaviors of the retarded.

When Kathy was placed in the special class, she thought she would get extra help there and would no longer be called dumb. She quickly learned that she was with all the "dumb" and "weird" kids, and that once there she was likely to stay throughout her school career.

While Kathy had difficulty doing the work assigned, she knew it was material she had had before, only there were fewer problems on each page and she was given more time to do them. In addition, she was always asked how things were alike or different, was read to by the teacher, and had much free time to color, draw, or work with puzzles. She earned tokens for each problem she got right and cashed them in for trinkets at the end of each day.

She now read at about a fifth grade level, but had no idea what would happen to her after high school. She had had no real prevocational training and at 18 would be ill-equipped to enter the job market.

Teaching approach

Kathy's teachers believed that she, as well as her retarded classmates, could not learn by making meaningful associations to material, was poor in reasoning, comprehension, and the ability to generalize or transfer, was inefficient in retention, and incapable of dealing with abstractions. She would learn best through automatic drill and repetitive practice. Rote memorization of the curriculum was encouraged, with a deemphasis on underlying meanings, conceptual understanding, and generalized principles. The material she was to learn was broken down into small steps, presented at a slow pace, and repeated often.

While Kathy did poorly in this program, it was all she was given. Since she learned so slowly, teachers had her spend more time on "basic" skills to make sure she learned them. Consequently, she had no time for school experiences such as safety patrol, library aide, art, or music. Watching Kathy slowly struggle to acquire the necessary sequential skills for achievement often strained her teacher's patience. Teaching the retarded was boring!

Just suppose Kathy's teachers ascribed to a developmental viewpoint of retardation. Just suppose that the retarded weren't turned off on learning before placement in a special class. Just suppose the brain-injured, disadvantaged, and familial retarded weren't all thrown together into a class and called educable retarded. Just suppose all the gadgets and gimmicks were thrown out of special education. Just suppose researchers examined how the retarded were similar to the normal rather than how they were different. How might things have gone differently for Kathy?

First, her teachers would know that material learned by rote is not easily transferred or generalized and requires frequent repetition for retention. They would not be surprised when students taught by rote methods easily forgot what they learned or failed to generalize to new situations what they did retain. Consequently, they would warn others that behaviors encouraged by restrictive teaching strategies can confirm the preconceptions that led to the strategies in the first place. They would ask whether the retarded's apparent inability to reason and comprehend was a real inability or the result of teaching which emphasized the rote and mechanical (Bauer & Yamamoto, 1972; Iano, 1971).

Second, Kathy's teachers would not view learning as the quantitative accumulation of knowledge or teaching as the primary means by which that knowledge is accumulated and academic progress made, but would stress the importance of maturational development in intellectual growth.

Third, her teachers would base their programs and methods on the pupil's assets rather than on largely untested generalizations about the learning characteristics of the retarded. They would avoid early placement in special programs, believing that retardation is not a static condition and aware that early placement may prevent a child from transferring back to regular classes.

Fourth, her teachers would teach the retarded in much the same manner as they would the normal, gearing their instruction to the developmental levels of the children. Discussion, individual and group projects, problem solving, and reasoning would all be included in the curriculum. When a child failed to progress to a higher level of achievement, they would not become bored but would find other significant educational activities to enrich the life of the child at this level (Bauer & Yamamoto, 1972; Iano, 1971).

Personality and environmental factors in learning proficiency

"Just supposes" are nice to think about, but they are just that—supposes! Unfortunately, the retarded expect to fail (MacMillan, 1971), the result of a lifetime of confronting tasks presented to them at the wrong time. Such a set to fail results in a style of problem solving in which motivation to avoid failure supersedes motivation directed toward achieving success (Cromwell, 1963). They also learn to distrust their own solutions to problems and thus look to others for direction.

The retarded have a strong desire for attention, praise, and encouragement. In normal development attention and praise as sought reinforcers are replaced with reinforcement inherent in being correct (Cromwell, 1963). Zigler and his associates believe that the retarded cares less about being correct than does the intellectually normal child of the same mental age. Retarded children who performed more poorly than normals of equal mental age when correctness was the only reinforcer, performed as well as normals when extrinsic rewards were provided (Zigler & deLabry, 1962).

To compound the picture, many retarded have negative self-concepts (Collins, Burger, & Doherty, 1970; Guthrie, Gorlow, & Butler, 1967; Schurr, Joiner, & Towne, 1970), a finding that may explain their greater susceptibility to countersuggestion (MacMillan & Carlson, 1971). These and other motivational differences between retarded and normal children suggest that learning inefficiency may not be responsible for the differences between these groups on learning tasks (Zigler, 1969; Zigler & Balla, 1971).

Community attitudes have added to the retarded's negative feelings about himself. Many popular misconceptions about the retarded result in their being rejected by their communities. In general, the retarded are viewed with degradation and denigration. The public seems to react more favorably toward the label slow learner than the label mentally retarded. By labeling, professionals, too, have added to these children's rejection (Hollinger & Jones, 1970; Jones, 1972).

These same attitudes influence those who enter the teaching profession. As a result, a disproportionately low number of very able students show interest in teaching the retarded. The field attracts many persons retired from other occupations and regular classroom teachers in the twilight of their professional careers. Many choose such teaching because they believe they can teach small classes of limited children without needing to know much and with little effort. In addition, the majority of personnel labeled teacher in classrooms for the mentally retarded have not completed the preservice preparation specified as necessary for professional competence (Davis, 1970).

Because of poor preparation and insincere interest, the teacher loss rate from such classes is believed to be much higher than from regular classrooms. Nevertheless, the children remain, and unlike the child in the regular classroom who moves to a new teacher each year, they feel each teacher's departure as a personal rejection. "No one wants to work with us!" Undoubtedly, this poor teacher preparation and large turnover has contributed to the retarded child's failure to learn. A 30-year span of research has demonstrated that, in most instances, retarded children who remain in regular classrooms do better than or as well as those placed in segregated settings (Blackman, 1967; Guskin & Spicker, 1968; Kirk, 1964; Zito & Bardon, 1969). Some believe that academic proficiency is less important than improvement in personal-social relationships. They state that at least when the retarded are grouped together, ridicule is reduced and they are able to form relationships with similarly rejected classmates. Unfortunately, this is not necessarily so (Iano, Ayers, Heller, McGettigan, & Walker, 1974). Although findings are not always consistent (Schurr et al., 1970), greater self-derogation exists among those placed in segregated classes than among those who remain in regular classrooms (Carroll, 1967; Meyrowitz, 1962). Perhaps the few classrooms where the opposite finding occurred should be scrutinized to discover the qualities that produced this favorable result.

Gozali (1972) asked 56 individuals how they felt about the EMR work-study program they participated in 8 years earlier. At that time, their average age was 15 and their average IQ was 69. The majority (85 percent) perceived their special class experience as degrading and useless. Ninety-one percent said they would not place their child in a special class because they "would like their children to really learn to read and write" or "to have friends and fun in schools." When asked about friendships and socialization with students from their special classes, the majority (87 percent) reported that they did not socialize with former classmates. They felt that special classes neither educated them nor provided them with a socialization support experience. We do not know, however, how these same youths would have felt had they remained in regular classes. If they expressed similar attitudes, then Gozali's findings reflect their attitudes about public school in general rather than their attitudes about experiences especially planned for them.

How should the retarded be taught?

"Like regular kids and maybe more so!" would be the developmentalist's answer to this question. Such theorists would stress emphasizing the similarities between the retarded and normal, particularly when matched on mental age, and deemphasizing the search for deficiencies. When a study fails to find a difference between retarded and normal children, sometimes its author is apologetic about the findings and questions the study's methodology rather than the assumption that the retarded are deficient. In addition, many of the studies that report significant differences between retarded children and normals fail to emphasize the extent of the differences. While statistically significant, many differences are quite small, meaning that they are probably of little practical importance. For example, a group of retarded children might learn a task in an average of 15 learning trials while a group of nonretarded learn it in an average of 13 trials. The difference of 2 may be statistically significant, meaning that its occurrence by chance is highly improbable, but in practical terms the degree of overlap between plots of the scores of the two groups probably would be so great that the teacher would have no need to differentiate between the two groups of children. In many studies the upper 10 or 20 percent of the normals and the lower 10 or 20 percent of the retarded account for the mean difference between the two groups. For all practical purposes the remainder perform alike. On some tasks allowing extra time for the slowest of the group may be all that is needed.

In a review of the literature up to 1967 Bracht and Glass (1967) cited only one study that examined the effects of instructional strategies on children with differing IQs. A programmed text in English was more effective with high-ability than low-ability students, while classroom instruction yielded better results with the low-ability group (Reed & Hayman, 1962). Since this review, several investigations have failed to reveal any significant interaction between instructional approach and mental ability (Gagne & Weigand, 1968; Katz, 1967; Tallmadge, 1968).

Keislar and Stern (1970), using children with average to above average IQs, found an interaction between mental age and instruction in the use of different problem solving strategies. Children with higher mental ages did relatively better using a complex but more efficient scanning strategy to solve problems requiring conceptual reasoning; those with lower mental ages did better with the use of a simpler strategy. In an earlier study (Stern & Keislar, 1967) these investigators found mental age was more strongly related to instructional strategy than was IQ.

Although retarded children were not used in either of these investigations the results suggest that many such children could be grouped with nonretarded children of the same mental age and taught by the same method. In other instances even mental age grouping might not be necessary.

Even if the retarded are slow learners (learn at a slower rate than normals), there is no strong evidence that they will forget the material more rapidly than fast learners once they have learned it well. An early study by Gillette (1936) implied that fast learners retain more than slow learners, and for many years this generalization was accepted as fact. More recently, however, other studies have indicated that fast and slow learners forget at about the same rate (Gregory & Bunch, 1959; Schoer, 1962; Shuell & Keppel, 1970; Stroud & Schoer, 1959; Underwood, 1954). These findings imply that it may not be necessary to repeat again and again the same material in order for the retarded to learn and retain it.

If more practice is necessary in order for the slow learner to acquire information, let us make sure that it is meaningful practice and that the learner is attentive to the instruction. Ross and Ross's (1972) finding that training in listening skills enhances the retarded's learning implies that many miss much of the material presented to them. We also know that memory is facilitated by learning to make many associations to the material to be recalled rather than by rote repetition of such material (Locascio & Ley, 1971). Reading ability in the retarded also correlates more closely with the ability to make associations to a picture than it does to other factors (Geller & Geller, 1971).

These findings strongly suggest that verbal elaboration training should replace the current practice of rote learning that exists in most classes for the retarded. These methods should facilitate vocabulary building, reading comprehension, and concept learning. Several investigators have made a start in this direction (Bender, Taylor, Riegel, & Turnure, 1972; Riegel, 1972; Williams, 1970).

At present little difference exists between the verbal interaction in special classes and that in regular classes; Stuck and Wyne (1971) found that special class and regular class teachers showed highly similar verbal behavior under quite different classroom conditions. Because verbal elaboration procedures would help both retarded and normal children, regular class teachers would need to adopt these procedures should the retarded remain in or return to their classes. Memory is also facilitated through verbal and visual elaboration training (e.g., make up a sentence about these two words, make up a picture about the two things doing something together). Mere repetition of two words is much less effective and allows for no transfer of learning (Taylor, Josberger, & Knowlton, 1972).

The deficit theorists have suggested that the retarded have a relatively inert verbal system and demonstrate some dissociation between speech and action. They therefore emphasize language enrichment for retarded groups (Luria, 1963). Other findings imply that the retarded use inefficient problem solving strategies, but also suggest that if they are taught to approach problems in the same manner as the nonretarded, their performance might improve (Das, 1972; Levitt, 1972). For example, McKinney (1972) demonstrated that retarded children with mental ages of 7–8 years can be taught effective problem solving strategies for the processing of information in a discovery learning task and that the learning of these strategies facilitated their subsequent concept attainment and problem solving efficiency. Ross (1971) gave retarded children long-term mediation training within the context of a music program emphasizing the principle and utility of mediational links. Post-training measures showed retention and transfer of the mediation training and marked improvement in nonverbal and verbal performance in a verbal learning task. Ross feels her findings support the notion that the performance deficits of the educable retarded are due to their inability to use their intellect effectively and that such inability is not an irreversible result of low intelligence, "but is due instead to the use of inappropriate training methods" (Ross, 1971, p. 326). Other studies have also found that training in the use of mediation strategies enhances the retarded's verbal learning (Borkowski & Kamfonik, 1972).

Classifications by learning potential score

Educators will undoubtedly continue to ask for predictions about a child's probability of success in school. Recently, an alternative to the intelligence test has been developed to determine whether those with low IQ scores actually are limited in reasoning and learning ability. This instrument is thought to measure learning potential (LP). Unlike the intelligence test, the assessment first tests the child on unfamiliar nonverbal reasoning problems, then instructs the child on task-relevant principles, and finally retests him on the original task. Those who both perform poorly on the pretest and fail to profit from instruction are considered less likely to learn than are others. The work of Budoff and his colleagues has established some validity for this procedure. Their results indicate that LP scores account for differences in classroom learning better than IQ or class assignment (Budoff, Meskin, & Harrison, 1971).

WHAT ELSE IS NEEDED?

Reinforcement in the classroom

Zigler and others have sensitized us to the motivational and emotional variables that depress the performance of retarded children. While research investigators have attempted to evaluate the relative contribution of motivation and cognitive variables, educators continue to stress the cognitive deficiencies of the retarded. As a result, teaching methods and curricula have emphasized cognitive rather than motivational techniques.

Because of the retarded's motivational problems, MacMillan (1971) feels the argument for or against special classes for the EMR is one with no practical value. He says the question to be answered is: "Which placement is most advantageous for which child?" He states (1971, p. 585),

Whether the low IQ, low social class, and/or minority child is placed in a self-contained class or a regular class, he is still likely to manifest a high expectancy for failure, positive and negative reaction tendencies, and outer-directedness. Unless these motivational factors are dealt with by the teacher, success for these children in school is unlikely.

The teacher's first task is to help the child reestablish a feeling of self-worth. Tasks should be given on which success is assured and large amounts of praise given for the success. The use of extrinsic rewards or tokens in order to communicate success can also be appropriate. Once a child comes to expect success, the teacher must help him to raise his lowered level of aspiration. Rewards must be made contingent on higher degrees of success. The gradual fading of teacher cues until only the cues inherent in the problem itself are present should help the child depend upon his own resources for problem solving rather than upon the teacher.

But we must not fall into the trap of assuming that all retarded children have motivational problems. There is as wide a variety of personality organization in the retarded as there is in the normal. And why not, since the retarded child is more child than retarded, and as such he is subject to the same environmental and family influences as are other children. A number of studies have demonstrated that retarded children with similar IQ scores vary considerably on personality measures and that personality variables correlate with achievement in retarded children just as they do in normals (Snyder, Jefferson, & Strauss, 1965). Nevertheless, let us examine the literature on reinforcement systems in the classroom.

Although a teacher's attention immediately following a desired behavior results in an increase in that behavior (Hulten & Kunzelmann, 1969), it is frequently difficult to attend to a child's appropriate behavior because the teacher cannot get to the child before he displays an inappropriate one. In addition, some children are not affected by praise. For these reasons, a number of teachers have utilized tokens to shape and maintain desirable behavior. Tokens are used when a teacher's attention does not control behavior. The token is usually preceded by some type of praise so that praise will eventually become a conditioned reinforcer.

Token reinforcers are objects or symbols which in and of themselves have little or no reinforcing value, but come to have value for the child because they can be exchanged, like money, for desired objects or priviileges. Tokens are superior to primary reinforcers, such as food, because they are independent of the deprivation state of the individual, can be saved until such time as a state of deprivation exists, and can be accumulated and exchanged for items which have more reinforcing value than food.

Grades traditionally have been the token reinforcement system of schools. However, the effectiveness of grades is often minimal since the amount of time between the desired behavior and reinforcement is too long to maintain such behavior. Children who work for grades usually do so because their parents reinforce their learning between marking periods and because they have learned to delay gratification. The advantage of the token is that it can be given immediately following a correct response.

Tokens have been used to decrease hyperactive and disruptive behavior (by dispensing them following periods when these behaviors do not appear), to increase instruction-following behavior, to increase study behavior, to shape and maintain academic and motor skills, and to improve reading, language, and conceptual behaviors. These various token reinforcement programs have been reviewed by Axelrod (1971) and O'Leary and Drabman (1971). Both reviews suggest that greater use be made of reinforcers already existing in the classroom rather than using candies or toys. Both also suggest that future studies should concentrate on devising means of withdrawing the token system so that other conditioned reinforcers, such as teacher attention or grades, can control behavior. Many teachers find it difficult to convince the child who has progressed that he should do more work to earn the same number of tokens (attempts both to increase level of aspiration and teacher control over behavior) or that he should be satisfied with just praise. Perhaps greater use of parents to provide back-up reinforcement would help achieve such an end.

Assistance from guidance staff

While changes within the classroom are helpful, other assistance is usually necessary. Both individual and group counseling have been employed to help raise the institutionalized retarded's self-concept, but public schools have made very little use of either procedure. After reviewing the literature concerned with the effectiveness of group counseling, Clarke and Clarke (1965, p. 426) concluded that counseling benefits the institutionalized retarded.

Group sessions provide an opportunity to relieve situational anxiety caused by misunderstood, or only half understood happenings. Questions freely answered by the therapist provide an opportunity for disseminating information, counteracting disturbing rumors, and for utilizing institutional incidents for concrete demonstrations of community demands and regulations. They make it possible to clarify misunderstandings on the spot, to dispel doubts, to reassure the insecure and to suggest solutions to the hesitant.

Children who received group counseling showed superior institutional adjustment, improved attitudes, and better work output (Clarke & Clarke, 1965).

There is no reason why group counseling could not achieve similar results with retarded children who are not institutionalized, particularly when they usually have more verbal skills than those who are institutionalized. Several studies have suggested that group counseling does have a measurable effect on the retarded (Humes, Adamczyk, & Myco, 1969; Mann, Beaber, & Jacobson, 1969). Counseled adolescents showed higher scores on personality inventories and a more positive self-concept than equivalent noncounseled groups. For example, the study by Mann and his colleagues revealed that 12 weekly sessions with a group of retarded boys increased their self-concept and reduced their general level of anxiety, their feelings of futility and anxiety about school, as well as their hostility toward school staff. In addition to these changes, the children's teachers rated their conduct, reading, and arithmetic as improved following counseling.

The self-report measures used in Mann's study to measure self-concept and anxiety serve as examples of the many personality inventories that have been used to assess change following counseling. Self-concept and anxiety were measured both before and after counseling through use of the Children's Self-Concept Scale (Lipsitt, 1958), The Way I Feel About Myself Scale (Piers & Harris, 1964), and the children's form of the Taylor Manifest Anxiety Scale (Castaneda, McCandless, & Palermo, 1956). In each of these scales the child either rates himself or circles Yes or No on various trait descriptions. Lawrence and Winschel (1973) feel that the validity and standardization of many self-report scales are unsatisfactory. Consequently, findings that emanate from their use are inconclusive. Hopefully, better measures will be employed in future studies of the effect of counseling on mildly retarded children.

In Mann's study each counseling session was structured around a particular topic introduced by the counselor, such as "dealing with authority figures" or "why special education?" Similarily, Humes and his colleagues (Humes et al., 1969) introduced topics to the group through the use of selected pictures from the Thematic Apperception Test and the Symonds Picture-Story Test. At each session the counselor presented one picture, which was intended to focus attention on typical adolescent problems. Perhaps the positive results of both these investigations was due to their structured technique since traditional unstructured approaches are often less effective with the retarded (Stern & Keislar, 1967). Group counseling may also be preferable to individual counseling because the more expressive members can serve as models for the others.

Direct training of social behavior has been employed to increase knowledge of social responses and to improve skill in logical reasoning. A group of young retarded children learned the correct social response in selected situations using doll play, live modeling, film slides, and puppets within a practical syllogism framework. The experimental group improved their social skills to a level higher than an intellectually normal group of the same age, while the controls showed no improvement (Ross, 1969).

Behavior therapy, which often takes the form of direct instruction, has been used with slow learners. A case presented by Mordock and Phillips (1971, pp. 232–233) illustrates the use of several behavioral techniques.

Sally, age 13, was referred for extremely immature behavior, characterized by poor impulse control, preoccupation with fantasy, and hyperactivity. She frequently refused to answer questions in class and annoyed others around her because of her restless behavior. Consequently, no one wanted to be seen with her and boys taunted and teased her. Relations with authority figures were extremely poor and teachers described her as an obnoxious brat.

Psychological evaluation by the school psychologist highlighted hysterical features in a girl with limited intellect (WISC verbal IQ 72, performance IQ 89). A male therapist was selected to treat her since continued exposure to him would serve as an *in vivo* desensitization to males. The target behavior selected was refusal to answer teacher initiated questions. Her science teacher was asked to cooperate with us since he was young and seemed less negative about her. He was instructed to ask no questions of Sally, but simply to bypass her when her turn came. Instead, he gave the therapist a list of questions which he would have asked her and which he ranked according to difficulty. These questions were then read to Sally by the therapist, starting with the easier items. At first, only a minimal answer was required, followed by elaboration. Sally, at first, would not cooperate in the training enterprise. Completion of the Reinforcement Survey Schedule revealed several things she wanted but, because of her poor behavior, they had been withheld from her by her parents. With their cooperation, Sally could acquire these privileges by accumulating points earned for answering the questions in therapy. She was not required to study the material, since her study habits were extremely poor, but to answer the questions from cards handed her. Concurrently, she was instructed to make a count of the number of notes she passed in class which asked students whether they were her friends, mad at her, etc. This behavior was reportedly annoying to other students or gave them reasons to ridicule her. She was then told that she could also earn points if she reported having passed less notes of this sort, following an explanation that friends were not gained by such behavior.

Behavior rehearsal was then introduced to help her initiate behaviors which would assist her to develop relationships with peers. A target girl was selected toward whom she could direct compliments. Practice in compliment giving was undertaken until she felt comfortable doing so, and then she was encouraged to initiate this behavior toward the girl selected, or toward others if she wished to do so. . . .

Following this phase, Sally was to answer questions in class and then to volunteer to answer pre-selected questions. During this period, Sally's grades in science improved from 55 to 75, while grades in her other five courses remained the same (50 to 60). Her restless behavior also diminished in science and she was reported to have several friends. Several weeks later other teachers noted improvement and, following her last marking period, she had improved in all courses. She also had a "best friend," which pleased her greatly. Sally was seen for a total of ten sessions. (*From* Psychotherapy: Theory, Research and Practice.)

Support from the community

The schools should not be the only agency providing services to the retarded. Retarded children, like all children, need to learn to occupy their leisure time. Special summer recreational facilities for the retarded are often provided by communities through support from local chapters of the National Association for Retarded Children. Although they provide summer fun, they do further isolate the retarded from his normal peers. However, since camps operated by churches and youth groups are leery about accepting members from special classes and discourage if not reject them, parents of the retarded have no choice but to fund and operate their own camps.

Not surprising, then, was Dinger's (1958) conclusion, after reviewing studies concerned with the community adjustment of retarded adults, that the retarded fail to participate in a community's civic and social life. Dinger's own investigation of the employed retarded revealed that their levels of industrial and domestic adjustment were much closer to normal than their leisure time activity.

The Jewish Community Centers Association of St. Louis (JCCA) has demonstrated that retarded children considerably more impaired than those discussed in this chapter can participate in activities designed for nonretarded children. Over a period of five years, 41 retarded children ranging in IQ from 48 to 78 joined numerous kinds of ongoing leisure time activities at the center. Although 30 of these youngsters had one or more physical handicaps, three-quarters of them did at least minimally well. Although center staff rated the social behavior of the retarded members as significantly different from normals in the same group, differences were manageable and often diminished with continued exposure to normal children (Pumphrey, Goodman, Kidd, & Peters, 1970).

JCCA staff also reported that children who began their agency experience before adolescence made a better adjustment than those who delayed joining until after this age-stage. Overactive adolescents in the lowest educable range were less successful than those with more withdrawn behavior patterns. JCCA staff also commented on the retarded's responses to their normal peers. At home or at school the EMRs learned to doubt all options but that of the authoritative adult. They had to learn to listen to and to follow the suggestions of other group members, as well as learn the current slang and fashion and to take the "kidding" of normal childhood. They also had difficulty in adjusting to new situations. Many, however, made marked progress in a short time. JCCA staff recommend that planned shifts in school routines might make entrance into the community less traumatic. The experience of JCCA staff suggests that many more EMRs should participate in normal community activities.

HOW DO THEY FARE?

In spite of ridicule and prejudice the mildly retarded do better than most of us would expect. They have done better in the past, however, than they are now doing. Follow-up studies in the 1920s and 1930s indicated that over 80 percent made a satisfactory adult adjustment (Anderson & Fearing, 1923; Beaman, 1932; Channing, 1932; Fairbank, 1933). More recent studies, however, place the figure at 50 to 60 percent

(Skaabrenk, 1971; Tobias, 1970). Unfortunately, as our society becomes more sophisticated in its approach to exceptionality, it becomes more sophisticated technologically as well. Having less need for unskilled and semiskilled workers and more need for the highly educated, there are less opportunities for the less bright.

Several follow-up studies (Titus & Travis, 1973; Tobias, 1970) revealed that the majority of mildly retarded males are employed by small businesses as laborers and shipping or mailing clerks. Females work primarily in institutional services as domestic or cafeteria help. Titus and Travis reported an average wage of $2.08 per hour, with a range from $1.40 to $3.45. Tobias reported a sizeable number as falling below minimum wages. He also reported that Puerto Ricans, employed primarily in manufacturing and clerical fields, have the best employment record, the white group an intermediate position, and blacks the worst record.

A substantial number also had higher IQ scores as adults. Tobias (1970) retested the IQs of 151 retarded subjects some 10 years after their original testing. Fifty-six percent of the Puerto Rican males achieved retest scores 10 or more points above their original scores, as did 41 percent of black males and 32 percent of white males. Among the women, where there were no racial differences in IQ change, 80 percent had retest scores within 10 points of their school IQs.

CONCLUDING REMARKS

From what we have reviewed, it appears that retardation is a transitory phenomenon; a child labeled retarded by the school may no longer be recognized as such in situations where academic competence is of minor importance. Compulsory school attendance and the school's stress on academic accomplishment have resulted in the school's labeling those individuals unsuccessful in school as retarded. The increasing complexity of society has decreased the opportunity for the less bright to obtain gainful employment. That many find employment in spite of poor schooling supports the notion that the retarded more easily meet the demands of society for vocational competence and social independence than they do the demands of school—change the demands of society and their retardation disappears! Wolfson (1970, p. 23) concludes;

The mentally retarded are people in their own right, in spite of their limited capacity for academic achievement. They have needs, wishes, and hopes which should be recognized and respected. The emphasis from supervision . . . should be changed to guidance and assistance when indicated to help these people to find themselves and lead their own lives.

What are their wishes? The same as yours and mine. With increasing age both retarded and normal children wish for abstract or intangible human conditions rather than for concrete or tangible possessions; they wish for things consistent with adult rather than child status and make altruistic wishes, benefiting others rather than themselves (Milgram & Riedal, 1969).

References

American Association on Mental Deficiency. *Manual on terminology and classification in mental retardation.* Washington, D.C.: American Association of Mental Deficiency, 1973.

Anderson, V. V., & Fearing, M. A. *A study of the careers of three hundred twenty-two feebleminded persons.* New York: National Committee for Mental Hygiene, 1923.

Axelrod, S. Token reinforcement programs in special classes. *Exceptional Children,* 1971, **37,** 371–379.

Bauer, D. H., & Yamamoto, K. Designing instructional settings for children labeled retarded: some reflections. *The Elementary School Journal,* 1972, **72,** 343–350.

Beaman, F. N. An experimental curriculum for special classes. Unpublished master's thesis, Northwestern University, 1932.

Bender, N. N., Taylor, A. M., Riegel, R. H., & Turnure, J. E. Variations of strategy pre-training for a strategy based approach for teaching EMR children in the United States. Paper presented at the annual meeting of the American Educational Research Association, Chicago, April 1972.

Blackman, L. S. The dimensions of a science of special education. *Mental Retardation,* 1967, **5**(4), 7–11.

Borkowski, J. G., & Kamfonik, A. Verbal mediation in moderately retarded children: effects of successive mediational experiences. *American Journal of Mental Deficiency,* 1972, **77,** 157–162.

Bracht, G. H., & Glass, G. V. The external validity of comparative experiments in education and the social sciences. (Research Paper No. 3) Boulder: Laboratory of Educational Research, University of Colorado, 1967.

Budoff, M., Meskin, J., & Harrison, R. H. Educational test of the learning-potential hypothesis. *American Journal of Mental Deficiency,* 1971, **70,** 159–169.

Carroll, A. W. The effects of segregated and partially integrated school programs on self-concept and academic achievement of educable mental retardates. *Exceptional Children,* 1967, **33,** 93–99.

Castaneda, A., McCandless, B. R., & Palermo, D. S. The children's form of the Manifest Anxiety Scale. *Child Development,* 1956, **27,** 318–326.

Cegelka, P. A., & Cegelka, W. J. A review of the research: reading and the educable mentally handicapped. *Exceptional Children,* 1970, **37,** 187–200.

Channing, A. *Employment of mentally deficient boys and girls.* (U.S. Children's Bureau Publication No. 210) Washington, D.C.: U.S. Government Printing Office, 1932.

Clarke, A. M., & Clarke, A. D. B. *Mental deficiency, the changing outlook.* (2nd ed.) New York: Free Press, 1965.

Collins, H. A., Burger, G. K., & Doherty, D. Self-concept of EMR and non-retarded adolescents. *American Journal of Mental Deficiency,* 1970, **75,** 285–289.

Cromwell, R. L. A social learning approach to mental retardation. In N. R. Ellis (Ed.), *Handbook of mental deficiency.* New York: McGraw-Hill, 1963.

Das, J. P. Patterns of cognitive ability in nonretarded and retarded children. *American Journal of Mental Deficiency*, 1972, **77**, 6–12.

Davis, F. R. Demand-degradable teacher standards: expediency and professional thanatos. *Mental Retardation*, 1970, **8**(1), 37–40.

Denny, M. R. Research in learning and performance. In H. A. Stevens & R. Heber (Eds.), *Mental retardation: a review of research.* Chicago: University of Chicago Press, 1964.

DeProspo, C. J. A suggested curriculum for the mentally handicapped. In M. E. Frampton & E. D. Gall (Eds.), *Special education for the exceptional.* Boston: Porter Sargent, 1956.

Dinger, J. C. *Post school adjustment of former special education pupils with implications for curricular revision.* (Doctoral dissertation, Pennsylvania University, No. 58-2669) Ann Arbor, Mich.: University Microfilms, 1958.

Ellis, N. R. (Ed.) *Handbook of mental deficiency.* New York: McGraw-Hill, 1963.

Fairbank, R. E. The subnormal child seventeen years after. *Mental Hygiene*, 1933, **17**, 177–208.

Gagne, R. M., & Weigand, V. K. Some factors in children's learning and retention of concrete rules. *Journal of Educational Psychology*, 1968, **59**, 355–361.

Garrison, I. K. Special programs for the mentally retarded in secondary school. In P. M. Halverson (Ed.), *Frontiers of secondary education.* Vol. 1. Syracuse, N.Y.: Syracuse University Press, 1956.

Garrison, M., & Hammill, D. D. Who are the retarded? *Exceptional Children*, 1971, **38**, 13–20.

Geller, E. S., & Geller, C. A. Performance variables related to the reading achievement of mentally retarded children. *Experimental Publication System*, 1971, **10** (Ms. No. 385–3).

Gillette, A. L. Learning and retention: a comparison of three experimental procedures. *Archives of Psychology*, 1936, **28**(198).

Gozali, J. Perception of the EMR special class by former students. *Mental Retardation*, 1972, **10**(1), 34–35.

Gregory, S. C., Jr., & Bunch, M. E. The relative retentive abilities of fast and slow learners. *Journal of General Psychology*, 1959, **60**, 173–181.

Gunzburg, H. C. Mental deficiencies. In B. B. Walman (Ed.), *Manual of child psychopathology.* New York: McGraw-Hill, 1972.

Guskin, S. L., & Spicker, H. H. Educational research in mental retardation. In N. R. Ellis (Ed.), *International review of research in mental retardation.* Vol. 3. New York: Academic Press, 1968.

Guthrie, G. M., Gorlow, L., & Butler, A. J. The attitude of the retardate toward herself: a summary of research at Laurelton State School and Hospital. *Pennsylvania Psychiatric Quarterly*, 1967, **7**, 24–34.

Hollinger, C. S., & Jones, R. L. Community attitudes toward slow learners and mental retardates: what's in a name? *Mental Retardation*, 1970, **8**(1), 19–23.

Hulten, W. J., & Kunzelmann, H. P. Teacher attention—a social consequence. *Mental Retardation*, 1969, **7**, 11–14.

Humes, C. W., Jr., Adamczyk, J. S., & Myco, R. W. A school study of group counseling with educable retarded adolescents. *American Journal of Mental Deficiency*, 1969, **74**, 191–195.

Iano, R. P. Learning deficiency versus developmental conceptions of mental retardation. *Exceptional Children*, 1971, **38**, 301–311.

Iano, R. P., Ayers, D., Heller, H. B., McGettigan, J. F., & Walker, V. S. Sociometric status of retarded children in an integrative program. *Exceptional Children*, 1974, **40**, 267–271.

Jastak, J. F., MacPhee, H. M., & Whitman, M. *Mental retardation: its nature and incidence.* New York: University Publishers, 1963.

Johnson, G. O. The education of mentally retarded children. In W. M. Cruickshank & G. O. Johnson (Eds.), *Education of exceptional children and youth.* (2nd ed.) Englewood Cliffs, N.J.: Prentice-Hall, 1967.

Jones, L. R. Labels and stigma in special education. *Exceptional Children,* 1972, **38,** 553–564.

Jordon, T. E. *The exceptional child.* Columbus, Ohio: Merrill, 1962.

Katz, P. Acquisition and retention of discrimination learning sets in lower class preschool children. *Journal of Educational Psychology,* 1967, **58,** 253–258.

Keislar, E. R., & Stern, C. Differentiated instruction in problem solving for children of different mental ability levels. *Journal of Educational Psychology,* 1970, **61,** 445–450.

Kirk, S. A. Research in education. In H. A. Stevens & R. Heber (Eds.), *Mental retardation: a review of research.* Chicago: University of Chicago Press, 1964.

Kirk, S. A., & Johnson, G. O. *Educating the retarded child.* New York: Houghton Mifflin, 1951.

Kohlberg, L. Early education: a cognitive-developmental view. *Child Development,* 1968, **39,** 1013–1062.

Lawrence, E. A., & Winschel, J. F. Self-concept and the retarded: research and issues. *Exceptional Children,* 1973, **39,** 310–319.

Levitt, E. Higher-order and lower-order reading responses of mentally retarded and nonretarded children at the first grade level. *American Journal of Mental Deficiency,* 1972, **77,** 13–20.

Lipsitt, L. P. A self-concept scale for children and its relationship to the children's form of the Manifest Anxiety Scale. *Child Development,* 1958, **29,** 463–472.

Locascio, D., & Ley, R. Associative reaction time in free recall. Paper presented at the annual meeting of the Eastern Psychological Association, New York, April 1971.

Luria, A. R. Psychological studies of mental deficiency in the Soviet Union. In N. R. Ellis (Ed.), *Handbook of mental deficiency.* New York: McGraw-Hill, 1963.

MacMillan, D. L. The problem of motivation in the education of the mentally retarded. *Exceptional Children,* 1971, **37,** 579–586.

MacMillan, D. L., & Carlson, J. S. Probability judgments by EMR and nonretarded children. II. A replication and extension. *American Journal of Mental Deficiency,* 1971, **76,** 82–86.

Mann, P. H., Beaber, J. B., & Jacobson, M. D. The effect of group counseling on educable mentally retarded boys' self-concepts. *Exceptional Children,* 1969, **35,** 359–366.

McKinney, J. D. Developmental study of the acquisition and utilization of conceptual strategies. *Journal of Educational Psychology,* 1972, **63,** 22–31.

Meyrowitz, J. H. Self-derogation in young retardates and special class placement. *Child Development,* 1962, **33,** 443–451.

Mercer, J. R. I.Q.: the lethal label. *Psychology Today,* 1972, **6,** 44–47, 95–97.

Milgram, N. A., & Riedal, W. W. Developmental and experiential factors in making wishes. *Child Development,* 1969, **40,** 763–771.

Mordock, J. B. Paired-associate learning in mental retardation: a review. *American Journal of Mental Deficiency,* 1968a, **72,** 857–865.

Mordock, J. B. Maze learning: the effects of variations in practice conditions, age, and intelligence. *American Journal of Mental Deficiency*, 1968b, **73**, 113–117.

Mordock, J. B. Distribution of practice in paired-associate learning. *American Journal of Mental Deficiency*, 1968c, **73**, 399–404.

Mordock, J. B., & Phillips, D. The behavior therapist in the schools. *Psychotherapy: Theory, Research and Practice*, 1971, **8**, 231–235.

O'Leary, K. D., & Drabman, R. Token reinforcement programs in the classroom: a review. *Psychological Bulletin*, 1971, **75**, 379–398.

Piers, E. V., & Harris, D. B. Age and other correlates of self-concept in children. *Journal of Educational Psychology*, 1964, **60**, 91–95.

Pumphrey, M. W., Goodman, M. B., Kidd, J. W., & Peters, E. N. Participation of retarded children in regular recreational activities at a community center. *Exceptional Children*, 1970, **36**, 453–458.

Reed, J. E., & Hayman, J. L., Jr. An experiment involving use of English 2600, an automated instruction text. *Journal of Educational Research*, 1962, **55**, 476–484.

Riegel, R. H. Measuring children's organizational strategies by sampling overt groupings. Paper presented at the annual meeting of the American Educational Research Association, Chicago, April 1972.

Robbin, C. School awards for EMR's? Yes! *Instructor*, 1970, **79**, 97–98.

Ross, D. Retention and transfer of mediation set in paired-associate learning of educable retarded children. *Journal of Educational Psychology*, 1971, **62**, 322–327.

Ross, D. M., & Ross, S. A. The efficacy of listening training for educable mentally retarded children. *American Journal of Mental Deficiency*, 1972, **77**, 137–142.

Ross, S. A. Effects of intentional training in social behavior on retarded children. *American Journal of Mental Deficiency*, 1969, **73**, 912–919.

Schoer, L. A. Effect of last length and interpolated learning on the learning and recall of fast and slow learners. *Journal of Educational Psychology*, 1962, **53**, 193–197.

Schurr, K. J., Joiner, L. M., & Towne, R. C. Self-concept research on the mentally retarded: a review of empirical studies. *Mental Retardation*, 1970, **8**(5), 39–43.

Shuell, T. J., & Keppel, G. Learning ability and retention. *Journal of Educational Psychology*, 1970, **61**, 59–65.

Skaarbrenk, K. J. A follow-up study of educable mentally retarded in Norway. *American Journal of Mental Deficiency*, 1971, **75**, 560–565.

Snyder, R., Jefferson, W., & Strauss, R. Personality variables as determiners of academic achievement of the mildly retarded. *Mental Retardation*, 1965, **3**(1), 15–18.

Stern, C., & Keislar, E. Acquisition of problem solving strategies by young children and its relation to mental age. *American Educational Research Journal*, 1967, **4**, 1–12.

Stroud, J. B., & Schoer, L. A. Individual differences in memory. *Journal of Educational Psychology*, 1959, **50**, 285–292.

Stuck, G. B., & Wyne, M. D. Study of verbal behavior in special and regular elementary school classrooms. *American Journal of Mental Deficiency*, 1971, **75**, 463–469.

Tallmadge, G. K. Relationships between training methods and learner characteristics. *Journal of Educational Psychology*, 1968, **59**, 32–36.

Taylor, A. M., Josberger, M., & Knowlton, J. Q. Mental elaboration and learning to EMR children. *American Journal of Mental Deficiency*, 1972, **77**, 69–76.

Titus, R. W., & Travis, J. T. Follow-up of EMR program graduates. *Mental Retardation*, 1973, 11(2), 24–26.

Tobias, J. Vocational adjustment of young retarded adults. *Mental Retardation*, 1970, 8(3), 13–17.

Underwood, B. J. Speed of learning and amount retained: a consideration of methodology. *Psychological Bulletin*, 1954, 51, 276–282.

Williams, E. H. Effects of readiness on incidental learning of EMR, normal and gifted children. *American Journal of Mental Deficiency*, 1970, 75, 117–119.

Wettingfeld, J. Library program for retarded children: with a bibliography to order. *Instructor*, 1970, 79, 73–74.

Wolfson, I. N. Adjustment of institutionalized mildly retarded patients twenty years after return to the community. *Mental Retardation*, 1970, 8(4), 20–23.

Zigler, E. Familial mental retardation: a continuing dilemma. *Science*, 1967, 157, 578–579.

Zigler, E. Developmental versus difference theories of mental retardation and the problem of motivation. *American Journal of Mental Deficiency*, 1969, 73, 536–556.

Zigler, E., & Balla, D. Luria's verbal deficiency theory of mental retardation and performance on sameness, symmetry, and opposition tasks: a critique. *American Journal of Mental Deficiency*, 1971, 75, 400–413.

Zigler, E., & deLabry, J. Concept-switching in middle class, lower class, and retarded children. *Journal of Abnormal and Social Psychology*, 1962, 65, 267–273.

Zito, R. J., & Bardon, J. I. Achievement motivation among Negro adolescents in regular and special education programs. *American Journal of Mental Deficiency*, 1969, 74, 20–26.

VI
Psychoeducation

The value of the help given to the exceptional child and his family depends upon the abilities of the professionals who deliver it. True, the effect of their skills is often minimized by the lack of interagency cooperation often existing in communities or by a family's inability to face its problems. However, we will focus on some of the variables that make for success in working with the exceptional child and will describe several specific programs dealing with children in difficulty.

Although we touched upon therapeutic approaches in our discussion of each disability, we hope to give the reader a more comprehensive grasp of psychoeducational remediation by devoting a full chapter to it. We feature the roles of the teacher, psychologist, and psychotherapist in the chapter, not because these professionals are more important than others in dealing with children, but because they are the professions most frequently involved in remediation in school settings. Although psychotherapy is infrequently used in the school, child guidance clinics are beginning to work more closely with schools. Many teachers only vaguely understand the purpose of psychotherapy and either over- or underestimate its influence, expecting the child to improve immediately once he is given therapy or dismissing it because the child "only plays with toys." Since many teachers, as well as psychologists, will work in institutional settings we devote some space to institutional programs.

It is not fair . . . children have to try to figure out the grown-ups all on their own, without any help from books or living people. Adults have all kinds of aids from researchers on how to understand boys and girls. We have to figure them *out with no clues at all.*
I wish there were a manual on mothers, daddys, and teachers.

—A 10-year-old

12
The exceptional child and the professional

By this time it should be clear that professionals working with exceptional children have differing opinions about how children should be handled. Some professionals who work with the psychotic attribute the disorder solely to family pathology and advocate removing the child from the family, while others view constitutional deficiencies as the source and advocate community support for the child's family. Experts on the deaf continue to debate the merits of the oral versus the manual approach to education. Those working with the disadvantaged argue about the relative importance of language deficiency and mediation processes. Psychotherapists argue about whether therapeutic intervention should deal only with observable behaviors or should attempt to elicit fantasies and change cognitions. Some teachers advocate teacher-centered approaches toward instruction while others advocate child-centered approaches.

The only way to resolve differences in opinion is to replace opinion with fact. As research evidence accumulates about an approach, opinion can give way to fact. Nevertheless, there are always those who are heavily committed to a particular approach and refuse to believe evidence contrary to their opinion. The same reluctance to give up a strongly held opinion characterizes professionals who have a particular belief about an individual child with whom they are working. In this chapter we will focus on three professionals who work with children—the teacher, the psychologist, and the psychotherapist. We will show how teachers differ in their ability to manage their classroom and will isolate some of the variables which relate to classroom control. We will then discuss the manner in which the school psychologist functions in his role as a consultant to teachers. Next, we will focus on the psychotherapist and his approach to children as well as the manner in which he and the teacher can work together for a child's benefit. Following our discussion of these three professionals and their interaction, we will describe various ways in which institutions have been organized to help a child when treatment requires temporary separation from his family.

THE TEACHER

Billy was in Mrs. Jones's class; for Mrs. Jones, Billy meant trouble. He daydreamed, talked without permission, poked other children, and made a general nuisance of himself. Worst of all, Mrs. Jones felt she had no time to assess adequately his strengths, weaknesses, and needs. She doubted that he had mastered the prerequisites necessary for placement in the third grade. In any case, Billy did very little work and resisted her efforts to evaluate his current level of achievement. Mrs. Jones had requested a conference with Bill's parents, but they both worked and couldn't come to school during the day. It was just as well, since she felt they wouldn't be of help anyway.

To try to diminish Billy's disruptive behavior, Mrs. Jones placed him in the back of the room, decreased her demands upon him for academic achievement, and let him draw or play, as long as he was quiet and well-behaved. Frequently, however, she had to stand near him to keep him in his seat. She believed that Billy was emotionally disturbed and, perhaps, needed special class placement. For this reason, she referred him for psychological testing.

Mrs. Jones taught in school A. Following the procedures established for referrals in this school, the psychologist administered an individual intelligence test and several measures of personality. He wrote a report emphasizing Bill's poor self-concept, his perception of reality as need-frustrating, and his unstable position in a difficult family situation. He concluded that Bill's measured intelligence was an underestimation of his ability, due to emotional factors that interfered with further development. Armed with this "increased understanding" of Bill, Mrs. Jones would either be satisfied that Bill's behavior was beyond her control or dissatisfied because no actual help was given. In other case, an "expert" had implied that no one could expect much from her because of Bill's difficulties.

If Mrs. Jones had taught in school B, things might have gone differently. In this school either a trained aide or the psychologist would observe Bill in the classroom and record the frequency of specific behaviors, such as talking out, hitting others, and remaining on task. Mrs. Jones would be asked to give Bill some informal tests to determine how many "problems" he could do in a delineated time period, how many words he should be expected to learn in a week, and so on. Mrs. Jones's behavior toward Bill would be observed and her style of interaction coded. Questions would be asked: "How many arithmetical facts does Bill know?" "What materials hold his interest?" "How do other children feel about him?" "Is he primarily a visual or auditory learner?" The psychologist in school B believes that Bill's environment can be programmed to bring him under control and that, with the selection of proper instructional materials and the introduction of more appropriate classroom or behavioral management techniques, Bill's classroom functioning will improve. Within this model report writing is secondary to continual involvement with each child referred. The teacher must be willing to modify both her classroom instruction and management techniques, and teacher aides must be available to assist in the preparation of instructional materials. In addition, the teacher, aide, and psychologist must meet frequently to discuss the child's progress. Teachers should also meet in small groups to discuss children with similar needs.

In school A the psychologist behaved as if his report would result in a change in the teacher's relationship with Billy. In school B the psychologist assumed that direct intervention of some sort was necessary to change Billy's behavior in the classroom. The teacher would have to change her behavior, her instructional or managerial approach, in order to change Billy. The psychologist would help her to do so by helping to formulate immediate goals and to outline steps needed to reach them. He would not tell the teacher exactly what to do, however, for he viewed their efforts as collaborative. Rather, he would suggest certain general approaches and leave the details to her. As we have seen, some behaviorally oriented psychologists give detailed instructions when helping teachers to change a child's behavior. Others feel such detailed guidance leads to dependency and blocks teacher growth.

What sort of person makes a good teacher of exceptional children? Mrs. Jones tried some techniques to control Billy but obviously didn't feel they would be of much help. If Mrs. Jones was to switch jobs and work in school B, she would have to function differently. She would have to learn a new set of skills and change her attitude about her own influence on children. But then, Mrs. Jones was a regular classroom teacher without specialized training in education of exceptional children. Whatever she knew about emotional disturbance or learning disabilities was learned from experience with several such children who had been in her regular classroom. She didn't consider herself an expert in dealing with exceptionality. After all, her major was elementary education not special education! The state education department had different certification requirements for special education teachers; obviously they were better equipped than she was to handle someone like Billy.

In Chapter 1, however, we emphasized that the trend was away from special class placement, that more exceptional children would be kept in the mainstream of education. Does this imply that the regular class teacher will need to take a number of courses in exceptionality and have some practice teaching experience with the exceptional child? It may, but many regular classroom teachers do quite well in managing exceptional children in their classroom, and they do so without much awareness of exceptionality. For example, research suggests that teachers who are successful in managing the behavior of nondisturbed children in their regular classroom are also successful in managing the behavior of disturbed children (Kounin, 1967; Kounin & Obradovic, 1968). A teacher's managerial success in the classroom was defined as the ability to induce work involvement and prevent deviance in the children in her class. Teachers who were effective in managing both the disturbed and nondisturbed child used group management techniques such as those embodied in the description of Miss Green below.

Group management techniques

Miss Green seemed to have eyes in the back of her head. She was able to ignore minor misbehavior and make timely interruptions of more serious misbehavior. She admonished children quickly and her reprimands rarely needed to be followed by punishments. She also was able to handle two issues at one time. While working with a reading group, she could still handle a disruptive child not doing his seatwork. Miss Green assigned a variety of seatwork during given time periods and used challenging material, material that required thought or creativity rather than rote or repetitive copying. She also instilled in the children a zest for upcoming tasks.

Miss Green communicated to her children that she knew what each was doing during a designated task. During recitation, she created some suspense by pausing after each question and looking around before selecting a child to recite. She selected them at random rather than in a predictable order, and she alerted children that they might be called upon to evaluate a reciter's performance.

She usually directed small groups of children or the entire class to perform an act rather than telling each student to perform that act. Consequently, movement between activities was orderly and proceeded smoothly. She also had a knack for being precise and giving the right amount of instructions when presenting new tasks.

Now, let us consider the description of Mrs. Blue, a teacher who had little success in maintaining student work involvement. Mrs. Blue always seemed to talk too much. When giving instructions, her discussion clearly exceeded that necessary to get the children to understand or participate in an activity. She usually dwelled too long on subactions, such as how to sit or where to put hands, or on "props" (pencils, crayons, books). Then she would direct individual children to do separately what a small group or the entire class could do at once. When a child misbehaved, she would preach or moralize to the child and sometimes to the entire class. She frequently initiated an activity and then left it dangling. She burst into children's activities with orders or questions without being sensitive to the child's or the group's readiness to receive her message. She reacted to many minor transgressions, but often ignored major ones, and when disciplining a child, she usually did so too late. For example, she scolded Mary for interrupting her when several other boys were poking each other and out of their seats. By the time she responded to their behavior, several other children had become involved.

In order to differentiate between the behaviors that characterize Miss Green and Mrs. Blue, Kounin and his colleagues have classified management techniques into eight major categories (Kounin & Obradovic, 1968), and control techniques into four categories (Kounin & Gump, 1958; Kounin, Gump, & Ryan, 1961). The teacher management techniques are as follows: slowdowns, smoothness, with-it-ness, overlappingness, group alerting, accountability, valence and challenge-arousal, seatwork variety-challenge.

Slowdowns refers to teacher-initiated friction that impedes a group's rate of movement. An example is the overdone behavior of Mrs. Blue, her tendency to give too many instructions and to overemphasize unimportant details. Smoothness applies to the manner in which a teacher initiates activities. Examples of lack of smoothness are Mrs. Blue's thrusting in on a child's activity in an untimely manner and not following through on activities. With-it-ness refers to Miss Green's ability to be tuned in on what is going on in her classroom. Overlappingness is a measure of the teacher's ability to attend to two issues simultaneously. Group alerting refers to the degree to which the teacher focuses on all the children in a group during transition periods and recitations. Miss Green's selecting children at random is an example of such behavior. Accountability refers to the degree to which the teacher communicates to the children knowledge of what each is doing in relation to the task assigned. Valence and challenge-arousal is the arousal of enthusiasm for an upcoming task, and seatwork variety-challenge refers to the number of changes in assigned seatwork during a given period of time to avoid overrepetitive work and to the use of a variety of materials requiring creative thought, not just rote accumulation of knowledge.

Control or desist techniques, that is, the manner in which a teacher attempts to control a disruptive child, were classified into four categories: threatening versus supportive, punishing versus reprimanding versus ignoring, clarity versus firmness versus roughness, and task focus versus approval focus. The threatening versus supportive category refers to the degree of warmth displayed by the teacher while intervening in a child's inappropriate behavior. Support was seen as more beneficial to the target child and to others watching. Of the three techniques—punishing (characterized by intensity and punitiveness), reprimanding (simple corrections), and ignoring—the simple reprimand was rated as having the best results, with ignoring and punishing following in that order. Clarity (defining deviancy and stating what to do to stop it) increased the conformance of the audience; firmness ("I mean it") decreased the deviancy of audience children interested in the deviancy; roughness (angry remarks, hostile looks) increased behavior disruption. Task focus techniques ("talking hurts arithmetic") were more effective in eliciting desirable behavior than approval focus techniques ("I don't like the boys who talk").

Specific controlling techniques, however, are not as critical as those relating to general classroom management. Kounin (1967, p. 227) remarks that classroom control "is a function of the techniques of creating an effective classroom ecology containing such variables as having a nonsatiating learning program, initiating and maintaining movement flow, and aiming teacher actions at appropriate targets."

While theoretically possible to train teachers to be more aware of their behavior and to make more use of general procedures rather than specific control techniques, Kounin's work implies that successful classroom management is a function of the teacher's personality style; that successful teachers are those who naturally make use of procedures that keep children involved in their work.

Another variable that relates to classroom management is the extent to which the teacher takes responsibility for the direction of her class and considers herself the source of all knowledge. Does the teacher create a climate where knowledge can be discovered by her pupils or does she dispense facts to be memorized. What kind of atmosphere or climate does she provide for learning?

Classroom climate

In the 1940s and 1950s there was considerable interest in classroom climate and the effects of the authoritarian, teacher-centered, dominative teacher compared to the democratic, child-centered, integrative teacher.

Anderson (1959) carried out an extensive critical review of studies concerning authoritarian and democratic leadership and learning. He reported that neither style of leadership was consistently related to better learning. He also concluded that the authoritarian-democratic construct was a grossly oversimplified dimension and inadequate for measuring leadership behavior. Later, Hyman (1964) reached a similar conclusion, although he did feel that teachers who were extreme examples of either style were less effective than other teachers.

More recently, investigators have examined differences in achievement between students taught by direct versus indirect methods. Although different investigators have defined these dimensions differently, behaviors identified as defining directive teaching approximate what others have called authoritarian, teacher-centered, or teacher-dominated approaches. Similarly, behaviors identified as defining indirective teaching approximate what others have called democratic, child-centered, or integrative approaches. (Although we consider the various terms denoting either approach interchangeable, in discussing research we will use the term selected by each author; the interested reader can refer to the original sources to examine subtle differences between the terms employed.)

Any approach to classroom teaching involves planning the course; organizing classroom, group, and individual activity; and dispensing factual knowledge. Classroom climate is rated direct or indirect according to the degree of formality and rigidity in handling these factors. Direct approaches tend to emphasize formal planning and structuring of the course, to minimize informal and group work and to structure what group activity is used, to structure rigidly individual and classroom activity, and to require factual knowledge from students based on an absolute source. Directive teachers also are seen as more impersonal toward students. They use more unconditional punishments, minimize the opportunity to make and learn from mistakes, maintain a more

A LEARNING CENTER

The selected students leave their rooms at math time and meet at the learning center for class. The learning center has carrels, is carpeted, and houses all the materials that the students need for this class. All students begin the class in the learning center, but if they want a quiet place to study they can always go to Miss Moore's classroom since it is empty at this time.

Miss Moore, as the group's teacher, has already contracted with the students for the specified work they are responsible for, so there are no assignments when the students enter. While some children sit at the tables, others go to study carrels, while still others take up places on the floor and begin to take out some of the math games.

There seems to be an almost infinite variety of materials available. A "Cyclo-teacher" offers different problems a child can solve. It also provides a chance for the children to make up their own problems.

Two students are playing a game making equations. They create their own equations with little number blocks or cubes. They are each given a certain number of cubes and have to create equations in a certain amount of time. "Pay the Cashier" is another game being played by four youngsters in the corner. One child gets a card which says to pay so much money to someone for a pizza. The child then learns to pay the exact amount or a larger amount and give the exact change back. The other students correct him if he makes a mistake.

Other activities include geoboards, pegboards, crossword puzzle work-books, slide rules, and an EDL (Educational Development Lab) machine which quickly flashes story problems to the children, who must immediately decide what math processes to use because the problem won't come up again. While many children are engaged in these activities, the others are doing assignments from workbooks or completing tests on their units of study. The teacher is correcting papers, talking with individual students, and occasionally joining some of the students in the games. The atmos-phere in the room seems quite free and the students change activities fre-quently, whenever they desire.

From Ernest R. House, Joe M. Steele, and Thomas Kerins. *The gifted classroom.* Center for Instructional Research and Curriculum Evaluation. Urbana: University of Illinois, June, 1971.

---

formal classroom atmosphere and a more formal relationship with stu-dents, and take absolute responsibility for grades (Tuckman, 1968). Indirect teachers accept and encourage student-initiated ideas more and make a more direct effort to build upon student ideas than do other teachers (Amidon & Giammatteo, 1965).

How do such atmospheres affect the student? Studies have demon-strated that students of teachers with authoritarian, in contrast to those with more democratic, attitudes are less involved in classroom activities, less cooperative, less active, less helpful, more nurturance seeking, and more concrete in responsiveness (Harvey, Prather, White, & Hoffmeister, 1968). They are also less critical thinkers (Measel & Wood, 1972) and dis-play less motivation to learn (Maehr & Stallings, 1972).

Perhaps the observational scoring system used most often to categorize teachers is the one developed by Flanders (1960) in cooperation with Amidon (Amidon & Flanders, 1971). Although these investigators feel the indirect approach is a better teaching strategy and offer support for this belief, Rosenshine (1968), in a review of 23 studies, concluded that investigators have not identified specific teacher behaviors that are associ-ated with achievement. He feels that research should focus on the cog-nitive strategies used by teachers, particularly the way they pursue ques-tions with individual children. In this vein, a study of the use of the discovery method in mathematics instruction indicated that teachers did not have appropriate strategies to ensure that all children made use of the discovery method (Hyman & Weltman, 1968).

One problem in assessing the effectiveness of different teaching approaches is in determining criteria of achievement. As indicated in Chapter 10, achievement tests measure amount learned and are heavily loaded with questions requiring convergent thinking. Rarely is diver-gent thinking ability required for successful performance on achievement tests. Consequently, the authoritarian or highly structured teacher may be expected to prepare students better to do well on such exams. That she doesn't is interesting. If children can learn factual material without overbearing direction from teachers, then maybe teachers can feel free to develop other roles.

A critical difference between direct and indirect teachers is that the indirect are better able to shift their behavior when necessary; they can be just as direct as any teacher in certain situations, but far more indirect in others. This ability, which is rarely found among direct teachers, means that the indirect teacher can adjust her own behavior to fit the situation of the moment (Amidon & Flanders, 1971). Later, when discussing consulting to teachers, we suggest that the autocratic teacher is unlikely to alter her behavior toward a child.

Fortunately, beginning teachers can be trained to be more indirect. Such training results in less use of criticism, less direction, more acceptance of student ideas, and more pupil-initiated talk (Amidon & Flanders, 1971). Very little is known, however, about the effects of such training on experienced teachers.

Because indirect teachers are more flexible, they can alter their style to that of the learner. Flexibility should be an essential requirement for teaching since students with different personality styles prefer particular types of teachers. For example, rather concrete and authoritarian students not only prefer an authoritarian, direct teacher (Harvey, 1970; Tuckman, 1968), but actually perform better under this teaching style (Domino, 1971). "The effective teacher must not be captive of his own acquired style: rather he must be able to react to student needs and circumstances of the moment. He must be able to radiate environments" (Tuckman, 1968, p. 69). Because exceptional children often show exaggerated learning styles, the less flexible teacher is probably less effective with them.

From this review we can tentatively conclude that a particular teaching approach, while not always affecting achievement test scores, may have an adverse effect on certain children. Consequently, the teacher with a more flexible style is probably better suited to teach children who are less able to alter their style to that of the teacher. Those with exaggerated learning styles, styles displayed by many exceptional children, would be better placed with the indirect teacher, the teacher who can modify his behavior in keeping with what each child brings to class.

Learning styles of students

A number of studies have examined the learning styles of different students. Several of these styles were discussed in Chapter 7 and were attributed to the child's social-learning history. We will briefly review these styles.

The rigid-inhibited style is characterized by concreteness, literal adherence to instructions, minimal creativity, poor problem solving ability, and a tendency to dichotomize events into black-white categories.

Anxious-dependent learners are somewhat similar but need continual reassurance from teachers. They are often inattentive and withdrawn, have high achievement anxiety and minimal creativity. In all probability, both of these styles would be maximally threatened by an indirect approach. As mentioned previously, indirect teachers were less preferred by the concrete student.

Some students, labeled the snipers, avoid failure, repress failure experiences, deny inadequacies, show pseudoindependence, and are prone to depression. We have discussed the possibility that many hysterics are an extreme example of this style.

Other children, sometimes referred to as the heroes, demonstrate intellectual inhibition, covert negativism, and contrariness; they are resentful of authority, rebellious, and erratic, yet ambivalent toward authority figures. Another group, the attention seekers, show socially oriented achievement, but do so in an overdriven manner.

Perhaps the child who gives teachers the most difficulty and who is placed most often in special class settings is the child displaying an undisciplined style. The undisciplined style is characterized by classroom disturbance, impatience, blaming others for errors, and irrelevant responsiveness. These youngsters seek immediate need gratification, behavior that leads to problems of control and management and eventually to poor relationships with authority figures.

Witkin and his colleagues (Witkin, Dyke, Faterson, Goodenough, & Karp, 1962) might describe the undisciplined child as an undifferentiated thinker, a child who perceives his environment in an unarticulated and global fashion. Researchers have used various terms to distinguish learning styles. The terms *undifferentiated* and *differentiated* are similar to *converger* and *diverger* (Hudson, 1966), *amorphous* and *analytic* (Wynne & Singer, 1963), and *ego-closed* and *ego-distant* (Voth & Mayman, 1963). Exceptional children most likely to display undifferentiated styles are the childhood schizophrenic, the blind, the child with a "severe conduct disorder," and the very dependent child.

Although we emphasized in Chapter 7 that a child's learning style results from his social-learning history, innate factors also interact with environmental influences to produce a unique learning style. Fries and Woolf (1953) proposed five congenital activity types, ranging from very active to very quiet. These activity patterns are said to influence parental attitudes and modes of relating. For example, a hyperactive infant may distress a quiet mother but be preferred by an active mother.

In their study of temperament and environmental stress, Thomas, Chess, and Birch (1968) refer to one particular group of children as difficult children or as mother killers. These children are characterized by irregularity in biological functions, negative responses to new stimuli, slowness in adapting to environmental changes, high frequency of negative mood, and predominance of intense reactions. They are recognizable early in life, and a disproportionately large number develop behavior disturbances. As infants these children sleep irregularly, awakening at unpredictable intervals, eat at irregular intervals, take varying amounts of food, and are difficult to toilet train since they are hard to anticipate. Many show withdrawal responses to all new aspects of the environment. This mother killer places undue strain on caretaking adults, and many parents react by developing inappropriate methods of handling.

The difficult child can develop along healthy lines, given "an optimally appropriate style of parental care." Some caretakers are able to remain consistently firm, often alternating in assuming responsibility for the child, thus avoiding one adult's becoming too weary and frustrated. Caretakers must be unusually tolerant and consistent, dealing with difficult periods with patience, good humor, persistence, and quiet firmness.

A second group isolated by Thomas and his colleagues were called easy children. They are almost ideal from a caretaker's point of view—positive in mood, highly regular, low or mild in intensity of reactions, readily adaptable, and usually positive in approaches to new situations. The majority do not develop behavior problems, but certain conditions may produce difficulties. The child's high adaptability may prove to be a difficulty, since he so readily adapts to the patterns taught at home. If the exceptions of peer groups or other groups conflict with parental standards, it may be exceedingly difficult for the child to resolve the conflict. Sometimes the conflicting interaction is between behavior approved when a child is young, but disapproved at a later age. So even the most desirable pattern of temperamental traits, under some conditions, may prove to be a liability. A child with this particular temperament might be affected more by protective-interdependent child rearing practices than would a child with a more active temperament. The child would, therefore, be more likely to develop a neurotic disorder when faced with severe stress.

Another cluster of traits that can result in later behavior disorder is the type Thomas describes as slow to warm up, characterized by low activity level, initial withdrawal responses, slow adaptability, low intensity of reactions, and relatively high frequency of negative mood responses. The significant theme is usually quiet withdrawal from new experiences and slow adaptation to them. The best approach to handling these children seems to combine patience with a willingness to wait. Impatient and quick-moving caretakers usually relate poorly to this child. Urging, coaxing, ordering, and propelling serve only to intensify the child's discomfort, and he may display quiet stubbornness, negativism, or great passivity in order to avoid painful situations. Yet, bowing to the child's behavior further complicates matters because the child is deprived of the kinds of experiences he needs to function autonomously.

Although Thomas and his colleagues do not describe how children with differing temperaments react to classroom environments, we would assume they would show differential reactions to learning experiences and would, therefore, display characteristic learning styles.

Kagan (1966) has identified two learning styles that he believes are manifestations of temperamental differences. He calls these styles the impulsive and the reflective. Impulsive children are those who respond rapidly in problem solving situations and who make frequent errors. Reflective children are those who respond after some deliberation and make few errors. Kagan believes these styles are due more to constitutional factors than to early learning experiences. Undoubtedly, the undisciplined group we spoke of earlier would have impulsive style children among its members.

Children with different styles have been found to differ on laboratory learning tasks. For example, analytic style children are superior to global style children on serial learning tasks (Long, 1962), on concept identification tasks (Davis, 1967; Ohnmacht, 1966), and on various problem solving tasks (Guetzkow, 1951). Nevertheless, very few investigators have studied the effects of learning style on learning in the classroom or on its interaction with instructional methods. Although investigators have offered some suggestions for managing children with different learning styles or temperaments (Mordock, 1968–1969; Rosenberg, 1968; Thomas et al., 1968), empirical support for these suggestions is lacking.

A study by Grieve and Davis (1971) does suggest that when global style students receive expository as opposed to discovery instruction, they have more difficulty applying knowledge to new situations. Outside of this study we know very little about the effects of different teaching strategies on children with different learning styles.

When a child displays a particular learning style, teachers who are uncomfortable with this style often expect inferior overall performance from the child rather than expecting uneven performance due to the strengths and weaknesses characteristic of that style. This "negative halo" effect leads us into a discussion of the influence of teacher expectancy upon children's academic performance.

Teacher expectancy

An experiment that received undue public attention was one claiming to demonstrate that "when teachers expected that certain children would show greater intellectual development, those children did show greater intellectual development" (Rosenthal & Jacobson, 1968, p. 83). Although the findings of this study have been rejected because of contradictory research, questionable experimental methodology, and inaccurate data interpretation and reporting (Mendels & Flanders, 1973; Thorndike, 1968), other studies have suggested a relationship between student learning style and teacher expectancy.

Teachers tend to overestimate the IQs of plungers, that is, children who unhesitatingly plunge into new activities. Children described as go-alongers, sideliners, and nonparticipators are viewed as less intelligent, in that order (Gordon & Thomas, 1967).

Brophy and Good (1970) noted that teachers systematically reinforce more correct responses of high than of low achievers. Those expected to function better receive more praise for correct responses and less criticism for incorrect responses than those not expected to perform well. In addition, when responding to an incorrect answer by a high achiever, teachers are more likely to repeat or rephrase the question and less likely to supply the answer or call on another child than when responding to an incorrect answer by a low achiever. Others also have noted that greater attention is paid to high than to low expectation students (Kester & Letchworth, 1972; Rothbart, Dalfen, & Barrett, 1971).

Seaver (1973) discovered that compared to controls, pupils who were taught by the same teacher as their older siblings performed better academically than those taught by a different teacher if their older siblings had been good students and worse if their siblings had performed poorly. Prior experience with an older sibling, therefore, resulted in teacher expectancies that influenced a child's academic performance.

Grieger (1970b) proposed the following model of the teacher expectancy effect: (1) the teacher forms differential expectations for children's performance; (2) she begins to treat children differentially in accordance with these expectations; (3) the children respond differentially to the teacher because they are being treated differentially; (4) when responding to the teacher, the child tends to exhibit behavior which complements and reinforces the teacher's expectations for him; (5) as a result, the general academic performance of some children is enhanced while that of others is depressed, with changes in the direction of teacher expectations; and (6) these results show up in achievement.

Special classes

What do classroom climate, learning style, and teacher expectancy have to do with the exceptional child? In Chapter 11 we discussed how placing a retarded child in a special class can result in a self-fulfilling prophecy. Because the child is retarded, we expect him to do poorly so we place him in a highly structured, teacher-directed classroom and lower our standards for him. When the child does not learn much, we say it is because he is retarded. What is even more discouraging, however, is that regular class teachers often are frightened by the word exceptional (Combs & Harper, 1967), feeling that they cannot teach children with this label. In reality, children removed from the regular classroom and labeled exceptional display the same learning styles as children who remain there; fears that they cannot be taught by the regular class teacher may be unwarranted.

Certain educational programs demand that the teacher employ some highly specific educational procedures (e.g., programs for the deaf, blind, or reading disabled); others, notably programs for the mentally retarded, emotionally disturbed, and culturally deprived, employ diversified procedures requiring a more general professional preparation. There is widespread agreement that special preparation is necessary in order to teach the exceptional child, preparation which differs from the requirements for elementary or secondary instruction. However, except for several areas of exceptionality, the search for these requirements has proved futile. A number of authors have lamented that special education lacks a model for teaching training or for evaluation of teacher effectiveness.

Many feel that the clinical teacher model is the fundamental model of special education; individualized instruction, based on diagnostic techniques, matches the learner and school tasks through the prescription of appropriate strategies and materials (Schwartz, 1967). The training based on this model is outlined in Figure 12.1.

Special education is often equated with special methods or special materials. Because of this emphasis, regular class teachers often believe they cannot teach exceptional children without an array of special methods and materials and without specialized training in their use. Shotel, Iano, and McGettigan (1972, p. 683) remark, "It is possible that special educators themselves are largely responsible for encouraging a mystique that will make it difficult to develop successful integrative programs for handicapped children."

Why do they say "mystique"? Primarily because regular class teachers know very little about what goes on in the special class or of the competencies needed to function there (Brooks & Bransford, 1971). Despite beliefs about the need for special materials, special training, and the clinical teacher model, there is no clear-cut evidence that special class teaching is a unique enterprise.

In a national survey of special classes for the emotionally disturbed, there was "an amazing lack of specific patterns and uniformity of approach" (Morse, Cutler, & Fink, 1964, p. 130). This finding highlights the need to find out just how "special" the special class is. "Is the special class, despite all traditional belief systems to the contrary, merely a smaller version of the regular classroom?" (Fink, 1972, p. 470). There is

CONTRACTS

Each week we have a different contract we have to fill out . . . like this week I will be doing a project on astronomy, but a couple of weeks ago, I was doing electricity. . . . I like this class because you can study anything you want to and not just have to study one thing. . . . In this class I think you're supposed to learn what a scientist does . . . like when someone put something in a box, you're supposed to take all the facts you

Figure 12.1 *The expanded teacher preparation model, showing the specific major tasks, enablers, and instructional options. (From L. Schwartz. A clinical teacher model for interrelated areas of special education. Exceptional Children, 1971, **37**, 565-571. Reprinted with permission of The Council for Exceptional Children.)*

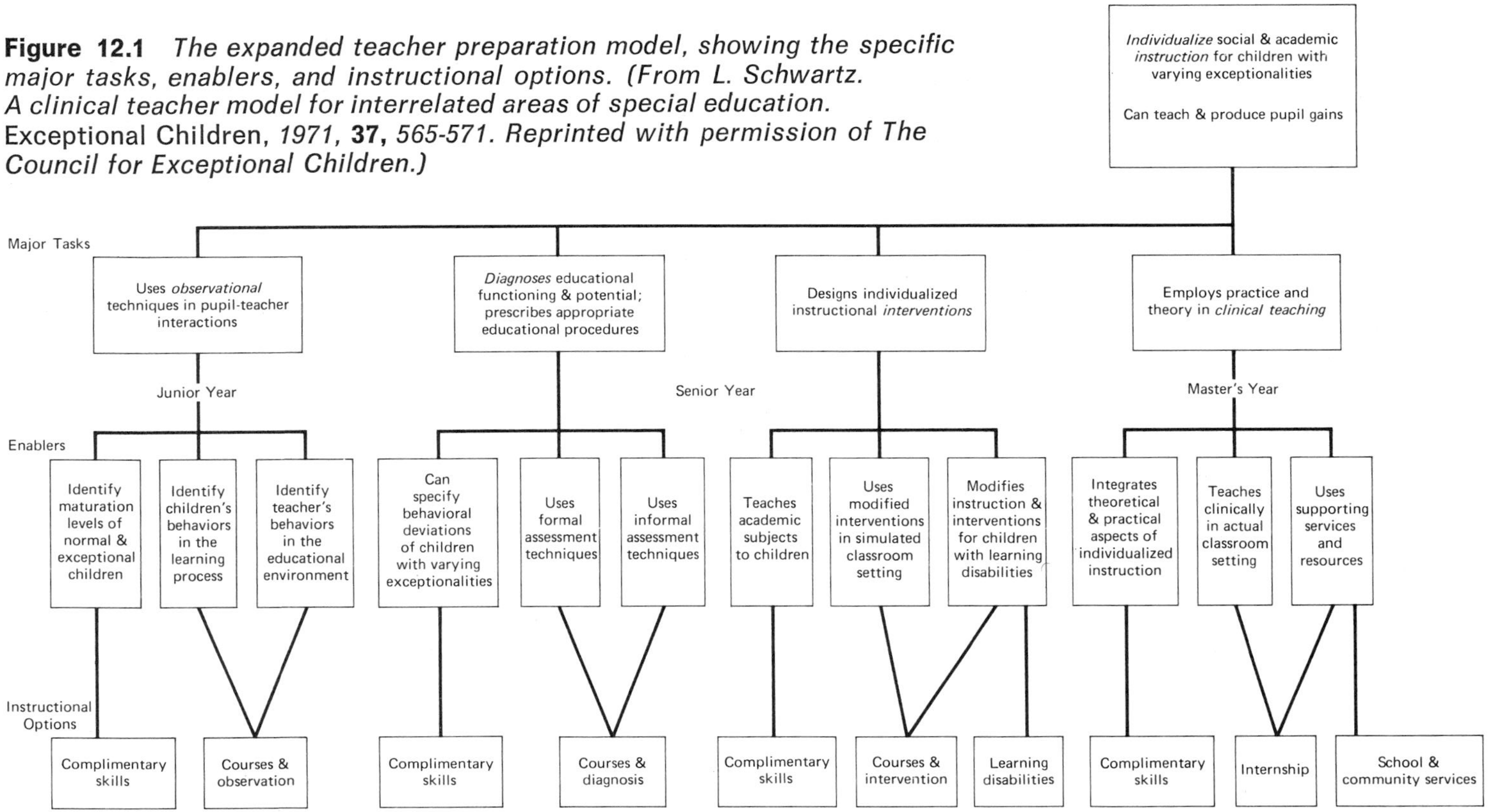

know about it and put them all together and then you can probably find out what it is. . . . I learn a lot from this science class because people are always bringing in different things like aviation, astronomy and chemistry. . . . In our regular 4th grade science class we have books but people know already what's in them and when teacher assigns us to read like unit 4 we're kind of bored with reading something we already know . . . but in this new science class you can be as advanced as you want.

From Ernest R. House, Joe M. Steele, and Thomas Kerins. *The gifted classroom.* Center for Instructional Research and Curriculum Evaluation. Urbana: University of Illinois, June, 1971.

---

some data suggesting that special class teachers of the disturbed spend more time controlling behavior, but the teacher control patterns utilized vary widely (Fink, 1972). Planned ignoring is used most frequently, a tactic commonly used by the regular classroom teacher!

A highly structured approach is effective when teaching reading vocabulary and attentional work behavior to emotionally disturbed children, but by structure is meant the systematic application of reinforcers (Gallagher, 1972).

Individualized and sequential programming also is considered a unique feature of special class education. Nevertheless, the open and ungraded approach to regular classroom instruction emphasizes these same features.

Nor is the personality of the special class teacher a unique one. Although many argue that the teacher's personality is the most significant variable in the classroom (Getzels & Jackson, 1963), very few studies have supported this assumption, nor have any demonstrated differences between regular and special class teachers. Ideally, the specialized needs of exceptional children should require teachers whose personal characteristics are as important as their professional competencies. Some special class children who perceive their teacher as understanding and as unconditionally accepting do perform better academically (Scheuer, 1971), but, then, regular class children may do likewise.

Dwyer (1972), a special class teacher with considerable experience, outlines features he considers essential for effective classroom performance. The teacher must hold three basic assumptions: (1) learning is dependent upon a certain level of controlled classroom behavior; (2) teacher behaviors influence children behaviors; and (3) teachers can set a classroom tone by intensifying or minimizing the children's entering behaviors.

Each teacher has a style whether he realizes it or not; it is what makes him the most comfortable. To analyze his style, each teacher should ask himself: (1) Does talking annoy me? (2) Does classroom traffic bother me? (3) Should everyone be working at the same time? (4) Do "off the subject" questions bother me? (5) Should all assigned work be completed? (6) Can children learn if it is noisy? (7) How do I feel about open displays of anger, including cursing? (8) How do I feel about a poorly conceived lesson? Should I see it through and then drop it or drop it immediately? (9) Are grades important? Because of the recent popularity of behavior modification techniques, the teacher should ask himself: (1) How do I feel about tokens and token systems? (2) Can I distinguish between bribes and rewards?

When these questions are answered honestly, the teacher should then decide which are the most important concerns and whether he could feel comfortable changing any of them. He should then encourage his principal to make an effort to match his style with the learning styles of children. For example, children who work well without pressure, cannot tolerate pressure, are poorly motivated, or are overly concerned with controls could be placed with the low-keyed teacher. Children placed with the high-keyed teacher could be those who need an atmosphere with few distractions, need all of their time accounted for, are impulsive but react to peer pressure, do not respect teachers who give them too much leeway, or are made anxious by having to plan their own activities.

Regarding management, Dwyer states that when he disciplines a child he is more successful when he is supportive than when he is threatening. "If you take him by the arm once, you'll have to every time!" Reprimanding is more successful than punishing, as is focusing on the inappropriate behavior rather than on the reprimand itself. A general explanation of consequences is preferable to teacher approval or judgmental statements. (Recall Hess and Shipman's work on the manner in which many lower class mothers reprimand their child.)

Dwyer feels that teachers serve as models for students. The questions children ask the teacher reveal that they consider him a model: Do you ever curse at home? Do you ever curse when you're angry? Did you get into trouble when you were a kid? Did you ever get a beating from your father? Did you steal? What are you going to do to your kid when he . . . ? Do you drink? Smoke?

The teacher's best weapons are social incentives (praise), ability to ignore behavior, and ability to model. His biggest pitfalls are personal anger and competition, faulty filtering of information, setting unrealistic goals, and lack of structure and direction. By structure Dwyer means the organization of a day with built-in flexibility. This organization should be spelled out to the class at each day's beginning. Subject matter should be diversified and options should be available at transition periods. There should be a list of tasks that must be done (find all the nouns on page 57, complete social studies workbook exercise on page 40), and a list of options (study for spelling, write a friendly letter). If the children have some planning ability, they can be given a schedule of what is planned for the day and they can organize a part of or all of it.

Since the teacher wants the children's full attention, he should give them his. He should move around the classroom, be available to provide help, and refrain from grading papers or planning lessons while the children are working.

Setting realistic goals for each child and operating in accordance with these goals is crucial. After determining each child's apparent strengths and weaknesses, the teacher should set up priorities and attack the easiest first, since success at this level may decrease the child's resistance to tackling more difficult tasks. Behavior should be viewed in relative terms —how is a child doing now compared to how he usually does? The norm for each child should be the guide.

Knowing a child's weaknesses allows the teacher to structure lessons so as to avoid a child's embarrassment. For example, the following approach can be employed with a poor reader: (1) have the child rehearse silently the parts he will read orally, (2) sit next to him and cue him when it is his turn, (3) check parts he has when the class reads a play, (4) point in your own book so he can follow, (5) assign small parts to allow participation, and (6) provide individual remediation such as token rewards for words learned.

OPINIONS

This is my best and favorite class!!! You don't have to memorize too much stuff. Just say what's on your mind. I like that because you can analyze every viewpoint and really never be wrong—9th grader.

. . .

It's just a good class and that's how I feel. Because this class understands feelings of humans—not for color, but for what you believe. It is good for us in the future for the rest of our lives—9th grader.

From Ernest R. House, Joe M. Steele, and Thomas Kevins. *The gifted classroom*. Center for Instructional Research and Curriculum Evaluation Urbana: University of Illinois, June, 1971.

Dwyer's students have listed what they like about class as follows: (1) to express their own opinion, (2) not being bothered when upset or in bad mood, (3) slow teaching, (4) extra chances, (5) lots of help, (6) humor in teaching, (7) trusting us, (8) fun experiences in learning, and (9) free-time learning activities. They don't like: (1) fooling around when they are in a bad mood, (2) too much humor gets us "high," (3) too much "write it out," and (4) having to do it over.

Note that nowhere in Dwyer's remarks is there mention of exceptionality. His comments seem equally appropriate for both the regular and the special class teacher. Nor are special materials given a high priority. Teacher-adapted materials are often sufficient and the materials frequently used are those found in regular classrooms, except that the special class should have materials that cover all grade levels.

Perhaps future research will demonstrate that teacher management techniques that are effective in the regular classroom (recall Kounin's work) are equally effective in the special class. If so, then effective regular class teachers might also teach the special classes or be given special incentives for working with special children. School systems vary in their attitudes about special classes. In some the regular class teacher is encouraged to take on a special class and is reinforced for doing so (Dinitz, 1971). In others teachers are actively discouraged from teaching special classes (Brown, 1971). School systems supporting the special class teacher have attracted better teachers into the field, teachers who appear to do well without formal training.

In summary, the importance of teacher expectancy for the child (recall that Mrs. Jones lowered rather than raised her expectations for Billy because she believed him too disturbed to learn), teacher style, and classroom climate seemed to be no different for successful special class teaching than for regular class teaching. Because some classes of children may vary little in learning style, the teacher can be less flexible. In other classes a greater variety of or more extreme examples of student learning styles may be present, calling for greater flexibility. Although research will undoubtedly continue in this area, hopefully the personality inventory and the preconceived observational schedule will be discarded and replaced with intensive study of individual teachers. Braun, Holzman, and Lasher (1969) have made a start in this direction. Findings, however, may always be inconclusive or elusive, primarily because our society's educational goals for the exceptional, as well as the normal, change with changes in society.

THE PSYCHOLOGIST IN THE SCHOOL

Although the psychologist may assume many functions in the school setting, we will focus on his role as consultant to teachers. A general model of the psychologist's role in the school is presented in Table 12.1. Although preventive and ameliorative assistance are listed separately, the line between them is not always clear. Most school psychologists consult regularly with teachers about children whom the teachers consider a problem. Often these children are never referred again, making it difficult to determine if consultation helped prevent the development of more serious problems, if the problem resulted from teacher-child incompatibility, or if the child would have improved spontaneously. The research is not clear in this area. Galvin (1972), for example, followed 43 children originally designated as having behavior problems. Four years later only 13 were so classified. None of the 43 received any therapeutic help during this period. On the other hand, Rubin and Balow (1971), in a study of 967 children in kindergarten through third

Table 12.1   A GENERAL SCHOOL PSYCHOLOGICAL SERVICES MODEL

Level of diagnostic-intervention services	Type of school population served	Major focus of diagnostic-intervention efforts	Some diagnostic-intervention strategies
Primary	Units of the school system (e.g., children in the elementary schools)	Developmental Preventive	Inservice (and preservice) training of teachers Incorporating psychological concepts into the curriculum
Secondary	Vulnerable sub-populations (e.g., black children in desegregated schools)	Ameliorative Compensatory	Diagnostic-intervention classes Use of teacher-psychological specialists
Tertiary	Subpopulations positively diagnosed as severe learning and/or behavior problems (e.g., school phobic children)	Remedial Therapeutic	Therapeutic tutoring Group counseling

From B. Phillips. The diagnosis-intervention class model: report of an effort at implementation. Paper presented at the annual convention of the American Psychological Association, Miami, Fla., September 1970.

grade, found that 41 percent were classified in one or more of the following categories: special class placement (2.3 percent), retention (11.6 percent), receipt of special services (18 percent), and problems of behavior and attitudes (28 percent). Rubin and Balow's findings raise serious questions regarding the ability of our present educational system to accommodate a significant proportion of children. However, 28 percent of the children were identified solely by teacher judgment. Considering Galvin's finding, many of these children might not be considered behavior problems at a later period in their development.

Reasons for teacher consultation

In spite of the difficulties in assessing the effects of consultation, studies suggest its potential value. One important reason for consultation is that teachers are not always able to identify correctly children's strengths and weaknesses—recall their difficulty in identifying the gifted. Von Valletta, Brantley, and Pryzwansky (1972) conducted an investigation of the accuracy of teachers' identification of problems in six areas

—vision, hearing, visual-motor integration, speech, verbal expression, and learning aptitude. Four first grade teachers rated 104 children across these areas. Validating instruments were administered subsequent to teacher ratings. The teacher could make two types of errors, failure to identify a problem (false negative) or false identification (false positive).

Teachers suspected that 12 of the 104 children had vision problems. The validating instrument, the Keystone telebinocular survey, selected 19. Of the 19 selected by the instrument, teachers had selected 4. They had failed to identify 15 (79 percent false negatives) and had made 8 false identifications (67 percent false positives).

In the area of hearing, teachers selected 16 children, while the Beltone audiometer selected 15. Six of the teacher's selections were validated by the audiometer's selection; 63 percent were false positives.

Teacher selections of speech problems were valid in 53 percent of the cases identified. They failed to identify 47 percent of the articulation problems and 71 percent of their selections were false identifications. In rating adequacy of verbal expression, the teachers agreed with the ITPA verbal expression subtest in 48 percent of their selections. Validity of teacher judgment was best in visual-motor integration, where 67 percent of their selections agreed with selection on the basis of scores on the Berry Developmental Test of Visual-Motor Integration.

In comparison to instrument selection, the teachers underselected in the area of learning aptitude. Fifty-seven percent of the children scored one or more standard deviations below the mean on the Primary Mental Abilities test, whereas teachers correctly identified 27 children (23 percent) and falsely identified 2. Judgments regarding learning aptitude may be directly related to factors that limit a teacher's exposure to a variety of types of children. For example, when teachers have been employed in one environment for several years, their perception of what is average may gradually increase or decrease as a function of the population with whom they work, without regard to any norm group external to the local environment.

These findings suggest that consultation with teachers is a needed service since without assistance from others, their expectations for children may be based on incorrect judgments.

A second reason for consultation is that teaching is a relatively lonely profession. Often teachers have no one to talk to about their children, except other teachers. Other teachers may be supportive, but they may lack the time to give assistance and cannot provide the viewpoint of a different perspective (Sarason, Levine, Goldenberg, Cherlin & Bennett, 1966). Faced with a difficult child, it is easy to lose objectivity. The help of a psychologist, provided it is offered in a positive, nondepreciative manner, may be the stimulus the teacher needs to make better use of her own resources.

The third reason, and the most important, is the children themselves. Decisions about children should be made by more than one person. Frequently, the psychologist serves as an advocate for the child in the school and community and helps the child's family to seek assistance for their difficulties. The school psychologist is usually the first mental health professional to whom parents are exposed. If he is supportive and helpful, they are more likely to seek further assistance and thereby help their child.

Assessing teacher style for effective consultation

Consulting to teachers often requires the same interview skills possessed by a therapist. Like the therapist, the consultant hopes to change the teacher's attitudes about and behavior toward the child referred. Consultation, therefore, hinges on the assumption that teachers are open to change. Unfortunately, this is not always the case. Mumford (1968) offers a typology of teacher roles, several of which are relatively closed to outside influence.

Mumford's *teacher-guide* views her job as helping the individual achieve total growth—intellectual, academic, and emotional. She does not consider herself an expert in personality or emotional problems and therefore feels comfortable in seeking assistance from another professional in dealing with her students. Mumford suggests that this type of teacher would respond best to frank give-and-take exchanges with the psychologist. Her involvement in the early stages of consultation would be greater than expected of other teacher types. Frequent discussion of progress and consultation about routine changes would be mandatory.

The *teacher-friend* is like the teacher-guide in viewing the total child as the target of the school, but takes basic satisfaction from befriending students. She feels that she has a special gift for empathizing with and understanding children. Therefore, having to seek professional help in dealing with a child appears to her to be an admission of failure, a lack of competence. When she does accept professional help, she is usually discouraged and desires to rid herself of the problem as quickly as possible as its presence serves as a continual reminder of her failure. With this type of teacher, it is best for the psychologist to emphasize the idea that some children come from backgrounds with sets of expectations different from hers. The problem is stated in terms of changing the child's expectations and his relevant contingencies, rather than focusing on her behaviors. Continual support and examples of differences between the child in question and others need to be given. Statements such as "Certainly this works well with others, but not with John," serve to reinforce her feelings of general competence with children.

The *teacher-authority* believes that the job of the school is simply to teach, and she finds evidence of her effectiveness in lack of problems in the classroom and the productivity of children. This teacher is not apt to ask for professional assistance in dealing with children because this would imply that she is ineffectual. The teacher-authority rarely calls for the psychologist's help; when she does, it is often for specific information such as test scores or background material.

Mumford suggests that the teacher-authority would respond best to didactically presented material. Perhaps the best approach to this teacher is to involve her as little as possible. For example, McNamara's (1968–1969) case (described in Chapter 7) was treated during recess when the remainder of the class was absent. Although this type of teacher will cooperate, it is often with a "show me" attitude. The psychologist would do well to take a more humble attitude than usual, stress the research aspect of the program rather than what the teacher will gain, and be prepared to do more listening than talking.

Mumford's descriptions of the teacher-authority corresponds to our descriptions of authoritarian personalities, individuals most likely to adopt an authoritarian approach toward teaching. How prevalent among teachers is the authoritarian personality? Harvey's (1970) research indicates that a large number of teachers (55 percent of his sample) display an authoritarian, concrete personality. In addition to the characteristics already listed when we discussed authoritarian teachers, concrete individuals tend to form generalized impressions of others from incomplete information (Ware & Harvey, 1967), are relatively insensitive to subtle and minimal cues and, hence, are susceptible to false but salient cues (Harvey, 1966), have a poor capacity to assume the orientation of others (Harvey, 1963; Harvey & Kline 1965), hold stereotypical solutions to complex and changing problems (Felknor & Harvey, 1963: Harvey, 1966), are intolerant of ambiguity (Harvey, 1966), and make extreme and polarized evaluations.

How will such a person react to information about a child that is dissonant from his own? Ware and Harvey (1967) report that the more abstract and cognitively complex individual seeks out more information than does the concrete individual before he forms an impression about a person. Concrete individuals consider a person who formerly manifested either socially desirable or undesirable behavior as less likely to subsequently evidence behavior of the opposite quality. This finding is consistent with an earlier one (Harvey, 1965) that concrete individuals are more disposed toward seeing "good" persons as all good, and "bad" as all bad.

When perceiving inconsistencies in a person's behavior, concrete individuals seek to neutralize the inconsistency by attributing it to temporal changes in the person, by giving fewer explanations of the inconsistencies, by giving poorly integrated accounts of the inconsistencies, by expressing explanations that merely reiterate the conflicting characteristics, and by using more stereotypical labels in their explanations (Harvey & Ware, 1967). These findings are consistent with Festinger's theory of cognitive dissonance presented in Chapter 10 (Festinger, 1957), except that the assumptions of dissonance theory are probably less valid for more abstractly functioning individuals (Harvey, 1967).

Harvey, Reich, and Wyer (1968) demonstrated that concrete individuals have a high level of arousal conditioned to stimuli about which they report intense attitudes. Under high arousal concrete individuals differentiate stimuli more poorly than when attitudes are low in intensity. Consulting efforts should be aimed, therefore, not only at imparting information but at decreasing arousal. For abstract individuals arousal is not a significant variable in stimulus differentiation.

This research helps clarify why the behavior of some teachers cannot be lastingly altered. Classifying teachers as to cognitive style and relating this variable to differential responsiveness to psychological services or to inservice training is a needed area of research. In any case, more energy should be directed toward developing effective consultative techniques with teacher types. Mumford (1968) has made a start in this direction.

Once the psychologist has gained the teacher's cooperation, the question of what teacher behaviors are relevant becomes of prime importance. What should the psychologist "tune in on" when observing the teacher's behavior in the classroom? Grieger, Mordock, and Breyer (1970, pp. 260–261) suggest several variables to examine when observing the teacher.

Perhaps most important is the teacher's reinforcer effectiveness. Do the children find her attention rewarding? Do they cue their behavior on her behaviors? Do they perform in order to acquire her attention or favor? If the answer is "no" to these and other similar questions, ways must be found to provide her with reinforcer value; one way being the institution of some concrete or token economy system.

A second variable is the degree of organization the teacher brings to her class. Is she organized in her efforts to teach and discipline her children? Most school psychologists have had experience with teachers who rarely plan their lessons, who typically react to the behaviors of children rather than initiate their behaviors, and who respond to children in an inconsistent fashion. Since a basic principle of learning theory is that behavior is determined by its consequences, it is important to organize her behavioral consequences. One way to do this is to instruct the teacher to cue on her own behaviors; to observe herself autocritically (i.e., have her ask herself how many times per day she praises appropriate behavior). Hopefully, she would see her own inconsistencies, and with assistance, find ways of ordering her behavior.

These authors go on to say that simply asking the teacher to report what she does or relying completely on her observations is not enough. Inaccuracies and distortions occur. For example, a teacher complained that her first grade children rarely raised their hands to respond, choosing instead to call out. Systematic observation noted that she typically recognized and responded to those who called out, often ignoring others who followed her request to raise their hands. Simple suggestions to ignore calling out behavior and to respond to hand raising resulted in a significant reduction in calling out behavior (Grieger, 1970a). Another teacher complained that the children in her classroom were rude to (e.g., hit, shoved, namecalled) one particular boy; behavioral counts, however, revealed that this youngster was the greatest offender. In light of similar experiences, direct observations appear necessary (Becker, Madsen, Arnold, & Thomas, 1967).

In addition to assessing the teacher's style, several research programs have identified an important dimension to consider when assessing the influence of teacher behavior on the behavior of children. Approximately 80 percent of the typical teacher's behavior toward her children is negatively oriented (e.g., giving after the fact reprimands, commands, threats) and only about 20 percent positively oriented (e.g., giving approval, expressing sympathy, asking questions). Since positive interactions significantly decrease negative and increase positive student behavior (Becker et al., 1967; Grieger et al., 1970), the degree to which teachers use positive techniques as opposed to negative ones is one relevant dimension for the psychologist to observe.

Behavioral, psychodynamic, and developmental approaches to consultation

Psychologists with a behavioral orientation see consultation as helping the teacher to pinpoint the actual behaviors of the child that she wants to change. Their goal is always to be specific, that is, to think in such terms as "Jack hits, pushes, and name calls," rather than "Jack is rude." Observation schedules are employed and the frequency noted of each designated behavior during a particular time period. Once the frequency of a behavior has been charted, specific recommendations are made geared both to eliminating undesirable behaviors and to supplanting them with desired ones. After an appropriate interval, behavioral frequencies are again obtained in order to evaluate the effectiveness of the recommended procedures (Grieger et al., 1970).

Psychodynamic consultants concentrate more on helping teachers understand the effects of stress upon performance, acquainting them with personality dynamics, and helping them to adopt more consistent attitudes and controls or to be more realistic in regard to a student's capacities and strivings.

The psychodynamic consultant considers the most important component of his role to be his relationship with the teacher. Teachers can feel guilty about their inability to deal with the aberrant child. The dynamic psychologist tries to reduce these guilt feelings and, in contrast to the behavioral approach, reassures the teacher as to her lack of personal responsibility. The psychologist's role must not be a threat to the teacher. The latter should see the former as a guide and counselor, a person who is aware of and appreciates the teacher's role and who wants to help her become more effective. The teacher is an expert in teaching; the psychologist the expert in dealing with psychological problems. Each is trained for competence in a specific area, and the association between the two must be one of respect, cooperation, and service to foster the child's optimal development.

The teacher is helped to realize that the psychologist performs no miracles. A physician handles an infection with penicillin and there is an immediate cure. There is no such easy solution with the withdrawn, the passive-aggressive, the schizoid child; some have been maladjusted for years. The teacher can be helped to handle the child more effectively, but there is no magic solution, no antibiotic dose. The psychologist can only offer suggestions that may—repeat, may—help the child in the classroom.

What percent of psychologists are behavioral as opposed to psychodynamic. Surveys indicate that the majority of school psychologists draw from both approaches and could be called eclectic (Andrews, 1971). Eclectics encourage teachers to adopt a variety of methods to deal with students and stress the use of flexible procedures. They focus on relieving the teacher's uneasy feelings, jointly defining the various aspects of the problem, planning together the steps to be taken, and setting realistic expectations regarding outcome. Ways in which other school personnel, as well as school and community resources, can be advantageously used also are a featured part of consultation (Handler, Gerston, & Handler, 1965). The eclectic uses both behavioral and psychodynamic techniques when he considers them applicable.

Perhaps school psychologists of the future will adopt a more developmental approach to consultation. Considering issues from within developmental theory, the psychologist would ask himself: At what stage of conceptual, social, or emotional development is the referred child? What conceptual system characterizes the thinking of his parents, teachers, principal, or even classroom or school, as the development of groups proceeds through similar stages (Bennis & Shepard, 1956)? What type of learning is characteristic of individuals at different levels of development, and what procedures can be employed to induce progression to a higher level? How can remedial tutoring, for example, be provided to a child excessively closed toward autonomy?

Since developmental theorists relate learning styles to antecedent training conditions, parent cooperation becomes important in intervention programs. The developmentalist would schedule conferences to help parents relate differently to children. Although only one formal research study could be found that investigated intervention with and without parent involvement (Duncan & Fitzgerald, 1969), the early childhood education programs reviewed in Chapter 9 stressed the importance of parental cooperation. Nevertheless, most of the school psychology and special education literature ignores parents as program participants. Practitioners frequently have little time for active parent involvement (and parents often don't cooperate or feel alienated from the school), but parent participation is often neglected for another reason. Many university trainers, categorize work with parents as clinical and feel that it is incongruent with the current effort to train school psychologists as "educational" consultants to school staff. Within developmental theory, educational efforts to induce progression must exist simultaneously with procedures aimed to decrease closedness or reduce compartmentalization (such efforts can be regarded as psychotherapeutic), otherwise the individual is not open to progression.

There is considerable evidence that differences in child rearing practices result in differential amounts of need for achievement, initiative, curiosity, creativity, language skill, etc. (see Chapters 7, 9, and 10). To assume that changes need take place only in the classroom is to ignore this wealth of data. Although behavior modification in the classroom is certainly effective, developmentalists would suggest that procedures to modify behavior should be directed toward a constellation of factors rather than toward specific behaviors; the child's total response hierarchy should be considered since this hierarchy would reflect his learning style. After studying the relationship of family interaction to the behavior of its members, Satir (in Richmond, 1971) remarks that no case was seen where learning problems existed in the absence of dysfunctional family communication. Whether the dysfunctional communication caused the learning problem or the learning problem caused the dysfunctional communication is another issue. The main point is that families cannot continue to be ignored in educational planning if significant changes in a child's achievement are to take place.

Psychological intervention needs to consider all the factors that can foster a child's progression from one developmental level to another. When functioning within a developmental framework, the goal of intervention is always clear—to foster developmental progression and to implement procedures designed to do so. Both Hewett (1968) and Klein (1972) derived a scheme of intervention from developmental theory for each of several levels of social development. We will present Klein's scheme later in the chapter.

THE PSYCHOTHERAPIST

We said earlier that efforts to induce progression in development must exist simultaneously with efforts to decrease closedness to progression. A child is usually closed to progression because he is in conflict. For example, a child who has strong tendencies to approach and avoid the same goal is said to have an approach-avoidance conflict (Dollard & Miller, 1950). Until this conflict is resolved, the child is unlikely to respond to efforts to get him to approach a goal by urging him to try harder. Urges to approach the goal only increase his fear and conflict. Many children in school are forced to chose between two undesirable alternatives, that is, they experience avoidance-avoidance conflicts (Dollard & Miller, 1950). For example, the child neither wants to do the school work, which he feels is beyond his ability, nor does he want to tell the teacher he cannot do it and incur the ridicule of others. The only way to escape vacillating in conflict is to adopt ways to get out of work—leave his seat, hit the child next to him, or visit the nurse. Although this conflict might be resolved by giving the child easier work, the child frequently refuses to do such work because he anticipates being embarrassed by not being able to do what other children can do.

Because the teacher is not always aware of the child's conflict and because awareness does not always mean that she can reduce the conflict, psychotherapeutic efforts are introduced to help the child resolve his conflicts. Most psychotherapies aim at reducing the fears that motivate avoidance. In later stages of therapy, when fear motivated avoidance is reduced, the child may be helped to approach the goal. We have seen how phobias are treated through procedures designed to keep anxiety at a minimum. We turn now to efforts directed at resolving conflicts that reduce closedness and allow a child to progress, efforts that are called psychotherapy.

Therapeutic approaches

By now we have learned that behavior therapists attempt to restructure malevolent aspects of a child's environment by changing the reinforcement contingencies to which he is exposed. They believe in doing (Phillips & Mordock, 1970, p. 2)

as much as can be done in as many of the patient's environmental situations as possible. . . . In order to accomplish such restructuring, the therapist must work in settings other than his office, particularly in the home and the classroom, and he must work with parents and teachers as well as with the child, himself.

The behaviorists believe that many children are isolated from others because of inappropriate behavior. Their bias is not to just talk about problems, but to do their best to change them. We saw in Chapter 11 that when Sally made several friends, her other inappropriate behaviors diminished since she was no longer preoccupied with obtaining attention. Consequently, her fantasies about making friends diminished, her study habits improved, and her "stupid answers" vanished. In behavioral terms a significant reduction in her inappropriate behavior elicited positive feedback from the environment, feedback that reinforced and maintained new behaviors and accelerated their generalization (Phillips & Mordock, 1970).

The insight oriented, or psychodynamic, therapist is interested in the child's thoughts, attitudes, and feelings rather than in his overt behavior. Efforts are directed at encouraging self-awareness and insight into the causes of his problems. Ideally, the medium for this discovery is verbal interaction between the child and the therapist. The child, however, is usually reluctant to talk about his feelings and instead reveals them through his play or his behavior. The child therapist frequently carries on extensive monologues in an effort to convey to the child that he understands his feelings and may have an explanation for them. The relationship between the child and therapist is of crucial importance. Usually the child relates to the therapist in a manner similar to his relations with other individuals. By pointing out to the child how he makes demands on and attempts to manipulate the therapist, the therapist can make him aware of how he relates to others and, at the same time, give him the opportunity to relate on different terms. Much of child therapy is a corrective emotional experience; the child is allowed to reexperience emotions, to be angry, sad, or depressed in the presence of a supportive person. The idea is to help the child face painful ideas, desires, and experiences that he has forgotten or repressed but that affect his behavior and make him unhappy. Grace's therapy, described in the section on conduct disorders in Chapter 9, was essentially a corrective emotional experience.

As we would suspect from our knowledge about parental influences on children's behavior, therapeutic efforts directed only at modifying the child are not always successful. The child's conflicts may be maintained by parental attitudes toward him. For example, if an obsessional child needs to be more assertive but his parents punish his assertive attempts, change in the child is unlikely. Similarily, a blind child who is babied by his parents is not likely to become more mature following individual psychotherapy. Many therapists, therefore, have turned to treating the child and his family together. This type of treatment is called family therapy. The reader is referred to Friedman (1965) and Mordock (1974) for case presentations that demonstrate technique in family therapy.

Although behavioral and dynamic therapists frequently debate the merits of each approach (Patterson, 1968), others see the two approaches as converging (Sloane, 1969). The developmentally oriented therapist sees value in both methods. A behavioral approach may be more effective for a child at one developmental level, while dynamically oriented therapy may be more appropriate for a child at another. The same orientation applies to families. Relatively undifferentiated fam-

ilies who are unreflective and impulsive may respond more favorably to
a behavioral approach, while more reflective families may prefer an approach that helps them straighten out their communication difficulties.

As mentioned in Chapter 11, the mentally retarded respond more favorably to therapeutic techniques that do not require much verbalization.
Leland and Smith (1965) have developed an approach that is based on
increasing the retarded child's cognitive clarity. Whenever the child
can convey to the therapist what he is doing, he can continue in the activity. Whenever he can't, the therapist interrupts the activity by verbal-
izing for the child. This therapy is a kind of cognitive stimulation designed to foster the organization of mental processes so that the child
can complete activities enabling him to function better outside the
therapy room. Sternlicht (1964) uses many nonverbal techniques to foster group discussion among retarded children. For example, each child
strokes a balloon against his cheek and is helped to find labels to describe the experience.

Glasser (1965) claims that delinquents respond best to an approach
he calls reality therapy. This therapy focuses on helping the delinquent
become more responsible so that he will be able to satisfy his needs
within the confines of reality.

The bright, motivated child responds well to client-centered therapy.
The theory of this nondirective approach is to provide a permissive atmosphere where the child verbalizes his feelings and the therapist reflects and clarifies the feelings for him. Eventually, the child comes to
see certain relationships between his feelings and his behavior. Perhaps
the best example of this approach is the case of Dibs reported by Axline
(1964).

Another form of therapy, which requires a certain level of intellectual ability, is called rational-emotive therapy (Ellis, 1962). This therapy is based on the assumption that irrational and self-defeating behavior results from internalization of irrational ideas communicated to
the child at a stage of life when rational modes of thinking were not
developed. Consequently, the disturbed individual is not aware of the
irrational ideas that sustain his emotional disturbance. The task of the
therapist is to get the child to disbelieve his illogical ideas, to change his
self-defeating attitudes. The therapist serves as a frank counterpropa-
gandist who directly contradicts and denies the self-defeating propa-
ganda that the child originally learned, and he encourages the child to
participate in activities that serve as forceful counterpropaganda against
the ideas believed.

The developmental therapeutic approach

Most therapy, be it dynamically or behaviorally oriented, is usually
considered without reference to age. Reinforcement principles in be-

havioristic therapy, reflection and clarification in client-centered, correction of misconceptions in rational-emotive, and interpretations in psychoanalytic are applied similarily to adults and children. Developmentally oriented therapists hope to apply methods according to their appropriateness for children at different developmental stages (Dusek, 1974). We saw in our discussion of school phobia in Chapter 7 that older school phobics did not respond favorably to the two treatment approaches that were successful with younger children. Similarly, approaches valid for older children might be invalid for younger.

To participate fully in the insight oriented therapies, the child's thinking skills have to be fairly well developed. An examination of stages of conceptual development reveals that children think differently at different ages. We have already discussed some of these differences in Chapter 5 when we described the child's reactions to physical disease.

The development of problem solving skill also proceeds through successive stages. Since therapy is essentially a problem solving activity, the therapist should be familiar with these stages. Problem solving skill proceeds through stages in which the child: (1) shows no mediation or verbal regulation of his behavior, (2) does not spontaneously produce relevant mediators, and (3) does not understand the essence of a problem in order to determine what mediators to produce. Problem solving, therefore, is viewed as a three-stage process of comprehension, production, and mediation; poor performance can result from a deficiency at any one of these stages (Bem, 1970).

Vygotsky (1962) asserted that internalization of verbal commands is the critical step in a child's development of control over his own behavior. A number of studies indicate that cognitive, self-guiding, private speech increases with age, as does the internalization of parental commands (Meichenbaum & Goodman, 1971). These results suggest a progression from external to internal control. Initially, the speech of adults controls a child's behavior; later, a child's own overt speech regulates his behavior; and finally, the child's covert speech assumes a regulatory role. Considering this knowledge, how might therapeutic procedures be modified in keeping with children's development through these stages? The work of Meichenbaum and Goodman (1971) provides some clues. Postulating that impulsivity results from a lack of sufficient self-regulatory behavior, these investigators trained impulsive children to talk to themselves, first overtly and then covertly, in order to modify their own behavior. They were taught to use their private speech for orienting, organizing, regulating, and self-rewarding functions. Results indicated that after such training, the impulsive children seemed to approach tasks differently. They took more time, talked to themselves, and improved their performance. The stability of these changes is currently being explored.

In addition to requiring mediation skills, the insight oriented therapies require that the child be able to plan, to be aware of potential obstacles, and to recognize the amount of time needed to reach a goal. In short, he has to have means-ends thinking. Not only young children lack such thinking; older disturbed children, children with personality disturbances and neuroses, also lack adequate means-ends thinking (Shure & Spivack, 1972). Training in means-ends thinking early in life might be more helpful than later application of treatment methods that require such thinking for a favorable response.

The therapist also has to be aware of other developmental changes that take place so as to modify therapeutic approaches accordingly. For example, role playing is likely to be ineffective in the child who has not progressed cognitively to the point where he can take the viewpoint of another. In addition, statements such as "How would you feel if Sally did this to you" are likely to be meaningless to a child still at an egocentric stage of development.

Adolescence also brings about changes that necessitate changes in therapeutic strategies. For example, boys who show a hearty appetite and stolidness (placidity and steadiness) in preadolescence and then display poor appetite and irritability at adolescence have the highest psychological health as adults. Similarly, girls who are relatively self-confident and controlled in preadolescence and who become whiny, dependent, explosive, and uncertain of themselves in adolescence have the highest adjustment in adulthood. In contrast, the preadolescent who shows no outer evidence of unrest at adolescence shows poor adjustment in adulthood (Livson & Peskin, 1967; Peskin, 1972). Healthy development, therefore, is not a linear progression. Anna Freud (1958, p. 275) stated, "The upholding of a steady equilibrium during the adolescent process is in itself abnormal." Since adolescence is an interruption of peaceful growth, children who show no changes at its onset have excessive defenses against these increases in physiological drive activity. Freud also remarks that an autonomous preadolescence allows a strengthened ego to express the affectivity of adolescence without untoward aggressions. From our discussion of autocratic and interdependent child rearing approaches in Chapter 7, we could speculate that children raised under either of these influences would not experience a normal adolescence.

Without knowledge of these changes, the therapist treating a child during the transition from preadolescence to adolescence might attribute changes in his client to his intervention. In addition, he might introduce techniques designed to return the adolescent to his preadolescent state and raise everyone's anxieties when these techniques are unsuccessful. Because in addition to helping the child the psychotherapist also has to help others understand a child's behavior, he must be able to distinguish changes in behavior due to development from those due to his therapeutic intervention. We turn now to a discussion of how the therapist and teacher can work together for the mutual benefit of a child.

Therapist and teacher

We saw in the behavioral treatment of Nancy in Chapter 11 that the teacher actively assisted the therapist in the program developed and that the behaviorist saw his role as fostering such participation. The dynamically oriented therapist also elicits the teacher's aid, but primarily as an informant. This role is seen in the therapist's treatment of Joan.

JOAN

Joan was a 10-year old black child who was out-of-touch with her own feelings. She denied having difficulties and claimed that everything was perfect in her family. In reality, her first three years in school were marked by hyperactivity, distractability, overtalkativeness, lying, incomplete work, and wanting all the teacher's attention. Her third grade teacher reported her desperate need for attention. Her mother described her as bright, yet vicious, moody, and nasty when not given her way. Clinic staff saw her mother as ungiving emotionally and as overcritical of Joan's behavior (perhaps an accelerating-autonomy mother). Consequently, Joan needed continual reassurance that she was functioning up to adult expectations.

The therapist's notes for the month of October and November describe her initial reaction to therapy.

October 1971

The initial therapy sessions with Joan were marked by a high level of apparently joyous activity, quickly moving from activity to activity, much directed toward entertaining me. The first signs that she anticipated some other kind of relationship came when she demanded that I help her with her problems, about which she did not choose to speak.

Gradually, her initial behavior has been replaced by a recurrent demand for a variety of favors.

November 1971

In the last month, Joan has become increasingly angry with me for not meeting all of her continual demands. She does not appear ready to look at this behavior objectively, nor has she been able to deal with any attempted explanation of its relationship to her mother's attitudes. Only briefly, just before the Thanksgiving vacation, did she quietly admit her ambivalent feelings toward her mother and her resentment of her mother's demands. This she quickly undid with, "But my mother's only doing what is good for me."

During this period Joan wrote the following essays in response to titles given to her by her classroom teacher.

Sometimes I Feel Happy
Sometimes I feel happy because I'm alive and can breathe. I can do things most people can't do. I have a nice house and a family. But most of all I have fun.

A Singer
If I were a singer, I would try my best to be very good at what I do and what I say. I would travel around the country and give food to the poor. I would always love my parents and thank God for what I have.

Each of these messages conveys the impression of a happy, trouble-free child. These themes correspond to the therapist's descriptions of her. Five months later her stories to titles were as follows.

Once Again
Once again I walk in the rain
Once again I try and try again
   but always fail to succeed.
I walk with love in my heart
   and run with winning in my heart
I'll die with my soul on fire once again.

How Come
How come
How come my heart trys to break,
   time and time again
I sleep with my heart on fire
How come

In response to pictures of a black couple and a young couple on the beach, she supplied her own titles and wrote:

A Black Divorce
Susan was a woman who decided to get married and she is now getting a divorce and she had no time to stay. Her husband is standing in back of her. She is crying. She had been talking to her lawyer. Her lawyer listened and was going to take her away because she had been crying for a long time. You see Blacks have many problems and she had a lot of them.

Young and in Love
Susan and Tom were in love and they wanted to get away so they went to the beach. "Oh, the water is pretty," said Susan. "I don't want to go home because my mother will be on my back." "Let's go to my house, but my father is at home. Let's go to a hotel. Let me put my pants on." "I have to go shopping." "Well, let's call your mother and tell her." "Let me go home and back. She won't say anything to me. I'll say I'm going to my friend's house. I love you. Let's go to sleep."

The teacher showed Joan's themes to the therapist. He saw in them evidence for therapeutic progress, progress simultaneously seen in therapy. His summary for March–April 1972 was as follows.

March–April 1972

Since the last report, I have been interpreting Joan's demands as reflecting underlying feelings of worthlessness and have, in addition, when appropriate, given in to these demands. As a consequence, Joan has become more trusting and more open, and she is able to discuss topics now that were previously taboo for her. Among these topics are her ambivalent feelings about her blackness, her returning home, and her sexual preoccupations.

Just prior to Joan's discharge from therapy and return to her mother, her stories again became superficial and unrevealing of feeling. Perhaps this regression was only a temporary setback, or perhaps therapy was terminated too soon.

Is psychotherapy effective?

Does psychotherapy help? This question has been answered affirmatively by some and negatively by others. Inconsistent findings have led to considerable debate between the protagonists and antagonists of psychotherapy. Some investigators conclude that spontaneous remission occurs as frequently as does remission in response to treatment, suggesting that treatment is irrelevant. Still others state that spontaneous remission is simply an artifact of experimental design. They state that improvement is not due to the passing of time but to cyclic manifestations of severity arising from internal and environmental factors (Subotnik, 1972). Studies that examine a group of individuals at any one

THE STUDENT-AIDE FACTOR

An integral part of the program, the student-aide, is an improvement on the teacher and counselor. *There is one student-aide for every three students.* Although the student-aide is a qualified teacher-psychologist, his or her duties have been modified from that of the teacher to co-exist in peaceful harmony with Project Discovery's main format of free-learning. Although there will be teachers (in the regular sense) to teach the State required courses, and those teaching the use of precision tools and delicate materials, for the free-learning courses, no teachers will exist. Their place will be taken by student-aides. A student-aide is a friend to his or her student "charges." The student-aide's duties are a cross between counselor, teacher, and personal psychologist for each of his or her three students. *The small ratio of aides to students enables aides and students to become closer, and for the aides to understand each of his or her "charges."*

The aide will discuss with each of his or her students each one's likes, dislikes, ambitions, study-format, etc. The student can always rely on help from his aide, and just as important—moral support, in times of individual "crises/disasters." Usually, a gifted child's ego must constantly be fed, or his morale becomes low, and incentive and performance drops. Thus, the duties of a student-aide will also include ego-boosting. Aides must be psychologists as well as educators also for the simple requirement of aides being able to administer tests, both psychological and educational. To match the right aide with a student, each student's psychological, mental as well as emotional profile must be matched (or nearly matched) with that of an aide so that both are compatible. This is necessary, because the project cannot afford a student that absolutely cannot get along with his aide.

From J. A. Merritt. Project Discovery: educating the gifted. Paper presented at the U.S. Office of Education Western Regional Conference—Hearing for the Educational Needs of the Mentally Gifted, Los Angeles, December 1970.

---

time rather than over a period of time may wrongly conclude that an individual is cured when in fact he is not. Children are usually referred for treatment because of a sudden onset of a new symptom or the worsening of existing symptoms. Usually, this exacerbation of symptoms is due to temporary changes in the child's environment, when he has adjusted to these changes the level of symptoms will usually recede, regardless of whether he received treatment or not. Treatment is beneficial only to the extent that the child has improved more permanently than would have been expected without treatment. Nevertheless, Robins (1970) questions whether treatment should even be evaluated in terms of improvement. He states that no one would think of evaluating the effectiveness of medical treatment by seeing how many patients in a medical clinic are well or have improved a year or two later in comparison with people who approached the clinic but were not treated (waiting-list control). He states (1970, p. 45) that: "The relevant question for such patients at follow up is neither cure nor improvement, as measured by current symptom level, but rather whether treatment has increased the proportion of the follow-up interval during which the patient has been able to function effectively."

Robins concludes that studies dealing with specific problems and using clearly defined goals have been unable to demonstrate the effectiveness of therapy. Most studies show that, except for psychotics who rarely improve, approximately two-thirds of treated and untreated groups show improvement. Considering that children are referred because of temporary changes in symptoms, such a result would be expected.

A problem that complicates evaluation of psychotherapy is the definition of success. Treatment is often evaluated in terms of the final outcome rather than in terms of change. The child who is less disturbed to begin with is often rated as having shown the greatest change when he usually has not (Mentz, 1972; Luborsky, Chandler, Auerbach, Cohen, & Bachrach, 1971). In other words, clinicians tend to judge treatment effects in terms of the final status of the client. Since the client with the best initial adjustment has the most favorable outcome (Mentz, 1972), his treatment is judged as more successful. Global outcome ratings, therefore, are self-fulfilling prophecies; the better the adjustment of the individual at the beginning of therapy the better is the outcome rating regardless of the amount of change.

In reality, more severely troubled clients tend to change more when quantitative measures of change are used (Luborsky et al, 1971). Because people, whether clinicians or not, tend to value the end result more, the changes that take place in severely disturbed patients are valued less.

Lazarus (1971), following up his adult patients, concluded that those who relapsed were more aggressive, oppositional, suspicious, perfectionistic, guarded, judgmental and conventionally religious, traits we have described as developing in an autocratic family atmosphere. Patients who maintained their gains were those exposed to a combination of treatments. The greater the amount of effort expended by the therapist, the more successful the treatment. These findings lead us into a discussion of milieu therapy, that is, treatment that attempts to modify the child's total environment.

MILIEU THERAPY

By now we have learned that behavior patterns are labeled maladjusted if they are unacceptable to the individual or to those around him and interfere with the normal course of development. When the maladjusted behavior is extreme or, in some cases, where the community lacks day facilities to provide necessary care, the individual may be enrolled in a residential center. A residential center has an advantage over other treatment methods because it provides the opportunity to modify the child's total environment and to introduce new learning experiences. The chief disadvantage is that the child is uprooted from familiar surroundings, an occurrence which may add to existing problems.

There are perhaps ten basic principles underlying milieu, or environmental, therapy (Carrick, 1968).

1. Milieu staff are familiar with the normal course of development and recognize what particular problems in development a child is having.
2. Satisfaction of the child's physical, social, emotional, and intellectual needs is mandatory.

3. The emotional life of the child is accepted. If he is angry or sad, these feelings are accepted rather than denied.
4. Graded opportunities for problem solving are provided.
5. Guidance is given in expressing feelings in socially appropriate ways.
6. There is a unified approach to treatment.
7. Both greater control and greater freedom than the child has experienced before can be provided, the goal being to help the child regulate himself.
8. The child is helped to clarify reality; safe opportunities are provided for the child to test reality for himself. Thinking, therefore, becomes less dominated by magical beliefs and more dominated by logical considerations.
9. The dynamics of the adjustment process for each child are weighed before direct attempts to change behavior are initiated. For example, before a child is required to give up an inappropriate method of self-assertion, he is taught an appropriate method.
10. Direct modification of behavior patterns is undertaken.

Although we have presented several children who were treated in residential centers, let us examine how these principles are put into practice in Holy Cross, a residential center for youthful drug addicts (12–18 years of age).

The Holy Cross program

Although the Holy Cross program employs mental health professionals, the philosophy of the program is not a medical one. Residents are not considered sick, but lacking adequate strategies to cope with stress; the Holy Cross philosophy emphasizes replacing maladaptive with acceptable behavior through an education and activity approach.

The program encompasses a variety of activities, but the adolescent addict participates only in those activities where he has demonstrated responsibility for self-management. Support for the development of increasing responsibility is provided by placement in what are called phase-levels. The first phase is the intake-orientation phase. Within this phase are four levels of responsibility.

The philosophy of the intake-orientation phase is based upon the assumption that the new resident has demonstrated, by past performance, an inability to handle responsibility. Therefore, the new resident is afforded the opportunity to begin demonstrating small and basic facets of responsibility, earning privileges as he progresses. When he has demonstrated responsible behavior at each of four levels within this intake-orientation phase, he moves to phase I.

A point system is an integral part of phase I. It helps to establish responsibility by having the adolescent pay points for certain privileges and earn points by performing the required tasks of life. Points also serve as reinforcers, allowing staff to react positively to the resident's appropriate behavior. In phase I business meetings are held by residents about house procedures, policies, or particular problems. Within phase I there are three levels of participation, each allowing more privileges but expecting more responsibility. At level III, the resident is allowed off grounds for coed supervised activities, may vote on cottage policies, may hold an elective office, and may receive visitors on the first Saturday of each month. After demonstrating responsibility at this level, the adolescent moves into phase II.

By the time a resident reaches phase II, he should be aware of the significant problems that brought him to Holy Cross and should be actively working with staff's support toward resolving these problems. Emphasis in this phase is placed on setting realistic goals for the future (careers, vocations, etc.). The resident is expected to be more community oriented (the Holy Cross community) and to participate in the orientation program for new residents.

There are two levels within phase II. Individual goals are more sharply focused and a work experience outside the cottage is required. At level II residents are allowed off grounds during daytime hours once a week, but are confined to local villages. Visitors can stay for the weekend. The residents then move into phase III where there are no levels.

Phase III residents may serve on an advisory council to the administration concerning programming. The point system is dropped in the hope that positive behavior has become self-reinforcing. Privileges afforded are similar to those found in normal home life. Residents participate in community programs conducted by Holy Cross, assist in orientation groups, attend their own treatment team meetings, and work off campus. At the end of this phase, they are ready to leave the campus (Kelly, 1972).

Although the Holy Cross program now functions relatively smoothly, the development of the program took lots of thought and hard work. A token system was tried before the phase-level system was introduced. The residents stole tokens from each other, ran away, or refused to cooperate. Initially, staff involved all residents in planning the direction of the program. Lacking responsibility and a background in decision making, the residents misused their freedom. Consequently, adult staff took back the authority they unwisely had relinquished and gave it to residents only after they had demonstrated the capability to handle it.

During his initial placement at Holy Cross, the adolescent is made to conform to the rules laid down by the adults in charge. Holy Cross staff adopted the approach after the residents displayed what was termed "irresponsibility." A second explanation is equally plausible. Studies have suggested that disturbed adolescents express a greater need than others for external control, and that they perceive permissiveness as indifference or disinterest (Mordock, Platt, & Dorney, 1968; Platt & Mordock, 1968). Studies of traits characteristic of staff admired by students indicate that the more sociable youngster responds more positively toward staff with more dominant qualities of temperament. Firmness in disciplining and aggressiveness were traits admired, except when they connoted threats of physical force, arousal of fear, or overcriticalness. Anxious fearful adolescents, however, are disturbed by staff who are either passive-silent or dominant-assertive. These findings support the notion not only that constant direction by adults is necessary, but also that differences in staff characteristics should be considered when fostering student-staff relationships.

In discussing the philosophy underlying their program for adolescents, Platt and Mordock remark (1968, pp. 8–9):

> Studies of the adolescent delinquent and the law have indicated that children imagine the law as a person in authority, not as a body of rules. The goal of their reeducation is to help the child form attitudes that are more conducive to his getting along without butting heads with society. The child often feels that authority is a weapon used against him, yet, at the same time, he wants rewarding relationships with authority figures. He must, therefore, learn how authority can work for him and how to trust in it and use it effectively.
>
> In our reality-oriented program, the student learns that adults in authority can be firm and yet warm and accepting. To the disturbed adolescent, the adult who works with him every day *is* the parent, the all-powerful authority figure, and this can be utilized in a constructive fashion. When crises occur—when a student explodes in rage, or becomes unduly depressed because of some real or imagined harm done to him—the teacher or the recreation instructor, on the spot, *cannot* defer his decision about how to act until he asks the physician. He *must* make a decision then and there, on the basis of his own knowledge and ideas. Disturbed adolescents need and want guidance. They learn to accept and to respect controls which the staff *must set* with requisite amount of firmness and consistency, and they learn to accept the flexibility required to help keep it reality-oriented. We are reminded of one youngster who remarked disparagingly, "My mother let me get away with anything and my father is a jerk; if I told the truth, like George Washington, then he let me off."

How relevant is the Holy Cross approach to the treatment of younger children? Helping adolescents develop responsibility prepares them to enter adulthood. Might we not be accelerating autonomy if we used a similar approach with younger children? Maybe. But the Holy Cross program focuses on developing coping strategies as much as it does on developing responsibility. Without adequate ways to cope with stress, the adolescent could not become responsible. The procedures the Holy Cross program uses to help the adolescent learn to cope are not unlike those used by Project Re-Ed for latency-aged children.

Project Re-Ed

As an attempt to cope with the professional manpower shortage, as well as to demonstrate that highly trained professionals are not always needed, George Peabody College for Teachers, in cooperation with the state of Tennessee, developed Project Re-Ed. Children in Re-Ed receive direct service from a corps of teacher-counselors who are college graduates, preferably with masters degrees, plus orientation training at a Re-Ed center. These individuals work with the children from the time they arise until the time they retire, except on weekends when the children return home. Their supervisors have similar training but more experience. The teacher-counselors are assisted by aides who have less than a college education. Testing and tutoring is provided by other teacher-counselors who have specialized in this area. Professional consultants are available on a part-time basis when requested by teacher-counselors.

While individual and group therapy are utilized at Holy Cross, the Re-Ed literature fails to note utilization of either form of psychotherapy. The philosophy of the Re-Ed approach is based upon the assumption that troubled children have acquired unacceptable habits that alienate them from their "ecology." By teaching ego-enhancing skills, the Re-Ed center hopes to replace the rejection by their ecology with approval and rewards for success. The goal is not to cure a child or to prepare him to cope with all possible life roles, but to restore to effective operation the small social system of which the child is an integral part. The goal is to seek a point of adequacy where the probability of successful functioning outweighs the probability of unsuccessful functioning (Hobbs, 1966, 1968).

Although 18-month post-discharge evaluations are standard policy of Re-Ed centers, published studies are of 6-month follow-ups only (Gamboa & Garrett, 1974; Weinstein, 1969). In Weinstein's study, referring agencies rated 89 percent of the children as moderately or greatly improved, while 83 percent of mothers and 78 percent of fathers reported the same degree of improvement. Should similar results be found after 18 months, the program can be considered effective.

Project Re-Ed is regarded by many professionals as a viable alternative to expensive residential treatment requiring an interdisciplinary staff. The Joint Commission on Mental Health for Children lauded the Re-Ed approach and recommended that at least one such school be established in each state to serve as a model for other programs.

Nevertheless, the effectiveness of any program must be evaluated in terms of the degree of maladjustment present in each child upon his admission to treatment. Unfortunately, descriptions of the children enrolled in Re-Ed centers are vague. Current literature describing reeducational centers specifies "mildly to moderately disturbed as appropriate candidates," but the degree of behavioral disorder is not clear, except that the children must be those "who can profit from short-term educational and behaviorally oriented programming in a relatively open group for whom projected community planning relative to school placement is already in progress." Obviously, then, the Re-Ed approach is probably not applicable to the more disturbed children described in Chapter 4 or the retarded children described in Chapter 3. It is also suspected that the program is not entirely appropriate for all children with conduct disorders (Chapter 9), since many have not profited by placement in child care institutions with approaches similar to those of the Re-Ed centers.

While it may be useful to try to demonstrate that relatively untrained individuals can run residential centers, traditional approaches that have proven effective should not be dismissed so lightly. For example, even within well-staffed residential centers, with philosophies not unlike those of the Re-Ed centers, group therapy improves a child's ability to relate to his peers (Johnson & Gold, 1971; Mordock, Ellis, & Greenstone, 1969).

In addition to rejecting traditional models, the Re-Ed designers concentrate their efforts on the child rather than on his family. By accepting the view that funds should be spent to help the child rather than his family, the philosophy of the Re-Ed centers is more traditional than they realize! That the Joint Commission lauded the Re-Ed centers so highly may be a reflection of the composition of the commission.

The Joint Commission on Mental Health for Children was composed of 89 M.D.s, 109 Ph.D.s, and only 14 social workers. Social workers have long been advocates of programs for the entire family and not just the child. Since many of the children enrolled in Re-Ed centers are from disorganized families, it seems unlikely that long-term effects can occur without more of a family emphasis and more interagency cooperation on behalf of the families of Re-Ed children.

The child welfare system in this country, in cooperation with voluntary agencies, has been operating child care institutions for some time with staffing patterns similar to those of Re-Ed centers. Without significant intervention on the behalf of families, the work with the child is often undone when the child returns home.

The Re-Ed approach has much to offer, some of which can be assimilated into already existing programs. It cannot, however, serve as a model for all programs. Magical wish fulfillment is not only characteristic of the young, it lingers on in many professionals who are disenchanted with tradition, who see newness as inherently good. Frequently, newer models of treatment based on newer theories are utilized as a panacea for all children. Each time someone invents a new method, it is always better than the old. Nevertheless, adopting new models of approach without adequate evaluation may produce, at some later time, an even greater number of disturbed children because of the wholesale adoption of an inadequate approach.

While the Holy Cross or Re-Ed approach may be adequate for some children, another type of residential program may be better suited for other children. At the present time, however, we know next to nothing about the differential impact of different social atmospheres upon different types of disturbed children. If we knew the relationships between the psychosocial elements of treatment environments and recovery from dysfunction, we could place children in settings more likely to facilitate recovery. Both American (Ellsworth, Maroney, Klett, Gordon, & Gunn, 1971; Kellam, Schmelzer, & Berman, 1966) and English (Moos & Houts, 1970; Moos & Schwartz, 1972) clinicians have been studying the different social atmospheres that prevail in psychiatric hospitals and have related dropout rate, release rate, and community tenure to hospital atmosphere, but their investigations are just beginning.

A DEVELOPMENTAL APPROACH TO EXCEPTIONALITY

Earlier in this chapter, we suggested that different psychotherapeutic approaches may be differentially effective with children at different age levels or with different learning styles. The same might be said for milieu treatment or for any treatment that attempts to restructure a child's environment. Before we can present what might be appropriate for children at different levels of development, however, we must briefly define what we mean by levels of development.

Throughout this book, reference has been made to the work of those who approach children's behavior from a developmental framework. In Chapter 4 we stated that much of the childhood schizophrenic's behavior was characteristic of the preschool child. The behavior seems bizarre chiefly because it is displayed by a much older youngster. The retarded child discussed in Chapter 11 was considered from a developmental rather than from a deficiency viewpoint. Children with self-defeating behavior (Chapter 7) were considered to display characteristics resembling those of younger children. For example, the very young child thinks in terms of "black" and "white" and feels that rules are sacrosanct. If the older child displays similar thinking, we would say that his cognitive development has not progressed beyond that of the younger child—that he shows arrested cognitive development.

Santostefano (1971) postulated that a child's cognitive functioning becomes organized in terms of cognitive controls during the first three or four years of life. The formation of cognitive controls develops through interaction between maturation and environmental stimulation. If the environment presents the child with stimulation appropriate for his cognitive age, then the organization of cognitive controls is fostered along normal lines. If, however, the environment presents him with stimulation that is inappropriate, then the dominant cognitive control of that developmental phase assumes a deviant organization in order to handle the atypical stimulation. Santostefano, as well as psychoanalytic theorists, assume that this deviant organization can persist even after the atypical stimulation, the stimulation originally responsible for the cognitive reorganization, has ceased. Santostefano (1971, p. 161) states:

For example, if a six-month-old is flooded by an aggressive, vigorous caretaker,

692
The other children

Table 12.2   IDEAL ENVIRONMENTS AT EACH OF FOUR AGE-STAGES

Age-stage	Optimal learning conditions	Teaching techniques
0–2	Maximum gratification and loving acceptance with minimal demands Create desire for teacher's approval and feeling of success	Concrete rewards Ample supplies, visual objects Teacher demonstrations Rote learning Minimal general discussions
2–3	Highly structured environment needed for external support so that rules can be learned Inconsistency to be avoided	Order and routine Few distractions Simple directions Short, definite tasks Labeling and sorting Emphasis on standing in relation to norms
3–5	Maximum opportunity for independent self-assertion Autonomy rather than enforced compliance	Discovery method Individual activities Free discussion Exploration to provide sensual gratification for eyes, ears, hands Experiences in all modalities—music, games, storytelling Use of child's real relationship with teacher for approval and disapproval
Over 6	Opportunity to achieve in accordance with internalized aims, interests, and values	Group projects Learning of information about the environment Mastery of skills with practical applications Use of peer competition and peer approval

Adapted from B. Klein. The Klein-Astor guide for developmental assessment. Unpublished paper, Astor Home, Rhinebeck, N.Y., 1972.

with stimulation excessive for his developmental status, we hypothesize that focal attention would be reorganized in response to this mismatch between organism and environment. Focal attention is the dominant cognitive strategy available to the infant at this phase in development. The reorganization could involve habitually directing attention passively and at only small segments of stimulation. While this reorganization enables the infant to maintain psychic equilibrium in

Milieu treatment implications	Milieu techniques
Needs met unreservedly, lovingly, consistently	Material gifts in abundance
Minimal demands for self-denial, sharing, etc.	Use of food as a highly personal and pleasurable experience, special dishes, feeding, etc.
Permanent one-to-one relationship with staff member	Much cuddling and touching
No volunteer visits with unfamiliar people; staff used instead	Enough staff so that maximum of individual attention can be given
	Counselors not specialized by talents but attached to one child
Use of approval and disapproval by the loved person to gain internal controls	Use of group and institutional rules as firm guidelines in absence of loved person
Reassurance without overprotection and external support of controls without letting the child control the environment	Food fads tolerated and sweets provided
Minimal punishment, impatience, and criticism	Maximum opportunity for individual, free, recreational activity leading to physical mastery, such as bike riding, roller skating
Tactful guidance toward acceptable impulse gratification	Neat collections and well-controlled paint and clay activity
Explanation and reassurance	Close contact with adults of both sexes, although child has relatively little need for mothering
Acceptance of masturbation within limits	
Nonacceptance of peer sex play	
Freedom and encouragement for initiative	Overemotional attitudes toward these adults tolerated
Approval of sexual characteristics and role	
Continued use of approval and disapproval by loved person with further demands for self-control	Encouragement of fantasy play, storytelling, and many individual creative projects
Use of shame for destructive or unethical behavior and logic to aid control	Trips and exposures to new experiences
Realistic expectations	High status for educational progress by admiration, interest, modeling
Compensatory experiences and skills	
Opportunities for practical achievement	Development of other ego skills and talents, particularly in the poorest school achievers
Moral attitudes consciously taught	
Acceptance of delay, frustration, and self-sacrifice demanded	Deemphasis of athletic prowess unless it is child's sole asset
	Real jobs made available
	Contributions to group living rewarded
	Use of discussion groups employing rationality and empathy to form character and resolve conflicts

his current stage of development, and in response to the environment with which he must deal, if this state of affairs persists beyond a critical point in time, or if the intensity of stimulation is beyond a critical point, then the deviantly organized focal attention control (that is, passive perceiving and limited scanning) would persist as an autonomous strategy and influence the emergence of cognitive controls to develop later.

In order to assess whether a child's development is proceeding normally, we need to know the behaviors or attitudes that are characteristic of particular age levels. Developmental theorists divide early childhood (ages 1–6) into four age-stages. In each of these stages there are basic tasks that the child has to master and particular behaviors that develop in order for him to do so. While the child also faces developmental tasks throughout childhood and adolescence, theorists have placed more emphasis on the successful mastery of the tasks faced in early childhood in order for development to proceed smoothly. Descriptions of these age-stages appear in the writings of Erikson (1950, 1959), A. Freud (1962), Fraiberg (1959), Piaget (see Flavell, 1963), Mahler (1968), and Sears (see Maier, 1965).

If a child at one age-stage displays behaviors characteristic of an earlier stage, we would suspect that he either experienced difficulty mastering the tasks at the earlier level or is experiencing difficulties at his present level, the extent of the difficulty depending upon how pervasive the arrestation. For example, a 6-year old's relationship with his mother can be more like a 4-year old's, but his sense of reality, peer relationships, eating attitudes, and other functions can be age-appropriate. Children whose parents are recently divorced frequently present this picture; their relationship with their mother returns to one characterized by marked dependency. If the 6-year old functions in many areas like a 4-year old, the arrestation would be considered more serious. Korner and Opsvig (1966) and Klein and Mordock (1974) both present a case illustration of a developmental approach to diagnosis.

Perhaps the most critical aspect of development is the relationship with the mothering figure. Studies of psychotic children indicate they frequently lack a consistent inner image of the mothering figure. Consequently, they are made extremely anxious when the mother figure is absent and display extreme jealousy of other children. Nevertheless, many psychotics reach much higher levels in other areas of functioning.

Table 12.2 presents the kind of environment Klein (1972) has postulated as necessary for successful mastery of the tasks demanded of the child at each age-stage. The optimal learning conditions and teaching techniques, adapted from Harvey et al. (1961) and Hewett (1968) describe ideal environments for the normal child at each age level. Milieu treatment implications and techniques are aspects of environment that Klein considers necessary to foster growth in the child whose development has been arrested at one of these stages.

At the present time developmental approaches to the treatment or management of children with developmental difficulties have arisen primarily from the works of psychoanalytic investigators. Hopefully, specialists in other areas of child development will join forces with those who work with exceptional children to develop more sophisticated approaches to children's management.

CONCLUDING REMARKS

We started and finished this book with discussions of cooperative ventures between professionals trained to work with children. And that is as it should be. No one group has all the answers, nor can one professional provide all the services necessary to help the exceptional child and his family. We say *his* because nearly three times as many males as females display the disorders presented in this book. Why this is so has yet to be determined.

The educator's and psychologist's roles have been featured throughout, because these two professionals usually work together more closely than other professionals involved in child study. Other disciplines need to follow their example, each coming to understand the other. Without such understanding, the exceptional child will be misunderstood. Although each profession may claim to have the correct model for understanding and managing developmental disorders, multiple models are needed to cope effectively with the variety of disorders presented in this book.

References

Amidon, E. J., & Flanders, N. A. *The role of the teacher in the classroom: a manual for understanding and improving teacher classroom behavior.* Minneapolis, Minn.: Association for Productive Teaching, 1971.

Amidon, E. J., & Giammatteo, M. C. The behavior of superior teachers. *Elementary School Journal,* 1965, **65,** 283–285.

Amidon, E. J., & Hough, J. B. (Eds.) *Interaction analysis: theory, research and application.* Reading, Mass.: Addison-Wesley, 1967.

Anderson, R. C. Learning in discussion: a resume of the authoritarian-democratic studies. *Harvard Educational Review,* 1959, **29,** 201–215.

Andrews, J. Theoretical orientations of practicing school psychologists: a report of a survey. Paper presented at the annual convention of the American Psychological Association, Washington, D.C., September 1971.

Axline, V. *Dibs: in search of self.* Boston: Houghton Mifflin, 1964.

Becker, W. C., Madsen, C. H., Jr., Arnold, C. E., & Thomas, D. R. The contingent use of teacher attention and praise in reducing classroom behavior problems. *Journal of Special Education,* 1967, **1,** 287–307.

Bem, S. The role of comprehension in children's problem-solving. *Developmental Psychology,* 1970, **2,** 351–358.

Bennis, W. G., & Shepard, H. A. A theory of group development. *Human Relations,* 1956, **9,** 415–537.

Braun, S. J., Holzman, M. S., & Lasher, M. B. Teacher of disturbed preschool children: an analysis of teaching styles. *American Journal of Orthopsychiatry,* 1969, **39,** 609–618.

Brooks, B. L., & Bransford, L. A. Modification of teachers' attitudes toward exceptional children. *Exceptional Children,* 1971, **38,** 259–260.

Brophy, J. E., & Good, T. L. Teacher communications of differential expectations for children's classroom performance: some behavioral data. *Journal of Educational Psychology,* 1970, **61,** 365–374.

Brown, M. A. Nonreinforcement for teachers: penalties for success. Paper presented at the annual convention of the American Psychological Association, Washington, D.C., September 1971.

Bullock, L. M., & Whelan, K. J. Competencies needed by teachers of the emotionally disturbed and socially maladjusted. *Exceptional Children,* 1971, **37,** 485–489.

Carrick, M. Milieu methods. *Devereux Schools Forum,* 1968, **4,** 57–65.

Combs, R., & Harper, J. Effects of labels on attitudes of educators toward handicapped children. *Exceptional Children,* 1967, **33,** 399–403.

Davis, J. K. *Concept identification as a function of cognitive style, complexity, and training procedure.* Madison: Wisconsin Research and Development Center for Cognitive Learning, University of Wisconsin, 1967.

Dinitz, E. Reinforcement for teachers: a program in which teachers ask for the "worst" class. Paper presented at the annual convention of the American Psychological Association, Washington, D.C.: September 1971.

Dollard, J., & Miller, N. E., *Personality and psychotherapy.* New York: McGraw-Hill, 1950.

Domino, G. Interactive effects of achievement orientation and teaching style in academic achievement. *Journal of Educational Psychology,* 1971, **62,** 427–431.

Duncan, L. W., & Fitzgerald, P. W. Increasing the parent-child communication through counselor-parent conferences. *Personnel and Guidance Journal,* 1969, **47,** 514–517.

Dusek, J. B. Implications of developmental theory for child mental health. *American Psychologist,* 1974, **29,** 19–24.

Dwyer, F. Teaching strategies appropriate for exceptional children. Lecture presented as part of a symposium on the maladjusted child, State University College of New Paltz, Center for Continuing Education, Astor Home for Children, Rhinebeck, N.Y., 1972.

Ellis, A. *Reason and emotion in psychotherapy,* New York: Lyle Stuart, 1962.

Ellsworth, R., Maroney, R., Klett, W., Gordon, H., & Gunn, R. Milieu characteristics of successful psychiatric treatment programs. *American Journal of Orthopsychiatry,* 1971, **41,** 427–441.

Erikson, E. H. *Childhood and society.* New York: Norton, 1950.

Erikson, E. H. *Identity and the life cycle.* New York: International Universities Press, 1959.

Felknor, E., & Harvey, O. J. *Cognitive determinants of concept formation and attainment.* (Technical Report No. 10, University of Colorado, Contract No. 1147 [07], National Institute of Mental Health) Boulder: University of Colorado, 1963.

Festinger, L. A theory of cognitive dissonance. New York: Harper & Row, 1957.

Fink, A. H. Teacher-pupil interaction in classes for the emotionally handicapped. *Exceptional Children,* 1972, **38,** 469–474.

Flanders, N. A. *Teacher influence, pupil attitudes and achievement.* (U.S. Department of Health, Education, and Welfare, Office of Education, Cooperative Research Project No. 397) Minneapolis: University of Minnesota, 1960.

Flavell, J. H. *The developmental psychology of Jean Piaget.* New York: Van Nostrand, 1963.

Fraiberg, S. H. *The magic years.* New York: Scribners, 1959.

Freud, A. Adolescence. *Psychoanalytic Study of the Child.* 1958, **13,** 255–278.

Freud, A. *Normality and pathology in childhood.* New York: International Universities, 1962.

Friedman, A. S. (Ed.). *Psychotherapy for the whole family.* New York: Springer, 1965.

Fries, M. E., & Woolf, P. J. Some hypotheses on the role of the congenital activity type in personality development. *Psychoanalytic Study of the Child,* 1953, **8**, 48–62.

Gallagher, P. A. Structuring academic tasks for emotionally disturbed boys. *Exceptional Children,* 1972, **38**, 711–720.

Galvin, J. P. Persistence of behavior disorders in children. *Exceptional Children,* 1972, **38**, 367–376.

Gamboa, A. M., & Garrett, J. E. Re-education: a mental health service in an educational setting. *American Journal of Orthopsychiatry,* 1974, **44**, 450–453.

Getzels, J. W., & Jackson, P. W. The teacher's personality and characteristics. In N. L. Gage (Ed.), *Handbook of research on teaching.* New York: Rand McNally, 1963.

Glasser, W. *Reality therapy: a new approach to psychiatry.* New York: Harper & Row, 1965.

Glavin, J. P. Persistence of behavior disorders in children. *Exceptional Children,* 1972, **38**, 367–376.

Gordon, E. M., & Thomas, A. Children's behavioral style and the teacher's appraisal of their intelligence. *Journal of School Psychology,* 1967, **5**, 292–300.

Grieger, R. N. Behavior modification with a total class: a case report. *Journal of School Psychology,* 1970a, **8**, 103–106.

Grieger, R. N. The effects of teacher expectancies on the intelligence of students and the behavior of teachers. Unpublished doctoral dissertation, Ohio State University, 1970b.

Grieger, R. N., Mordock, J. B., & Breyer, N. General guidelines for conducting behavior modification programs in public school settings. *Journal of School Psychology,* 1970, **8**, 259–266.

Grieve, T. D., & Davis, J. K. The relationship of cognitive style and method of instruction to performance in ninth grade geography. *Journal of Educational Research,* 1971, **65**, 137–139.

Guetzkow, H. Analysis of the operation of set in problem-solving behavior. *Journal of General Psychology,* 1951, **45**, 219–244.

Handler, L., Gerston, A., & Handler, B. Suggestions for improved psychologist-teacher communication. *Psychology in the Schools,* 1965, **2**, 77–81.

Harvey, O. J. *Cognitive determinants of role playing.* (Technical Report No. 3, University of Colorado, Contract No. 1147 [07], National Institute of Mental Health) Boulder: University of Colorado, 1963.

Harvey, O. J. Some situational and cognitive determinants of dissonance resolution. *Journal of Personality and Social Psychology,* 1965, **1**, 349–355.

Harvey, O. J. System structure, flexibility and creativity. In O. J. Harvey (Ed.), *Experience, structure and adaptability.* New York: Springer, 1966.

Harvey, O. J. Conceptual systems and attitude change. In C. W. Sherif & M. Sherif (Eds.), *Attitude, ego involvement and change.* New York: Wiley, 1967.

Harvey, O. J. Beliefs and behavior: some implications for education. *The Science Teacher,* 1970, **37**(9).

Harvey, O. J., Hunt, D. E., & Schroder, H. M. *Conceptual systems and personality organization.* New York: Wiley, 1961.

Harvey, O. J., & Kline, J. A. *Some situational and cognitive determinants of role playing: a replication and extension.* (Technical Report No. 15, University of Colorado, Contract No. 1147 [07], National Institute of Mental Health) Boulder: University of Colorado, 1965.

Harvey, O. J., Prather, M., White, B. J., & Hoffmeister, J. K. Teachers' beliefs, classroom atmosphere and student behavior. *American Educational Research Journal,* 1968, **5**, 151–166.

Harvey, O. J., Reich, J. W., & Wyer, R. S. Effects of attitude direction, attitude intensity and structure of beliefs upon differentiation. *Journal of Personality and Social Psychology*, 1968, **10**, 472–478.

Harvey, O. J., & Ware, R. Personality differences in dissonance resolution. *Journal of Personality and Social Psychology*, 1967, **7**, 227–230.

Harvey, O. J., White, J. B., Prather, M. S., Alter, R. D., & Hoffmeister, J. K. Teachers' belief systems and preschool atmospheres. *Journal of Educational Psychology*, 1966, **57**, 373–381.

Hewett, F. *The emotionally disturbed child in the classroom*. Boston: Allyn & Bacon, 1968.

Hobbs, N. Helping disturbed children: psychological and ecological strategies. *American Psychologist*, 1966, **21**, 1105–1115.

Hobbs, N. Reeducation, reality, and community responsibility. In J. W. Carter, Jr. (Ed.), *Research contributions from psychology to community mental health*. New York: Behavioral Publications, 1968.

Hudson, L. *Contrary imaginations: a psychological study of the young student*. New York: Schocken, 1966.

Hyman, I. Some effects of teaching style on pupil behavior. Unpublished doctoral dissertation, Rutgers University, 1964.

Hyman, I., & Weltman, L. A research approach to the selection of a modern mathematics series. *Research Bulletin: New Jersey School Development Council*, 1968, **12**, 4–8.

Johnson, D. L., & Gold, S. R. An empirical approach to issues of selection and evaluation in group therapy. *International Journal of Group Psychotherapy*, 1971, **21**, 456–469.

Kagan, J. Developmental studies in reflection and analysis. In A. H. Kidd & J. H. Rivoire (Eds.), *Perceptual and conceptual development in children*. New York: International Universities Press, 1966.

Kellam, J., Schmelzer, J., & Berman, A. Variations in the atmospheres of psychiatric wards. *Archives of General Psychiatry*, 1966, **14**, 561–570.

Kelly, R. E. Memo to staff. Holy Cross Campus, February 10, 1972.

Kester, S. W., & Letchworth, G. A. Communication of teacher expectations and their effects on achievement and attitude of secondary school students. *Journal of Educational Research*, 1972, **66**, 51–54.

Klein, B. The Klein-Astor guide for developmental assessment. Unpublished paper, Astor Home, Rhinebeck, N.Y., 1972.

Klein, B., & Mordock, J. B. A guide for differential developmental diagnosis, with a case demonstrating its use. Paper presented at the Eighth International Congress of the International Association for Child Psychiatry and Allied Professions, Philadelphia, July, 1974.

Korner, A. F., & Opsvig, P. Developmental considerations in diagnosis and treatment: a case illustration. *Journal of the American Academy of Child Psychiatry*, 1966, **5**, 594–616.

Kounin, J. An analysis of teachers' managerial techniques. *Psychology in the Schools*, 1967, **4**, 221–227.

Kounin, J. S., & Gump, P. V. Ripple effect in school discipline. *Elementary School Journal*, 1958, **59**, 158–162.

Kounin, J. S., Gump, P. V., & Ryan, J. J., III. Explorations in classroom management. *Journal of Teacher Education*, 1961, **12**, 235–246.

Kounin, J. S., & Obradovic, S. Managing emotionally disturbed children in regular classrooms. *Journal of Special Education*, 1968, **2**, 1–8.

Lazarus, A. A. Notes on behavior therapy, the problem of relapse and some tentative solutions. *Psychotherapy*, 1971, **8**, 192–194.

Leland, H., & Smith, D. E. *Play therapy with mentally subnormal children*. New York: Grune & Stratton, 1965.

Livson, N., & Peskin, H. Prediction of adult psychological health in a longitudinal study. *Journal of Abnormal Psychology*, 1967, **72**, 509–518.

Long, R. I. Field-articulation as a factor in verbal learning and recall. *Perceptual and Motor Skills*, 1962, **15**, 151–158.

Luborsky, L., Chandler, M., Auerbach, A., Cohen, J., & Bachrach, H. Factors influencing the outcome of psychotherapy: a review of quantitative research. *Psychological Bulletin*, 1971, **75**, 145–185.

Maehr, M. L., & Stallings, W. M. Freedom from external evaluation. *Child Development*, 1972, **43**, 177–185.

Mahler, M. S. *On human symbiosis and the vicissitudes of individuation.* New York: International Universities, 1968.

Maier, H. W. *Three theories of child development: the contributions of Erik H. Erikson, Jean Piaget, and Robert Sears and their applications.* New York: Harper & Row, 1965.

McNamara, J. R. Behavior therapy in the classroom: a case report. *Journal of School Psychology*, 1968–1969, **7**, 48–51.

Measel, W., & Wood, D. W. Teacher verbal behavior and pupil thinking in the elementary school. *Journal of Educational Research*, 1972, **66**, 99–102.

Meichenbaum, D. H., & Goodman, J. Training impulsive children to talk to themselves: a means of developing self-control. *Journal of Abnormal Psychology*, 1971, **77**, 115–126.

Mendels, G. E., & Flanders, G. E. Teacher expectations and pupil performance. *American Educational Research Journal*, 1973, **10**, 202–212.

Mentz, J. What is "success" in psychotherapy? *Journal of Abnormal Psychology*, 1972, **80**, 11–19.

Moos, R., & Houts, P. Differential effects of the social atmospheres of psychiatric wards. *Human Relations*, 1970, **23**, 47–60.

Moos, R., & Schwartz, J. Treatment environment and treatment outcome. *Journal of Nervous and Mental Disease*, 1972, **6**, 264–275.

Mordock, J. B. The use of behavioral rating scales in the inservice training of teachers. *Journal of School Psychology*, 1968–1969, **7**, 10–12.

Mordock, J. B. Sibling sex fantasies in family therapy: a case report. *Journal of Family Counseling*, 1974, **2**, 60–65.

Mordock, J. B., Ellis, M. E., & Greenstone, J. Effects of group and individual psychotherapy on sociometric choice of disturbed institutionalized adolescents. *International Journal of Group Psychotherapy*, 1969, **9**, 510–517.

Mordock, J. B., Platt, H., & Dorney, J. F. A comparison of the child-rearing attitudes of three groups of emotionally disturbed adolescents and their parents. *Pennsylvania Psychiatric Quarterly*, 1968, **8**, 18–22.

Morse, W. C., Cutler, R. L., & Fink, A. H. *Public school classes for the emotionally disturbed: a research analysis.* Washington, D.C.: The Council for Exceptional Children, 1964.

Mumford, E. Teacher response to school mental health programs. *American Journal of Psychiatry*, 1968, **125**, 75–81.

Ohnmacht, F. W. Effects of field independence and dogmatism in reversal and nonreversal shifts in concept formation. *Perceptual and Motor Skills*, 1966, **22**, 491–497.

Patterson, C. H. Relationship therapy and/or behavior therapy. *Psychotherapy: Theory, Research, and Practice*, 1968, **5**, 226–233.

Peskin, H. Multiple prediction of adult psychological health from preadolescent and adolescent behavior. *Journal of Consulting and Clinical Psychology*, 1972, **38**, 155–160.

Phillips, D., & Mordock, J. B. Behavior therapy with children: some general guidelines and specific suggestions. Paper presented at the annual convention of the American Association of Psychiatric Services for Children, Philadelphia, November 1970.

Platt, H., & Mordock, J. B. Dynamic psycho-educational intervention for the intellectually and emotionally impaired. Paper presented at the annual convention of the American Psychological Association, San Francisco, September 1968.

Richmond, J. B. Epidemiology of learning disorders. In J. H. Menkes & R. J. Schain (Eds.), *Learning disorders in children. Report of the Sixty-first Ross Conference on Pediatric Research.* Columbus: Ross Laboratories, 1971.

Rist, R. C. Student social class and teacher expectations: the self-fulfilling prophecy in ghetto education. *Harvard Educational Review,* 1970, **40,** 411–451.

Robins, L. N. Follow-up studies investigating childhood disorders. In E. H. Hare & J. K. Wing (Eds.), *Psychiatric epidemiology.* London: Oxford University Press, 1970.

Rosenberg, M. B. *Diagnostic teaching.* Seattle: Special Child Publications, 1968.

Rosenshine, B. Teaching behaviors related to pupil achievement. Paper presented at the meeting of the National Council for the Social Studies, Washington, D.C., 1968.

Rosenthal, R., & Jacobson, L. *Pygmalion in the classroom.* New York: Holt, Rinehart & Winston, 1968.

Rothbart, M., Dalfen, S., & Barrett, R. Effects of teacher's expectancy on student-teacher interaction. *Journal of Educational Psychology,* 1971, **62,** 49–54.

Rubin, R., & Balow, B. Learning and behavior disorders: a longitudinal study. *Exceptional Children,* 1971, **38,** 293–299.

Salter, A. *Conditioned reflex therapy.* New York: Capricorn, 1961.

Santostefano, S. Beyond nosology: diagnosis from the viewpoint of development. In H. E. Rie (Ed.), *Perspectives in child psychopathology.* New York: Aldine-Atherton, 1971.

Sarason, S. B., Levine, M., Goldenberg, I. I., Cherlin, D. C., & Bennett, E. M. *Psychology in community settings,* New York: Wiley, 1966.

Scheuer, A. L. The relationship between personal attitudes and effectiveness in teachers of the emotionally disturbed. *Exceptional Children,* 1971, **37,** 723–731.

Schwartz, L. Preparation of the clinical teacher for special education: 1866–1966. *Exceptional Children,* 1967, **34,** 117–124.

Schwartz, L. A clinical teacher model for interrelated areas of special education. *Exceptional Children,* 1971, **37,** 565–571.

Seaver, W. B. Effects of naturally induced teacher expectancies. *Journal of Personality and Social Psychology,* 1973, **28,** 333–342.

Shotel, J. R., Iano, R. P., & McGettigan, J. F. Teacher attitudes associated with the integration of handicapped children. *Exceptional Children,* 1972, **38,** 677–683.

Shure, M. B., & Spivack, G. Means-ends thinking, adjustment, and social class among elementary-school-aged children. *Journal of Consulting and Clinical Psychology,* 1972, **38,** 348–353.

Sloane, R. B. The converging paths of behavior therapy and psychotherapy. *American Journal of Psychiatry,* 1969, **125,** 877–885.

Sternlicht, M. Establishing an initial relationship in group psychotherapy with delinquent retarded male adolescents. *American Journal of Mental Deficiency,* 1964, **69,** 39–41.

Subotnik, L. Spontaneous remission: fact or artifact. *Psychological Bulletin,* 1972, **77,** 32–48.

Thomas, A., Chess, S., & Birch, H. G. *Temperament and behavior disorders in children.* New York: New York University Press, 1968.

Thorndike, R. Review of *Pygmalion in the classroom*. *American Educational Research Journal*, 1968, 5, 708–711.

Tuckman, B. W. A study of the effectiveness of directive versus nondirective vocational teachers as a function of student characteristics and course format. (Project No. 6-2300, U.S. Office of Education, Bureau of Research) New Brunswick, N.J.: Rutgers University, 1968.

Von Valletta, J., Brantley, J. C., & Pryzwansky, W. B. Multiphasic screening of first grade children. Paper presented at the annual convention of the American Psychological Association, Honolulu, September 1972.

Voth, H. M., & Mayman, N. A dimension of personality organization. *Archives of General Psychiatry*, 1963, 6, 288–293.

Vygotsky, L. S. *Thought and language*. New York: Wiley, 1962.

Ware, R., & Harvey, O. J. A cognitive determinant of impression formation. *Journal of Personality and Social Psychology*, 1967, 5, 38–44.

Weinstein, L. Project Re-Ed schools for emotionally disturbed children: effectiveness as viewed by referring agencies, parents and teachers. *Exceptional Children*, 1969, 35, 703–711.

Witkin, H. A., Dyke, R. B., Faterson, H. F., Goodenough, D. R., & Karp, S. A. *Psychological differentiation*. New York: Wiley, 1962.

Wolpe, J. P. *The practice of behavior therapy*. New York: Pergamon, 1969.

Wynne, L., & Singer, M. Thought disorder and family relations of schizophrenics. II. A classification of forms of thinking. *Archives of General Psychiatry*, 1963, 9, 199–206.

Glossary

ABSTRACTION   Process of elimination of details in order to move from the particular to the general, to grasp essential qualities rather than concrete characteristics. (See also GENERALIZATION)

ACALCULIA   Loss of ability to perform mathematical functions.
- dyscalculia: disturbance or impairment in the ability to do simple arithmetic.

AGITOGRAPHIA   Writing disability characterized by rapid writing movements and the omission or distortion of letters, words, or parts of words.

AGNOSIA   Inability to identify familiar objects through a particular sense organ.
- astereognosia: inability to recognize size relationships between objects or to conceive of their form when feeling or handling them.
- auditory agnosia (nonverbal): inability to identify object by sound (e.g., cannot recognize the ring of the telephone).
- auditory-verbal agnosia: inability to comprehend the meaning of words heard.
- color agnosia: inability to name and sort colors.
- geometric form agnosia: inability to make correct form discrimination.
- picture agnosia: inability to perceive pictures correctly.
- tactile agnosia: inability to recognize objects by touch.
- tactile-verbal agnosia: inability to trace a word or read braille.
- visual or optic agnosia: inability to recognize objects, persons, or places by sight.

AGRAMMALOGIA, AGGRAMMATISM   Inability to recall the structure of sentences.

AGRAPHIA   Inability to recall the kinesthetic patterns involved in writing, i.e., inability to relate the mental images of words to the motor movements necessary for writing them.

ALEXIA   Loss of ability to deal with visual language symbols while vision and intelligence remain intact; aphasia in the form of total word blindness or complete nonreading state.
- dyslexia: partial inability to read or to understand what one reads silently or aloud; usually but not always associated with brain dysfunction.

AMBIDEXTROUS   No lateral preference; also to function equally with left or right side in all activities.

AMETROPIA   Abnormality of the eye that results in light rays being focused in front of (myopia) or behind (hyperopia) rather than on the retina when the eye is at rest; commonly called nearsightedness and farsightedness, respectively.

AMUSIA   Loss of ability to produce or to comprehend musical sounds.

ANARTHRIA   Loss of ability to form words accurately due to brain lesion or damage to peripheral nerves that carry impulses to the articulatory muscles.
*   dysarthria: partial impairment of the above.

ANGIOGRAPHY   X-ray of the blood vessels of an area following the injection of an artery with a suitable contrast medium; useful in demonstrating intracranial tumors, vascular malformations, and blood clots.

ANGULAR GYRUS   Posterior portion of the lower parietal region; the left angular gyrus is associated with speech functions.

ANOXIA   See ASPHYXIA.

APHASIA   General term for various types of language disorders; loss of ability to comprehend, manipulate, or express words in speech, writing, or signs; usually associated with injury or dysfunction in brain centers controlling such processes. (See also ALEXIA)
*   auditory aphasia: inability to comprehend spoken words; also known as word deafness and receptive aphasia.
*   expressive aphasia: inability to remember the pattern of movements required to speak words even though the words are known; confusion in relationships and tenses rather than in words themselves (e.g., Betty give I present).
*   nominal aphasia: inability to recall the names of objects.
*   paraphasia: substitution of inappropriate words that maintain a structural relationship to words replaced; severe paraphasia is called jargon aphasia. Substitution of inappropriate parts of words is called garbled speech.

APRAXIA   Loss of ability to perform purposeful movements.

ARTICULATORY DEFECTS   Defects of speech characterized by substitutions, omissions, or distortions of sounds, which ordinarily render speech difficult if not impossible to understand; may be of organic, psychogenic, or functional origin.

ASPHYXIA   Decrease in the amount of oxygen and increase in the amount of carbon dioxide in the body as a result of respiration difficulty.

ASSOCIATIVE LEARNING DISABILITY   Difficulty in making and retaining associations between meanings and symbolic representations of these meanings; occurs most frequently as difficulty in connecting meanings (from background of experience) and the oral language to express these meanings with visual symbols (word forms).

ASTEREOGNOSIA   See AGNOSIA.

ASTIGMATISM   Abnormality of the eye due to variability in the refraction of light in the various axes resulting in hazy vision.

ASYMBOLIA   Loss of ability to use or understand symbols, such as those used in mathematics, chemistry, music, etc.

ASYMMETRY   Lack of symmetry of parts or organs on opposite sides of the body.

AUDING   Listening, recognizing, and interpreting spoken language as differentiated from merely hearing and responding to sounds.

AUDITORY DISCRIMINATION   Differentiation of sounds, speech or nonspeech; may involve differentiation of tone, rhythm, volume, or direction of sound. Discrimination of speech sounds depends on the ability to detect likenesses and differences in speech sounds and to recognize the component sounds in a word and their order.

AUDITORY IMPERCEPTION   Inability to understand oral verbal communication; inability to understand the significance of familiar sounds.

AUDITORY PERCEPTION   Ability to receive sounds and understand their meaning.

AVOIDANCE BEHAVIOR   Behavior that results in the avoidance of an aversive stimulus (e.g., child stays away from a feared object).

BABINSKI RESPONSE   Reflex action, the backward extension of the big toe, sometimes accompanied by slight spreading of other toes, elicited by stroking the lateral aspect of the sole of the foot. Presence of the reflex in children beyond the age of 5 years can be sign of pyramidal tract involvement.

BASE LINE RATE   Rate of a response, i.e., how many times in a given period of time does a particular behavior occur. Determined prior to introduction of an intervention procedure.

BEHAVIOR SHAPING   Development of a particular response by reinforcing approximations of the desired response.

BLINDNESS   "Central visual acuity of 20/200 or less in the better eye with correcting glasses; or central visual acuity of more than 20/200 if there is a field defect in which the peripheral field has contracted to such an extent that the widest diameter of visual field substands an angular distance no greater than 20 degrees" (*National Association for the Prevention of Blindness*).

BODY IMAGE   Awareness by the individual of his own body (conscious mental picture or subconscious knowledge of the body's position in space and time); includes the impressions received from internal signals as well as feedback.

CENTRAL DOMINANCE   Control of activities by the brain, with one hemisphere considered dominant over the other. Confusion in control may be indicative of neurological damage. Measurement of central dominance is made through outward performance, but in situations that have not become familiar to the individual through practice.

CENTRAL NERVOUS SYSTEM (CNS)   Brain and spinal cord.

CEREBELLUM   Portion of the brain involved in control of skeletal muscles; plays an important role in the coordination of voluntary muscle movements.

CEREBRUM   Largest part of the brain, consisting of two hemispheres separated by a deep longitudinal fissure.

CHILD BEHAVIOR RATING SCALE   Series of behavioral descriptions to isolate and rate various behavioral factors such as distractibility, poor coordination, proneness to emotional upset, emotional detachment, and social isolation; each behavioral item is rated and ratings are summed across items to obtain a factor score that can be compared with a group norm.

CHOREIFORM MOVEMENTS   Sudden spasmodic or jerky movements of short duration that occur irregularly and arhythmically in different muscles.

CLASSICAL CONDITIONING   Conditioning of respondent behavior, exemplified by the Pavlovian paradigm, through the pairing of a new stimulus (conditioned stimulus) with an existing stimulus (unconditioned stimulus): e.g., food elicits salivation in hungry dog; when bell (conditioned stimulus) is presented in temporal contiguity with food (unconditioned stimulus) it will come to elicit salivation (respondent behavior). Similarly, if a child is made anxious by some stimulus in a room, other stimuli in the room may come to elicit anxiety.

CLASSIFICATION   To group or arrange objects or ideas in terms of some essential similarity; to form inclusive or general labels for groups of items (e.g., boys and girls are classified as children, men and women as adults, all as people).

CLONUS   Spasmodic alteration of muscle contraction and relation; opposite of tonus.

CLOZE PROCEDURE   Technique used in testing, practice work, and determination of readability; words in a text are replaced by blank spaces, testee fills in the blanks, and measurement is done by scoring the number of blanks that are filled correctly.

COGNITIVE STYLE Individual's characteristic approach to problem solving and cognitive tasks (e.g., analytical style is characterized by perception of separate parts of a whole; wholistic style by perception of things in their entirety with little awareness of components).

COMMUNICATION Process of transmission and reception of ideas, information, reactions, etc., through the use of words or other signs and symbols; may be direct (as in the exchange of words or gestures) or delayed (as in the use of written language or graphic representation) .

COMMUNICATION HANDICAP Any problem involving hearing or speech and which results in impairment of communication.

COMPULSIVENESS Insistence on performing or doing things in habitual ways.

CONCRETISM Style of thinking in terms of immediate experience, specific objects, and particular situations; absence of the ability to generalize to perceive similarities among objects, situations, or ideas.

CONDITIONED AVERSIVE STIMULUS Neutral stimulus that comes to function as an aversive stimulus after being paired with a negative (or aversive) stimulus (e.g., when a bell is paired with shock, the bell becomes a conditioned aversive stimulus).

CONDITIONED REINFORCER Neutral stimulus that comes to function as a reinforcing stimulus for a behavior through classical conditioning.

CONTINGENCY MANAGEMENT Technique to increase a response that has a low independent rate (A) by following its occurrence with a response that has a high independent rate (B) so that B serves to reinforce A (e.g., child can play with toy cars, a response with high independent rate, after he does three arithmetic problems, a response with low independent rate).

CONVERGENT THINKING Ability to select from accumulated knowledge the item needed to answer a question correctly; the thought process required to produce a specified response, such as the answer to the question "When was George Washington born?"

CORRELATION Extent of mutual relationship between two or more things.

CORRELATION COEFFICIENT A measure of correlation, called r, having a value of $+1$ for a perfect positive linear correlation (child who ranks 3 on test A also ranks 3 on test B when B is given to the same group), -1 for a perfect negative correlation (child who ranks 1 out of 30 on test A ranks 30 out of 30 on test B when B is given to the same group), and 0 for a complete lack of correlation.

CRANIAL NERVES Twelve pairs of nerves that have their origin in the brain. Lesions in these nerves give rise to loss or disturbance in sensation as well as facial paralysis, difficulty in swallowing or talking, or drooping of the shoulder, depending upon which nerve is affected.

CULTURALLY DEPRIVED Children whose background is so extremely limited that they appear to have failed to absorb the culture of any racial, religious, or ethnic group.

CULTURALLY DIFFERENT See CULTURALLY HANDICAPPED.

CULTURALLY DISADVANTAGED See CULTURALLY HANDICAPPED.

CULTURALLY HANDICAPPED Children who find the cultural environment of the school radically different from that in which they have grown and developed. Differences in racial, religious, language, etc., background may be at the root of the problem. The term culturally different or culturally disabled is sometimes applied to this group. Also, limitations of background, as in the group known as culturally deprived, may constitute the handicap.

DEAF Having no functional hearing, although some residual hearing may remain; usually defined as hearing losses greater than 60 decibels.

DEEP TENDON REFLEX Involuntary action of a deep structure of the body; a tendon reflex as opposed to a superficial or skin reflex (e.g., the knee jerk elicited by a blow with a patellar hammer).

DEVELOPMENTAL LAG   See MATURATIONAL LAG.

DEXTRAL   Consistently right-sided in lateral preference.

DIAGNOSIS   Process by which a deficit in the perceptive, integrative, or expressive processes is specified.

DISCRIMINATION   Process of detecting differences. (See also AUDITORY DISCRIMINATION, VISUAL DISCRIMINATION)

DISINHIBITION   1. Removal of a conditioned inhibition (in terms of classical conditioning, reconditioning to extinguish a previously conditioned response that blocked an unconditioned response). 2. Sometimes used by educators to mean impulsivity; lack of ability to restrain oneself from responding to stimuli regardless of situation (e.g., a child's inability to inhibit his responses to distracting stimuli in a classroom setting).

DISSOCIATION   Inability to see things as a whole, a unity, or a Gestalt; tendency to respond to a stimulus in terms of parts or segments; also difficulty in bringing two or more parts together into a relationship to complete the whole.

DISTRACTIBILITY   Tendency to be drawn to extraneous stimuli or to focus on minor details with a lack of attention to major aspects; often used synonymously with short attention span, although the latter suggests an inability to concentrate on one thing for very long even without distractions.

DIVERGENT THINKING   Ability to generate a number of possible alternative solutions to a problem presented; thought processes required to produce an unspecified response, such as the answer to the question "How many ways can you use a brick?"

DIZYGOTIC TWINS   Twins originating from two fertilized ova and thus having different genetic makeups; fraternal twins.

DYSDIADOCHOKINESIS   Inability to perform repetitive movements, such as tapping with the finger.

DYSGRAPHIA   Partial inability to express ideas by means of writing or written symbols; usually associated with brain dysfunction.

DYSKINESIA   Partial impairment of voluntary movement, resulting in incomplete movements, poor coordination, and clumsy behavior.

DYSLALIA   Speech impairment due to defects in the organs of speech; not the same as slovenly speech.

DYSLEXIA   See ALEXIA.

DYSNOMIA   Inability to recall a word at will when the word is known and can be recognized.

DYSPHAGIA   Difficulty in swallowing; often found in cerebral palsied children.

DYSPHASIA   Impairment of speech resulting from brain dysfunction.

DYSPHEMIA   Stammering.

DYSPHONIA   Difficulty in speaking due to hoarseness.

DYSPNEA   Air hunger resulting in labored or difficult breathing and usually accompanied by pain; normal when due to vigorous exercise.

DYSPRAXIA, DYSPRASIA   Difficulty or pain in performing any function.

DYSTONIA   Impairment of muscle tone.

DYSTROPHY   Degeneration of an organ or structure.

ECHOLALIA, ECHOPHRASIA   Apparently uncontrollable response of repeating a word or sentence just heard.

EDUCATIONAL RETARDATION   Measure of the difference between a child's intellectual capacity and his level of achievement in academic areas.

ELECTROCARDIOGRAM   Graphic record of the electrical activity of the heart.

ELECTROENCEPHALOGRAM (EEG)   Graphic record of the electrical activity of the brain, especially of the cerebral cortex. The electrical impulses are detected by means of wires attached to the scalp and are recorded graphically in waves.

ELECTRORETINOGRAM   Graphic record of the electrical activity of the retina made by placing one electrode upon the cornea and the other on the optic nerve.

EMOTIONAL BLOCKING   Inability to think or make satisfactory responses due to excessive emotion; usually related to fear.

EMOTIONAL LABILITY   Tendency toward cyclic emotional behavior characterized by sudden unexplainable shifts from one emotion to another.

ENDOGENOUS MENTAL DEFICIENCY   Condition or defect based on hereditary factors; also known as primary mental deficiency or subnormality.

ENURESIS   Lack of control of discharge of urine; nighttime bedwetting.

ESCAPE BEHAVIOR   Behavior that results in the removal or weakening of an aversive stimulus (e.g., child shuts eyes in presence of feared object).

ETIOLOGY   Assignment of cause; in medicine, the theory of the causes of a disease.

EXCEPTIONAL CHILD   Child who deviates significantly from the norm; may be exceptional by virtue of unusually high or low intelligence, physical disabilities, etc.

EXOGENOUS MENTAL DEFICIENCY   Condition or defect resulting from environmental factors, including trauma, infection, etc.; also known as secondary mental deficiency or subnormality.

EXTINCTION   Elimination of a conditioned response by repeated presentation of a conditioned stimulus without the presence of the unconditioned stimulus.

FACTOR ANALYSIS   Statistical procedure whereby factors (elements that contribute to bringing about any given result) are extracted from a given set of data through intercorrelational procedures (e.g., items on a test of motor ability actually measure different abilities or factors, such as balance with vision, coordination in the distal segments of the body, or balance without vision; a child with good balance with vision will usually perform well on all items that involve that factor but might do poorly on items measuring other factors).

FALLOPIAN TUBE   Tube that conveys the ovum from the ovary to the uterus and spermatozoa from the uterus toward the ovum.

FALSE POSITIVE   Diagnosis finding that a condition is present when it is not.

FALSE NEGATIVE   Diagnosis finding that a condition is not present when it is.

GALVANIC SKIN RESPONSE (GSR)   Use of a galvanometer, an instrument that measures current by electromagnetic action, to measure autonomic nervous system arousal through the amount of perspiration (the more perspiration, the better the electrical conductivity).

GARBLED SPEECH   See APHASIA, PARAPHASIA.

GENERALIZATION   Process of determining essential similarities among individual objects or ideas; disregarding the differences among the individual ideas and operating in terms of the similarities; requires moving from a group of ideas or objects to a broader group including the original one. On the verbal level, it is the ability to state the common element in, or to provide a label for, a group of individual items.

GENERALIZED REINFORCER   Conditioned reinforcer that is paired with one or more primary reinforcers (e.g., tokens).

GENETIC   Having to do with the principles of heredity and variation in animals and plants of the same or related kinds.

GERSTMANN'S SYNDROME   Combination of disabilities including finger agnosia, right-left disorientation, acalculia, and agraphia.

GESTALT   Term used to express any unified whole whose properties cannot be derived by adding the parts and their relationships; a whole that is more than the sum of its parts (e.g., wheelbarrow is more than just a wheel + handles + basket).

GRAPHESTHESIA Sense by which outlines, numbers, words, or symbols traced or written on the skin are recognized.

HAPTIC Pertaining to touch; tactile. Sometimes used to signify spatial perception through touch with the term tactile restricted to simply perception of tactual sensation.

HARD-OF-HEARING Having defective but still functional hearing; usually defined as hearing losses of 20 to 60 decibels.

HEARING COMPREHENSION LEVEL Reading level at which child is able to comprehend 75 percent of graded materials read to him and displays an oral vocabulary of a level commensurate with that used in the selection (sometimes questionably referred to as the capacity level).

HEMIANOPIA Condition in which one has only half of the field of vision in one or both eyes.

HEMISPHERICAL DOMINANCE Dominant control of body movements by one cerebral hemisphere, resulting in the preferred use of left or right (laterality).

HYPERACTIVITY Level of activity above the norm; inability to restrict activity to a level appropriate to situation.

HYPERKINETIC Excessive motor function or activity.

HYPERKINETIC BRAIN DAMAGE Disruption of normal development of the nervous system, although intelligence usually normal or above normal; characterized by impulsivity, sensory or motor dysfunction, hyperactivity, low frustration tolerance, uneven developmental profile, perseveration. Often erroneously diagnosed as emotional disturbance or mental retardation when the real problem has gone undetected over a long period of time.

HYPEROPIA See AMETROPIA.

HYPOACTIVITY Pronounced absence of physical activity; level of activity below the norm.

HYPOKINESIS Diminished motor function or activity, often appearing as listlessness.

HYPOTHALAMUS Part of the brain stem directly below the thalamus, containing centers for regulation of metabolism, body temperature, hunger, thirst and emotional behavior; the chief subcortical center for regulation of sympathetic and parasympathetic reactions, "the fight or flight" reactions.

IDIOGLOSSIA, IDIOLALIA Phenomenon of "invented language" caused by the omission, substitution, distortion, and transposition of speech sounds.

IMPERCEPTION Lack of ability to interpret sensory information correctly; a cognitive impairment rather than a sensory impairment.

IMPULSIVENESS Tendency to act on impulse, to respond without thinking.

INFORMAL READING INVENTORY (IRI) Means of appraising reading level and strengths and weaknesses in reading. Child reads selections of increasing difficulty; through observation and evaluation of oral reading of vocabulary words, silent reading of passages, oral reading of passages, and responses to comprehension questions, the examiner analyzes the child's current achievement in reading and his capacity level.

INITIAL TEACHING ALPHABET (i.t.a.; I.T.A.) Notation system, devised by Sir John Pitman and originally known as an augmented Roman alphabet, which uses the conventional symbols of English plus others designed to represent particular sounds that are variably represented in English; intended to reduce the confusion, at the beginning stages of learning to read, which is apt to rise out of the inconsistencies of English orthography.

INTELLIGENCE TESTS Tests supposed to measure the individual's mental endowment or capacity for learning. Factors actually tapped by tests are those that investigators have felt were the components of intelligence. The intelligence quotient or mental age derived from such a test is the current functioning level of intelligence and may be depressed, relative to innate capacity, by limitations of experience, emotional disturbances, organic factors, etc.

INTONATION Pattern of pitch, stress, and juncture in language.

KINESTHESIA Sense by which movements of the body or of its several members are perceived.

KINESTHETIC METHOD Method of treating reading disability through the systematic incorporation of muscle movement (such as tracing the outline of words) to supplement visual and auditory stimuli.

KINETIC REVERSAL Reversal of elements of a word characterized by their being moved from one part of the word to another (saw/was, left/felt).

LATERAL CONFUSION Tendency to perform some acts with a right side preference and others with a left or to shift from right to left for one type of activity.

LATERALITY Preferred use of left or right side of body determined by hemispherical dominance. (See also CENTRAL DOMINANCE, PERIPHERAL DOMINANCE)

LEARNING DISABILITY Specific deficit in perceptual, integrative, or expressive processes that severely impairs learning efficiency.

LIMBIC SYSTEM Term used to include all of the limbic lobe (lobe on the medial surface of the cerebral cortex) as well as associated subcortical nuclei, such as the septal nuclei, hypothalamus, and parts of the basal ganglia; believed to control emotions so that damage to parts of the system could result in abnormal emotional reactions (e.g., aggressiveness, hyperactivity).

MATURATIONAL LAG (1) Degree to which a child's neurological age is lower than his chronological age. (2) Concept of differential development of areas of the brain and of personality which mature according to recognized patterns.

MEMORY SPAN Measure of the amount of material that can be grasped and retained on one presentation. No general measure of memory span can be made, since the amount an individual can retain may vary greatly according to the kind of material (digits, letters, related words in sentences, pictures, etc.) and the mode of presentation (oral or visual stimuli). Success on these tests is highly dependent on the degree of attention and concentration.

MENINGITIS Inflammation of the membranes of the brain or spinal cord usually caused by disease.

MENTAL AGE Child's intellectual age in years and months; based on calculations comparing child's test scores to group norm for scores at different chronological ages.

MENTAL RETARDATION "Mental retardation refers to subaverage general intellectual functioning, which originates during the developmental period and is associated with impairment in one or more of the following: (1) maturation, (2) learning, and (3) social adjustment" (*American Association on Mental Deficiency*).

MIOSIS Cell division that results in cells with half the number of chromosomes present in the original cell; process by which germ cells multiply.

MITOSIS Indirect cell division; indirect division of both the nucleus and the cell body, resulting in cells with the same number of chromosomes as in the original cell; process by which all somatic cells of multicellular organisms multiply.

MIXED CEREBRAL DOMINANCE Theory that language disorders may be due wholly or partly to the fact that one cerebral hemisphere does not consistently lead the other in the control of bodily movements, i.e., hemispherical dominance is not adequately established.

MONOZYGOTIC TWINS Twins originating from a single fertilized ovum and thus having identical genetic makeup; identical twins.

MORO REFLEX Defensive reflex in response to loud noises present in the infant and disappearing with increasing age; consists of the drawing of the infant's arms across its chest in an embracing manner.

MUSCLE POWER Strength of a muscle.

MYOCLONIA Intermittent spasm or twitching of a muscle(s).

MYOPIA See AMETROPIA.

NATAL Pertaining to birth.

NEGATIVE REINFORCEMENT Withdrawal of an event that then causes an increase in the probability of a response (e.g., removal of shock causes animal to press a bar more frequently, removal of threat causes child to learn more readily). Often inappropriately used interchangeably with terms punishment, removal of positive reinforcement, or aversive stimulus.

NEGATIVISM Extreme opposition and resistance to suggestions or advice; normally observed in late infancy and sometimes exaggerated in psychotic conditions.

NEONATAL Pertaining to the period from birth through the first month of life.

NEURAL Pertaining to a nerve or to the nerves.

NEUROLOGICAL Pertaining to the nervous system; neurological problems are those arising from disease, damage, or dysfunction of the nervous system.

NEUROLOGICAL EXAMINATION Examination of sensory or motor responses, especially of the reflexes, to determine whether there are localized impairments of the nervous system.

NEUROLOGICAL HANDICAP Some impairment of the central nervous system.

NEUROLOGY Discipline that studies the structure and function of the nervous system.

NYSTAGMUS Constant, involuntary, cyclical movement of the eyeball in any direction; may be due to cerebellar dysfunction, inner ear disease, or amblyopia (reduced vision).

OPERANT BEHAVIOR Responses emitted by the organism, which need not be related to any particular stimulus; rate of response and number of responses are used as measures of operant strength.

OPERANT CONDITIONING Application of reinforcements to increase or decrease an operant behavior.

ORGANIC Pertaining to internal organs; organic involvement in a disability means that the problem arises from or is complicated by disease or dysfunction within the body system, particularly the brain.

ORGANICITY Degree to which a condition can be attributed to central nervous system impairment.

PARTIALLY SIGHTED Visual acuity of 20/70 or less in the better eye with correcting glasses, but still some functional sight. (See also BLINDNESS)

PATHOGNOMONIC SIGN Sign of a disorder that definitely establishes its presence.

PERCEPTION Interpretation of sensory information; mechanism by which the intellect recognizes and makes sense out of sensory stimulation; accurate mental association of present stimuli with memories of past experiences.

- perception of position in space: accurate interpretation of an object as being behind, before, above, below, or to the side.
- perception of spatial relationships: comprehending the position of two or more objects in relation to oneself and in relation to each other.
- perceptual constancy: accurate interpretation of objects as being the same in spite of their being sensed in various ways (being turned, partially concealed, etc.) .

figure-ground perception: selection from the mass of incoming stimuli of stimuli as focuses of attention; these selected stimuli form the figure in the person's perceptual field, while the majority of stimuli form a dimly perceived ground. Disturbances in figure-ground perception may take the form of confusion between or reversal of figure and background, or inability to see any difference between figure and ground.

PERFORMANCE TEST   Test composed of items that do not involve the use of language, either oral or visual, except for the interpretation and following of directions. Even directions may be given without words if necessary. Such test items are essential when measuring the functional intelligence of children with reading disabilities or of deaf children.

PERINATAL   Pertaining to the period immediately before, during, or immediately after birth.

PERIPHERAL DOMINANCE   Handedness, eyedness, etc., and the relationships among them; factors of laterality which are observable in outward activities.

PERSEVERATION   Persistance of a previous response in spite of its lack of application to the present situation; may be evidenced in repetition of words that occurred in an earlier situation, repetition of words before continuing to speak, repetition of patterns of thought that previously satisfied a purpose different from the present one, bringing up an idea repeatedly, or repetition of patterns of movement, such as continuing to write a letter or symbol across a page.

PNEUMOENCEPHALOGRAM   X-ray examination of the brain after injecting air or gas into the cerebral ventricles.

PHONEME   In linguistics, basic sound units of speech. There are forty-four phonemes in the English language.

PHONICS   Study of orthographic representations of speech sounds.

PHYLOGENETIC   Concerning the race history of a given class of organisms, while ontogenetic refers to the life history of an individual organism.

POSITIVE REINFORCEMENT   Application of an event that increases the probability of a response.

PRENATAL   Pertaining to the period before birth.

PRESCRIPTION   Process by which a program of remediation for a specific learning disability is outlined.

PRIMARY READING RETARDATION   Particular type of reading disabilities defined by Rabinovitch as an impairment 'of the ability to deal with letters and words as symbols and thus to integrate the meaningfulness of written material, with no definite evidence of brain damage but rather an apparent basic disturbance in pattern of neurological organization.

PROGNOSIS   Prediction about child's eventual course of development or response to treatment.

PROGRAMMED LEARNING   System of self-instruction in which the pupil is presented with material for learning, a question or questions to be answered, and then the correct answer or answers. Materials are so planned that they occur in logical sequence with increasing difficulty and provide for active pupil participation and immediate reinforcement of learning.

PROPRIOCEPTOR   Organ that is sensitive to the position and movement of the body and its members; found in the vestibule of the inner ear and the semicircular canals, and in the muscles, tendons, and joints.

PROTOCOL   Overall pattern of a child's handicap and his diagnosis; all that is known about a particular child.

PSYCHONEUROLOGY   Term suggested to designate the area of study concerned with the behavioral and conceptual disorders associated with brain dysfunctions in human beings.

PSYCHOTHERAPEUTIC   Designed to provide treatment for emotional problems.

PUNISHMENT

- positive: application of an event, causing a decrease in the probability of a response (e.g., animal is shocked during bar pressing and ceases to press bar; child is hit during play with a toy and ceases to play with the toy).
- negative: withdrawal of positive reinforcement, resulting in a decrease in the probability of a response (e.g., an animal not rewarded by food after pressing a bar is less likely to press the bar; removal of parental response to a child's whining decreases the probability of whining behavior).

PYRAMIDAL TRACT   One of three descending tracts of the spinal cord; consists of fibers arising from the giant cells of the motor area of the cerebral cortex.

READINESS   Possession of prerequisite behaviors necessary to perform a task.

READING RETARDATION   Measure of the difference between a child's capacity for achievement and his current achievement in reading.

REAUDITORIZATION   Ability to recall the name or sound of visual symbols (letters).

REFRACTIVE ERROR   Defect in the shape of the eyeball or in the refracting media in the eye such that parallel rays of light are not brought to focus upon the retina.

RESPONDENT BEHAVIOR   Behavior elicited by certain stimuli. The strength of respondent behavior is a function of stimulus characteristics such as intensity, frequency, or duration.

RETICULAR ACTIVATING SYSTEM (RAS)   Mass of nuclei and fibers in the core of the brain stem just above the spinal cord; responds to fibers coming down from the various higher centers, suppressing some sensory messages and facilitating others; acts as a general arousal system for the higher centers in response to impulses from fibers coming upward to it.

RIGIDITY   Maintaining an attitude or behavioral set when such a set is no longer appropriate.

SATIATION   Loss of effectiveness of a primary reinforcer.

SEPTUM   Membranous wall dividing two cavities.

SINISTRAL   Consistently left-sided in lateral preference.

SKEWED DISTRIBUTION OF SCORES   Frequency distribution that deviates from bilateral symmetry.

- positively skewed: distribution in which the median score falls to the right of the mean score (many low scores with relatively few high scores, as in a distribution of IQ scores from a sample of retarded children).
- negatively skewed: distribution in which the median score falls to the left of the mean score (many high scores with relatively few low scores, as in a distribution of IQ scores from a sample of gifted children).

SOFT NEUROLOGICAL SIGN   Equivocal sign in diagnosis of neurological dysfunction (e.g., poor performance on a voluntary activity may suggest neurological dysfunction but may also be due to factors such as lack of practice or muscle weakness).

SPECIFIC LANGUAGE DISABILITY   Term usually applied to difficulties in learning to read and spell where intelligence and arithmetic abilities are within normal range.

SPECIFIC READING DISABILITY   Inability to acquire reading ability where there is no mental retardation or serious visual deficiency; labeled by Morgan in 1896 as congenital word blindness.

SPIKE   Abnormal exaggerated electrical discharge recorded on the electroencephalogram.

STATIC REVERSAL   Reversal of an element of a word characterized by a change of its orientation rather than movement to another part of the word as in a kinetic reversal (b/d, p/b, bat/pat, bin/din).

STRABISMUS Disorder of the eye in which the optic axes of both eyes cannot be directed to the same point; term means "a squinting," where one eye deviates from the other when they turn to look at an object.

STREPHOSYMBOLIA Perception of visual stimuli, especially words, in reverse order but without the reversal of the individual letters characteristic of mirror perception; sometimes called "twisted symbols."

SUBCORTICAL REGIONS OF THE BRAIN Brain stem, containing the thalamus, hypothalamus, and reticular activating system.

SYNDROME Group of symptoms or signs that, when considered together, characterizes a handicap, disorder, disability, etc.

TACHISTOSCOPE Apparatus that exposes to view letters or words for a selected period of time.

TACTUAL EXTINCTION Complete inhibition of a conditioned tactual response. If it occurs rapidly, it is suggestive of neurological dysfunction; extinction to double simultaneous tactile stimulation is often felt to signify a developmental delay.

THALAMUS Part of the brain stem that receives sensory impulses, with the exception of the olfactory impulses, and relays them through thalamocortical radiations to specific cortical areas; also receives impulses from the cortex and relays them to visceral and somatic effectors.

TIME-OUT FROM REINFORCEMENT Removal of a child whenever he displays inappropriate behavior in a situation where appropriate behavior has been receiving accelerating consequences.

UNCONDITIONED AVERSIVE STIMULUS Any naturally aversive stimulus to an organism (e.g., strong shock, loud noises, pain).

VAK Word learning technique that makes use of visual, auditory, and kinesthetic stimulation. Child sees, hears, writes, and reads words he has a need to learn. Frequently used by remedial cases after the need for tracing disappears; may be necessary in more severe corrective cases.

VAKT Word learning technique which makes use of visual, auditory, kinesthetic, words pronounced as they are written for him, and so on. Words are selected from his own oral language background to satisfy present needs. Generally and tactile stimulation. Child traces words that he pronounces himself, hears used by remedial cases and some of the most severe corrective.

VERBALISM Use of language, either oral or written, without adequate understanding of the concepts represented by the language; frequently evidenced by ability to give the right words in response to questions but inability to interpret these words or act in terms of them.

VERBAL TEST Test composed of items that involve the manipulation of language in oral or written form.

VISUAL DISCRIMINATION Ability to differentiate between and see similarities in visual patterns, such as letter forms, word patterns, etc., as well as gross forms (pictures, geometric patterns, etc.).

VISUAL EXTINCTION Complete inhibition of a conditioned visual response. If occurs rapidly is suggestive of neurological dysfunction.

VISUAL TRACKING Ability to follow moving visual target and keep it within the visual field; also known as visual pursuit.

WORD BLINDNESS See SPECIFIC READING DISABILITY.

WORD PERCEPTION Associating meaning with a word form.

WORD RECOGNITION Process of reassociating the meaning of the word and its oral language counterpart with the printed form.

Index of names

Index of subjects